THERAPEUTIC EXERCISE

FOUNDATIONS AND TECHNIQUES

Second Edition

THERAPEUTIC EXERCISE

FOUNDATIONS AND TECHNIQUES

Second Edition

CAROLYN KISNER, M.S., P.T.

Assistant Professor
The Ohio State University
School of Allied Medical Professions
Physical Therapy Division
Columbus, Ohio

LYNN ALLEN COLBY, M.S., P.T.

Assistant Professor
The Ohio State University
School of Allied Medical Professions
Physical Therapy Division
Columbus, Ohio

ILLUSTRATIONS BY JERRY L. KISNER, M.S.

F. A. DAVIS · PHILADELPHIA

Library of Congress Cataloging-in-Publication Data

Kisner, Carolyn.
    Therapeutic exercise: foundations and techniques / Carolyn Kisner, Lynn Allen Colby. — 2nd ed.
        p.   cm.
    Includes bibliographical references.
    ISBN 0-8036-5372-7
    1. Exercise therapy.   I. Colby, Lynn Allen.   II. Title.
RM725.K53   1990   89-25674
615.8′2—dc20   CIP

PREFACE TO THE SECOND EDITION __

We are pleased that the first edition of this textbook has been widely accepted as an instructional tool by entry level students as well as a reference book by practicing health professionals. The realm of therapeutic exercise and the expected expertise of practitioners continue to grow. Recent research in the basic and clinical sciences has provided new and expanded information for substantiation and explanation of many exercise procedures. We feel it is important for health professionals to incorporate this information into their clinical practice. With this in mind, we offer the changes and additions in this second edition.

• One area of the book that has been extensively revised and expanded is the material dealing with the response of soft tissue to injury and therapeutic intervention. We address basic properties of soft tissue, biomechanics of stress and strain, acute and chronic inflammation, and the use and effectiveness of appropriate exercises during the healing process.

• Since the first edition was written, research has provided more background information and rationale in approaches to neck and back care, the use of isokinetics, and the management of surgical and cardiopulmonary patients. Additions and clarifications have been made to many of the chapters to reflect the rapid growth of information in these areas. Appropriate changes or additions of illustrations have also been included.

• A new chapter, "Principles of Exercise for the Obstetric Patient," has been included in this edition to reflect the involvement of health professionals in evaluation and treatment of women during the childbearing year. The contributing author has had considerable education and experience in this area.

• Other new sections within the book include TMJ dysfunction, self-traction and positional traction techniques, continuous passive motion, and aerobic conditioning in patients with special conditions.

It is our hope that this revised edition will continue to provide a foundation for designing creative and appropriate therapeutic exercise programs.

PREFACE TO THE FIRST EDITION _____

Therapeutic exercise is one of the key tools that a physical therapist uses to restore and improve a patient's musculoskeletal or cardiopulmonary well being. Every therapist needs to have a foundation of knowledge and skills that can be used to manage the majority of patient problems seen. The therapist can then build upon the basic knowledge and progress into specialty areas as interest and patient population dictate. This book has been designed to provide a foundation of appropriate exercise principles and techniques based on current rationale to be used as an instructional tool for the student in the classroom and laboratory setting. It can also be used as a reference for the therapist and other practitioners using exercise in a clinical setting. The scope is inclusive of all basic approaches to exercise including joints, muscles, and other soft-tissue and cardiopulmonary conditions. This book does not deal with neuromuscular facilitation techniques because there are many excellent books that specifically address the problems and treatment approaches for the neurologically involved patient. A number of advanced musculoskeletal therapeutic techniques, such as spinal mobilization and manipulation as well as extremity manipulation, have also been excluded from this textbook. We feel a solid foundation in basic skills is necessary prior to learning these advanced skills.

Within this book the reader is directed in the choice of exercise techniques according to the problems presented by the patient and the goals for treatment, not on diagnosis. The book is not a cookbook of exercise routines and protocols for various conditions, because we believe that to learn *how* but not *why* or *when* to apply exercise techniques does not serve the interest of the patient. This book is divided into three major sections to provide a useful foundation in the *how to,* as well as the rationale in the *when* and *why* of therapeutic exercise.

In Part 1, the first chapter begins by drawing together information on a basic approach to evaluation and program development using a simplified problem-solving method and summarizing the typical goals for therapeutic exercise intervention. The remaining four chapters in Part 1 describe the rationale and techniques of therapeutic exercise including range of motion, strengthening procedures, soft-tissue stretching, relaxation techniques, and peripheral joint mobilization techniques.

Part 2 presents information on when to apply therapeutic exercise techniques. The section begins with Chapter 6, in which information is presented on soft-tissue injury, the repair process, and typical clinical problems. Treatment goals and a general plan of care, based on the clinical problems described, are used to summarize each stage of healing as well as the conditions of rheumatoid arthritis, osteoarthritis, post-fracture management, and surgical management. The goals and plans of care can be used as a foundation for establishing any exercise program and are used as the basis for describing approaches to exercise for each region of the body in the remaining chapters in this section.

The remaining chapters in Part 2 are designed to accomplish three purposes. The first purpose is to provide a review of anatomy, joint mechanics, and muscle function for the region of the body to be treated. This material has been included to help the reader recall important facts that are necessary in designing exercises to restore normal anatomic and biomechanical relationships. The second purpose is to present management approaches in the treatment of joint, soft-tissue, and vascular problems common to the region of the body being discussed. The presentation is not comprehensive but is inclusive of enough problems to provide a foundation in treatment approach. The information is not presented as a protocol but rather as a guideline of what to consider for treatment. Patient condition and response to evaluation should be the deciding factors in the choice of techniques. Within each chapter, additional exercise techniques, unique to the region, are described. The third purpose is to include information on the therapeutic exercise management of common surgical procedures. For background information, a brief overview of a variety of surgical procedures is given. Numerous references are provided for in-depth descriptions of surgical procedures if further study is desired. Emphasis is placed on the use of therapeutic exercise in postoperative management by outlining the guidelines, precautions, and progression of the plan of care.

Part 3 includes therapeutic exercise principles and techniques in the specialty areas of chest physical therapy and aerobic exercise. The concluding chapter provides a process for the analysis of physical fitness programs.

We believe the integrated approach used in this book, emphasizing identification of patient problems through skillful evaluation, establishing realistic goals based on the problems, and then deciding on a plan of care to meet the goals, decreases the emphasis on establishing cookbook treatments. This format allows the therapist the challenge of creatively designing an exercise program to best meet the needs of each individual patient. The approach goes beyond the technical doing and allows the therapist to be a thinking contributor to health care.

ACKNOWLEDGMENTS FOR THE SECOND EDITION _____

We wish to thank the following people for their help with this revision:

Cathy Konkler—for her contributing chapter on exercise for the childbearing year.

Mike, Deanna, and Craig—who patiently posed for the pictures in the second edition.

Leonard Elbaum, PT; Jennifer Barbee Ellison, MHS, PT; Steven M. Freers, MS, PT; Holly Herman, MS, RPT; Gary Lentell, MS, PT; Glenn N. Scudder, MS, PT; and Susan Roehrig, Ph.D, PT for their careful review and constructive suggestions of the new material in the second edition.

The staff at F. A. Davis, Don Freggens, Jr; Herb Powell, Jr.; Jean-François Vilain; and Nancee Vogel, for their efficient shepherding of this second edition.

ACKNOWLEDGMENTS FOR THE FIRST EDITION _____

We wish to acknowledge the many people who have had an influence on us and helped us to develop our foundations and skills in therapeutic exercise and, specifically, to express our appreciation to those who have had an influence on the development of this book.

Dorothy Pinkston, Ph.D., P.T.—the original mentor who instilled a love for therapeutic exercise in her students.

Richard Earhart—who challenged our minds and hands to develop new skills in the area of joint mobilization.

Freddie Kaltenborn—who skillfully organized and refined our knowledge and skills in the Norwegian school of thought of joint mobilization and who has been such a monumental influence on the progress of manual therapy. His teachings provided the foundation for Chapter 5.

The diligent leaders, educators, and authors in the developing specialty areas of orthopedic physical therapy who have instilled a sense of challenge and pride in physical therapists.

Florence Kendal, M.S., P.T.—for her critical analysis of exercises and muscle function and for her influence on our understanding of posture for the well being of the individual.

Robin A. McKenzie, M.N.Z.S.P., M.N.Z.M.T.A.—for revolutionizing our evaluation and understanding of the function of the intervertebral disk and helping us recognize the importance of involving patients in the responsibility and management of their own spinal problems. His teachings influenced portions of Chapters 14 and 15.

Carolyn Burnett, M.S., P.T.—for her contributing chapter on aerobic exercise and conditioning and for her keen eye and photographic skills in the composition of the slides that were the basis for the illustrations for this book.

Jerry Kisner, M.S.—for his creative and technical talents in the development of the illustrations in this text.

John, Brian, and Cydney—who posed so patiently for the many photographs.

The reviewers who looked critically at the strengths and weaknesses of our original and revised manuscripts and provided many constructive suggestions.

Frank Pierson, M.S., P.T., Director, Division of Physical Therapy, School of Allied Medical Professions, The Ohio State University—for his constant support during the intensive preparation of the manuscript.

Gladys Woods, Professor Emeritus and former Director, Division of Physical Therapy, The Ohio State University—for her encouragement and dreams.

CONTENTS_____

PART 2. APPLICATION OF THERAPEUTIC EXERCISE TECHNIQUES TO REGIONS OF THE BODY

PART 3. SPECIAL AREAS OF THERAPEUTIC EXERCISE

PART ——————————————— 1

GENERAL CONCEPTS AND TECHNIQUES

CHAPTER ——————————————— 1

Introduction to Therapeutic Exercise

The ultimate goal of any therapeutic exercise program is the achievement of symptom-free movement and function. In order to effectively administer therapeutic exercise to a patient, the therapist must know the basic principles and effects of treatment, must be able to do a functional evaluation of the patient, and must know the interrelationships of the anatomy and kinesiology of the part, as well as have an understanding of the state of the disability and its potential rate of recovery, complications, precautions, and contraindications. Material in this book is presented with the assumption that the reader has had a foundation in human anatomy, physiology, medical kinesiology, and evaluation procedures (including posture evaluation, goniometric measurements, manual muscle testing, and systematic orthopedic evaluation procedures), and that the reader possesses basic information about the pathology of orthopedic and cardiopulmonary medical conditions.

OBJECTIVES

After studying this chapter, the reader will be able to:
1. outline a standard approach to patient evaluation and program development related to goals and plan of care.
2. describe the goals of therapeutic exercise and define related terminology.

I. APPROACH TO PATIENT EVALUATION AND PROGRAM DEVELOPMENT[39]

Patient care is a problem-solving process.[41] Simply depicted, it is a feedback loop (Figure 1-1)[39] and is compatible with the problem-oriented medical records approach.[16] A complete evaluation of the patient avoids the pitfall of overlooking some important contributing factor and allows for defining the functional limitations of the patient. This section outlines an evaluation process for orthopedic and related problems. The reader is referred to several sources for in-depth study of evaluation procedures and techniques.[8–12,21,24,27–29,34–36,47]

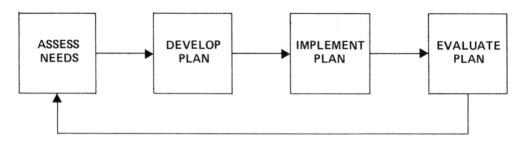

FIGURE 1–1. A simplified feedback loop depicting a problem-solving approach to patient care. (From: Pierson, Burnett and Kisner,[39] with permission.)

A. Assess Needs

The first step is to assess the patient's needs by using an evaluation process that gathers subjective information and objective data about the patient and the problem.

1. Subjective information (the case history)

Ask questions to get the patient to:
a. describe how he perceives his symptoms.
   (1) Establish the location, type, and nature of the pain or symptoms.
   (2) Determine if the pain and symptoms fit into a pattern related to segmental reference zones, nerve root patterns, or extrasegmental reference patterns such as dural reference, myofascial pain patterns, peripheral nerve patterns, or circulatory pain.
b. describe the behavior of the symptoms through a 24-hour period.
   (1) Identify which motions or positions cause and influence the symptoms.
   (2) Determine how severe or how limiting the problem is.
   (3) Determine how irritable the problem is by how easily the symptoms are evoked and how long they last.
c. briefly describe his general health, medications being taken, and whether any x-ray studies have been done.
d. describe any previous history of the condition. Find out if there has been previous treatment for the problem and what the results of the treatment were.
e. describe related history, such as any medical or surgical intervention. Determine whether the problem affects the patient's occupation, family, social life, or other environmental situations.

2. Objective data (the clinical evaluation)

Systematically administer tests that will define the anatomic structure(s) involved[10,11] and the functional limitations of the patient.
a. **Inspection**
   Make observations of activities and appearance of body parts. Evaluate:
   (1) activities of daily living (ADL) such as gait; patient's ability to sit, stand, or dress himself; and general ease of movement.
   (2) use of any adaptive aids.

(3) posture.

(4) shape of body parts such as contour changes, swelling, atrophy, hypertrophy, and asymmetry.

(5) appearance of skin, such as scars and discoloration.

b. **Function**

Use the principle of selective tension by administering specific tests in a systematic manner to determine if the lesion is within an inert structure (joint capsule, ligaments, bursae, fascia, dura mater, and dural sheaths around nerve roots) or a contractile unit (muscle with its tendons and attachments).[10] Additional joint integrity tests are used to verify problems within the joint.[27] Then, if possible, identify the anatomic structure involved and its state of pathology[10] so that an appropriate therapeutic exercise program can be designed (see Chapter 6). Functional tests include:

(1) active range of motion (ROM)

The patient is asked to move the body parts related to the symptoms through their range of motion. From the way he moves and the amount of motion, determine if the patient is able and willing to move the part. Since both contractile and inert structures are influenced by active motion, specific problems are not isolated. Anything abnormal in the movement, any experience of pain, or any changes in sensation are noted.

(2) passive range of motion

The same movements that the patient did actively are repeated passively. When the end of the available range is reached, pressure is applied in order to get a feel of the resistance of the tissues; the pressure is called OVERPRESSURE and the feel is called END-FEEL. With the muscles relaxed, only inert structures are being stressed. Note if any of the tests provoke the patient's symptoms.

(a) Measure the ROM and compare it with the active ROM. Determine if the limitation follows a pattern of restriction typical for that joint when joint problems exist. (These patterns are described for each peripheral joint under the respective sections on joint problems in Chapters 7 through 12.)

(b) Describe the *end-feel* (the feel the evaluator experiences at the end of the range when overpressure is applied). Decide if the feel is soft (related to compressing or stretching soft tissues), firm (related to stretching joint capsules and ligaments), or hard (related to a bony block), or if there is no end-feel (empty) because the patient will not allow movement to the end of the available range (related to an acutely painful condition in which the patient inhibits motion). Decide if the end-feel is normal or abnormal for that joint.

Abnormal end-feels include:

—springy (intra-articular block such as a torn meniscus or articular cartilage).

—muscle guarding (involuntary muscle contraction in response to acute pain).

—muscle spasm (prolonged muscle contraction in response to circulatory and metabolic changes).

—muscle spasticity (increased tone and contraction in muscle in response to central nervous system influences).

—any end-feel that is different than normal for that joint, or at a different part of the range than normal for the joint being tested.

(c) Determine the *stage of pathology* by observing when pain is experienced relative to the range of motion. Is the pain or muscle guarding experienced before the end-feel (acute), concurrent with the end-feel (subacute), or after application of overpressure (chronic)?

(d) Determine the *stability and mobility* of the joint. Record, using the following grades:

Ankylosed	0
Hypomobile	
Considerable limitation	1
Slight limitation	2
Normal	3
Hypermobile	
Slight increase	4
Considerable increase	5
Unstable	6

(e) Note if there is a *painful arc*, which is pain experienced with either active or passive motion somewhere within the ROM. It indicates that some sensitive structure is being pinched during that part of the range of motion. Sometimes pain-sensitive structures are pinched at the end of the range. This is not a painful arc, although such pain should be noted.

(3) joint integrity tests

These are passive tests, used to rule out or confirm joint or capsule lesions prior to testing for muscle (contractile) lesions.[27] The tests include:

(a) traction

Separate the joint surfaces and note if the pain increases or decreases and how easily the bones move apart.

(b) compression

Approximate the joint surfaces and note if the pain increases or decreases. If the pain increases, the compressive force of muscle contraction may also cause increased pain. The source of the pain then is known to be some structure within the joint and not a muscle lesion.

(c) gliding

Glide one of the joint surfaces on the other and note the quality and quantity of the joint play movement (how easily the bones move and whether or not the joint movement causes pain).

(4) resisted tests

Resist the related muscles so that they contract isometrically in midrange in order to determine if there is pain or decreased strength in the contractile units. Mid-range isometric contractions are used so that there is minimal movement or stress to the noncontractile structures around the joint. Initially the tests are performed on groups of muscles; then if a problem is noted, each muscle potentially involved is isolated and tested.

c. **Palpation**

Palpate, if possible, structures that are incriminated as the source of the problems. Usually palpations are best done after the functional tests in order not to increase the irritability of the structures prior to testing. Include:

(1) skin and subcutaneous tissue; note temperature, edema, and texture.
(2) muscles, tendons, and attachments; note tone, tenderness, trigger points, and contractures.
(3) tendon sheaths and bursae; note tenderness, texture, and crepitus.
(4) joints; note effusion, tenderness, changes in position or shape, and associated areas such as ligaments.
(5) nerves and blood vessels; note presence of neuroma and pulse.

d. **Neurologic tests**

Any indication of motor weakness or change in sensation directs the evaluator to specific tests to determine nerve, nerve root, or central nervous system involvement. Evaluate:

(1) key muscles
Determine strength and reflexes of muscles related to specific spinal levels and nerve patterns.
(2) motor ability
Determine central versus peripheral control of muscles.
(3) sensory testing
Note changes in temperature, perception, superficial and deep pressure, pain patterns, and proprioception.
(4) nerve trunk
Determine if there is pain on pressure or stretching of the trunks.
(5) cranial nerve integrity

e. **Additional tests**

(1) Special tests, unique to the specific tissue in each region, are carried out if necessary in order to confirm or rule out the structures in question.
(2) Tests performed by physicians or other health personnel may be necessary to identify the source of referred pain patterns and medical disorders.

Note: To this point, the outline has addressed a common approach to evaluating orthopedic lesions. Many patients require other specific testing procedures, depending on their disability.[4]

f. **Cardiovascular status**

(1) endurance testing such as determining a target heart rate and then monitoring the pulse before, during, and after exercise
(2) circulatory integrity such as monitoring a lower extremity pulse, color, and edema
(3) monitor symptoms such as syncope

g. **Respiratory capacity and function**

(1) auscultation
(2) breathing pattern, including rate and rhythm
(3) ability to cough effectively
(4) functional limitations or restrictions
(5) vital capacity and flow rates
(6) chest mobility

h. **Cortical integration and control**

(1) two-point discrimination
(2) stereognosis

(3) body awareness of limbs and trunk
(4) spatial awareness
(5) perception of vertical alignment
(6) associated reactions, synergies, synkinesis
(7) postural, righting, protective, and balance reflexes
(8) fine and gross motor control: tremor, acceleration, deceleration, direction, distance, stability, reciprocal motion, manipulative skills

i. **Functional ability or capacity**
   (1) wheelchair assessment: kind, skills, and care
   (2) dressing, personal hygiene, feeding, and safety assessments
j. **Developmental level for children**

3. Assessment

Once the subjective and objective data about the patient are gathered, the information is then integrated to determine an overall assessment of the patient and the presenting problems.

a. List the problem areas
   When appropriate, state the problems as they relate to the involved anatomic structure.

b. Determine major versus minor problems
   Identify problems that can be dealt with directly by using physical therapy procedures versus those that should be referred to other specialties.

B. Develop Plan

After assessing the patient's needs, the next step is to plan the treatment, which involves establishing Goals of Treatment and developing a Plan of Care.

1. Goals or objectives of treatment[6,16,39]

a. The goals or objectives are based on:
   (1) The problems identified in the evaluation and assessment
   (2) The psychologic status, such as the patient's adjustment to the problem, motivation, and personality
   (3) Socioeconomic and cultural reactions and expectations
   (4) Home or alternative care; the physical and emotional environment; family reaction, cooperation, and responsibilities
   (5) The patient's vocational plans and goals

b. Each goal should be operationalized to include:
   (1) A measurable outcome
   (2) Specific conditions or tests used
   (3) The time expected to accomplish the goal

c. Long-term goals:
   (1) Are a final measurable outcome expected at the conclusion of a therapeutic or rehabilitation program, or at the conclusion of one phase of a program
   (2) Are often described in functional terms

d. Short-term goals (these are often stated as behavioral objectives):
   (1) Reflect the component skills needed to attain the long-term goals
   (2) Are helpful in directing the decision-making process

Note: Throughout this textbook lists of treatment goals and plan of care are included. They are written in general terms, not as described here with measurable outcome, tests, and time, because of the global nature of information they refer to. The therapist should use the lists as guidelines and operationalize the goals for each patient according to his or her condition and need as described in this section.

2. Plan of care
   a. Determine what therapeutic approaches will most appropriately meet the goals; consider resources available to the patient's situation.
   b. Select techniques or therapeutic modalities that will fulfill the plan and meet the goals.
   c. Determine what modes of evaluation will be used to document the change reflected in the goals.
   d. Anticipate the length of treatment and plan for discharge; consider any alternate services for treatment.

C. Implement Plan

Once the plan of care is established, use procedures and techniques that will fulfill the plan and meet the goals.

D. Evaluate Plan

Frequently evaluate and reassess the effectiveness of the procedures and techniques and modify them or the treatment plan whenever indicated.
1. Compare original data with current data at frequent intervals.
2. Identify goals that have been met, those that need modification, or new goals according to changes in the patient or his life-style.

E. Home Program

A home program should be viewed as an extension of the treatment plan of care.
1. Early identification of the patient's home or alternative care setting, family reactions, social and economic capabilities, equipment needed, and vocational plans provide a foundation for anticipating adjustment to and compliance with a home exercise program.
2. Identify who could and would work with the patient at home.
   a. Involve that person early in the program in order to make the transition easier.
   b. Teach the person what to do; observe his or her techniques and schedule a follow-up visit to review techniques and answer questions.
3. A home, school, or job visit prior to discharge is advisable in any situation in which there are questions of adaptation or compliance. Using an in-home physical therapy service can assist greatly in the transition from hospital to home and can provide follow-up care if necessary.
4. Motivation and compliance are two situations difficult to control. The following are some suggestions that may influence the patient.
   a. Have early involvement of the family and patient when establishing goals and assisting with the treatment plan. Teaching a home program on the day of discharge and expecting understanding and follow-through is unrealistic. The home program should consist of previously learned activities.
   b. Convey the importance of the program with enthusiasm; include open communication and follow-up.
   c. Provide the patient with simple drawings and clearly written instructions of exercises, indicating frequency, duration, and number of repetitions.

Be realistic; provide the least amount of exercises to accomplish the goals. Avoid long, tedious routines.

d. Work with the patient and family to fit the program into their anticipated daily schedule. It may require that some of the exercises be done at one time of day, and others at another time.

e. Provide checkpoints for the patient so he can see progress or note results of maintenance.

f. Schedule the patient for re-evaluation at appropriate intervals and revise the program according to the new level of performance. Project a termination date if possible.

5. Maintain a copy of the home program in the patient's records.

II. GOALS OF THERAPEUTIC EXERCISE

Following an evaluation of the patient and identification of the problems, the goals of treatment are developed and the plan of care is established. What needs to be done next is to determine whether therapeutic exercise can be used to meet the goals and plan of care that have been established.

The positive effects of therapeutic exercise include the prevention of dysfunction as well as the development, improvement, restoration, or maintenance of normal:

—strength

—endurance and cardiovascular fitness

—mobility and flexibility

—relaxation

—coordination and skill

It is well known that the human body and the individual body systems react and develop in response to the forces and stresses placed upon them. Gravity is a constant force that affects the neuromuscular, musculoskeletal, and circulatory systems.

Wolff's law states that growing bone adapts to the forces placed upon it.[3] In the developing human, gravitational stresses, particularly those that occur in weight-bearing (antigravity) positions, contribute to the growth of the skeletal system.[42] Every normal muscular contraction also places a normal stress on bone and affects its shape and density.[3,42] The muscular and cardiopulmonary systems also develop strength and endurance as stresses are placed upon them during any movements involved in daily activity.

The absence of normal stresses on the body systems can lead to deformity and injury. For example, the absence of normal weight bearing, associated with prolonged bed rest, and the absence of normal muscle pull on bone, as seen in flaccid paralysis, will cause osteoporosis and muscle atrophy.[3,5] Prolonged inactivity will also lead to decreased efficiency of the respiratory and circulatory systems.[5,44] The presence of abnormal stresses, such as the abnormal pull of muscle seen in spastic cerebral palsy, will lead to bone deformity in the immature skeletal system.[42] Repeated and undue stress on the muscular or skeletal systems can cause pain and dysfunction[5]

In therapeutic exercise, stresses and forces are placed on the body systems in a positive, progressive, and appropriately planned manner to ultimately improve the overall function of the individual to meet the demands of daily living.

A. Strength

A major goal that can be achieved through therapeutic exercise is the development, enhancement, or maintenance of strength. Strength is the ability of a muscle or muscle group to produce tension and a resulting force in one maximal effort, either dynamically or statically, in relation to the demands placed upon it.[13,17,22,38]

Throughout the course of normal growth and development, the child and the adult develop normal muscle strength needed for daily activities. Normal strength may refer to adequate, typical, or average strength of a single muscle, of a person, or of a general population group.[28,30] In manual muscle testing, normal is a standard and is defined as that amount or degree of strength of a muscle that allows that muscle to contract against gravity and hold against maximum resistance.[12,28]

As a muscle contracts and develops tension, a force is exerted by that muscle. The amount of force produced depends on a wide variety of biomechanical, physiologic, and neuromuscular factors.

1. **Factors that influence the strength of normal muscle**
   a. Cross-sectional size of the muscle—the larger the diameter, the greater the strength.[17,24,37]
   b. Length-tension relationship of a muscle at the time of contraction—a muscle produces the greatest tension when it is slightly lengthened at the time of contraction.[18,33]
   c. Recruitment of motor units—the greater the number of motor units firing, the greater the force output.[13,14,17,33]
   d. Type of muscle contraction—a muscle produces the most force output when contracting eccentrically (lengthening) against resistance. The muscle produces slightly less force when contracting isometrically (holding) and the least force when contracting concentrically (shortening) against a load.[17,33]
   e. Speed of contraction—greater torques are produced at lower speeds probably because of greater opportunity for recruitment.[17,30,33]
   f. Motivation of the patient[2,17]—a patient must be willing to put forth a maximum effort in order to generate maximum strength.

2. **Changes in the neuromuscular system that lead to increased strength are**
   a. Hypertrophy[2,17,22,37]
      The strength capacity of a muscle is directly related to the physiologic cross-sectional area of the muscle fiber. The diameter of a muscle fiber is related to muscle bulk. With exercise specifically designed to develop strength, the size of myofibrils can be increased. This is called *hypertrophy*. The factors that contribute to hypertrophy are complex but include (1) an increase in the amount of protein in the muscle fiber; (2) an increase in the density of the capillary bed; and (3) biochemical changes in the muscle fiber.

      Although there is only limited evidence, it has been suggested that the strength of muscle may also be increased with exercise that causes hyperplasia, an increase in the *number* of muscle fibers. This increase may be caused by longitudinal fiber splitting.[15,19,23] Fiber splitting has been observed in laboratory animals subjected to heavy resistance exercise over a period of time. These findings have been difficult to replicate, and this phenomenon has not yet been observed in normal human beings. The observed fiber splitting may be the result of how the tissue was prepared for analysis rather than biologic changes in the muscle fibers.[40]

    b. Recruitment[13,14,17,22,37]

Another important factor that affects a muscle's capacity to increase strength is the recruitment of increased numbers of motor units during exercise. The greater the number of motor units firing, the greater the force output of a muscle. It has been shown that strength can be increased without muscle hypertrophy.[20] Rapid gains in strength in the very early phases of resistance exercise programs are probably the result of recruitment rather than hypertrophy.[14]

3. General guidelines for strength exercises

    a. The Overload Principle

In order to increase strength, a load that exceeds the metabolic capacity of the muscle must be used during exercise. This will lead to hypertrophy and recruitment and therefore to an increase in strength of the muscle.[22]

    b. The capacity of a muscle to produce tension can be improved by exercising against a high load or a low load.[13]

    c. In both cases, the muscle must be exercised to the point of fatigue in order for adaptive increases in strength to occur.[17]

    d. Variations in the type and structure of exercise programs, designed to increase strength, will be discussed in Chapter 3.

B. Endurance and Cardiovascular Fitness

Muscular endurance or total body endurance can also be improved or maintained with therapeutic exercise. Endurance is necessary for performing repeated motor tasks in daily living and carrying on a sustained level of functional activity, such as walking or climbing stairs. Both types of endurance refer to work performed over a prolonged period of time.

1. Types of endurance

Although they are interrelated, endurance of a single muscle or muscle group and endurance of the total body, particularly as it relates to the cardiovascular and pulmonary systems, will be defined separately.

    a. Muscular endurance

The ability of a muscle to contract repeatedly or generate tension and sustain that tension over a prolonged period of time. As endurance increases, a muscle will be able to perform a greater number of contractions or hold against a load over an extended period of time.[13,17]

    b. General (total) body endurance

The ability of an individual to sustain low-intensity exercise, such as walking, jogging, or climbing, over an extended period of time.[1,2,13] Endurance exercise, also called aerobic exercise, or conditioning is done to enhance the cardiovascular or pulmonary fitness of an individual.[1,2,17,25]

2. Changes in the muscular, cardiovascular, and pulmonary systems that lead to increased endurance

    a. Immediate changes during exercise[2]

        (1) Increased blood flow to muscle because of increased demands for oxygen

        (2) Increased heart rate

        (3) Increase in arterial pressure with heavy exercise. This is due to in-

creased stroke volume, increased cardiac output, increased heart rate, and increased peripheral resistance to blood flow.

(4) Increased oxygen demand and consumption

(5) Increased rate and depth of respiration; secondary muscles of respiration contract to assist the respiration process

b. Adaptive (long-term) changes[2,17]

(1) Muscle changes

The vascularization of the muscle or the density of the capillary bed increases. When a muscle contracts at low intensity for many repetitions to the point of fatigue, aerobic activity occurs in the muscle to provide energy for muscle contraction. Oxygen is necessary for this process to occur. Greater amounts of oxygen can be made available to the muscle as the capillary bed becomes more dense and blood supply to the muscle increases.

(2) Cardiac and vascular changes[1,2,17]

(a) Cardiac output and stroke volume increase. This leads to an increase in the efficiency of the working capacity of the heart.

(b) Resting heart rate decreases. During exercise, of course, the heart rate increases, but as endurance improves, the heart rate returns to a resting level more rapidly after exercise.

Note: It must be noted that cardiac reserve (the difference between the capacity to do work and the demand for cardiac work) decreases with age and with heart and lung disease. Therefore, the implementation and progression of a conditioning program for the normal young individual versus the patient with cardiopulmonary and circulatory disease will vary greatly (see Chapter 21).

3. Guidelines for endurance exercise[1,2,13,17]

a. Muscular endurance

Active exercise performed repeatedly against a moderate load to the point of fatigue will increase the endurance of a muscle. An increase in muscle endurance will also occur in exercise programs designed to increase strength.

b. General endurance[1,2,13,17]

The aerobic capacity of an individual is related to the effective transport of oxygen and maximal oxygen uptake. Exercises that challenge the oxygen transport system will increase endurance, aerobic capacity, and overall cardiopulmonary fitness. Conditioning programs and cardiac rehabilitation programs are designed to meet these goals. These programs often follow these general guidelines:

(1) Exercise is usually directed to large muscle groups, as in walking, running, swimming, and cycling.

(2) Exercise is prolonged and performed for 15 to 45 minutes or more.

(3) The frequency of the exercise varies (every other day, 5 days a week, and so forth), but adequate time for rest is important.

(4) Details of conditioning and aerobic exercises can be found in Chapter 21.

C. Mobility and Flexibility

In addition to strength and endurance, mobility of soft tissues and joints is necessary for the performance of normal functional movements. When an individual with normal neuromuscular control carries out activities of daily living, soft tissues and joints continually elongate and/or shorten, and their appropriate length is maintained. If normal motion of body parts is restricted in any way, adaptive shortening (tightness) of soft tissues and joints will occur. Disease or trauma to soft tissue and joints, which can cause pain, weakness, or inflammation, can impair mobility. Tightness should be prevented, if possible, but if tightness does occur, mobility exercises may be used to restore the involved structures to their appropriate length.

1. Soft-tissue mobility

Soft tissue refers to muscles, connective tissue, and skin. Each will be considered separately.

a. Muscle

Because of the contractile and elastic properties of a muscle, it shortens when stimulated and relaxes after contraction, and it can also be stretched passively. If a muscle is immobile for a period of time, it loses its flexibility and assumes the shortened position in which it has been held. This is often referred to as a *contracture.*[32,44]

In order to restore full flexibility through therapeutic exercise, consideration must be given to the neurophysiologic properties of muscle, such as the function of the muscle spindle, the Golgi tendon organ, and the process of relaxation, and to the passive elastic properties of muscle. The procedures for lengthening shortened muscles may be done actively or passively.

b. Connective tissue[32,44]

Normal connective tissue is primarily composed of a network of collagen and ground substance. Although it is inert and has no contractile properties, it is somewhat supple and will elongate slowly with a maintained stretch and will adaptively shorten if immobilized.

A denser form of connective tissue is found in scars; it develops when injured soft tissue is immobilized during the healing process. This dense form of connective tissue does not yield to stretch and has no resilient properties.

Prolonged immobilization of soft tissue must be avoided, if possible, to prevent the formation of this dense fibrotic tissue and irreversible contractures. Procedures for maintaining mobility of connective tissue are done passively.

c. Skin

The normal mobility of skin must also be maintained if normal movement is to occur. The suppleness of skin allows it to yield to stretch during active or passive movements of the body.

Skin may develop tightness and cause limitation of motion when scar tissue is formed after severe burns, incisions, or lacerations. Scars do not yield easily to stretch. Early movement, when possible, will minimize tightness from scarring.

2. Joint mobility[27]

In order for any normal motion to occur, proper joint kinematics are necessary. Adequate capsule laxity is necessary to allow normal roll-gliding to occur between the bony surfaces within the joint.

Any restriction of the capsule or faulty relationship of the joint surfaces will interfere with normal motion. Normal mobility can be restored by either general or specific joint mobilization techniques.

3. Types of mobility exercises

a. Passive stretching

Manual, mechanical, or positional stretch to soft tissues, in which the force is applied opposite to the direction of shortening

b. Active inhibition

A reflex inhibition and subsequent elongation of muscles, using neurologic principles to reduce tension and lengthen the contractile elements within muscles[28,46]

c. Flexibility exercise

A general term used to describe exercises performed by a person to passively or actively elongate soft tissues without the assistance of a therapist.

d. Joint mobilization[27]

Passive traction and/or gliding movements to joint surfaces that maintain or restore the joint play normally allowed by the capsule, so that the normal roll-glide mechanics can occur as a person moves.

Specific procedures, techniques, and precautions for stretching and joint mobilization will be discussed in Chapters 4 and 5.

D. Relaxation

Relaxation refers to a conscious effort to relieve tension in muscles.[29,31] Through therapeutic exercise an individual can become aware of prolonged muscle tension and can be taught to control or inhibit it.

Prolonged muscle tension can cause pain, which leads to muscle spasm, which causes more pain. Tension headaches and muscular pain in the region of the cervical spine are often associated with prolonged muscle tension.[29] Patients with severe chronic pulmonary disease often experience tension in the muscles of the upper trunk, which decreases their ability to breathe deeply and efficiently.[31] Pain associated with childbirth may be increased because of increased tension in muscles and the inability of the woman in labor to relax. All of these clinical problems can be diminished by relaxation exercises.

1. Therapeutic basis of relaxation exercises[18,26,29,31,43]

a. After an active contraction of skeletal muscle, a reflex relaxation occurs. The stronger the contraction, the greater the subsequent relaxation of that muscle. In addition, as a muscle is contracting, its corresponding antagonistic muscle is inhibited (Sherrington's law of reciprocal innervation).

b. Conscious thought can also affect tension in muscle. This has been demonstrated in biofeedback and transcendental meditation. Exercise to promote relaxation is based on the therapeutic use of these reflexive and conscious processes, used separately or in combination.

2. Guidelines for relaxation exercises[26,29,31,43]

a. The patient is placed in a comfortable position, with all body parts well supported. The patient is taught to progressively contract and relax musculature.

b. This process is often coupled with deep breathing exercises to further promote relaxation. Specific procedures are outlined in Chapters 4 and 14.

E. Coordination and Skill[7,31,45,46]

1. General discussion

Coordination and gross or fine motor skills are a highly complex aspect of normal motor function. Coordination refers to using the right muscles at the right time with correct intensity. Extensive organization within the central nervous system is necessary to guide motor patterns. Coordination is the basis of smooth and efficient movement, which often occurs automatically.

Coordination develops from the fetal period throughout the early years of life. Motor skills are initially dependent on primitive reflex activity and later evolve into refined movement. Voluntarily and cortically controlled movements can develop into automatic reactions through motor learning, which involves constant repetition and reinforcement of those movements.

It is assumed that in order to acquire normal coordination one must have an intact neuromuscular system. A balance of normal reciprocal innervation and co-contraction, leading to smooth reciprocal movements and appropriate stability, is necessary in carrying out a motor skill. Sensory input and sensory feedback are an essential part of that mechanism. Lesions of the central nervous system, such as cerebrovascular accidents, cerebral palsy, and multiple sclerosis, and a wide range of other neurologic disorders, will obviously interrupt coordination. Normal movements needed in gross and fine motor activities, ranging from locomotion to writing, will be impaired.

2. Therapeutic exercise approaches for the improvement of neuromuscular coordination

a. General principles of coordination exercises involve[31]
 (1) Constant repetition of a few motor activities
 (2) Use of sensory cues (tactile, visual, proprioceptive) to enhance motor performance.
 (3) Increase of speed of the activity over time.
b. Many different approaches to therapy have been developed. These include
 (1) Frenkel's exercises
 (2) Proprioceptive Neuromuscular Facilitation (Knott and Voss)
 (3) Neurodevelopmental Treatment (Bobath)
 (4) Neurophysiological Basis of Development (Rood, Randolph)
 (5) Sensory Integrative Therapy (Ayres).
 This book is not designed to deal in depth with therapeutic exercise as it relates to disorders of the neurologic systems and their effects on movement. Extensive information may be found by referring to the above-mentioned authors.

III. SUMMARY

This chapter presented a brief outline of an approach to patient program development, using a simplified problem-solving process as the basis and integrating it with an evaluation and assessment process. It is recommended that the reader have a course in evaluation techniques prior to using this book and attempting to choose and administer exercise techniques to patients.

The general goals that can be achieved by the broad scope of therapeutic exercise were also discussed. Each of these goals will be expanded and explained in much greater detail in the remaining chapters of this book.

REFERENCES

1. Allman, FL: *Exercises in sports medicine.* In Basmajian, JV (ed): *Therapeutic Exercise,* ed. 3. Williams & Wilkins, Baltimore, 1978.
2. Astrand, P and Rodahl, K: *Textbook of Work Physiology.* McGraw-Hill, New York, 1977.
3. Bassett, CAL: *Effect of force on skeletal tissue.* In Downey, JA and Darling, RC: *Physiological Basis of Rehabilitation Medicine.* WB Saunders, Philadelphia, 1971.
4. Bohman, I and Jaeger, D: *Guidelines for patient evaluation.* Phys Ther 53:1067, 1973.
5. Browse, NL: *The Physiology and Pathology of Bed Rest.* Charles C Thomas, Springfield, IL, 1965.
6. Burnett, CB: *Course Syallbus, PT 585.02.* The Ohio State University, Division of Physical Therapy, Columbus, 1987.
7. Carr, JH, et al: *Movement and Science: Foundations for Physical Therapy in Rehabilitation.* Aspen Publishers, Rockville, MD, 1987.
8. Cookson, J: *Orthopedic manual therapy—An overview part II: The spine.* Phys Ther 59:259, 1979.
9. Cookson, J and Kent, B: *Orthopedic manual therapy—An overview part I: The extremities.* Phys Ther 59:136, 1979.
10. Cyriax, J: *Textbook of Orthopaedic Medicine, Vol 1. Diagnosis of Soft Tissue Lesions,* ed 8. Bailliere and Tindall, London, 1982.
11. Cyriax, J and Cyriax, O: *Illustrated Manual of Orthopaedic Medicine.* Butterworth, Boston, 1983.
12. Daniels, L and Worthingham, C: *Muscle Testing: Techniques of Manual Examination,* ed 4. WB Saunders, Philadelphia, 1980.
13. Delateur, BJ: *Therapeutic exercise to develop strength and endurance.* In Kottke, FJ, Stillwell, GK, and Lehmann, JF (eds): *Krusen's Handbook of Physical Medicine and Rehabilitation,* ed 3. WB Saunders, Philadelphia, 1982.
14. Delorme, TL and Watson, AL: *Progressive Resistance Exercise.* Appleton-Century, New York, 1951.
15. Edgerton, V: *Morphology and histochemistry of the soleus muscle from normal and exercised rats.* Am J Anat 127:81, 1970.
16. Feitelberg, S: *The Problem Oriented Records System in Physical Therapy.* University of Vermont, Burlington, 1975.
17. Fox, E and Matthews, D: *The Physiological Basis of Physical Education and Athletics,* ed 3. Saunders College Publishing, Philadelphia, 1981.
18. Glowitzke, BA and Milner, M: *Understanding the Scientific Basis of Human Movement,* ed 2. Williams & Wilkins, Baltimore, 1980.
19. Gonyea, WJ, Ericson, GC, and Bonde-Petersen, F: *Skeletal muscle fiber splitting induced by weightlifting exercise in cats.* Acta Physiol Scand 99:105, 1977.
20. Gordon, EE, Kowalski, K, and Fritts, M: *Protein changes in quadriceps muscle of rat with repetitive exercises.* Arch Phys Med Rehab 48:296, 1967.
21. Grieve, G: *Common Vertebral Joint Problems.* Churchill-Livingstone, New York, 1982.
22. Hellebrandt, RA and Houtz, SJ: *Mechanisms of muscle training in man: Experimental demonstration of the overload principle.* Phys Ther Rev 36:371, 1956.
23. Ho, K, et al: *Muscle fiber splitting with weightlifting exercise.* Med Sci Sports 9(1):65, 1977.
24. Hoppenfeld, S: *Physical Examination of the Spine and Extremities.* Appleton-Century-Crofts, New York, 1976.
25. Irwin, S and Tecklin, JS: *Cardiopulmonary Physical Therapy.* CV Mosby, St Louis, 1985.
26. Jacobson, E: *Progressive Relaxation.* University of Chicago Press, Chicago, 1938.
27. Kaltenborn, F: *Mobilization of the Extremity Joints: Examination and Basic Treatment Techniques,* ed 3. Norway, 1980.
28. Kendall, FP and McCreary, EK: *Muscles: Testing and Function,* ed 3. Wiliams & Wilkins, Baltimore, 1983.
29. Kessler, R and Hertling, D: *Management of Common Musculoskeletal Disorders.* Harper & Row, Philadelphia, 1983.
30. Knutgren, HG: *Neuromuscular Mechanisms for Therapeutic and Conditioning Exercise.* University Park Press, Baltimore, 1976.

31. Kottke, FJ: *Therapeutic exercise to develop neuromuscular coordination.* In Kottke, FJ, Stillwell, GK, and Lehmann, JF (eds): *Krusen's Handbook of Physical Medicine and Rehabilitation,* ed 3. WB Saunders, Philadelphia, 1982.
32. Kottke, FJ: *Therapeutic exercise to maintain mobility.* In Kottke, FJ, Stillwell, GK, and Lehmann, JF (eds): *Krusen's Handbook of Physical Medicine and Rehabilitation,* ed 3. WB Saunders, Philadelphia, 1982.
33. Lehmkuhl, LD and Smith, LK: *Brunnstrom's Clinical Kinesiology,* ed 4. FA Davis Company, Philadelphia, 1983.
34. Magee, D: *Orthopedic Physical Assessment.* WB Saunders, Philadelphia, 1987.
35. Maitland, G: *Peripheral Manipulation,* ed 2. Butterworth, Boston, 1977.
36. Maitland, G: *Vertebral Manipulation,* ed 4. Butterworth, Boston, 1977.
37. Moritani, T and DeVries, HK: *Neural factors vs. hypertrophy in the time course of muscle strength gain.* Am J Phys Med 58:115, 1979.
38. Ostering, L: *Isokinetic and isometric torque force relationships.* Arch Phys Med Rehab 58:254, 1977.
39. Pierson, F, Burnett, C, and Kisner, C: *A Problem Solving Process.* The Ohio State University, Division of Physical Therapy, Columbus, 1986.
40. Rose, SJ and Rothstein, JM: *Muscle mutability, part I. General concepts and adaptations to altered patterns of use.* Phys Ther 62:1773, 1982.
41. Schenek, J: *The Problem Solving Systems.* Workshop Notes, The Ohio State University, March 1979.
42. Sharrard, WJW: *The hip in cerebral palsy.* In Samilson, RL (ed): *Orthopedic Aspects of Cerebral Palsy.* JB Lippincott, Philadelphia, 1975.
43. Sinclair, JD: *Exercise in pulmonary disease.* In Basmajian, JV (ed): *Therapeutic Exercise,* ed 3. Williams & Wilkins, Baltimore, 1978.
44. Vallbona, C: *Bodily responses to immobilization.* In Kottke, FJ, Stillwell, GK and Lehmann, JF (eds): *Krusen's Handbook of Physical Medicine and Rehabilitation.* WB Saunders, Philadelphia, 1982.
45. Umphried, DA (ed): *Neurological Rehabilitation.* CV Mosby, St Louis, 1985.
46. Voss, DE, Ionta, MK, and Myers, BJ: *Proprioceptive Neuromuscular Facilitation,* ed 3. Harper & Row, Philadelphia, 1985.
47. Zohn, D and Mennell, J: *Muskuoskeletal pain: Principles of Physical Diagnosis and Physical Treatment.* Little, Brown & Company, Boston, 1976.

CHAPTER ———————————— 2

Range of Motion

Movement of a body segment takes place as muscles or external forces move bones. Bones move with respect to each other at the connecting joints. The structure of the joints as well as the integrity and flexibility of the soft tissues that pass over the joints affect the amount of motion that can occur between any two bones. The full motion possible is called the RANGE OF MOTION (ROM). When moving a segment through its range of motion, all structures in the region are affected: muscles, joint surfaces, capsules, ligaments, fascia, vessels, and nerves. Range of motion activities are most easily described in terms of joint range and muscle range. To describe joint range, terms such as flexion, extension, abduction, adduction, and rotation are used. Ranges of available joint motion are usually measured with a goniometer and recorded in degrees.[15–18] Muscle range is related to the functional excursion of muscles.

Functional excursion is that distance that a muscle is capable of shortening after it has been elongated to its maximum.[14] In some cases the functional excursion, or range of a muscle, is directly influenced by the joint it crosses. For example, the range for the brachialis muscle is limited by the range available at the elbow joint. This is true of one-joint muscles (muscles whose proximal and distal attachments are on the bones on either side of one joint). For two- or multi-joint muscles (those muscles that cross over two or more joints), their range goes beyond the limits of any one joint they cross over. An example of a two-joint muscle functioning at the elbow is the biceps brachii muscle. If it contracts and moves the elbow into flexion and the forearm into supination while simultaneously moving the shoulder into flexion, it will shorten to a point known as active insufficiency, where it can shorten no more. This is one end of its range. The muscle is lengthened full range by extending the elbow, pronating the forearm, and simultaneously extending the shoulder. When fully elongated it is in a position known as passive insufficiency. Two- or multi-joint muscles normally function in the mid portion of their functional excursion, where ideal length-tension relationships exist.[14]

In order to maintain normal range of motion, the segments must be moved through their available ranges periodically, whether it be the available joint range or muscle range. It is recognized that many factors can lead to decreased ROM, such as systemic, joint, neurologic, or muscular diseases; surgical or traumatic insults; or simply inactivity or immobilization for any reason. Therapeutically, range of motion activities are administered to maintain existing joint and soft-tissue mobility, which will minimize the effects of contracture formation.[3]

OBJECTIVES

After studying this chapter, the reader will be able to:
1. describe range of motion and what affects it.
2. define passive, active, and active-assistive range of motion.
3. identify indications and goals for passive and active range of motion activities.
4. identify limitations of passive and active range of motion activities.
5. identify contraindications to range of motion.
6. describe procedures for applying range of motion techniques.
7. apply techniques for joint and muscle range of motion using anatomic planes of motion.
8. apply techniques for combined ranges of motion.
9. apply techniques of range of motion using self-assistance and mechanical assistance including wand, finger ladder, pulley, shoulder wheel, powder (skate) board, and suspension devices.
10. describe the benefits and procedures for use of continuous passive motion (CPM) equipment.

I. DEFINITIONS OF RANGE OF MOTION EXERCISES

A. Passive

Movement within the unrestricted ROM for a segment that is produced entirely by an EXTERNAL FORCE; there is no voluntary muscle contraction. The external force may be from gravity, a machine, another individual, or another part of the individual's own body.[5] Passive ROM and passive stretching are not synonymous; see Chapter 4 for definitions and descriptions of passive stretching.

B. Active

Movement within the unrestricted ROM for a segment that is produced by an active contraction of the MUSCLES crossing that joint.

C. Active-Assistive

A type of active ROM in which assistance is provided by an outside force, either manually or mechanically, because the prime mover muscles need assistance to complete the motion.

II. INDICATIONS AND GOALS FOR RANGE OF MOTION

A. Passive ROM

1. When a patient is not able to or not supposed to actively move a segment or segments of the body, as when comatose, paralyzed, or on complete bed rest, or when there is an inflammatory reaction and active ROM is painful, controlled passive ROM is used to decrease the complications of immobilization in order to[5]
   a. maintain joint and soft-tissue integrity.
   b. minimize the effects of the formation of contractures.
   c. maintain mechanical elasticity of muscle.

        d. assist circulation and vascular dynamics.

        e. enhance synovial movement for cartilage nutrition and diffusion of materials in the joint.

        f. decrease or inhibit pain.

        g. assist with the healing process following injury or surgery.

        h. help maintain the patient's awareness of movement.

   2. When a therapist is evaluating inert structures (see Chapter 1), passive ROM is used to determine limitations of motion, to determine joint stability, and to determine muscle and other soft-tissue elasticity.

   3. When a therapist is teaching an active exercise program, passive ROM is used to demonstrate the desired motion.

   4. When a therapist is preparing a patient for stretching, passive ROM is often used preceding the passive stretching techniques. Techniques to increase the range of motion when there is restricted motion are described in Chapters 4 and 5.

B. Active and Active-Assistive ROM

   1. When a patient is able to actively contract his muscles and move a segment either with or without assistance, and when there are no contraindications, active ROM is used to:

        a. accomplish the same goals of passive ROM with the added benefits that result from muscle contraction.

        b. maintain physiologic elasticity and contractility of the participating muscles.

        c. provide sensory feedback from the contracting muscles.

        d. provide stimulus for bone integrity.

        e. increase circulation and prevent thrombus formation.

        f. develop coordination and motor skills for functional activities.

   2. When a patient has weak musculature (poor to fair minus muscle test grade), active-assistive ROM is used to provide enough assistance to the muscles in a carefully controlled manner so that the muscle can function at its maximum level and progressively be strengthened.

   3. When a patient is placed on an aerobic conditioning program, active-assistive or active ROM can be used to improve cardiovascular and respiratory responses if it is done with multiple repetitions and the results are monitored (see Chapter 21).

C. Special Considerations

   1. When a segment of the body is immobilized for a period of time, ROM is used on the regions above and below the immobilized segment to:

        a. maintain the areas in as normal a condition as possible.

        b. prepare for new activities, such as walking with crutches.

   2. When a patient is on bed rest, ROM is used to avoid the complications of decreased circulation, bone demineralization, and decreased cardiac and respiratory function.

III. LIMITATIONS OF RANGE OF MOTION

A. Limitations of Passive Motion

   1. True passive relaxed range of motion may be difficult to obtain when muscle is innervated and the patient is conscious.

   2. Passive motion WILL NOT:

    a. prevent muscle atrophy.
    b. increase strength or endurance.
    c. assist circulation to the extent that active, voluntary muscle contraction will.

B. Limitations of Active ROM

1. For strong muscles, it will not maintain or increase strength (see Chapter 3).
2. It will not develop skill or coordination except in the movement patterns used.

IV. PRECAUTIONS AND CONTRAINDICATIONS TO RANGE OF MOTION

A. Both passive and active ROM are contraindicated under any circumstance when motion to a part is disruptive to the healing process, yet complete immobility leads to adhesion and contracture formation, sluggish circulation, and prolonged recovery time. In light of research by Salter,[23] early continuous passive range of motion within a pain-free range has been shown to be beneficial to the healing and early recovery of many soft tissue and joint lesions (see Section IX, A). Historically ROM has been contraindicated immediately following acute tears, fractures, and surgery, but since the benefits of controlled motion have demonstrated decreased pain and an increased rate of recovery, early controlled motion is used as long as the patient's tolerance is monitored. It is imperative that the therapist recognize the value as well as potential abuse of motion and stay within the range, speed, and tolerance of the patient during the acute recovery stage.[5] Additional trauma to the part is contraindicated. Signs of too much or the wrong motion include increased pain and increased inflammation (greater swelling, heat, and redness). (see Chapter 6 for principles of when to use various types of passive and active motion therapeutically.)

B. Active ROM is contraindicated when the cardiovascular condition of a patient is unstable and active exercise would jeopardize the patient's life, such as immediately following a myocardial infarction. In such circumstances, passive ROM may be initiated to the major joints along with some active ROM to the ankles and feet to avoid venous stasis and thrombus formation. Individualized activities are initiated and progress gradually as the patient tolerates.[4,29]

C. Range of motion is not synonymous with stretching. For precautions and contraindications to passive and active stretching techniques, see Chapters 4 and 5.

V. PROCEDURES FOR APPLYING RANGE OF MOTION TECHNIQUES

A. Based on an evaluation of the patient's level of function, determine patient goals and whether passive, active-assistive, or active range of motion will meet the goals.

B. Place the patient in a comfortable position that will allow you to move the segment through the available ROM. Be sure he has proper body alignment.

C. Free the region from restrictive clothing, linen, splints, and dressings. Drape the patient as necessary.

D. Position yourself so that proper body mechanics can be used.

E. To control movement, grasp the extremity around the joints. If the joints are painful, modify the grip, still providing support necessary for control.

   F. Support areas of poor structural integrity such as a hypermobile joint or a recent fracture site or where there is paralysis.

   G. Move the segment through its complete pain-free range. Do not force beyond the available range. If you force motion, it becomes a stretching technique. (For principles and techniques of stretching, see Chapter 4.)

   H. Do the motions smoothly and rhythmically, five to ten repetitions. The number of repetitions depends on the objectives of the program and the patient's condition and response to the treatment.

   I. If the PLAN OF CARE includes the use of PASSIVE ROM:

     1. the force for movement is external, being provided by a therapist or mechanical device. When appropriate, a patient may provide the force and be taught to move the part with a normal extremity.

     2. no active resistance or assistance is given by the patient's muscles crossing the joint. If so, it becomes an active exercise.

     3. the motion is done within the free range of motion, that is, the range that is available without forced motion or pain.

   J. If the PLAN OF CARE is the use of ACTIVE-ASSISTIVE OR ACTIVE ROM:

     1. demonstrate to the patient the motion desired using passive ROM, then ask him to perform the motion. Have your hands in position to assist or guide the patient if needed.

     2. assistance is given only as needed for smooth motion. When there is weakness, assistance may be required only at the beginning or end of the ROM.

     3. the motion is done within the available range of motion.

   K. ROM techniques may be performed in the

     1. anatomic planes of range of motion (frontal, sagittal, transverse).

     2. muscle range of elongation (antagonistic to the line of pull of the muscle).

     3. combined patterns (combined movements incorporating several planes of motion).

     4. functional patterns (motions used in activities of daily living).

   L. Monitor the patient's general condition during and following the procedure. Note whether vital signs are affected, any change in the warmth and color of the segment, and any change in the range of motion, pain, or quality of movement.

   M. Document observable and measurable reactions to the treatment.

   N. Modify or progress the treatment as necessary.

VI. TECHNIQUES FOR JOINT AND MUSCLE ROM USING ANATOMIC PLANES OF MOTION[7,13,27]

The following descriptions are, for the most part, with the patient in the supine position. Alternate positions for many motions are possible and for some motions are necessary. For efficiency, do all motions possible in one position, then change the patient's position and do all appropriate motions in that position, progressing the treatment with minimal turning of the patient. Individual body types or environmental limitations might necessitate variations of the suggested hand placements. Use of good body mechanics by the therapist while applying proper stabilization and motion to the patient to accomplish the goals and avoid injury to weakened structures is the primary consideration.

Note: The term upper or top hand means the hand of the therapist that is toward the patient's head; bottom or lower hand refers to the hand towards the patient's foot. Antagonistic ranges of motion are grouped together for ease of application.

A. Upper Extremity

1. Shoulder: flexion and extension (Figure 2-1A and B)

HAND PLACEMENT AND MOTION

Grasp the patient's arm under the elbow with your lower hand. With the top hand, cross over and grasp the wrist and palm of the patient's hand. Lift the arm through the available range and return.

Note: For normal motion, the scapula should be free to rotate upward as the shoulder flexes. If motion of the glenohumeral joint only is desired, the scapula is stabilized as described in the section on stretching (Chapter 4).

2. Shoulder: extension (hyperextension) (Figure 2-2)

ALTERNATE POSITIONS

Extension past zero is possible if the patient's shoulder is at the edge of the bed when supine, or if the patient is positioned side-lying or prone.

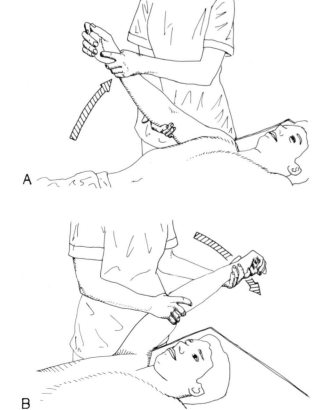

A

B

FIGURE 2–1. Hand placement and positions for initiating (*A*) and completing (*B*) shoulder flexion.

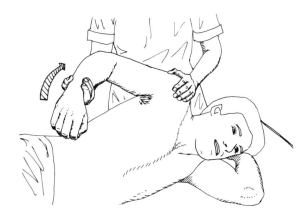

FIGURE 2–2. Hyperextension of the shoulder with the patient side-lying.

3. Shoulder: abduction and adduction (Figure 2-3)

HAND PLACEMENT AND MOTION

Use the same hand placement as with flexion, but move the arm out to the side. The elbow may be flexed.

Note: To reach full range of abduction there must be external rotation of the humerus and upward rotation of the scapula.

4. Shoulder: internal (medial) and external (lateral) rotation (Figure 2-4)

INITIAL POSITION OF THE ARM

If possible, the arm is abducted to 90 degrees, the elbow is flexed to 90 degrees, and the forearm is held in neutral position. Rotation may also be done with the patient's arm at the side of thorax, but full internal rotation will not be possible.

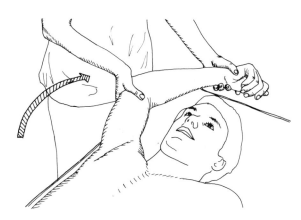

FIGURE 2–3. Abduction of the shoulder with the elbow flexed.

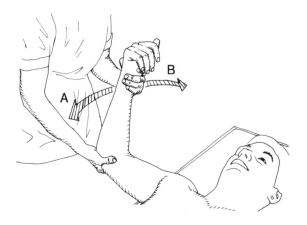

FIGURE 2–4. Position for initiating internal (*A*) and external (*B*) rotation of the shoulder.

HAND PLACEMENT AND MOTION
Grasp the hand and the wrist with your index finger between the patient's thumb and index finger. Place your thumb and the rest of your fingers on either side of the patient's wrist, thus stabilizing the wrist. With the other hand, stabilize the elbow. Rotate the humerus by moving the forearm like a spoke on a wheel.

5. **Shoulder: horizontal abduction (extension) and adduction (flexion) (Figure 2-5A and B)**

POSITION OF THE ARM
To reach full horizontal abduction, the shoulder must be at the edge of the table. Begin with the arm either flexed or abducted 90 degrees.

HAND PLACEMENT AND MOTION
Hand placement is the same as with flexion, but the therapist turns her body and faces the patient's head as his arm is moved out to the side and then across his body.

6. **Scapula: elevation/depression, protraction/retraction, and upward/downward rotation**

POSITION OF PATIENT
Prone, with the patient's arm at his side (Figure 2-6) or side-lying, with the patient facing the therapist and the patient's arm draped over the therapist's bottom arm (see Figure 5-23).

HAND PLACEMENT AND MOTION
Cup the top hand over the acromion process, and place the other hand around the inferior angle of the scapula. For elevation, depression, protraction, and retraction, the clavicle also moves as the scapular motions are directed at the acromion process. For rotation, direct the scapular motions at the inferior angle.

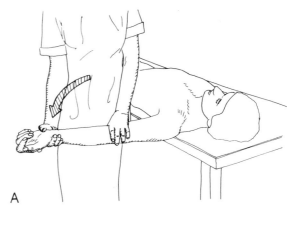

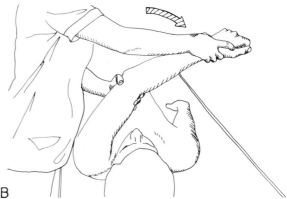

FIGURE 2–5. Horizontal abduction (*A*) and adduction (*B*) of the shoulder.

7. **Elbow: flexion and extension (Figure 2-7)**

HAND PLACEMENT AND MOTION
Hand placement is the same as with shoulder flexion except the motion occurs at the elbow as it is flexed and extended.
Note: Control forearm supination and pronation with your fingers around the wrist. Do elbow flexion and extension with the forearm pronated as well as supinated. The shoulder should not protract when the elbow extends; this disguises the true range.

8. **Elongation of two-joint muscles crossing the shoulder and elbow**
   a. **Biceps brachii muscle** (Figure 2-8)

   POSITION OF PATIENT
   Supine, with the shoulder at the edge of the treatment table so that the shoulder can be extended past the neutral position.

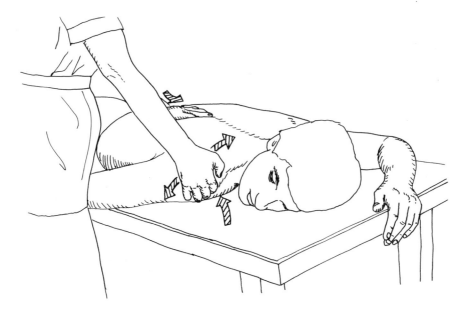

FIGURE 2–6. Scapular motions with the patient prone.

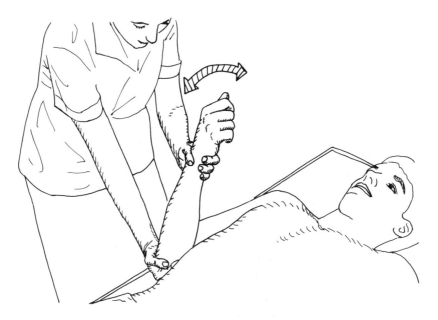

FIGURE 2–7. Elbow motions with the forearm supinated.

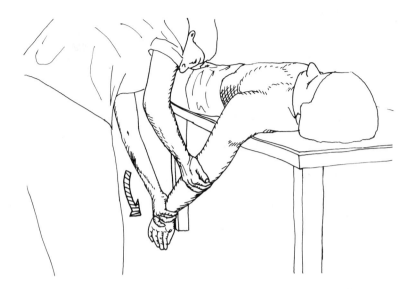

FIGURE 2–8. End range of motion for the biceps brachii muscle.

HAND PLACEMENT AND MOTION
First pronate the patient's forearm by grasping around the wrist, and extend the elbow by supporting under the elbow. The shoulder is then extended (hyperextended) until the patient experiences discomfort in the anterior arm region. At this point, full available lengthening of the two-joint muscle is reached.

b. **Long head of the triceps brachii muscle** (Figure 2-9)

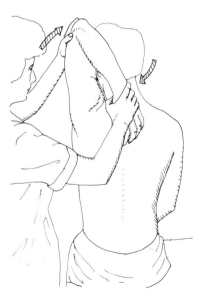

FIGURE 2–9. End range of motion for the long head of the triceps brachii muscle.

POSITION OF PATIENT

When near normal range of this muscle is available, the patient needs to be sitting or standing to reach the full ROM. If there is marked limitation in muscle range, ROM can be done in the supine position.

HAND PLACEMENT AND MOTION

First flex the patient's elbow full range with one hand on the distal forearm, then flex the shoulder by lifting up on the humerus with the other hand under the elbow. Full available range is reached when discomfort is experienced in the posterior arm region.

9. Forearm: pronation and supination (Figure 2-10)

HAND PLACEMENT AND MOTION

Grasp the patient's wrist, supporting the hand with the index finger and placing the thumb and the rest of the fingers on either side of the distal forearm. The motion is a rolling of the radius around the ulna, done at the distal radius. Stabilize the elbow with the other hand.

ALTERNATE HAND PLACEMENT

Sandwich the patient's distal forearm between the palms of your two hands.

Note: Pronation and supination should be done with the elbow both flexed and extended.

Caution: Do not stress the wrist by twisting the hand; control the pronation and supination motion by moving the radius around the ulna.

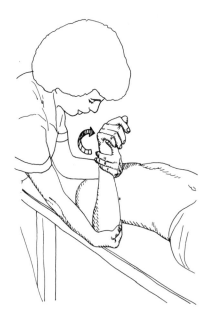

FIGURE 2-10. Pronation of the forearm.

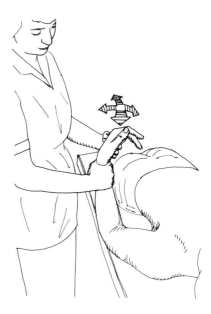

FIGURE 2–11. ROM activities at the wrist.

10. **Wrist: flexion (palmar flexion) and extension (dorsiflexion), radial and ulnar deviation (Figure 2-11)**

    HAND PLACEMENT AND MOTION
    For all wrist motions, grasp the patient's hand just distal to the joint with one hand, and stabilize the forearm with the other hand.
    Note: The range of the extrinsic muscles to the fingers will affect the range at the wrist if tension is placed on them. To get full range of the wrist joint, allow the fingers to move freely as you move the wrist.

11. **Hand: cupping and flattening the arch of the hand at the carpometacarpal and intermetacarpal joints (Figure 2-12)**

    HAND PLACEMENT AND MOTION
    Face the patient's hand; place the fingers in the palms of the patient's hand and the thumbs on the posterior aspect. Roll the metacarpals to increase the arch, then flatten it.

    ALTERNATE HAND PLACEMENT
    One hand is placed on the posterior aspect of the patient's hand with the fingers and thumb cupping around the metacarpals.
    Note: Extension and abduction of the thumb at the carpometacarpal joint are important in maintaining the web space for functional movement of the hand. Isolated flexion-extension and abduction-adduction ROM of this joint should be done as described in number 12.

12. **Joints of the thumb and fingers: flexion and extension and abduction and adduction (of the metacarpophalangeal joints of the fingers) (Figure 2-13A and B)**

    HAND PLACEMENT AND MOTION
    Each joint of the patient's hand can be moved individually by stabilizing the

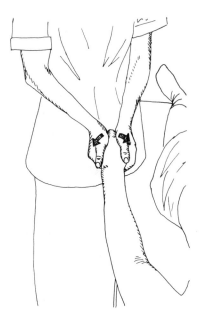

FIGURE 2–12. ROM to the arch of the hand.

proximal bone with the index finger and thumb of one hand, and moving the distal bone with the index finger and thumb of the other hand. Depending on the position of the patient, the forearm and hand can be stabilized on the bed or table, or against the therapist's body.

ALTERNATE METHOD
Several joints can be moved simultaneously if proper stabilization is provided. Example: To move all the metacarpophalangeal joints of digits 2

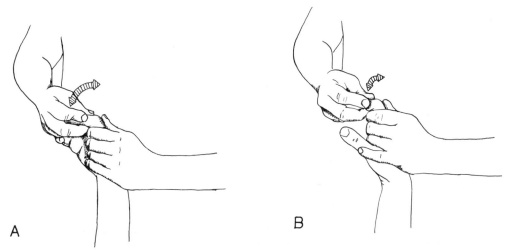

A   B

FIGURE 2–13. ROM to the metacarpophalangeal joint of the thumb (*A*), and interphalangeal joint of a finger (*B*).

through 5, stabilize the metacarpals with one hand and move all the proximal phalanges with the other hand.

Note: To accomplish full joint range of motion, do not place tension on the extrinsic muscles going to the fingers. Tension on the muscles can be relieved by altering the wrist position as the fingers are moved.

13. **Elongation of extrinsic muscles of the wrist and hand**

GENERAL TECHNIQUE

Elongate the muscles over one joint at a time, stabilize that joint, then elongate the muscle over the next joint until the multi-joint muscles are at maximum length. To minimize joint compression of the small joints of the fingers, begin the motion with the distal-most joint.

a. **Flexor digitorum profundus and superficialis muscles** (Figure 2-14A)

HAND PLACEMENT AND MOTION

First extend the distal interphalangeal joints, stabilize them, then extend the proximal interphalangeal joints. Hold these joints then extend the metacarpophalangeal joints.

Stabilize all the finger joints and begin to extend the wrist. When the patient feels discomfort in the forearm, the muscles are fully elongated.

b. **Extensor digitorum muscles** (Figure 2-14B)

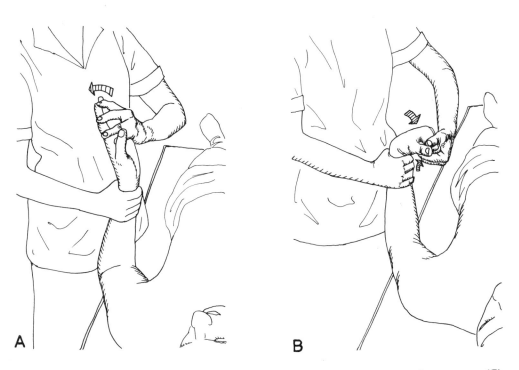

A

B

FIGURE 2–14. End of the range for the extrinsic finger flexors (*A*) and extensors (*B*).

HAND PLACEMENT AND MOTION

First flex the patient's distal interphalangeal joints, hold them, and flex the proximal interphalangeal joints, then the metacarpophalangeal joints. While stabilizing all these joints in the flexed position, begin to flex the wrist until the patient feels discomfort on the dorsum of the hand.

B. Lower Extremity

1. Hip and knee: simultaneous flexion and extension (Figure 2-15A and B)

HAND PLACEMENT AND MOTION

Support the patient's leg with the fingers of the top hand under the patient's knee, and the lower hand under the heel. As the knee flexes full range, swing the fingers to the side of the thigh.

Note: To reach full range of hip flexion, the knee must also be flexed in order to release tension on the hamstring muscle group. To reach full range of knee flexion, the hip must be flexed in order to release tension on the rectus femoris muscle (see number 3).

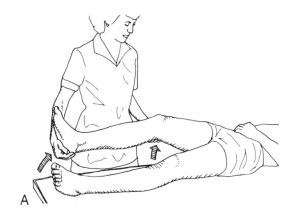

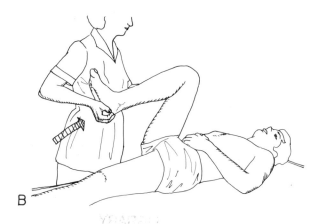

FIGURE 2-15. Initiating (*A*) and completing (*B*) combined hip and knee flexion.

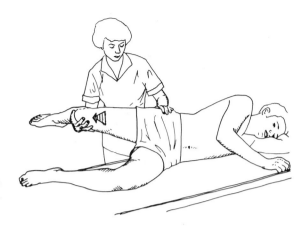

FIGURE 2–16. Hand placements to complete full range of hip extension with the patient side-lying.

2. **Hip: extension (hyperextension) (Figure 2-16)**
ALTERNATE POSITIONS
Prone or side-lying must be used if the patient has near normal or normal motion.

HAND PLACEMENT AND MOTION
If prone, lift with the bottom hand under the patient's knee; stabilize the pelvis with the top hand or arm. If side-lying, bring the bottom hand under the patient's thigh and place the hand on the anterior surface; stabilize the pelvis with the top hand.
Note: If the knee is flexed full range, the rectus femoris muscle is placed on a stretch, and full hip range into extension is limited by tension on the muscle (see number 3, part b to follow).

3. **Elongation of two-joint muscles crossing the hip and knee**
   a. **Hamstring muscle group** (Figure 2-17)

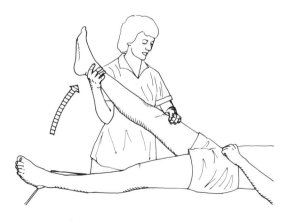

FIGURE 2–17. Range of motion to the hamstring muscle group.

HAND PLACEMENT AND MOTION

Place the lower hand under the patient's heel and the upper hand across the anterior aspect of the patient's knee. Keep the knee in extension as the hip is flexed.

VARIATION

If the hamstrings are so tight as to limit the knee from going into extension, the available range of the muscle is reached simply by extending the knee as far as the muscle allows and not moving the hip.

ALTERNATE HAND PLACEMENT

If the knee requires support, cradle the patient's leg in your lower arm with your elbow flexed under the calf and your hand across the anterior aspect of the patient's knee. The other hand provides support or stabilization where needed.

b. **Rectus femoris muscle**

POSITION OF PATIENT AND MOTION

Supine with knees flexed over the edge of the treatment table. Continue to flex the patient's knee until discomfort is experienced in the anterior thigh, which means the full available range is reached.

ALTERNATE POSITION AND MOTION

Prone; flex the patient's knee until discomfort is felt in the anterior thigh (see Figure 4-18). If the patient has a lot of flexibility, the hip may have to be extended after the knee is flexed full range (similar to Figures 2-16 and 4-9, except the knee is flexed full range before extending the hip).

4. **Hip: abduction and adduction (Figure 2-18)**

HAND PLACEMENT AND MOTION

Support the patient's leg with the upper hand under the knee and the lower hand under the ankle. For full range of adduction, the opposite leg needs to be in a partially abducted position. Keep the patient's hip and knee in extension and neutral to rotation as abduction and adduction are done.

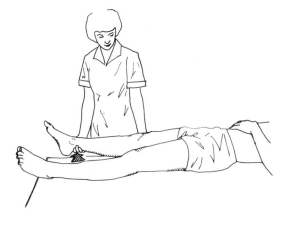

FIGURE 2–18. Abduction of the hip, maintaining the hip in extension and neutral to rotation.

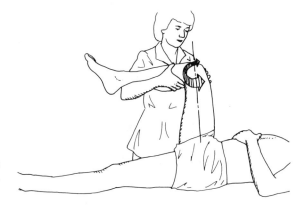

FIGURE 2–19. Rotation of the hip with the hip positioned in 90 degrees flexion.

5. **Hip: internal (medial) and external (lateral) rotation**

   HAND PLACEMENT AND MOTIONS WITH THE HIP AND KNEE EXTENDED
   Grasp just proximal to the patient's knee with the top hand and just proximal to the ankle with the bottom hand. Roll the thigh inward and outward.

   HAND PLACEMENT AND MOTIONS WITH THE HIP AND KNEE FLEXED (FIGURE 2-19)
   Flex the patient's hip and knee to 90 degrees; support the knee with the top hand. Cradle the thigh with the bottom arm, and also support the proximal calf with the bottom hand. Rotate the femur by moving the leg like a pendulum. This hand placement provides some support to the knee but still should be used with caution if there is knee instability.

6. **Ankle: dorsiflexion (Figure 2-20)**

   HAND PLACEMENT AND MOTION
   Stabilize around the malleoli with the top hand. Cup the patient's heel with the bottom hand and place the forearm along the bottom of the foot. Pull

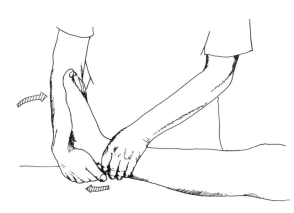

FIGURE 2–20. Dorsiflexion of the ankle.

the calcaneus distalward with the thumb and fingers while pushing upward with the forearm.
Note: If the knee is flexed, full range of the ankle joint can be obtained. If the knee is extended, the lengthened range of the two-joint gastrocnemius muscle can be obtained, but the gastrocnemius will limit full range of dorsiflexion. Dorsiflexion should be done in both positions of the knee to provide range to both the joint and the muscle.

7. Ankle: plantarflexion

HAND PLACEMENT AND MOTION
Place the top hand on the dorsum of the foot and push it into plantarflexion; the other hand supports the heel.
Note: In bed-bound patients the ankle tends to assume a plantarflexed position from the weight of the blankets and pull of gravity, so this motion may not need to be done.

8. Subtalar (lower ankle) joint: inversion and eversion (Figure 2-21A and B)

HAND PLACEMENT AND MOTION
Place the thumb medial and the fingers lateral to the joint on either side of the heel; turn the heel inward and outward.
Note: Supination of the forefoot may be combined with inversion, and pronation may be combined with eversion.

9. Transverse tarsal joint: supination and pronation (Figure 2-22)

HAND PLACEMENT AND MOTION
Stabilize the patient's talus and calcaneus with the top hand. With the bottom hand, grasp around the navicular and cuboid. Gently raise and lower the arch.

10. Joints of the toes: flexion and extension and abduction and adduction (metatarsophalangeal and interphalangeal joints) (Figure 2-23)

HAND PLACEMENT AND MOTION
With one hand, stabilize the bone proximal to the joint that is to be moved

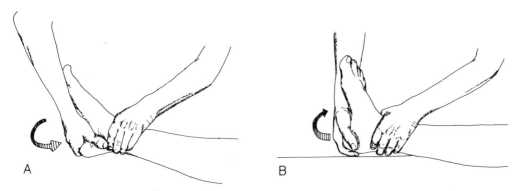

A   B

FIGURE 2–21. End position for inversion (A) and eversion (B) of the subtalar joint.

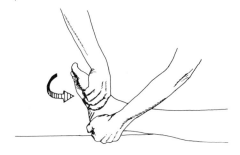

FIGURE 2–22. End position for supination of the transverse tarsal joint.

and move the distal bone with the other hand. The technique is the same as with ROM of the fingers.

ALTERNATE METHOD
Several joints of the toes can be moved simultaneously if care is taken not to stress any structure.

C. Cervical Spine

POSITION OF THERAPIST AND HAND PLACEMENT
Standing at the end of the treatment table, securely grasp the patient's head by placing both hands under the occipital region (Figure 2-24).

1. Flexion (forward bending)

MOTION
Lift the head as though it were nodding.

2. Extension (backward bending or hyperextension)

MOTION
Tip the head backward.
Note: If supine, the patient's head must clear the end of the table. The patient may also be prone or sitting.

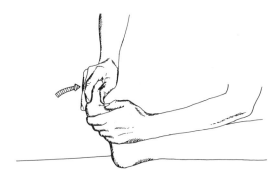

FIGURE 2–23. Extension of the metatarsophalangeal joint of the large toe.

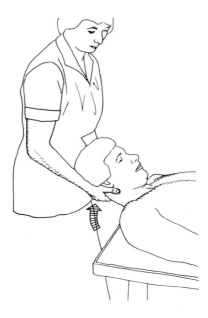

FIGURE 2–24. Hand placement for cervical motions, illustrating flexion.

3. Lateral flexion (side bending)

MOTION
Maintain the cervical spine neutral to flexion and extension as you direct it into side bending and approximate the ear toward the shoulder.

4. Rotation (Figure 2-25)

MOTION
Rotate the head from side to side.

D. Lumbar Spine

1. Flexion (Figure 2-26)

HAND PLACEMENT AND MOTION
Bring both of the patient's knees to his chest by lifting under the knees (hip and knee flexion). Flexion of the spine occurs as the hips are flexed full range and the pelvis starts to rotate posteriorly. Greater range of flexion can be obtained by lifting under the patient's sacrum with the lower hand.

2. Extension

POSITION OF PATIENT
Prone

HAND PLACEMENT AND MOTION
With hands under the thighs, lift the thighs upward until the pelvis rotates anteriorly and the lumbar spine extends.

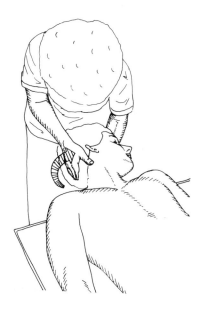

FIGURE 2–25. Hand placement and end of range for cervical rotation to the left.

3. Rotation (Figure 2-27)

POSITION OF PATIENT
Hook-lying.

HAND PLACEMENT AND MOTION
Push both of the patient's knees laterally in one direction until the pelvis on the opposite side comes up off the treatment table. Stabilize the patient's thorax with the top hand. Repeat in the opposite direction.

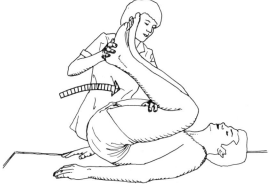

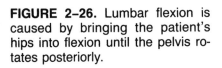
FIGURE 2–26. Lumbar flexion is caused by bringing the patient's hips into flexion until the pelvis rotates posteriorly.

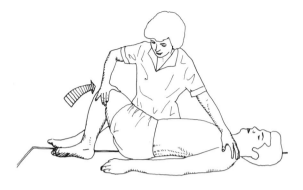

FIGURE 2–27. Rotation of the lumbar spine is caused when the thorax is stabilized and the pelvis lifts off the table as far as allowed.

VII. TECHNIQUES FOR ROM USING COMBINED PATTERNS OF MOTION

Effective and efficient ROM can be administered by combining several joint motions that transect several planes. The following examples include portions of patterns similar to the proprioceptive neuromuscular facilitation (PNF) patterns of movement.[26,28] By using such patterns for passive or active ROM, the goals and program can easily be progressed to facilitation techniques. For explanation and progression of the PNF techniques, the reader is referred to several texts.[26,28] Other patterns can also be developed by the therapist, based on appropriate goals.

A. Upper Extremity

1. Position of patient is supine or sitting. Begin with the patient's shoulder extended, abducted, and internally rotated and the forearm pronated. As you flex the patient's shoulder, simultaneously adduct and externally rotate it and supinate the forearm. Then return the arm to the starting position.
2. Begin the same as in 1, except have the shoulder adducted instead of abducted. As you flex the patient's shoulder, simultaneously abduct and externally rotate it and supinate the forearm. Then return the arm to the starting position.
3. The patterns in 1 and 2 can be done with the elbow flexed or extended, or the elbow can move from one position to the other as the shoulder goes through the ROM.

B. Lower Extremity

1. Position of patient is supine. Begin with the patient's hip extended, abducted, and internally rotated. As you flex the patient's hip, simultaneously adduct and externally rotate it. Then return the lower extremity to the starting position.
2. Begin with the hip extended, adducted, and externally rotated. As you flex the patient's hip, simultaneously abduct and internally rotate it. Then return to the starting position.
3. The patterns in 1 and 2 can be done with the knee flexed or extended, or the knee can move from one position to the other as the hip goes through the ROM.

VIII. TECHNIQUES OF ROM USING SELF-ASSISTANCE AND MECHANICAL ASSISTANCE

A. Self-Assistance

When a patient has unilateral weakness or paralysis, he can be taught to use his normal extremity to move the involved extremity through ranges of motion.[25,27]

1. Arm and forearm

Instruct the patient to reach across his body with his normal extremity and grasp his involved extremity around the wrist, supporting the wrist and hand.

a. Shoulder flexion and extension

The patient lifts the involved extremity over his head and returns it to his side (Figure 2-28A).

b. Shoulder horizontal abduction and adduction

Beginning with his arm abducted 90 degrees, the patient pulls his extremity across his chest and returns it out to the side (Figure 2-28B).

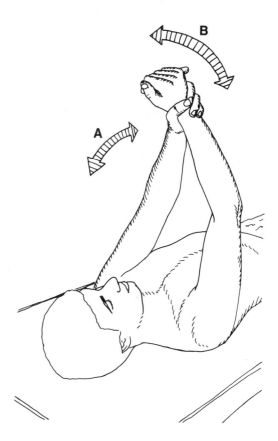

FIGURE 2–28. Patient giving self-assisted ROM to shoulder flexion and extension (*A*) or horizontal abduction and adduction (*B*).

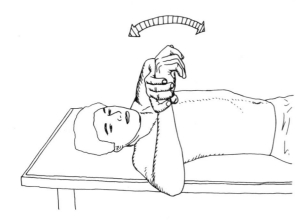

FIGURE 2–29. Arm position of patient for giving self-assisted ROM to internal and external rotation of shoulder.

  c. **Shoulder rotation**
    Beginning with the arm abducted 90 degrees and elbow flexed 90 degrees, the patient rotates his forearm (Figure 2-29).
  d. **Elbow flexion and extension**
    The patient bends his elbow until the hand is near the shoulder, then moves the hand down toward the side of his leg.
  e. **Pronation and supination of the forearm**
    Beginning with his forearm resting across his body, the patient rotates the radius around the ulna. Emphasize to the patient not to twist the hand at the wrist joint.

2. **Wrist and hand**
  The patient's normal thumb is moved to his involved hands with his normal fingers along the dorsum of his hand.
  a. **Wrist flexion and extension and radial and ulnar deviation**
    The patient moves his wrist in all directions, applying no pressure against the fingers (Figure 2-30).
  b. **Finger flexion and extension**
    The patient uses his normal thumb to extend his involved fingers, and cups his normal fingers over the dorsum of the involved fingers to flex them (Figure 2-31).
  c. **Thumb flexion with opposition and extension with reposition**
    The patient cups his normal fingers around the radial border of the thenar eminence of his involved thumb and places his normal thumb along the palmar surface of the involved thumb to extend it (Figure 2-32). To flex and oppose his thumb, he cups his normal hand around the dorsal surface of the involved hand and pushes the first metacarpal toward the little finger.

3. **Hip and knee**
  The patient is supine; he is instructed to slide his normal foot under the knee of the involved extremity (Figure 2-33).
  a. Hip and knee flexion
    Instruct the patient to initiate the motion by lifting his involved knee up with the normal foot. He then can grasp the knee with his normal hand and bring the knee up toward his chest.

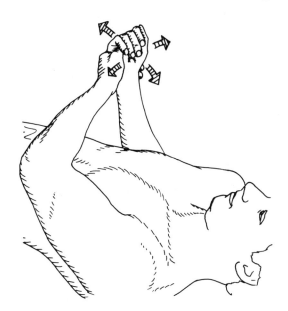

FIGURE 2-30. Patient applying self-assisted wrist motions.

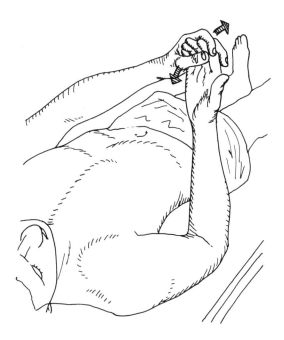

FIGURE 2-31. Patient applying self-assisted finger flexion and extension.

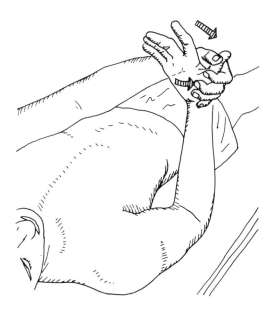

FIGURE 2–32. Patient applying self-assisted thumb extension.

    b. Hip abduction and adduction
        Instruct the patient to slide his normal foot from the knee down to his ankle and then move the involved extremity from side to side.

  4. Ankle and toes
    The patient sits with the involved extremity crossed over the normal so that the distal leg rests on the normal knee. With the normal hand, the involved ankle can be moved into dorsiflexion and plantarflexion, inversion and eversion, and toe flexion and extension (Figure 2-34).

B. Wand Exercises

When a patient has voluntary muscle control in an involved upper extremity but needs guidance or motivation to complete the ranges of motion in the shoulder or elbow, a dowel rod (cane, wooden stick, or similar object) can be used to provide assistance.

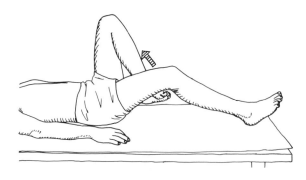

FIGURE 2–33. Position of patient's foot for initiating self-assisted ROM to the hip.

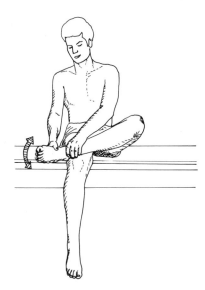

FIGURE 2–34. Position of patient and hand placement for self-assisted ankle motions.

PROCEDURE

Initially, guide the patient through the proper motion for each activity to ensure that he does not use substitute motions. The patient grasps the wand with both hands; the normal extremity guides the involved extremity. He may be standing, sitting, or supine.

1. Shoulder flexion and return (Figure 2-35)

The wand is grasped with the hands a shoulder-width apart. The wand is lifted forward and upward through the available range, with the elbows kept

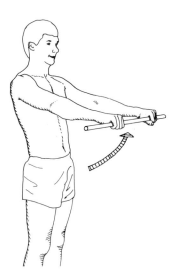

FIGURE 2–35. The patient using a wand for self-assisted shoulder flexion.

in extension if possible. There should be smooth scapulohumeral motion; do not allow scapular elevation or trunk twisting.

2. Shoulder horizontal abduction and adduction

The wand is lifted to 90 degrees flexion (same as in Figure 2-35). Keeping the elbows in extension, the patient pushes and pulls the wand back and forth across his chest through the available range. Do not allow trunk rotation.

3. Shoulder internal and external rotation (Figure 2-36)

The patient's shoulders are abducted 90 degrees and his elbows flexed 90 degrees. For external rotation, the wand is moved toward the patient's head; for internal rotation, the wand is moved toward his waistline.

ALTERNATE POSITION

The patient's arms are at his sides and the elbows are flexed 90 degrees. Rotation of the arms is accomplished by moving the wand from side to side across the trunk while maintaining the elbows at the side. The rotation should occur in the humerus; do not allow elbow flexion and extension.

4. Elbow flexion and extension

The patient's forearms may be pronated or supinated; the hands grasp the wand, shoulder-width apart. Instruct the patient to flex and extend the elbows.

5. Shoulder hyperextension

The patient may be standing or prone. He places the wand behind his buttocks, grasps the wand with hands, shoulder-width apart, and then lifts the wand backward away from the trunk. He should avoid trunk flexion.

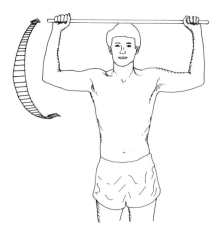

FIGURE 2–36. The patient using a wand for self-assisted shoulder rotation.

6. Variations and combinations of movements

For example, the patient begins with the wand behind his buttocks (as in number 5), then moves the wand up his back to achieve scapular winging, shoulder internal rotation, and elbow flexion.

C. Finger Ladder

The finger ladder (or wall climbing) is a device that can provide the patient with objective reinforcement and therefore motivation for doing shoulder range of motion.

Precaution: The patient must be taught the proper motions and not allowed to substitute with trunk side bending, toe raising, or scapular elevation.

1. Shoulder flexion

The patient stands, facing the finger ladder an arm's length away, and places the index or middle finger on a step of the ladder. The arm is moved into flexion by climbing with the fingers. The patient steps closer to the ladder as the arm is elevated.

2. Shoulder abduction (Figure 2-37)

The patient stands sideways, with the affected shoulder toward the ladder an arm's length away. The patient needs to externally rotate the shoulder as he abducts with elevation.

D. Overhead Pulleys

If properly taught, pulley systems can be effectively used to assist an involved extremity in performing ROM.

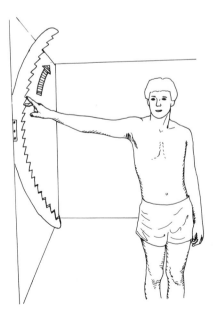

FIGURE 2–37. Shoulder abduction using a finger ladder.

PULLEY SET-UP

Two pulleys are attached to an overhead bar or to the ceiling approximately shoulder-width apart. A rope is passed over both pulleys, and a handle is attached to each end of the rope. The patient may be sitting, standing, or supine, with the shoulders aligned under the pulleys.

1. **Shoulder flexion (Figure 2-38A) and abduction (Figure 2-38B)**

    Instruct the patient to hold one handle in each hand, then with the normal hand, pull the rope and lift the involved extremity, either forward (flexion) or out to the side (abduction). The elbow should be kept in extension if possible. The patient should not shrug the shoulder (scapular elevation) or lean the trunk. Guide and instruct the patient so there is smooth motion.

    Precaution: Assistive pulley activities for the shoulder are easily misused by the patient, resulting in compression of the humerus against the acromion process. Continual compression will lead to pain and decreased function. Proper patient selection and appropriate instruction can avoid this problem. If a patient cannot learn to use the pulley with proper shoulder mechanics, it should not be done. With increased pain or decreased mobility, discontinue this activity (see Chapter 7).

2. **Shoulder internal and external rotation (Figure 2-39)**

    Position the patient with the shoulder abducted 90 degrees and the elbow flexed 90 degrees. Have the arm supported on the back of a chair if sitting,

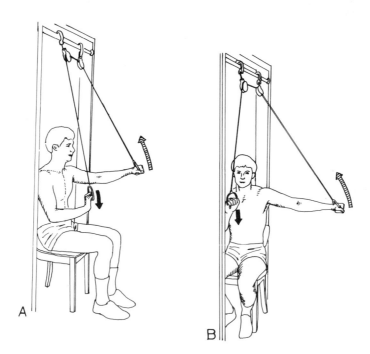

FIGURE 2–38. Shoulder flexion (*A*) and abduction (*B*) using overhead pulleys to assist the motion.

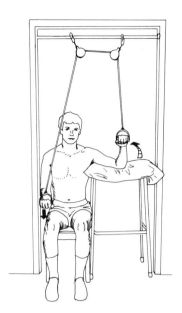

FIGURE 2–39. Position for shoulder rotation using overhead pulleys to assist the motion.

or on the treatment table if supine. The patient then lifts the forearm with the pulley, causing rotation in the arm.

3. Elbow flexion

With the patient's arm stabilized along the side of his trunk, he lifts his forearm and bends his elbow.

E. Shoulder Wheel

With proper instruction, the shoulder wheel can be used to motivate a patient to do active ROM activities at the shoulder. Resistance can also be added to the wheel for strengthening procedures.

SET-UP

A shoulder wheel is permanently attached to a wall. Usually it can be adjusted to various heights and arm lengths.

PROCEDURE

The patient is positioned so that his shoulder joint is at the axis of the wheel and the motion desired is in the arc of the wheel. The patient should not feel the need nor be instructed to move the wheel through its entire arc (for example, through the full circle) for any one motion. To avoid this, do not allow him to twist or turn his body. The range of the shoulder joint and arc of the bone should direct how far the patient moves.

1. Abduction and adduction (Figure 2-40)

The patient stands facing the wheel or with his back to it. The axis of the shoulder joint is matched to the axis of the wheel. The handle is adjusted to match the length of his arm. He then grasps the handle and moves his arm clockwise or counterclockwise to the limit of his range of motion. When

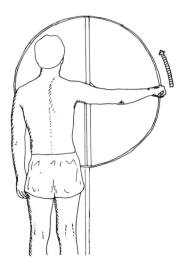

FIGURE 2–40. One position for shoulder abduction using a shoulder wheel for assistance.

elevating the arm above the horizontal plane, the patient should externally rotate the shoulder.

2. Flexion and extension

The patient stands sideways with the involved shoulder toward the wheel. He then moves the wheel forward and backward to the limits of his range of motion.

3. Internal and external rotation (Figure 2-41)

The patient's shoulder is abducted to 90 degrees and his elbow flexed to 90 degrees. He stands sideways with his elbow placed at the axis of the wheel.

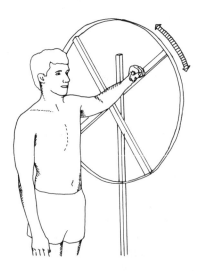

FIGURE 2–41. Position for shoulder rotation using a shoulder wheel for assistance.

The handle is adjusted so his hand can grasp it; he then turns his arm to the limits of his range of motion.

F. Skate Board; Powder Board

These devices are usually used following surgical procedures to the hip to encourage ROM (see Chapter 10). Proper instructions make them useful, but just telling the patient to move his leg often results in faulty movement or lack of interest.

PROCEDURE
Place the board under the involved extremity. If available, strap a skate to the foot. If there is no skate, place powder or a towel under the extremity to lower the friction of the leg moving on the board.

1. Hip abduction and adduction

POSITION OF PATIENT
The patient is supine. The foot should be pointing upright to keep the hip neutral to rotation. Do not allow the leg to roll outward as the patient moves it from side to side.

2. Hip flexion and extension

POSITION OF PATIENT
The patient is supine. He slides his foot up and down the board, allowing the knee to also flex and extend. The hip should not rotate, abduct, or adduct.

ALTERNATE POSITION
The patient is side-lying, with the affected hip up. The board is placed between the legs and supported with pillows if necessary. The skateboard can also be placed on an elevated platform.
Precaution: If side-lying is used following hip surgery, the affected hip must not fall into adduction.

G. Suspension

This technique is used to free a body part from the resistance of friction while it is moving. The part is suspended in a sling attached to a rope that is fixed to an appropriate point above the body segment.[7,8]

1. Two types of suspension

a. Vertical fixation
The point of attachment of the rope is over the center of gravity of the moving segment. The part can then move like a pendulum, describing an arc (Figure 2-42). Usually the movement is small range, so this type of suspension is primarily used for support.
b. Axial fixation
The point of attachment of all ropes supporting the part is above the axis of the joint to be moved (Figure 2-43). The part will move on a flat plane, parallel to the floor. This type of fixation allows for maximum movement of a joint.

2. Benefits of suspension for ROM exercises[8]

a. Active participation is required, thus the patient learns to use the appropriate muscles for the desired movement.

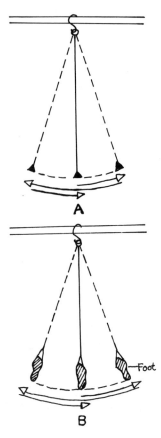

FIGURE 2–42. Vertical fixation: Movement of a pendulum (*A*). Attachment of the rope over the center of gravity of the extremity results in the foot moving like a pendulum (*B*). (Redrawn from Hollis,[7] p. 71, with permission.)

    b. Relaxation is promoted through secure support and smooth rhythmic motion.

    c. Little work is required of stabilizing muscles because the part is supported.

    d. Modifications can be made to the system to provide grades of exercise resistance.[7–11]

    e. After instruction, the patient can often work independently of a therapist.

3. Examples for active ROM using axial fixation suspension

For extensive descriptions of suspension set-ups, refer to the sources listed in references 7 through 11.

    a. Shoulder abduction and adduction with axial fixation (Figure 2-44)

    b. Hip flexion and extension with axial fixation (Figure 2-45)

H. Reciprocal Exercise Unit

This device can be set up to provide some hip and knee flexion and extension to an involved lower extremity by using the strength of a normal lower extremity. The device is mobile in that it can be attached to a patient's bed, wheel-

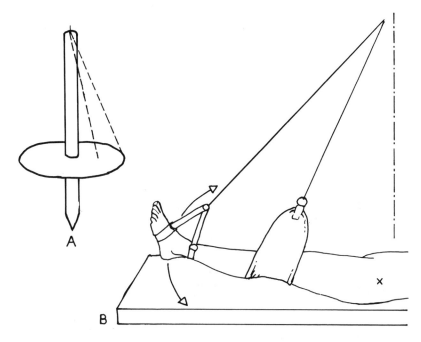

FIGURE 2–43. Axial fixation: A pencil through a circle of paper demonstrates that the paper moves parallel to the floor when the pencil is pivoted (*A*). Attachment of all ropes above the joint results in the extremity moving parallel to the floor (*B*). (Redrawn from Hollis,[7] p. 72, with permission.)

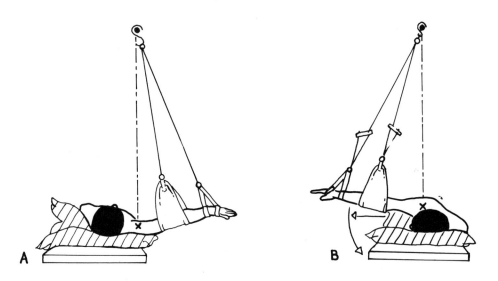

FIGURE 2–44. Shoulder abduction and adduction in axial fixation (_ . _ . axial line) supine (*A*) and prone (*B*). This position may be used for protraction and retraction of the scapula. (Redrawn from Hollis,[7] p. 76, with permission.)

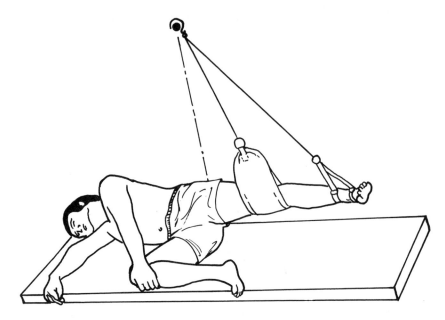

FIGURE 2–45. Flexion and extension of the hip joint in axial fixation (_ . _ . axial line). (Redrawn from Hollis,[7] p. 75, with permission.)

chair, or standard chair. The circumference of motion as well as excursion of the lower extremities can be adjusted. A reciprocal exercise unit has additional exercise benefits in that it can be used for reciprocal patterning, endurance training, and initiating a strengthening program. (See Chapter 3, Figure 3-30.)

I. Applications

The variety of applications of mechanical devices for assistive ROM is potentially endless, being limited only by the imagination and resources of the therapist. Whenever using equipment, the primary concerns must be:

1. Goals

Does the motion accomplish the goals?

2. Proper mechanics of the moving segment

Is proper stabilization provided and has proper instruction been given to avoid substitute motions?

3. Patient comfort and safety

Are all hazards to the patient from faulty equipment or improper instruction eliminated?

IX. CONTINUOUS PASSIVE MOTION (CPM)

Continuous passive motion (CPM), in contrast to intermittent passive motion, is motion that is uninterrupted for extended periods of time.[5] It is usually applied by a mechanical device that moves a desired joint continuously through a controlled range of motion without patient effort for as long as 24 hours a day, for 7 or more successive days. The motion is passive so that muscle fatigue does not interfere with the motion. A machine is used because an individual would not be able to apply the controlled motion continually for the extended periods of time. The treatment technique is based on the research and protocols developed by Robert Salter.[23]

A. Benefits of CPM[5,19-24]

1. CPM is effective in lessening the negative effects of joint immobilization in conditions such as arthritis, contractures and intra-articular fractures; in decreasing the frequency of postoperative complications; and in improving the recovery rate and range of motion following a variety of surgical procedures.
2. CPM has been shown to:
   a. prevent development of adhesions and decrease contracture formation
   b. decrease postoperative pain
   c. enhance nutritional status of the extremity by improving the circulation through the continuous pumping action
   d. increase synovial fluid lubrication of the joint
   e. decrease joint effusion and wound edema, thus improving wound healing
   f. increase the rate of intra-articular cartilage healing and regeneration
   g. provide a quicker return of the range of motion

B. Procedure[1,6,23]

Note: a variety of protocols have been developed based on individual surgeon's experience. Patient response, surgical procedure, or disease entity may necessitate modifying the range, time, and duration of CPM application.

1. The device may be applied to the involved extremity immediately following surgery while the patient is still under anesthesia, or at least within 3 days after surgery if bulky dressings prevent early motion.
2. The size and position of the motion arc for the joint is determined. A low arc of 20 to 30 degrees may be used immediately after surgery. The degrees are readjusted daily or at an appropriate time interval in order to progress the patient's range as tolerated.
3. The rate of motion is determined; usually 1 cycle per minute or per 2 minutes is well tolerated.
4. The amount of time on the CPM machine may vary for different protocols; anywhere from continuous for 24 hours to continuous for 1 hour 3 times a day.[6,23] The longer periods of time per day reportedly result in a shorter hospital stay, fewer postoperative complications, and greater range of motion at discharge,[6] although no significant difference was found in a study that compared 5 hours per day with 20 hours per day of CPM.[1]
5. Physical therapy treatments are usually initiated during periods when the patient is not on CPM, including active assistive or sling exercises.
6. Duration minimum is usually 1 week or when a satisfactory range of motion is reached. A therapeutic exercise program of active exercises is continued until the patient attains appropriate functional goals.

C. Equipment (Figure 2-46)

Several different companies now manufacture CPM machines. They are designed to be adjustable, easily controlled, versatile, and portable. Some are battery operated to allow the individual to wear the device for up to 8 hours

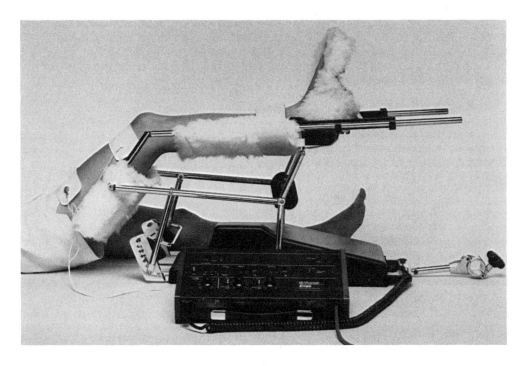

FIGURE 2–46. CM-100 Continuous Motion Device. (Courtesy of Empi Inc., St. Paul, MN)

while functioning with daily activities. The batteries are then recharged while the person sleeps. Machines have been developed for just about every peripheral joint.

X. RANGE OF MOTION THROUGH FUNCTIONAL PATTERNS

To accomplish motion through functional patterns, first determine what pattern of movement is desired, then move the extremity through that pattern using manual assistance, mechanical assistance if it is appropriate, or self-assistance from the patient. Functional patterning can be beneficial in initiating the teaching of activities of daily living (ADL) as well as in instructing the blind in functional activities.[12]

XI. SUMMARY

The benefits, limitations, indications, contraindications, and techniques of both passive and active range of motion exercises have been described. Techniques included manual ROM using anatomic planes and combined patterns, self-assisted ROM, and mechanical-assisted ROM.

REFERENCES

1. Basso, DM and Knapp, L: *Comparison of two continuous passive motion protocols for patients with total knee implants.* Phys Ther 67:360, 1987.
2. Bonner, CD, Johnson, M, and Lynford, BE: *A portable sling suspension apparatus.* Phys Ther 49:47, 1969.

3. Donatelli, R and Owens-Burckhart, H: *Effects of immobilization on the extensibility of periarticular connective tissue.* JOSPT 3:67, 1981.
4. *Exercise Testing and Training of Individuals with Heart Disease or at High Risk for its Development: A Handbook for Physicians.* American Heart Association, The Committee on Exercise, 1975.
5. Frank, C, et al: *Physiology and therapeutic value of passive joint motion.* Clin Orthopaed Rel Res 185:113, 1984.
6. Gose, J: *Continuous passive motion in the postoperative treatment of patients with total knee replacement.* Phys Ther 67:39, 1987.
7. Hollis, M: *Practical Exercise Therapy.* Blackwell Scientific Publications, London, 1976.
8. Johnson, MM and Bonner, CD: *Sling suspension techniques demonstrating the use of a new portable frame. Part I: Introduction, definitions, equipment and advantages.* Phys Ther 51:524, 1971.
9. Johnson, MM and Bonner, CD: *Sling suspension techniques demonstrating the use of a new portable frame. Part II: Methods of progression in an exercise program: The upper extremity.* Phys Ther 51:1092, 1971.
10. Johnson, MM and Bonner, CD: *Sling suspension techniques demonstrating the use of a new portable frame. Part III: Treatment of motor disabilities: The lower extremity.* Phys Ther 51:1288, 1971.
11. Johnson, MM, Ehrenkranz, C, and Bonner, CD: *Sling suspension techniques demonstrating the use of a new portable frame. Part IV: Treatment of motor disabilities: Neck and trunk.* Phys Ther 53:856, 1973.
12. Kennedy, C: *Is there any rational basis for the theory that repetitive passive movement can contribute to voluntary motion?* Phys Ther 48:256, 1968.
13. Kisner, C and Allen, L: *Therapeutic Exercise I: Course Syllabus and Laboratory Manual.* The Ohio State University, Division of Physical Therapy, Columbus, 1981.
14. Lehmkuhl, LD and Smith, L: *Brunnstrom's Clinical Kinesiology,* ed 4. FA Davis, Philadelphia, 1983.
15. *Manual of Orthopaedic Surgery.* American Orthopaedic Association, Chicago, 1972.
16. Minor, MD and Minor, SD: *Patient Evaluation Methods for the Health Professional.* Reston Publishing Co, Reston, VA, 1985.
17. Moore, ML: *Clinical assessment of joint motion.* In Basmajian, JV (ed): *Therapeutic Exercises,* ed 3. Williams & Wilkins, Baltimore, 1978.
18. Norkin, CC and White, DJ: *Measurement of Joint Motion: A Guide to Goniometry.* FA Davis, Philadelphia, 1985.
19. Salter, RB, Simmens, DF, and Malcolm, BW: *The biological effects of continuous passive motion on the healing of full thickness defects in articular cartilage.* J Bone Joint Surg (Am) 62:1232, 1980.
20. Salter, RB: *The prevention of arthritis through the preservation of cartilage.* J Can Assoc Radiol 31:5, 1981.
21. Salter, RB, Bell, RS, and Keely, FW: *The protective effect of continuous passive motion on living cartilage in acute septic arthritis.* Clin Orthop 159:223, 1981.
22. Salter, RB: *Textbook of Disorders and Injuries of the Musculoskeletal System,* ed 2. Williams & Wilkins, Baltimore, 1983.
23. Salter, RB, et al: *Clinical application of basic research on continuous passive motion for disorders and injuries of synovial joints.* J Orthop Res 1:325, 1984.
24. Stap, LJ and Woodfin, PM: *Continuous passive motion in the treatment of knee flexion contractures: A case report.* Phys Ther 66:1720, 1986.
25. *Strike Back at Stroke.* American Heart Association, New York.
26. Sullivan, P, Markos, P, and Minor, M: *An Integrated Approach to Therapeutic Exercise: Theory and Clinical Application.* Reston Publishing Co., Reston, VA, 1982.
27. Tookey, P and Larson, C: *Range of Motion Exercise: Key to Joint Mobility.* Rehabilitation Publication No. 703. American Rehabilitation Foundation, Minneapolis, 1968.
28. Voss, DE, Ionta, MK, and Myers, BJ: *Proprioceptive Neuromuscular Facilitation,* ed 3. Haper & Row, Philadelphia, 1985.
29. Wenger, N and Hillerstein, H: *Rehabilitation of the Coronary Patient.* John Wiley & Sons, New York, 1978.

Resistance Exercise

If resistance is applied to a muscle as it contracts, the muscle will become stronger over a period of time. Adaptive changes can occur in muscle through the use of therapeutic exercise if the metabolic capabilities of the muscle are progressively overloaded.[38] Muscle, which is contractile tissue, becomes stronger as the result of hypertrophy of muscle fibers and an increase in the recruitment of motor units in the muscle.[17,26,35,55,58,93] As the strength of a muscle increases, the cardiovascular response of the muscle improves so that muscular endurance and power also increase.

Many factors, such as disease, disuse, and immobilization, may result in muscle weakness.[14,71,87] The therapeutic use of resistance in an exercise program, whether applied manually or mechanically, is an integral part of a patient's PLAN OF CARE when the ultimate goal is to improve strength, endurance, and overall physical function.

OBJECTIVES

After studying this chapter, the reader will be able to:
1. define resistance exercise.
2. describe the goals and indications for resistance exercise and differentiate strength, endurance, and power.
3. explain the precautions and contraindications of resistance exercise.
4. describe and differentiate between isotonic, isometric, and isokinetic resistance exercise.
5. explain the similarities and differences between manual and mechanical resistance exercise.
6. explain the principles of application of manual resistance exercise.
7. describe appropriate techniques of manual resistance exercise, using the anatomic planes of motion.
8. define mechanical resistance exercise.
9. describe specific regimens of resistance exercise.
10. discuss the variables found in resistance exercise programs.
11. identify and explain the use of various types of equipment used in resistance exercise.

I. DEFINITION OF RESISTANCE EXERCISE

Resistance exercise is any form of active exercise in which a dynamic or static muscular contraction is resisted by an outside force.[43] The external force may be applied manually or mechanically.

A. Manual Resistance Exercise

Manual resistance exercise is a type of active exercise in which resistance is provided by a therapist or other health professional. Although the amount of resistance cannot be measured quantitatively, this technique is useful in the early stages of an exercise program when the muscle to be strengthened is weak and can overcome only mild to moderate resistance. It is also useful when the range of joint movement needs to be carefully controlled. The amount of resistance given is limited only by the strength of the therapist.

B. Mechanical Resistance Exercise

Mechanical resistance exercise is a form of active exercise in which resistance is applied through the use of equipment or a mechanical apparatus. The amount of resistance can be measured quantitatively and progressed over time. It is often used in specific resistance exercise regimens. It is also useful when amounts of resistance greater than the therapist can apply manually are necessary.

II. GOALS AND INDICATIONS OF RESISTANCE EXERCISE

The overall purpose of resistance exercise is to improve physical function. The specific goals are to:

A. Increase Strength

1. Strength refers to the force output of a contracting muscle and is directly related to the amount of tension a contracting muscle can produce.[38,41,56,79]
2. In order to increase the strength of a muscle, the muscle contraction must be loaded or resisted so that increasing levels of tension will develop due to hypertrophy and recruitment of muscle fibers (see Chapter 1).

B. Increase Muscular Endurance

1. Endurance is the ability to perform low-intensity repetitive exercise over a prolonged period of time.[17,26]
2. Muscular endurance is improved by performing exercise against mild resistance for many repetitions.[13]
3. It has been shown that in most exercise programs designed to increase strength, muscular endurance also increases.[17]
4. In certain clinical situations it may be more appropriate to implement a resistance exercise program that will increase a patient's muscular endurance rather than his strength. For example, it has been shown that after many acute or chronic knee injuries, dynamic exercises, carried out for a high number of repetitions against light resistance, are more comfortable

and create less joint irritation than dynamic exercises performed against heavy resistance.[60,89]

5. Total body endurance also can be improved with prolonged low-intensity exercise. This will be discussed in detail in Chapter 21.

C. Increase Power

1. Power is also a measure of muscular performance and is defined as work per unit of time[13,37,56,58] (force × distance/time). Force times velocity is an equivalent definition.[58,69,77,78,79]

2. The rate at which a muscle contracts and develops force throughout the range of motion and the relationship of speed and force are both factors that affect power.[6,68]

3. When exercise is performed dynamically against resistance over a specified interval of time, power will increase.

   a. Power can be increased by moving either a very high load for a low number of repetitions or a low load for a high number of repetitions to the point of muscular fatigue.[79]

   b. In some of the literature in sports medicine and physical education the term power is used to describe a burst of high-intensity muscle activity that occurs for a very short period of time (10 to 20 seconds) to the point of muscular fatigue.[11,31] Although this may be descriptive of certain physical activities, it is inappropriate to limit the use of the term power to explosive high-effort muscle activity only.[79]

   c. Some authors[13,26] call high-intensity exercise carried out over a short interval of time anaerobic power, and low-intensity exercise sustained over a long period of time aerobic power. (The terms aerobic power and endurance are often used interchangeably.)

      (1) This distinction is made because[26,77,79]

         (a) Type II (phasic fast-twitch) muscle fibers, which generate a great amount of tension in a short period of time, are geared toward anaerobic metabolic activity and tend to fatigue quickly.

         (b) Type I (tonic, slow-twitch) muscle fibers generate a low level of muscle tension but can sustain the contraction for a long time. These fibers are geared toward aerobic metabolism and are very slow to fatigue.

      (2) Muscles are composed of both phasic and tonic fibers.

         (a) Some muscles have a greater distribution of tonic fibers and others have a greater distribution of phasic fibers.

         (b) This leads to differentiation and specialization in muscles. For example, a heavy distribution of Type I tonic fibers is found in postural muscles in which low-level, sustained muscle tension constantly holds the body erect against gravity.

            A high proportion of Type II phasic motor units is found in muscles that produce a great burst of tension to enable a person to lift his entire body weight when climbing a flight of stairs or propelling himself forward on crutches.

4. Resistance exercise programs can be designed to selectively recruit different fiber types in muscles by controlling the intensity and speed of exercise.

There is no question that strength, endurance, and power are all related and can all be improved with resistance exercises. It is important that the therapist evaluate each clinical situation and design exercise programs that will meet the specific needs of each patient.

III. PRECAUTIONS FOR AND CONTRAINDICATIONS TO RESISTANCE EXERCISE

Although manual and mechanical resistance exercises have significant value, there are a number of precautions and contraindications that a therapist must consider before implementing and while carrying out a resistance exercise program.

A. Precautions

1. **Cardiovascular precautions**[47]

   a. The Valsalva's maneuver, which is an expiratory effort against a closed glottis, must be avoided during resistance exercise. When a person is exerting a strenuous and prolonged effort, the phenomenon can occur.

   b. Description of the sequence

      (1) Deep inspiration

      (2) Closure of the glottis

      (3) Contraction of abdominal muscles

      (4) Increase in intrathoracic and intra-abdominal pressures that leads to decreased venous blood flow to the heart. Decreased venous return leads to a decreased cardiac output, which, in turn, causes a temporary drop in arterial blood pressure. This decrease in arterial pressure leads to an increase in the heart rate.

      (5) When the expiratory effort is *released* and expiration occurs, there is a pronounced *increase* in blood pressure up to 200 mm Hg or higher. This is due to rapid venous blood flow into the heart and leads to a forceful contraction of the heart.

   c. Significance in exercise

      (1) The Valsalva's maneuver should be avoided during exercise so that abnormal stress on the cardiovascular system and the abdominal wall can be avoided.

      (2) High-risk patients

         (a) Patients with a history of cardiovascular poblems (cerebrovascular accident, myocardial infarction, or hypertension)

         (b) Geriatric patients

         (c) Patients who have had abdominal surgery or herniation of the abdominal wall

   d. Prevention of the Valsalva's maneuver during exercise[25,47]

      (1) Caution the patient about holding his breath.

      (2) Have the patient exhale when performing a motion.

      (3) Ask the patient to count or talk or breathe rhythmically during exercise.

      Note: The Valsalva's maneuver is most commonly seen when a patient is performing isometric[25] or heavy resistance exercise[16]. Patients with a history of cardiovascular problems should be monitored closely and may have to avoid isometric or heavy resistance exercises completely.[16,25]

2. **Fatigue**

   Fatigue is a complex phenomenon that affects functional performance and must be considered in a therapeutic exercise program. Fatigue has a variety of definitions, which are based on the type of fatigue being discussed.[14]

   a. Local muscle fatigue is the diminished response of a muscle to a repeated stimulus.[7] This is a normal physiologic response of muscle and is characterized by a decrease in the amplitude of the motor unit potentials.[14]

(1) Muscle fatigue can occur during either dynamic or static muscular contractions and whenever high-intensity or low-intensity exercise is performed over a period of time.

(2) The diminished response of the muscle is due to a combination of factors which include[26,83,93]

    (a) disturbances in the contractile mechanism of the muscle itself because of a decrease in energy stores, insufficient oxygen, and a build-up of lactic acid.

    (b) inhibitory (protective) influences from the central nervous system.

    (c) possibly a decrease in the conduction of impulses at the myoneural junction, particularly in fast-twitch fibers.

(3) Muscle fatigue is associated with an uncomfortable sensation within the muscle or even pain and spasm. When fatigued, the response of the muscle may be slower or the range of movement performed by the muscle will be less.[42]

b. General muscular (total body) fatigue is the diminished response of a person during prolonged physical activity such as walking or jogging.

(1) General fatigue with very prolonged but relatively low-intensity exercise is probably due to[26,34]

    (a) a decrease in blood sugar (glucose) levels.

    (b) a decrease in glycogen stores in muscle and liver.

    (c) a depletion of potassium, especially in the elderly patient.

(2) This is an important consideration in endurance and conditioning programs and will be discussed further in Chapter 21.

c. Fatigue associated with specific clinical diseases[14]

(1) Fatigue may occur more rapidly or at predictable intervals in certain diseases associated with neuromuscular or cardiopulmonary dysfunction.

    (a) In multiple sclerosis the patient usually awakens rested and functions well in the early morning. By mid-afternoon the patient reaches a peak of fatigue and becomes notably weak. Then by early evening fatigue diminishes and strength improves.

    (b) Patients with cardiac disease, peripheral vascular dysfunction, and pulmonary disease all have deficits that compromise the oxygen transport system. These patients fatigue more rapidly and require a longer period of time for recovery from fatigue.

(2) The therapist must be aware of the patterns of fatigue that occur in specific diseases and gear the exercise program accordingly.

3. Recovery from fatigue

Adequate time for recovery from fatigue must be built into every resistance exercise program. After vigorous exercise, the body must be given a period of time to restore itself to a state that existed prior to the exhaustive exercise.[5,26]

a. Changes that occur in muscle during recovery[26,57]

(1) Energy stores are replenished.

(2) Lactic acid is removed from skeletal muscle and blood in approximately 1 hour after exercise.

(3) Oxygen stores are replenished in muscles.

(4) Glycogen is replaced over several days.
b. It has been shown that if light exercise is performed during the recovery period, recovery from fatigue will occur more rapidly than with total rest.[10,26,32]
c. Only if a patient is allowed to recover from fatigue after each exercise session will long-term physical performance (strength, power, or endurance) improve.

4. Overwork

a. Resistance exercise programs for patients with certain neuromuscular diseases must be progressed very cautiously to avoid a problem known as overwork.
b. Overwork is a phenomenon that actually causes temporary or permanent deterioration of strength as a result of exercise. Simply stated, ". . . it is not always true that if a little exercise is good, then more exercise must be better."[61] The cause of overwork is not fully understood.
c. Fatigue and overwork are not synonymous terms. Because of the sensation of discomfort that accompanies fatigue in the person with an intact neuromuscular system, exercise is rarely performed to the point of overwork.
d. A progressive deterioration of strength from overwork has been observed clinically in patients with nonprogressive, lower motor neuron disease who participated in vigorous resistance exercise programs.[93]
e. This phenomenon has also been produced in laboratory animals. One study[36] demonstrated that when strenuous exercise was begun soon after a peripheral nerve lesion, the return of functional muscle strength was retarded. It was suggested that this could be due to an excessive protein breakdown in the denervated muscle.
f. Overwork can be avoided if the intensity, duration, and progression of exercise are conservative.
g. Careful and periodic re-evaluation of a patient's strength will help the therapist determine whether a patient's strength is improving as the result of the resistance exercise program.

5. Substitute motions

a. If too much resistance is applied to a contracting muscle during exercise, substitute motions can occur.
b. When muscles are weak because of fatigue, paralysis, or pain, a patient will attempt to carry out the desired movements, which those weak muscles normally perform, by any means possible.[73] For example, If the deltoid or supraspinatus muscles are weak or abduction of the arm is painful, a patient will elevate his scapula (shrug his shoulder) and laterally flex his trunk to the opposite side. It may appear that the patient is abducting the arm, but in fact he is not.
c. In order to avoid substitute motions in an exercise program, an appropriate amount of resistance and correct stabilization must be applied either manually or with equipment. Specific points of stabilization during resistance exercise will be outlined later in this chapter.

6. Osteoporosis

a. Osteoporosis (bone atrophy) is a condition of bone that leads to a loss of bone mass. It is often the result of prolonged immobilization or bed rest and associated musculoskeletal or neuromuscular disease.[87] In addition to the loss of bone mass, there is also narrowing of the bone shaft and widening of the medullary canal. These changes make the bone highly susceptible to pathologic fracture.[8] A pathologic fracture is a fracture of bone already weakened by disease. Very minor stresses on the skeletal system can then cause a fracture.

  (1) Patients with flaccid paralysis as the result of neuromuscular disease or trauma develop bone atrophy rapidly because of the loss of normal muscle pull on bone and loss of weight bearing.[8]

  (2) Patients who have had rheumatoid arthritis for many years will develop osteoporosis in the bones near the affected joints. This may be due to prolonged immobilization, decreased use, or lack of weight bearing caused by joint pain and inflammation.[87]

  (3) Patients receiving systemic steroid therapy also tend to develop osteoporosis and are at higher risk for pathologic fracture.[8]

  (4) Postmenopausal women are at high risk for developing osteoporosis, particularly affecting the neck of the femur and the vertebral bodies.

  b. If a patient with osteoporosis is involved in a strengthening or endurance exercise program, resistance must be applied and progressed very cautiously to avoid the possibility of causing a pathologic fracture.

7. **Muscle soreness associated with exercise**[24,26,28]

  a. Immediate muscle soreness often develops during or directly after strenuous exercise, performed to the point of fatigue.

    (1) This response occurs as a muscle becomes fatigued because of lack of adequate blood flow and oxygen (ischemia) and a temporary build up of metabolites such as lactic acid and potassium in the exercised muscle.[23]

    (2) The muscle pain or soreness experienced during intense exercise is transient and subsides quickly after exercise when adequate blood flow and oxygen are restored to the muscle.

  b. Delayed muscle soreness develops 24 to 48 hours after vigorous exercise and slowly diminishes within a week.[24,26,28]

    (1) The possible causes of delayed muscle soreness have been investigated for many years.

      (a) One early theory was that an accumulation of lactic acid in muscle caused delayed as well as immediate muscle soreness after exercise. This theory has been disproved recently[90] and in earlier studies.[3,57] Studies have shown that it requires only about 1 hour of rest after exercise to exhaustion to remove almost all lactic acid from skeletal muscle and blood.[27,48]

      (b) In 1961 deVries[22] proposed the theory that acute muscle pain caused by ischemia during exercise also caused muscle spasm, which in turn caused more ischemia and pain and, therefore, more muscle spasm. It was thought that a reflex pain-spasm cycle was the cause of delayed muscle soreness several days after exercise. The spasm theory is not well supported in the literature as attempts to replicate deVries's results have not been successful.[1,2]

      (c) The torn tissue theory suggests that delayed muscle soreness is due to microscopic tearing of muscle during vigorous exercise and a resulting degeneration and necrosis of these fibers.[24,29]

(d) The connective tissue theory[2] suggests that connective tissues (including tendons), rather than muscle fibers, are damaged during strenuous exercise and result in delayed muscle soreness.

(2) Today the consensus is that exercise-induced delayed muscle soreness is caused by a combination of microtrauma to both connective tissue and myofibrils.[2,29]

c. Delayed muscle soreness appears to be more severe and occurs more frequently after eccentric exercise than after concentric exercise, when both are performed against resistance.[30,87] There may be more tearing of muscle fibers and connective tissue when a muscle lengthens against resistance than when it shortens against resistance.[22,24,26,84]

d. Delayed muscle soreness can be decreased or prevented if resistance exercise is preceded by performing light warm-up activities, by stretching the muscles to be strengthened, and by *gradually* increasing the amount of resistance in an exercise program.[21,26]

B. Contraindications

1. Inflammation

Resistance exercises are not indicated when a muscle or joint is inflamed or swollen. The use of resistance can lead to increased swelling and more damage to muscles or joints.

2. Pain

If a patient experiences severe joint or muscle pain during resistance exercise or for more than 24 hours after exercise, resistance should be either entirely eliminated or substantially reduced. A careful evaluation of the cause of pain must be made by the therapist.

IV. TYPES OF RESISTANCE EXERCISE

Resistance can be applied to either dynamic or static muscle contractions. Resistance exercises can be carried out isotonically (with either concentric or eccentric muscle contractions), isokinetically, and isometrically.[17,26,29,43,58,78] In all cases the ultimate goal is to improve physical function through the development of increased muscular strength, endurance, or power.

A. Isotonic Resistance Exercise

Isotonic resistance exercise is a dynamic form of exercise that is carried out against a constant or variable load as a muscle lengthens or shortens through the available range of motion.[26,40,58] Dynamic strength, muscular endurance, and power can be developed with isotonic exercise.

1. Manual or mechanical resistance

Isotonic exercise can be performed against manual or mechanical resistance, depending on the needs and abilities of the patient. Both manual and mechanical resistance exercises will be discussed extensively in this chapter.

2. Constant versus variable resistance

a. Traditionally isotonic resistance exercise has been performed using a fixed load such as free weights.

b. The term isotonic literally means same or constant tension. But, in fact, when a muscle contracts dynamically against a fixed load (resistance), the tension produced in the muscle varies as it shortens or lengthens through the available range of motion. Maximum muscle tension actually develops at only one point in the range of motion with isotonic exercise performed against a fixed load.[15,26,40]

c. Variable Resistance Exercise
   (1) When isotonic exercise is carried out by using variable resistance equipment, such as the Eagle or Nautilus systems, the contracting muscle is subjected to varying amounts of resistance through the range to more effectively load the muscle at multiple points in the range.
   (2) When an isotonic muscle contraction is resisted manually, the therapist can vary the resistance appropriately to meet the changing strength capabilities of the muscle throughout the range of motion.[58]

3. **Concentric versus eccentric exercise**[15,58]
   a. Isotonic resistance exercise can also be performed *concentrically, eccentrically,* or both. That is, resistance can be applied to a muscle as it shortens or lengthens.
   b. Concentric and eccentric exercise can be carried out against manual or mechanical resistance.
   c. Most isotonic resistance exercise programs involve a combination of concentric and eccentric exercise, depending on a patient's strength capabilities and functional needs.
      (1) When a muscle contracts maximally and shortens (concentric contraction), it cannot generate as much tension as when it contracts maximally and lengthens (eccentric contraction).
      (2) Therefore, in the very early stages of an exercise program when a muscle is very weak, eccentric exercise against light manual resistance may be most appropriate.
      (3) As strength improves, concentric exercises against manual resistance can be added in a strengthening program.
      (4) Then, as a patient continues to progress, he can perform eccentric or concentric exercise against mechanical resistance.
   d. *Precautions for Eccentric Exercise*
      (1) There is the potential for excessive stress on the cardiovascular system (i.e., increased heart rate) when eccentric exercise is performed against heavy resistance.[16] Therefore, eccentric exercise may be contraindicated for some patients.
      (2) Greater delayed muscle soreness can develop more easily as the result of vigorous eccentric exercise as compared with concentric exercise.[15,16,24,26,28,30,54] The explanation for this may be that
         (a) greater microtrauma to myofibrils and connective tissue occurs when a muscle lengthens against resistance than when it shortens.
         (b) a greater amount of resistance is necessary to overload a muscle performing an eccentric contraction as compared with a concentric contraction.
      (3) Appropriate pacing and progression of an isotonic resistance exercise program can minimize or prevent delayed muscle soreness.[29,30]

B. Isokinetic exercise

Isokinetic exercise is a form of dynamic exercise in which the velocity of muscle shortening or lengthening is controlled by a rate-limiting device that controls (limits) the speed of movement of a body part.[15,40,67]

1. If the patient is well motivated and performing maximally, the muscle is maximally loaded, and near-maximal tension is produced throughout the range of joint motion.
2. Since the velocity of limb movement allowed is constant, the resistance, which the isokinetic exercise unit provides, will vary. For this reason, isokinetic exercise is sometimes referred to as *accommodating resistance exercise.*[15,40,67,68]
3. Isokinetic exercise can be performed concentrically on all rate-limiting devices and eccentrically on some. In both forms of exercise the velocity of limb movement is constant.
4. Only with isokinetic exercise can a patient safely train at very fast speeds of limb movement.
5. Several authors have indicated that isokinetic exercise strengthens muscles more efficiently than isotonic resistance exercise.[15,40,78,82]

C. Isometric Resistance Exercise

Isometric resistance exercise is a static form of exercise that occurs when a muscle contracts without an appreciable change in the length of the muscle or without visible joint motion.[4,15,17,41,58,74] Although there is no physical work done (force × distance), a great amount of tension and force output are produced by the muscle.[13,58,67] A muscle can generate greater tension with a maximum isometric contraction than with a maximum concentric contraction, but not as much as with a maximum eccentric contraction.[58]

1. Strength will increase if an isometric contraction is sustained against resistance. It has been shown that an isometric contraction should be held against resistance for at least 6 seconds. This allows time for peak tension to develop and metabolic changes to begin to occur in the muscle.[26,93] Isometric resistance exercise will not improve muscle endurance as effectively as dynamic exercise.
2. During isometric training it is sufficient to use an exercise load (resistance) of 60 to 80% of the muscle's force-developing capacity in order to gain strength.[51,65]
3. Since there is no joint movement, strength will develop only at the position in which the exercise is performed. In order to develop strength throughout the range of motion, resistance must be applied when the joint is in several positions.[26,62]
4. The length of a muscle at the time of contraction directly affects the amount of tension that can be produced at a specific point in the range of motion.[4,41,58,92] Therefore, the amount of resistance against which the patient will be able to hold will vary at different points in the range.
5. Resistance can be applied either manually or mechanically by having the patient hold against a heavy load or push against an immovable object.
6. *Muscle setting exercises* are also a form of isometric exercise but are not performed against any appreciable resistance.
   a. In this book, muscle setting will be used to describe gentle, static muscle contractions used to maintain mobility between muscle fibers and to decrease muscle spasm and pain.[50] Two common examples are quadriceps setting and gluteal setting.

b. Since muscle setting exercises are not performed against resistance, they will not appreciably increase muscle strength.

c. Setting exercises *may* retard atrophy in the very early stage of rehabilitation of a muscle or joint when immobilization is necessary.

V. MANUAL RESISTANCE EXERCISE

A. Definition

Manual resistance exercise is a form of active resistance exercise in which the resistance force is applied by the therapist to either a dynamic or static muscular contraction.

1. When joint motion is permissible, resistance is usually applied throughout the range of motion as the muscle shortens. Controlled resistance may also be applied to cause a lengthening contraction of a muscle.

2. Exercise is carried out in the anatomic planes of motion or in diagonal patterns known as proprioceptive neuromuscular facilitation (PNF) techniques.[88]

3. A specific muscle may also be strengthened by resisting the action of that muscle, as described in manual muscle testing procedures.[12,49]

B. Principles of Applying Manual Resistance Exercise

1. Prior to initiating the exercise

a. Evaluate the patient's range of motion and strength. Manual muscle testing will help the therapist establish a qualitative baseline level of strength against which progress can be measured. It will also help the therapist determine the appropriate amount of resistance that should be given in the exercise program.

b. Explain the exercise plan and procedures to the patient.

c. As with range of motion (ROM) exercise (see Chapter 2), place the patient in a comfortable position. Assume a position next to the patient where proper body mechanics can be used. Ensure that the region of the body where the exercise is to be done is free of restrictive clothing.

d. Demonstrate the desired motion to the patient by passively moving the patient's extremity through the desired motion.

e. Explain to the patient that he must perform the exercise with maximum effort.

f. Ensure that the patient does not hold his breath during the maximum effort to avoid the Valsalva's maneuver.[47]

2. During manual resistance exercise

a. Consider the site of application of resistance.

Resistance is usually applied to the distal end of the segment where the muscle to be strengthened attaches. Distal placement of resistance generates the greatest amount of external torque with the least amount of effort from the therapist. For example, to strengthen the anterior deltoid, resistance is applied to the distal humerus as the patient flexes his shoulder (Figure 3-1).

(1) The site of application of resistance will vary depending on the strength of the patient and the therapist as well as the stability of the segment.

(2) Resistance may be applied across an intermediate joint if that joint is

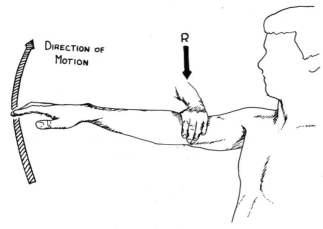

FIGURE 3–1. Resistance (R) is applied at the distal end of the segment being strengthened and in the direction opposite to the direction of movement of the arm.

stable and pain free and if there is adequate muscle strength supporting the joint.

  b. Determine the direction of resistance.

    Resistance is applied in the direction directly opposite to the desired motion (see Figure 3-1).

  c. Provide stabilization.

    In order to avoid substitute motions when strengthening a specific muscle, appropriate stabilization must be applied by the therapist or with equipment such as splints or belts. Stabilization of a segment is generally applied at the proximal attachment of the muscle to be strengthened. For example, in the case of the biceps brachii muscle, stabilization should occur at the anterior shoulder as elbow flexion is resisted (Figure 3-2).

  d. Apply the appropriate amount of resistance.

    The desired response from the patient should be a maximum pain-free effort. In dynamic exercise performed against resistance the motion should be smooth, not tremulous. The resistance applied should equal the abilities of the muscle at all points in the range of motion.

  e. Revise the site of application of resistance or decrease the amount of resistance if

    (1) the patient is unable to complete the full range of motion.

    (2) the site of application of resistance is painful.

    (3) muscular tremor develops.

    (4) substitute motions occur.

  f. Establish the number of repetitions.

    (1) In general, 8 to 10 repetitions of a specific motion will take the patient to a point of muscular fatigue.

    (2) Additional repetitions may be carried out after an adequate period of rest is allowed for recovery from fatigue.

VI. TECHNIQUES OF MANUAL RESISTANCE EXERCISE

Consistent with Chapter 2, the majority of exercises described and illustrated in this section are done with the patient in a *supine position*. Alternate positions will be de-

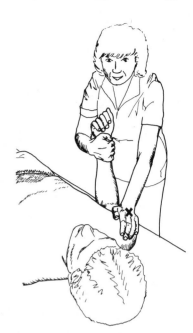

FIGURE 3–2. Stabilization is applied at the proximal attachment of the muscle being strengthened. In this illustration, the proximal humerus is stabilized as elbow flexion is resisted.

scribed when appropriate or necessary. In all illustrations the direction in which resistance (R) is applied is indicated with a solid arrow.

Opposite motions, such as flexion/extension and abduction/adduction, are often alternately resisted in an exercise program where strength in both an agonist and an antagonist is desired. Manual resistance exercises described in this chapter are for the upper and lower extremities. Additional exercises for increasing strength in the extremities can be found in Chapters 7 through 12. Resistance exercises for the cervical, thoracic, and lumbar spine will be described and illustrated in Chapters 14 and 17.

A. The Upper Extremity

1. **Flexion of the shoulder (Figure 3-3)**
   a. Resistance is applied to the anterior aspect of the distal arm or to the distal portion of the forearm if the elbow is stable and pain free.
   b. Stabilization of the scapula and trunk is provided by the treatment table.

2. **Extension of the shoulder**
   a. Resistance is applied to the posterior aspect of the distal arm or the distal portion of the forearm.
   b. Stabilization of the scapula is provided by the table.

3. **Hyperextension of the shoulder**
   a. The patient may be in the supine position, close to the edge of the table, side-lying, or prone so that hyperextension can occur.
   b. Resistance is applied in the same manner as with extension of the shoulder.
   c. Stabilization is applied to the anterior aspect of the shoulder if the patient is supine. If the patient is side-lying, adequate stabilization must be given to the trunk and scapula. This can usually be done if the therapist

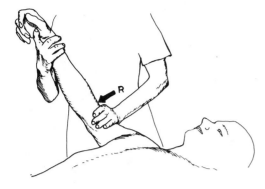

FIGURE 3–3. Resisted shoulder flexion.

places the patient close to the edge of the table and stabilizes the patient with her lower trunk.

4. **Abduction and adduction of the shoulder**
   a. Resistance is applied to the distal portion of the arm with the patient's elbow flexed to 90 degrees. To resist abduction (Figure 3-4) give resistance to the lateral aspect of the arm; to resist adduction give resistance to the medial aspect of the arm.
   b. Stabilization (although not pictured in Figure 3-4) is applied to the superior aspect of the shoulder if necessary to prevent elevation of the scapula during abduction.

5. **Internal and external rotation of the shoulder**
   a. Flex the elbow to 90 degrees and abduct the shoulder to 90 degrees.
   b. Resistance is given to the distal portion of the forearm during internal rotation (Figure 3-5) and external rotation.
   c. Stabilization is applied to the anterior portion of the shoulder during internal rotation. The back and scapula are stabilized by the table during external rotation.

6. **Horizontal abduction and adduction of the shoulder**
   a. Flex the shoulder and elbow to 90 degrees and place the shoulder in neutral rotation.
   b. Resistance is applied to the distal portion of the arm just above the elbow during horizontal adduction and abduction.
   c. Stabilization is applied to the anterior aspect of the shoulder during horizontal adduction. The table will stabilize the scapula and trunk during horizontal abduction.
   d. In order to resist horizontal abduction from 0 to 45 degrees, the patient must be close to the edge of the table while supine, or be placed side-lying or prone.

7. **Elevation and depression of the scapula**
   a. The patient should be in a sitting position.

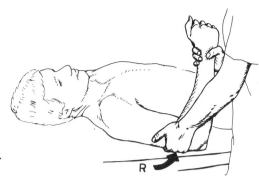

FIGURE 3–4. Resisted shoulder abduction.

    b. Resistance is applied along the superior aspect of the shoulder girdle just above the clavicle during scapular elevation (Figure 3-6).

    c. In order to resist scapular depression, have the patient attempt to reach down toward his feet and push his hand into the therapist's hand. When the patient has adequate strength, have him sit on the edge of a low table and lift his body weight with both his hands.

8. Protraction and retraction of the scapula

    a. Resistance is applied to the anterior portion of the shoulder at the head of the humerus to resist protraction and to the posterior aspect of the shoulder to resist retraction. Resistance may also be applied to the scapula.

    b. Stabilization is applied to the trunk to prevent trunk rotation.

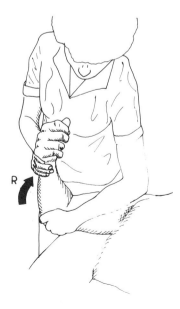

FIGURE 3–5. Resisted shoulder internal rotation.

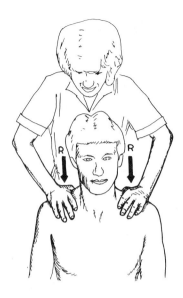

FIGURE 3–6. Elevation of the shoulders (scapulae), resisted bilaterally.

9. Flexion and extension of the elbow

a. To strengthen the elbow flexors, resistance is applied to the anterior aspect of the distal forearm (Figure 3-7). The forearm may be positioned in supination, pronation, and neutral to resist individual flexor muscles of the elbow, that is, the brachialis, brachioradialis, and biceps brachii.

b. To strengthen the elbow extensors, place the patient prone (Figure 3-8) or supine and apply resistance to the distal aspect of the forearm.

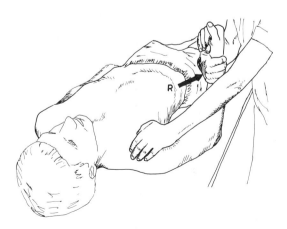

FIGURE 3–7. Resisted elbow flexion with proximal stabilization.

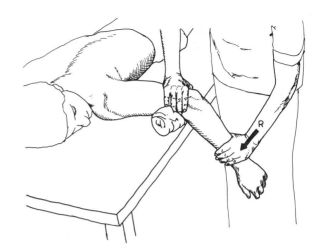

FIGURE 3–8. Resisted elbow extension.

    c. Stabilization is applied to the upper portion of the humerus during both motions.

10. **Pronation and supination of the forearm (Figure 3-9)**
    a. Resistance is applied to the radius of the distal forearm with the patient's elbow flexed to 90 degrees.

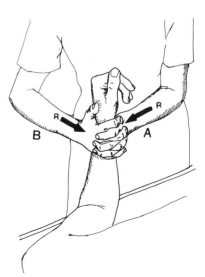

FIGURE 3–9. (*A*), Resisted pronation; (*B*), resisted supination of the forearm.

b. Stabilization may need to be applied to the humerus to prevent motion of the shoulder.

11. Flexion and extension of the wrist (Figure 3-10)

a. Resistance is applied to the volar and dorsal aspects of the hand at the level of the metacarpals to resist flexion and extension, respectively.
b. Stabilization is applied to the volar or dorsal aspect of the distal forearm.

12. Radial and ulnar deviation of the wrist

a. Resistance is applied to second and fifth metacarpals alternately to resist radial and ulnar deviation.
b. Stabilization is applied to the distal forearm.

13. Motions of the fingers (Figure 3-11) and thumb (Figure 3-12)

a. Resistance is applied just distal to the joint that is moving. Resistance is applied to one joint motion at a time.
b. Stabilization should occur at the joints proximal and distal to the joint to be strengthened.

B. The Lower Extremity

1. Flexion of the hip with knee flexion (Figure 3-13)

a. Resistance is applied to the anterior portion of the distal thigh. Simultaneous resistance to knee flexion may be applied at the distal and posterior aspect of the lower leg, just above the ankle.
b. Stabilization is applied to the pelvis and lumbar spine by keeping the patient's opposite hip in extension.

2. Extension of the hip (Figure 3-14)

a. Resistance is applied to the posterior aspect of the distal thigh with one hand and to the inferior and distal aspect of the heel with the other hand.
b. Stabilization of the pelvis and lumbar spine is provided by the table.

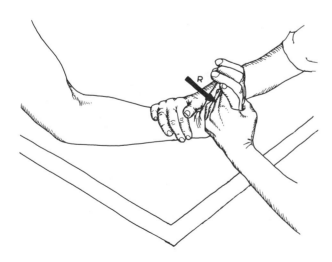

FIGURE 3–10. Resisted wrist flexion and stabilization of the forearm.

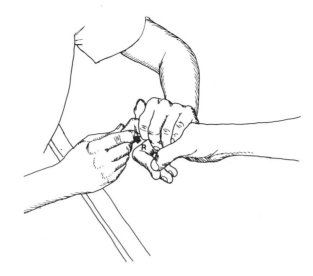

FIGURE 3–11. Resisted flexion of the proximal interphalangeal (PIP) joint of the index finger with stabilization of the MCP and DIP joints.

3. **Hyperextension of the hip (Figure 3-15)**
   a. The patient is placed prone.
   b. Resistance is given to the posterior aspect of the distal thigh.
   c. Stabilization is applied to the posterior aspect of the pelvis in order to avoid motion of the lumbar spine.

4. **Abduction and adduction of the hip (Figure 3-16)**
   a. Resistance is applied to the lateral and the medial aspects of the distal thigh to resist abduction and adduction, respectively, or to the lateral and medial aspects of the distal leg just above the malleoli if the knee is stable and pain free.
   b. Stabilization is applied
      (1) to the pelvis to avoid hip hiking from substitute action of the quadratus lumborum.

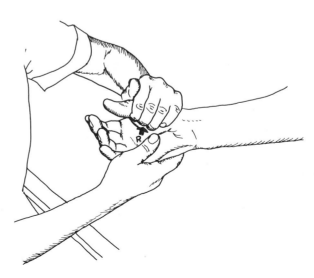

FIGURE 3–12. Resisted opposition of the thumb.

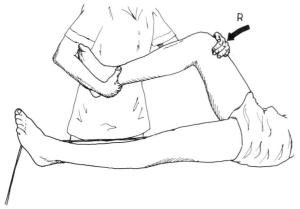

FIGURE 3–13. Resisted flexion of the hip with the knee flexed.

(2) to keep the thigh in neutral to prevent external rotation of the femur and subsequent substitution by the iliopsoas.

5. **Internal and external rotation of the hip**
    a. With the patient supine and the hip and knee extended
       (1) resistance is applied to the lateral aspect of the distal thigh to resist external rotation and to the medial aspect of the thigh to resist internal rotation.
       (2) stabilization is applied to the pelvis.
    b. With the patient supine and the hip and knee flexed (Figure 3-17)
       (1) resistance is applied to the medial aspect of the lower leg just above the malleolus during external rotation and to the lateral aspect of the lower leg during internal rotation.
       (2) stabilization is applied to the anterior aspect of the pelvis as the thigh is supported to keep the hip in 90 degrees flexion.

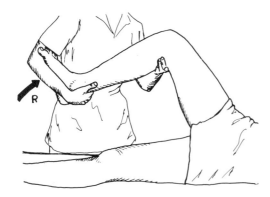

FIGURE 3–14. Resisted hip and knee extension with hand placement at the popliteal space to prevent hyperextension of the knee.

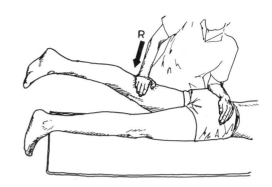

FIGURE 3–15. Resisted hyperextension of the hip with stabilization of the pelvis.

        c. With the patient prone, with the hip extended and the knee flexed (Figure 3-18)
           (1) resistance is applied to the medial and lateral aspects of the lower leg.
           (2) stabilization is given to the pelvis by applying pressure across the buttocks.

    6. Flexion of the knee
        a. Resistance to knee flexion may be combined with resistance to hip flexion as described earlier with the patient supine.
        b. With the patient prone and the hip extended (Figure 3-19),
           (1) resistance is given to the posterior aspect of the lower leg just above the heel.
           (2) stabilization is given to the posterior pelvis across the buttocks.
        c. The patient may also be sitting at the edge of a table with the hips and knees flexed and the trunk supported and stabilized.

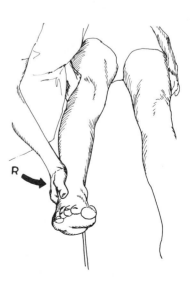

FIGURE 3–16. Resisted hip abduction.

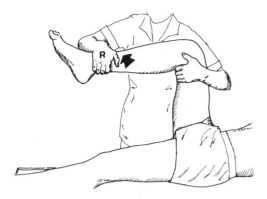

FIGURE 3–17. Resisted external rotation of the hip with the patient supine.

7. **Extension of the knee**
   a. Resistance is applied to the anterior aspect of the lower leg.
      (1) If the patient is lying supine on a table, the hip must be abducted and the knee flexed so the lower leg is over the side of the table. This position should not be used if the rectus femoris or iliopsoas is tight, because it will cause an anterior tilt of the pelvis and place stress on the low back.
      (2) If the patient is prone, a rolled towel should be placed under the anterior aspect of the distal thigh. This will allow the patella to glide normally during knee extension.
   b. Stabilization of the femur and pelvis is necessary.
   c. The sitting position is often used for vigorous strengthening of the knee extensors. If this position is used, trunk and back stabilization is necessary for optimum performance.[75]

8. **Dorsiflexion and plantarflexion of the ankle**
   a. Resistance is applied to the dorsum of the foot just above the toes to resist dorsiflexion (Figure 3-20A) and to the plantar surface of the foot at the metatarsals to resist plantarflexion (Figure 3-20B).
   b. Stabilization is applied to the lower leg.

9. **Inversion and eversion of the ankle**
   a. Resistance is applied to the medial aspect of the first metatarsal to resist inversion and to the lateral aspect of the fifth metatarsal to resist eversion.
   b. Stabilization is applied to the lower leg.

10. **Flexion and extension of the toes**
    a. Resistance is applied to the plantar and dorsal surfaces of the toes as the patient flexes and extends the toes.
    b. Stabilization should occur at the joints above and below the joint that is moving.

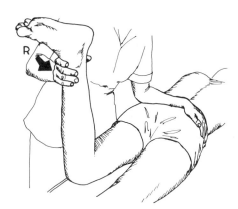

FIGURE 3–18. Resisted internal rotation of the hip with the patient prone.

C. Summary of Manual Resistance Exercise

These suggested techniques and methods of application of manual resistance exercise should be varied by the therapist to suit the individual abilities and needs of the patient. Variations in the therapist's position and hand placements may be necessary, depending on the size and strength of the therapist and patient. The therapist may also build variety and interest into a strengthening program by combining manual resistance and mechanical resistance in the exercise program.

VII. MECHANICAL RESISTANCE EXERCISE

A. Definition

Mechanical resistance exercise is any form of exercise in which resistance (the exercise load) is applied by some type of equipment. Various terms are used to

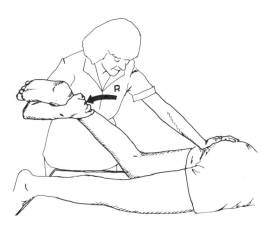

FIGURE 3–19. Resisted knee flexion with stabilization of the hip.

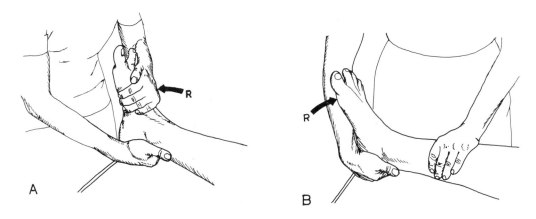

FIGURE 3–20. (*A*), Resisted dorsiflexion; (*B*), resisted plantarflexion of the ankle.

describe this type of exercise. They include *progressive resistive exercise (PRE),*[18,19] *active-resistive training,*[78] *overload training,* and *load-resisting exercise.*[18,19,80]

Mechanical resistance exercises are used to increase muscular strength, power, or endurance in rehabilitation or conditioning programs. In order to improve muscular function, the muscle must be progressively overloaded by increasing the resistance or the number of repetitions the exercise is performed. Then, as adaptation to the increased demands occurs, more load must be placed on the muscle or more repetitions must be performed.

Mechanical resistance can be used in place of manual resistance so that a patient can exercise independently or when the strength of the patient becomes greater than the therapist can control.

B. Specificity of Exercise[17,26,51,68,86]

It is very difficult to compare the effectiveness of one exercise program with that of another because of the number of variables that exist in resistance exercise programs. What is important is that an exercise program be designed to meet the specific needs of each patient. More and more emphasis is being placed on the necessity for specificity of training to be built into every exercise program.

It should be obvious that specificity of exercise implies that the muscle groups strengthened in a resistance exercise program must be the same muscles that require strength during a specific functional activity. Specificity in training programs can also relate to the speed at which an exercise is performed, the type of muscle contraction elicited, the intensity of the exercise, or the part of the range in which the exercise is performed. All these variables must match the requirements and demands placed upon the patient during specific functional activities.

C. Variables in Mechanical Resistance Exercise Programs

Many variables can be built into a mechanical resistance exercise program, depending on the ultimate goals of the exercise program. These variables may include the exercise load, or how much weight is lifted or lowered; the number of repetitions, or how many times the weight is lifted or lowered; the number of sets or bouts of exercise performed; and the frequency of exercise, or how many times a week the exercise is carried out. Other variables are the type of exercise performed and the speed at which the exercise is done, the intensity of the exercise, and the arc of limb movement.

1. **The exercise load and number of repetitions**
   a. One way to progressively overload a muscle is to gradually increase the *exercise load* (amount of resistance) used in an exercise program. Generally, in exercise programs that are designed to improve muscular strength, the weight a person lifts, lowers, or holds a specified number of times is progressively increased.[38,80]
      (1) It is always difficult to determine how much weight a person should use when beginning a resistance exercise program. One early method, devised by DeLorme,[18,19] was to determine a *repetition maximum (RM)*. A repetition maximum is the greatest amount of weight (load) a muscle can move through the range of motion a specific number of times. DeLorme used 10 RM as a baseline and measurement of the improvement in muscle strength. That is, he determined the greatest amount of weight a subject could move through the range exactly 10 times. Other investigators have recommended a baseline of 6 RM to a 15 RM to improve strength.[26,66,78,80]
      (2) A repetition maximum is not easy to calculate and is not the most accurate method available today to measure strength before or after a resistance training program. Isokinetic dynamometers and myometers give a more accurate measure of strength. But a repetition maximum is still one way to determine the amount of resistance a person should use to initiate a weight-training program.
   b. Another variable in a mechanical resistance exercise program is the *number of repetitions* that an exercise is performed against resistance. If the number of repetitions is progressively increased, the muscle will be continually overloaded and adaptive changes in muscle will occur. Exercise programs that are designed to improve muscle endurance often involve increasing the number of times a person does an exercise against a constant load.[15,78]
   c. In some programs the amount of resistance and the number of repetitions are both progressively increased to improve strength and endurance. No specific progression of resistance or number of repetitions has been determined to be the most efficient means of improving muscular strength or endurance.

2. **Bouts and frequency of exercise**[15,26,55]
   a. Bouts are the number, or sets, of a repetition maximum performed during each exercise session. Usually several bouts of a specific RM are carried out with the patient resting after each bout.
      (1) Many combinations of sets and repetitions effectively improve muscular strength and endurance. Strength gains have occurred in programs in which 3 bouts of a 6 RM, 2 bouts of a 12 RM, and 6 bouts of a 3 RM, as well as many other variations have been used.[26,78]
      (2) Strength gains have even occurred when a 1 RM was used.[76] Although a 1 RM is not practical in clinical settings, as long as a mus-

cle is progressively overloaded, strength, endurance, or both will increase.

b. Frequency is the number of times exercise is done within a day or within a week. Most exercise programs are performed every other day or 4 to 5 times a week.[26] Adequate time must be allowed for recovery from fatigue if improvement is to occur.

3. Duration of exercise

Duration is the total number of days, weeks, or months during which an exercise program is performed. In order to significantly increase strength, a program must be at least 6 weeks in duration.[19,26]

4. Speed of exercise[6,15,44,58,68,77,85,86,91]

a. The speed at which a muscle contracts significantly affects the tension that the muscle produces. As the velocity of muscle shortening increases, the force that the muscle can generate decreases. Electromyogram (EMG) activity and torque decrease as a muscle shortens at faster contractile velocities, because the muscle does not have sufficient time to develop peak tension. The reverse is true during lengthening (eccentric) contractions performed against resistance. An *increase* in the speed of contracting and lengthening against a heavy load generates *greater* tension in the muscle. It has been suggested that this increase in tension may be a mechanism for protecting a muscle when it is excessively loaded.

b. During isotonic resistance exercise (using free weights or variable resistance units), only the patient controls the speed of limb movement. Usually isotonic resistance exercises are done at slow speeds so that momentum does not become a significant factor during exercise and to ensure safety for the patient.

c. Isokinetic exercise devices provide accommodating resistance to limb movement at very slow (15 degrees/second) to very fast (500 degrees/second) velocities in rehabilitation, conditioning, and athletic training programs.

d. *Speed-specific isokinetic training*

(1) In the early 1970s the concept of the specificity of speed of exercise was introduced by Moffroid.[67,68] This study and others suggested that if isokinetic exercise was performed at a slow speed, strength gains over time would occur at slow speeds only. But if isokinetic exercise was performed at fast speeds, strength gains would occur at velocities equal to or less than the training speed.

(2) In later studies it was reported that training at slow speeds could lead to strength gains at faster speeds.[44,81,86]

(3) The consensus today is that there is some but not an extensive amount of physiologic carry-over from one training speed to another. Therefore, it is now suggested that isokinetic exercise should be performed at a variety of velocities in a training program. This is called *Velocity Spectrum Training*.[15,44,78,81]

(4) The speed of exercise selected in any isokinetic training program should be comparable to the speed of movement required in a specific functional activity.

5. **Type of muscle contraction**
   a. It has already been mentioned that resistance exercises can be performed dynamically or statically and concentrically or eccentrically.
   b. The force output (strength) of a muscle will vary with the type of muscle contraction performed.[17,26,77]
      (1) The greatest tension in a muscle is generated during an eccentric (lengthening) contraction performed against supramaximal resistance.
      (2) Slightly less force can be produced in a muscle when it contracts isometrically against resistance.
      (3) The least force is generated when a muscle contracts concentrically (shortens) against a load.
   c. With this in mind, the types of muscle contractions performed during an exercise program will depend on the condition of the patient and the ultimate goals of the exercise program.
      (1) Consistent with the concept of the specificity of exercise, a therapist will want to choose resistance exercises to meet the functional needs of a patient. If static strength is required for a specific functional activity, then isometric muscle contractions should be an important aspect of the exercise program. If dynamic strength is necessary, then concentric or eccentric contractions can be incorporated into the training program.
      (2) In the early stages of a rehabilitation program following a musculoskeletal injury, isometric resistance exercises may be initiated when a limb is immobilized or when a patient cannot tolerate resisted range of motion.
      (3) Eccentric exercise may be indicated when limb movement against resistance is desired but the tension-developing capacity of the muscle is very poor. Eccentric exercise can be performed against manual resistance or with isotonic or isokinetic equipment.
      (4) An eccentric muscle contraction may also be more comfortable if a concentric contraction produces pain in the early stages of soft tissue healing.[9]
      (5) As a patient progresses, a combination of eccentric and concentric exercise is usually performed because most functional activities require a combination of eccentric and concentric strength.
   d. The very nature of most mechanical resistance equipment, such as free weights and weight-pulley systems, builds both concentric and eccentric exercise into a training program (see Figure 3-26).
      (1) When a weight is lifted against gravity, a concentric muscle contraction occurs.
      (2) When a weight is then lowered, an eccentric contraction of the same muscle occurs to control the descent of the weight.
   Note: Studies suggest that the magnitude of adaptive strength gains is comparable after eccentric and concentric regimens despite the fact that a muscle has greater tension-developing capacity eccentrically than concentrically. This may be the result of inhibition of the muscle secondary to pain or soreness associated with eccentric exercise.[24,26,30,45,46,54,84]

6. **Submaximal versus maximal exercise**
   Resistance exercise can be performed as a patient exerts either a submaximal or a maximal effort. The goals of the exercise program, the stage of

healing after injury, or the patient's condition will help the therapist deter-mine whether exercise should be carried out against maximal or submaxi-mal resistance.

   a. Submaximal or maximal exercise can be done in an isometric, isotonic, or isokinetic program.
   b. A submaximal exercise program is often established[15]
      (1) when the goal of the exercise is to increase muscular endurance where many repetitions of the exercise are done.
      (2) during the early stages of rehabilitation to protect healing tissues or avoid soft tissue pain.
      (3) when isokinetic exercise is performed at very slow speeds.[15]
   c. Exercise is performed against maximum resistance to improve muscu-lar strength and power.

   Precaution: When dynamic muscle contractions are performed against heavy resistance isotonically or at slow speeds with maximum effort on an isokinetic unit, excessive joint compression or pain can occur.

7. **Range of movement—short-arc versus full-arc exercise**

   Resistance exercises may be done through the entire range of motion (full-arc exercise) or through a limited range (short-arc exercise). For example, after surgery for repair of the anterior cruciate ligament, full knee extension is often contraindicated during the early and intermediate stages of rehabili-tation. Therefore, resistance exercises are carried out in only a limited arc of movement. Gradually, resistance is applied through the complete (full-arc) range of motion to prepare for functional activities.

8. **Position of the patient**

   The position a patient assumes when strengthening a particular muscle group will affect the tension-developing capacity of the muscle, the amount of weight the patient can control, and the carry-over of the exercise to func-tional activities.

   a. The same muscle, if exercised with the patient in different positions and with the muscle in different degrees of lengthening, will produce differ-ent amounts of muscle tension because of the relationship between length and tension that exists in muscle. Peak tension develops in a muscle when it is in a slightly lengthened position at the time of contrac-tion.[33,58,63,92]
   b. The therapist should also consider whether strength is necessary in an open or a closed kinematic chain during a specific functional activity and have the patient train accordingly. For example, if the hip and knee ex-tensors are strengthened by having the patient stand and lift his body weight on steps (closed chain), there may be better functional carry-over to stair-climbing than if the patient only strengthens the hip or knee ex-tensors by lifting or lowering weights with the lower limb moving freely in space (open chain).

VIII. SPECIFIC EXERCISE REGIMENS

As investigators have looked at various approaches to exercise designed to develop strength and/or endurance, a number of formats have evolved. Some early studies advo-cated isotonic exercise, whereas others described the value of isometric exercise. More recently, studies have been carried out to evaluate the effectiveness of isokinetic exercise. An overview of these variations of mechanical resistance exercise programs follows.

A. Isotonic Regimens

1. DeLorme technique[18,19,66,78]

a. Originally this technique was called heavy resistance exercise, but DeLorme later developed the term progressive resistive exercise (PRE) to describe his approach to strengthening exercise.

b. Procedure
   (1) Determine the 10 RM.
   (2) The patient then carries out:
       10 repetitions at $1/2$ of the 10 RM.
       10 repetitions at $3/4$ of the 10 RM.
       10 repetitions at the full 10 RM.
   (3) The patient performs all 3 bouts at each exercise session with a brief rest between bouts.
   (4) The approach builds in a warm-up period because the patient initially lifts only $1/2$ and $3/4$ of the 10 RM.
   (5) The 10 RM is increased weekly as strength increases.

2. The Oxford technique[94]

a. This is the reverse of the 3-bout DeLorme system. It was designed to diminish resistance as muscle fatigue develops.

b. Procedure
   (1) Determine the 10 RM.
   (2) The patient then performs:
       10 repetitions at the full 10 RM.
       10 repetitions at $3/4$ of the 10 RM.
       10 repetitions at $1/2$ of the 10 RM.

c. This technique attempts to decrease the detrimental effects of fatigue.

d. A general, nonspecific warm-up period of active exercise is advocated prior to beginning the bouts of resistance exercise.

3. Daily adjustable progressive resistance exercise—the DAPRE technique[52,53]

a. The DAPRE technique was developed by Knight to more objectively determine when to increase resistance and how much to increase the resistance in an exercise program.

b. Procedure
   (1) Determine an initial *working weight* (Knight suggests a 6 RM).
   (2) The patient then performs
       Set No. 1: 10 repetitions of $1/2$ the working weight.
       Set No. 2: 6 repetitions of $3/4$ the working weight.
       Set No. 3: as many repetitions as possible of the full working weight.
       Set No. 4: as many repetitions as possible of the *adjusted working weight*. The *adjusted working weight* is based on the number of repetitions of the full working weight performed during Set No. 3.
   (3) The number of repetitions done in Set No. 4 is used to determine the working weight for the next day.

c. Guidelines for adjustment of the working weight

Number of Repetitions Performed During Set No. 3	Adjustment to Working Weight for	
	Set No. 4	Next Day
0–2	Decrease 5–10 lb and repeat set	Decrease 5–10 lb
3–4	Decrease 0–5 lb	Same weight
5–6	Keep weight the same	Increase 5–10 lb
7–10	Increase 5–10 lb	Increase 5–15 lb
11	Increase 10–15 lb	Increase 10–20 lb

Knight points out that the "ideal" maximum number of repetitions (when the patient is asked to perform as many repetitions as possible) is 5 to 7 repetitions.
- d. The DAPRE system eliminates the arbitrary determination of how much weight should be added in a resistance exercise program on a day-to-day basis.
- e. This system can be used with free weights or weight machines.

4. **Circuit weight training**[78]

Another approach to isotonic resistance exercise is circuit weight training. Resistance exercises are carried out in a specific sequence using a variety of exercises for total body conditioning. Exercises can be done using free weights or weight training units such as the Universal, Nautilus, or Eagle systems.
- a. Exercises could include 8 to 10 RMs of:
  - (1) bench press
  - (2) leg press
  - (3) situps
  - (4) shoulder press
  - (5) squats
  - (6) curls
- b. A rest period (usually 30 seconds to 1 minute) is taken between each bout of exercise.
- c. Many examples of circuit weight training regimens can be found in the athletic training and sports medicine literature.

B. Isometric Regimens

1. **Brief maximal isometric exercise**
   - a. In the 1950s, Hettinger and Muller[39] studied and advocated isometric exercise as an optimal means for increasing muscle strength.
   - b. Procedure
     - (1) The patient performs a *single* isometric contraction of the muscle to be strengthened against a fixed resistance. The contraction is held for 5 to 6 seconds.
     - (2) This is done once a day, 5 to 6 times per week.
   - c. This study was both upheld and refuted by later studies.

2. **Brief repetitive isometric exercise (BRIME)**[60]
   - a. This is a refinement of the earlier isometric study. Five to ten brief but maximum isometric contractions are performed against resistance 5 days per week.

b. This repetitive approach was found to be more effective and maintained the subject's level of motivation better than using a single maximum contraction.

3. **Current use of isometrics in rehabilitation and conditioning**
   a. These early studies documented that isometric resistance exercise can be an effective means of improving muscle strength.
   b. Although isometric exercise can improve muscular endurance, the effect is minimal; dynamic (isotonic and isokinetic) exercises are a more effective means of increasing muscle endurance.
   c. *Multiple angle isometrics* are necessary if the goal of exercise is to improve strength throughout the range of motion. Gains in strength will only occur at or closely adjacent to the training angle.[15,62] Physiologic overflow only occurs a total of 20 degrees from the training angle (10 degrees in either direction).[51]
      (1) Resistance should be applied at least every 20 degrees through the range.
      (2) Davies[15] suggests 10 sets of 10 repetitions of 10-second contractions every 10 degrees in the range of motion. (A 10-second contraction may be preferable to a 6-second contraction, as recommended earlier in this chapter, if your patient counts quickly!)

C. Isokinetic Regimens

1. **Velocity spectrum rehabilitation**[15]

   Most isokinetic exercise programs designed to develop strength, endurance, or power involve performing exercises on an isokinetic unit at slow, medium, and fast velocities.
   a. A minimum of 3 contractile velocities is usually chosen for a training program. A common exercise bout might include training at 60, 120, and 180 degrees/second or 60, 150, and 240 degrees/second.
   b. It has been suggested that the effects of training only carry over 15 degrees/second from the training velocity.[15,44] Therefore, some clinicians may choose to set up programs with as many as 8 to 10 training velocities.
   c. In the early stages of an isokinetic exercise program, it is useful to begin with submaximal isokinetic exercise at intermediate and slow speeds so the patient gets the "feel" of the isokinetic equipment and still protects the muscle. As the patient progresses, he may exert maximal effort at intermediate speeds. Slow-speed training is usually eliminated when the patient begins to exert maximal effort.
   d. During the later stage of a rehabilitation program, it is beneficial to exercise maximally at faster contractile velocities for several reasons.[15,82]
      (1) Since the speed of limb movement during specific functional motor activities, such as walking and running, occurs at fast velocities, high-speed exercise may better prepare the patient for these activities.
      (2) At faster velocities, muscles generate less torque and less compressive forces on joints.
   e. Finally, specificity of training applies to the velocity at which exercises are done. It is important to choose training speeds that are similar to the speed of movement during a specific functional activity.

2. As with isotonic and isometric programs, no one regimen of isokinetic exercise has been proven to be the best.[26] The number of repetitions, sets, frequency, and duration in the program will vary.

IX. USE OF EQUIPMENT WITH RESISTANCE EXERCISE

A wide variety of mechanical apparatus and equipment is available for resistance exercise programs. A simple hand-held weight may adequately meet the needs of a patient carrying out an exercise program at home, whereas a sophisticated isokinetic exercise unit may better suit the needs of another patient.

There are a number of advantages for choosing mechanical resistance over manual resistance in an exercise program. When mechanical equipment is used, the therapist can quantitatively measure a patient's baseline strength prior to initiating the exercise program. The therapist also has an objective measurement of a patient's improvement of strength over time. The patient too can see measurable progress in an exercise program. The level of resistance applied during a given exercise is not limited by the strength of the therapist. The use of equipment also adds variety to an exercise program even in the early stages of rehabilitation when a patient's strength may still be quite limited.

There is an enormous selection of equipment on the market today, specifically for use in resistance exercise programs. The equipment ranges from simple to complex, small to large, and inexpensive to expensive. The choice of equipment used in a resistance exercise program primarily depends on the individual needs and abilities of the patient carrying out the exercise. The selection of equipment also depends on the availability of the equipment, the cost of purchase of the equipment by a facility or by a patient, and the space requirement for the equipment at home or in a clinical setting.

A. General Principles for the Use of Equipment

In order to use equipment effectively and safely in a resistance exercise program, the therapist must consider the following:

1. Evaluate the patient's strength, range of motion, bone or joint deformities, pain, and integrity of the skin before using the equipment.
2. Determine the most advantageous types of exercise that could be used to strengthen the involved muscle groups, and choose the appropriate equipment.
3. Adhere to all safety precautions when applying the equipment.
   a. Be sure all attachments, cuffs, collars, and buckles are securely fastened and adjusted to the individual patient prior to the exercise.
   b. Apply padding for comfort, if necessary, especially over bony prominences.
   c. Stabilize or support appropriate structures to prevent unwanted movement and to prevent undue stress on body parts.
4. Be certain that the full available range of motion is completed during dynamic exercise without the use of substitute motions.
5. When the exercise has been completed
   a. Disengage the equipment and leave it in proper condition for future use.
   b. Never leave broken or potentially hazardous equipment for future use.
6. Observe and re-evaluate the patient to determine how the exercise program was tolerated by the patient. Record observations and objective data as soon as possible.

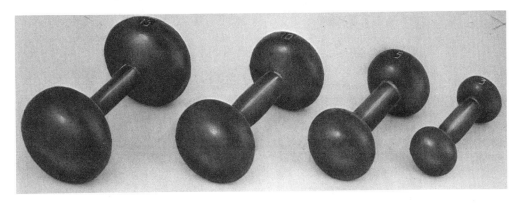

FIGURE 3–21. Graduated dumbbell weights. (Courtesy of J.A. Preston Corporation, Clifton, NJ)

B. Isotonic Resistance Exercise Equipment

1. Free weights

Free weights are graduated weights that are hand held or applied to the upper or lower extremity and include
a. barbells.
b. dumbbells (Figure 3-21).
c. cuff weights with Velcro closures (Figure 3-22).
d. sandbags.
e. weight boots (Figure 3-23).
The variety of free weights available is extensive. The therapist must select equipment for a department that will meet the needs of many patients. Each type of free weight has its advantages and disadvantages. For example, dumbbells, Velcro cuff weights, and sandbags have fixed poundage.

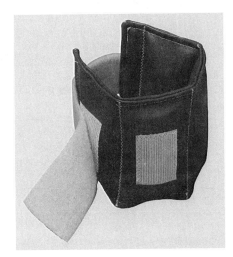

FIGURE 3–22. The Cuff®, a cuff weight with Velcro closure. (Courtesy of the Dipsters Corporation, Scarsdale, NY)

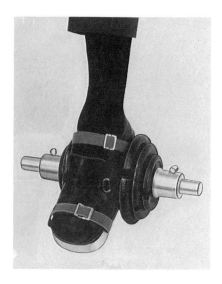

FIGURE 3–23. Assembled quadriceps weight boot with interchangeable weights. (Courtesy of J.A. Preston Corporation, Clifton, NJ)

Therefore, a series of increasing weights and sizes are necessary to adequately progress a patient as his strength increases. On the other hand, barbells and weight boots have interchangeable weights but require time to assemble and adjust to each patient.

2. Elastic resistance devices (see Figure 7-3A)
   a. Elastic resistance materials such as Thera-Band and Rehabilitation Xercise Tubing are available in several grades or thicknesses. The thicker the elastic material, the greater the resistance applied to the contracting muscle.
   b. The elastic material can be cut to different lengths and set up so that upper and lower extremity or trunk musculature can be strengthened.

3. Pulley systems
   Pulley systems (with weights or springs) can be used for upper or lower extremity strengthening. These include
   a. free-standing or wall-mounted pulley-weight systems (Figure 3-24)
      (1) A variety of systems are available from several manufacturers.
      (2) These are often attached to a wall or doorframe.
      (3) Permanent or interchangeable weights are available.
      (4) The patient can be set up in many positions, such as sitting in a wheelchair or lying prone on a cart. Many muscle groups may be strengthened by repositioning the patient.
      (5) Free-standing, multiple-station units, such as the Universal system, allow the patient to exercise multiple muscle groups by moving from one station to another.
   b. Elgin Exercise Unit (Figure 3-25)
      (1) This system uses a series of interconnected cables and independent weights and pulleys that make it possible for a patient to perform isotonic or isometric exercises using many different muscle groups.

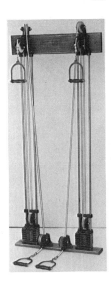

FIGURE 3-24. Wall pulley weight system. (Courtesy of J.A. Preston Corporation, Clifton, NJ)

    (2) Weak and strong muscles can be exercised by load-assisting or load-resisting methods on the Elgin table.

    (3) In addition to strengthening exercises, the Elgin table can also be used to apply a prolonged mechanical stretch force. (See Chapter 4.)

Note: When free weights, elastic resistance material, or pulley systems are used as a source of mechanical resistance, strengthening of a muscle often occurs both concentrically and eccentrically. For example, when a patient is holding a weight and strengthening the elbow flexors (Figure 3-26), the muscle is contracting both concentrically and eccentrically against resistance as he lifts and lowers the weight. This needs to be considered when determining the number of repetitions carried out in the exercise program and when evaluating a patient's rate of fatigue and level of delayed muscle soreness.

4. Isotonic torque arm units

    a. Exercise equipment, such as the N-K Unit (Figure 3-27) provides constant resistance through either a hydraulic force plate friction mechanism or an interchangeable weight-resistance system.

    b. These units are primarily designed to provide resistance to the knee joint but can also be used to strengthen hip and shoulder musculature.[72]

        (1) Resisted knee flexion and extension is carried out with the patient sitting or prone.

        (2) Resisted hip flexion or extension is carried out with the patient lying or standing.

5. Variable resistance equipment

    a. Some weight-cable equipment systems such as the Eagle (Figure 3-28) or Nautilus and Universal DVR systems are designed to provide variable resistance throughout the range of motion as a muscle contracts concentrically and eccentrically.

        (1) A cam device in the weight-cable system varies the load applied to

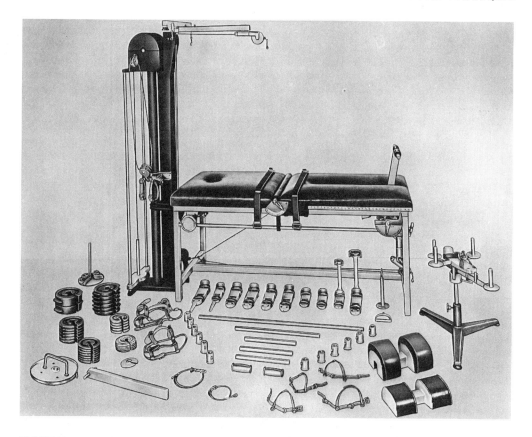

FIGURE 3–25. Elgin Exercise Unit Model A–1500. (Courtesy of the Elgin Exercise Equipment Company, Sandwich, IL)

the contracting muscle, even though the weight selected is constant.

(2) The cam shaft, in theory, is designed to replicate the torque curve of the muscle being exercised.

b. Other variable resistance units, such as the Keiser Cam II system, use pressurized pneumatic resistance that varies the resistance applied to the muscle through the range of motion.

c. A variety of units are available. Each unit is designed for exercise of a specific muscle group in the trunk or extremities. For example, a patient may do squats on one machine and leg curls on another machine to strengthen the lower extremities.

d. The main advantage of variable resistance equipment over the use of free weights is that the contracting muscle is loaded maximally at multiple points rather than at just one point in the range of motion.

e. The main disadvantage of variable resistance equipment is that a great amount of space is needed to set up multiple units so that many muscle groups can be strengthened.

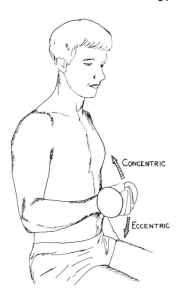

FIGURE 3–26. Concentric and eccentric strengthening of the elbow flexors occurs as the patient lifts and lowers the weight.

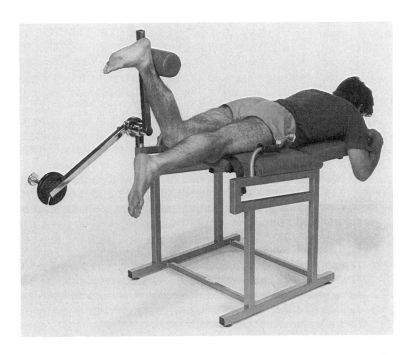

FIGURE 3–27. N-K Exercise Unit with torque arm and interchangeable weights. (Courtesy of N-K Products Company, Inc., Soquel, CA)

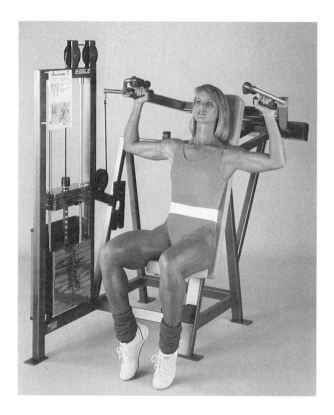

FIGURE 3–28. The Cybex®/Eagle Fitness Systems shoulder press provides variable resistance throughout the range of motion. (Courtesy of Cybex, Division of Lumex, Ronkonkoma, NY)

6. **Exercise bicycle**

   The stationary exercise bicycle is used to increase lower extremity strength and endurance (Figure 3-29). Resistance can be graded with an adjustable friction device. Distance, speed, or duration of exercise can also be monitored.

   The exercise bicycle provides resistance to muscles during repetitive, reciprocal movements of the lower extremities. It is particularly appropriate for low-intensity–high-repetition exercises designed to increase muscular or cardiovascular endurance.

7. **Resistive reciprocal exercise units**

   a. A number of resistive exercisers are available and are used for repetitive reciprocal exercise (Figure 3-30). They are most often used to improve lower extremity endurance, strength, or reciprocal coordination and a person's cardiopulmonary fitness. Many units can also be wall mounted and adapted for upper extremity exercise.

   b. A resistance mechanism adjusts to provide light or heavy resistance.

   c. These units are attached to a sturdy straightback chair or wheelchair and are an alternative for patients who cannot safely use a stationary bicycle.

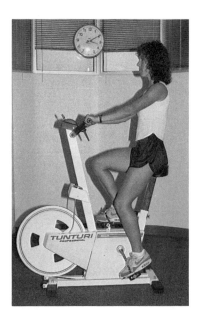

FIGURE 3–29. Exercise bicycles are used to increase muscular endurance and cardiopulmonary fitness.

8. **Isotonic equipment—constant versus variable resistance**
   a. Equipment such as free weights, standard weight-pulley systems, or elastic materials that impose a fixed load on a contracting muscle maximally strengthen a muscle at only one point in the range of motion when a patient is in a particular position. The weight that is lifted or lowered through the range of motion can be no greater than what the muscle can lift at the *weakest* point in the range. During isotonic exercise performed against constant resistance, a patient will be working maximally at only one small portion of the range of motion.
   b. When using free weights it is possible to vary the point in the range of motion at which the maximum resistance load is experienced by changing the patient's position with respect to gravity, or the direction of the resistance load. For example, shoulder flexion may be resisted with the patient standing or supine and holding a weight in his hand.
      (1) Patient standing (Figure 3-31)
          Maximum resistance is experienced and maximum torque is produced when the shoulder is at 90 degrees of flexion. Zero torque is produced when the shoulder is at 0 degrees of flexion. Torque again decreases as the patient lifts the weight from 90 to 180 degrees of flexion.
      (2) Patient supine (Figure 3-32)
          Maximum resistance is experienced and maximum torque is produced when the shoulder is at 0 degrees of flexion. Zero torque is produced at 90 degrees of shoulder flexion. The shoulder flexors are not active between 90 and 180 degrees of shoulder flexion. Instead, the shoulder extensors must contract eccentrically to control the descent of the arm and weight.

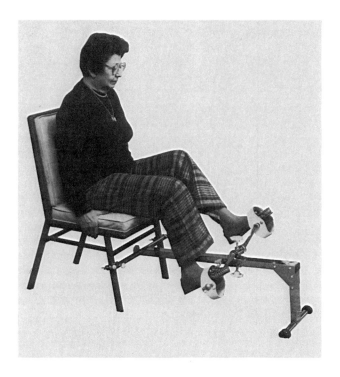

FIGURE 3–30. The Can-Do® Exerciser, a resistive reciprocal exerciser. (Courtesy of the Dipsters Corporation, Scarsdale, NY)

    (3) Therefore, the therapist must determine at which portion of the patient's range of movement maximum strength is needed and must choose the optimum position in which the exercise should be performed.

  c. Standard weight-pulley systems provide maximum resistance when the angle of the pulley is at right angles to the moving bone.

  d. With elastic resistance material, the muscle will receive the maximum resistive force when the material is angled 90 degrees to the moving bone. The therapist should determine where in the range of maximum resistance is desired and anchor the elastic material so it is at right angles in that portion of the range. When the material is at an acute angle to the moving bone, there will be less resistance and more joint compressive force.

  e. With variable resistance equipment, the contracting muscle can be maximally loaded at multiple points in the range of motion without changing the patient's position. The design of each unit dictates the position in which the patient will perform the exercise.

  f. With both constant and variable isotonic resistance equipment, exercises are done slowly to ensure patient safety and minimize momentum and acceleration. One exception is variable resistance equipment that uses pneumatic pressure as a source of resistance. Faster training speeds can be used safely with this type of equipment. There may be limited carry-over to functional activities when resistance exercises are only done slowly.

  g. Neither constant nor weight-cable variable isotonic resistance equipment can accommodate to a painful arc as a patient moves through the

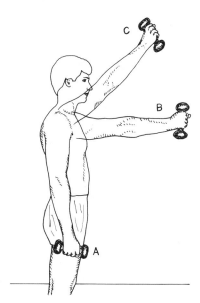

FIGURE 3–31. When the patient is standing and lifting a weight: (*A*), Zero torque is produced in the shoulder flexors when the shoulder is at 0 degrees flexion, (*B*), Maximum torque is produced when the shoulder is at 90 degrees flexion. (*C*), Torque again decreases as the arm moves from 90 to 180 degrees of shoulder flexion.

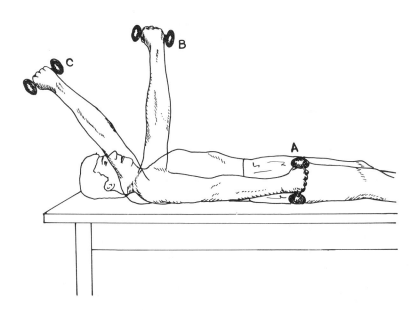

FIGURE 3–32. When the patient is supine and lifting a weight: (*A*), Maximum torque is produced at 0 degrees of shoulder flexion. (*B*), Zero torque is produced at 90 degrees shoulder flexion. (*C*), The shoulder extensors are active and contract eccentrically against resistance from 90 to 180 degrees shoulder flexion.

range of motion. Only pneumatic pressure variable resistance equipment and isokinetic equipment have this capability.

C. Equipment Used With Isometric Exercise

1. Many pieces of equipment designed for dynamic strengthening exercises can also be modified for use in an isometric strengthening program.
   a. When a patient attempts to lift a weight that provides resistance greater than the force the muscle can generate, an isometric contraction occurs.
   b. Many of the free weights and weighted pulley systems can be adapted for isometric use.
   c. Most isokinetic devices can be set up with the speed set at 0 degrees/ second at a variety of joint angles for isometric resistance.
   d. Many isometric exercises can be performed against resistance without any equipment. For example, a patient can strengthen the shoulder flexors, abductors, and rotators by pushing his arm against a wall (see Figure 7-13A, B, and C).

2. **Procedure for use of equipment**
   a. Determine the point in the range of motion at which the muscle contraction is to occur and set the patient up accordingly.
   b. To avoid substitute motions, appropriate stabilization is absolutely necessary.
   c. Instruct the patient to contract the muscle, hold at least 6 seconds,[4,80] then relax and repeat.
   d. To increase strength throughout the range of motion, have the patient carry out the exercise at several points in the range where strength is desired.[26]
   e. Make sure the patient exhales (counts, talks, or so forth) while exerting his maximum effort during isometric resistance exercise to minimize the effect on the cardiovascular system.[25]

D. Isokinetic Exercise Equipment

Several manufacturers offer isokinetic dynamometers or rate-limiting devices that control the velocity of motion and provide accommodating resistance during dynamic exercise to the extremities or trunk. The equipment provides resistance proportional to the force generated by the person using the machine. The pre-set rate (degrees/second) cannot be exceeded no matter how vigorously the person pushes against the force arm. Therefore, the muscle contracts to its maximum capacity at all points in the range of motion.

1. **Isokinetic training and testing equipment**
   a. The range of isokinetic equipment available for either training or testing seems to increase daily. New product lines and improvements in existing equipment are continually being developed. The best source of current information on equipment capabilities are brochures distributed by the manufacturer or product demonstrations at professional meetings.
   b. Some isokinetic exercise systems are designed for both testing and training extremity or trunk musculature. They include the Cybex II + (Figure 3-33), the KIN/COM, the Brodex, the Lido, and the Merac. Some systems are designed exclusively for testing or training trunk musculature (Figure 3-34). Each of these systems has its unique advantages and capabilities.

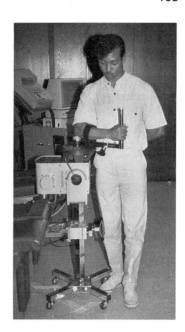

FIGURE 3–33. The Cybex® II+. The isokinetic dynamometer is used for exercise or testing musculature of the extremities.

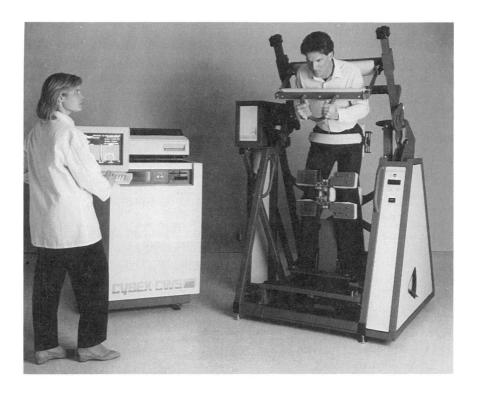

FIGURE 3–34. Cybex®'s Back-to-Work Clinic allows assessment and rehabilitation of the back. (Courtesy of Cybex, Division of Lumex, Ronkonkoma, NY)

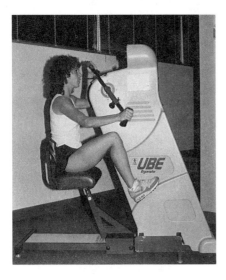

FIGURE 3-35. The Upper Body Exerciser®
(UBE) is used for upper extremity strength and
endurance training.

c. Other isokinetic units such as the Orthotron II (UBE) and the Upper
Body Exerciser (Figure 3-35) are designed for training only.
d. Concentric or eccentric resistance exercise can be performed on isokinetic equipment. Some equipment systems have only a concentric
mode for exercise, whereas others have both concentric and eccentric
modes.
e. The range of training and testing velocities available varies from 0 degrees per second to as high as 500 or 1000 degrees per second.
f. Full-arc or short-arc exercise can be done by controlling the range of
movement available with a computer or range-limiting device.

2. **Isokinetic equipment—advantages and disadvantages**
a. Advantages
(1) Isokinetic equipment can provide maximum resistance at all points
in the range of motion as a muscle contracts.
(2) Both high-speed and low-speed training can be done safely and effectively.
(3) The equipment accommodates for a painful arc of motion.
(4) As a patient fatigues, exercise can still continue.
(5) Reciprocal exercise against resistance can be performed, allowing
one muscle group to rest while its antagonist contracts. This minimizes muscle ischemia.
b. Disadvantages
(1) The equipment is large and expensive.
(2) Set-up time and assistance from personnel are necessary if a patient is to exercise multiple muscle groups.
(3) The equipment cannot be used for a home exercise program.

X. SUMMARY

This chapter on resistance exercise has included definitions of manual and mechanical resistance exercise, including isotonic, isometric, and isokinetic exercise. The goals and indications of resistance exercise were outlined, and the concepts of strength, power, and endurance were explained. Precautions to be considered during resistance exercises were also summarized. They are fatigue, recovery from fatigue, overwork, cardiovascular precautions, muscle soreness, substitute motions, and osteoporosis. Two contraindications—severe pain and acute inflammation—were listed. Principles of manual resistance exercise and techniques for properly applying resistance and stabilization manually during exercise were also explained.

The use of mechanical resistance exercise was described, and possible variables in programs were outlined. These variables included repetitions, exercise load, bouts, frequency, duration, and speed of exercise. Finally, an overview of mechanical equipment and exercise apparatus was discussed. Advantages and limitations of several pieces of equipment were explained for use in isotonic, isometric, and isokinetic exercise programs.

REFERENCES

1. Abraham, WM: *Exercise-induced muscle soreness.* Phys Sports Med 7(10):57, 1979.
2. Abraham, WM: *Factors in delayed muscle soreness.* Med Sci Sports 9:11, 1977.
3. Asmussen, E: *Observations on experimental muscle soreness.* Acta Rheumatol Scand 1:109, 1956.
4. Asmussen, E: *Muscular performance.* In Rodahl, K and Howath, S: *Muscle as a Tissue.* McGraw-Hill, New York, 1962.
5. Astrand, P and Rodahl, K: *Textbook of Work Physiology.* McGraw-Hill, New York, 1977.
6. Barnes, W: *Relationship between motor unit activation to muscular contraction at different contractile velocities.* Phys Ther 60:1152, 1980.
7. Basmajian, JV: *Muscles Alive,* ed 3. Williams & Wilkins, Baltimore, 1974.
8. Bassett, CAL: *Effect of force on skeletal tissue.* In Downey, JA and Darling, RC (eds): *Physiological Basis of Rehabilitation Medicine.* WB Saunders, Philadelphia, 1971.
9. Bennett, JG and Stauder, WT: *Evaluation and treatment of anterior knee pain using eccentric exercise.* Med Sci Sports Exerc 18:526, 1986.
10. Bonen, A and Belcastro, AN: *Comparison of self-directed recovery methods on lactic acid removal rates.* Med Sci Sports 8(3):176, 1976.
11. Considine, WJ and Sullivan, WJ: *Relationship of selected tests of leg strength and leg power in college men.* Res Quar 44:404, 1973.
12. Daniels, L and Worthingham, C: *Muscle Testing: Techniques of Manual Examination,* ed 4. WB Saunders, Philadelphia, 1980.
13. Darling, RC: *Exercise.* In Downey, and Darling, RC (eds): *The Physiological Basis of Rehabilitation Medicine.* WB Saunders, Philadelphia, 1971.
14. Darling, RC: *Fatigue.* In Downey, J and Darling, RC (eds): *The Physiological Basis of Rehabilitation Medicine.* WB Saunders, Philadelphia, 1971.
15. Davies, GJ: *A Compendium of Isokinetics in Clinical Usage and Rehabilitation Techniques,* ed 2. S & S Publishing, La Crosse, WI 1985.
16. Dean, E: *Physiology and therapeutic implications of negative work: A review.* Phys Ther 68:233, 1988.
17. DeLateur, BJ: *Therapeutic exercise to develop strength and endurance.* In Kottke, FJ, Stillwell, GK, and Lehmann, JF (eds): *Krusen's Handbook of Physical Medicine and Rehabilitation,* ed 3. WB Saunders, Philadelphia, 1982.
18. Delorme, TL and Watkins, A: *Progressive Resistance Exercise.* Appleton-Century, New York, 1951.
19. Delorme, T and Watkins, A: *Technics of progressive resistance exercise.* Arch Phys Med Rehabil 29:263, 1948.

20. DeVine, K: *EMG activity recorded from an unexercised muscle during maximum isometric exercise of contralateral agonists and antagonists.* Phys Ther 61:898, 1981.
21. DeVries, HA: *Electromyographic observations on the effects static stretching has on muscular distress.* Res Quar 32:468, 1961.
22. Devries, HA: *Quantitative electromyographic investigation of the spasm theory of muscle pain.* AM J Phys Med 45:119, 1966.
23. Dorpat, TL and Holmes, TH: *Mechanisms of skeletal muscle pain and fatigue.* Arch Neurol Psychol 74:628, 1955.
24. Evans, WJ: *Exercise-induced skeletal muscle damage.* Physician Sports Med 15:89, 1987.
25. Fardy, P: *Isometric exercise and the cardiovascular system.* Phys Sports Med 9:43, 1981.
26. Fox, E and Matthews, D: *The Physiological Basis of Physical Education and Athletics,* ed 3. Saunders College Publishing, Philadelphia, 1981.
27. Fox, EL, Robinson, S, and Wiegman, D: *Metabolic energy sources during continuous and interval running.* J Appl Physiol 27:174, 1969.
28. Francis, KT: *Delayed muscle soreness: A review.* JOSPT 5(1):10, 1983.
29. Friden, J, Sjostrom, M, and Ekblom, B: *A morphological study of delayed muscle soreness.* Experimentia 37:506, 1981.
30. Friden, J, Sjostrom, M, and Ekblom, B: *Myofibrillar damage following intense eccentric exercise in man.* Int J Sports Med 4:170, 1983.
31. Gettman, LR and Polluck, ML: *What makes a superstar? A physiological profile.* Phys Sports Med 5:64, 1977.
32. Gisolti, C, Robinson, S, and Turrell, ES: *Effects of aerobic work performed during recovery from exhausting work.* J Appl Physiol 21:1767, 1966.
33. Glowitzke, BA and Milner, M: *Understanding the Scientific Basis of Human Movement,* ed 2. Williams & Wilkins, Baltimore, 1980.
34. Gollnick, P, et al: *Glycogen depletion patterns in human skeletal muscle fibers during prolonged work.* J Appl Physiol 34:615, 1973.
35. Gordon, EE, Kowalski, K, and Fritts, M: *Protein changes in quadriceps muscle of rat with repetitive exercises.* Arch Phys Med Rehabil 48:296, 1967.
36. Herbison, GJ, Jaweed, MM, Ditunno, JF, et al: *Effect of overwork during reinnervation of rat muscle.* Exper Neurol 41:1, 1973.
37. Hellebrandt, FA and Houtz, SJ: *Methods of muscle training: The influence of pacing.* Phys Ther Rev 38:319, 1958.
38. Hellebrandt, FA and Houtz, SJ: *Mechanisms of muscle training in man: Experimental demonstration of the overload principle.* Phys Ther Rev 36:371, 1956.
39. Hettinger, T and Muller, EA: *Muskelliestung and Muskeltraining.* Arbeitsphysiol 15:111, 1953.
40. Hislop, HJ and Perrine, J: *The isokinetic concept of exercise.* Phy Ther 47:114, 1967.
41. Hislop, HJ: *Quantitative changes in human muscular strength during isometric exercise.* Phys Ther 43:21, 1963.
42. Hollis, M: *Practical Exercise Therapy.* Blackwell Scientific Publications, Oxford, 1976.
43. Huddleston, OL: *Therapeutic Exercises: Kinesiotherapy.* FA Davis, Philadelphia, 1961.
44. Jenkins, WL, Thackaberry, M, and Killan, C: *Speed-specific isokinetic training.* J Orthop Sports Phys Ther 6:181, 1984.
45. Johnson, BL, et al: *A comparison of concentric and eccentric muscle training.* Med Sci Sports 8(1):35, 1976.
46. Johnson, BL: *Eccentric vs. concentric muscle training for strength development.* Med Sci Sports 4:111, 1972.
47. Jones, H: The Valsalva procedure: Its clinical importance to the physical therapist. J Am Phys Ther Assoc 45:570, 1965.
48. Karlsson, J and Saltin, B: *Oxygen deficits and muscle metabolites in intermittent exercise.* Acta Physiol Scand 82:115, 1971.
49. Kendall, H and Kendall, F: *Muscle Testing and Function.* Williams & Wilkins, Baltimore, 1949.
50. Kessler, R and Hertling, D: *Management of Common Musculoskeletal Disorders.* Harper & Row, Philadelphia, 1983.
51. Knapik, JJ, Mawadsley, RH and Ramos, MU: *Angular specificity and test mode specificity of isometric and isokinetic strength training.* J Orthop Sports Phys Ther 5:58, 1983.

52. Knight, KL: *Knee rehabilitation by the daily adjustable progressive resistive exercise technique.* Am J Sports Med 7:336, 1979.
53. Knight, KL: *Quadriceps strengthening with DAPRE technique: Case studies with neurological implications.* Med Sci Sports Exerc 17:636, 1985.
54. Knuttgren, HG: *Human performance in high intensity exercise with concentric and eccentric muscle contractions.* Int J Sports Med 7:6, 1986.
55. Knuttgren, HG: *Neuromuscular Mechanisms for Therapeutic and Conditioning Exercise.* University Park Press, Baltimore, 1976.
56. Laird, CG and Rozier, CK: *Toward understanding the terminology of exercise mechanics.* Phys Ther 59:287, 1979.
57. Lamb, D: *Physiology of Exercise.* Macmillan, New York, 1978.
58. Lehmkuhl, LD and Smith, LK: *Brunnstrom's Clinical Kinesiology,* ed 4. FA Davis, Philadelphia, 1983.
59. Lesmes, GR, Costill, DL, Coyle, EF, and Fink, WJ: *Muscle strength and power changes during maximal isokinetic training.* Med Sci Sports Exerc 10:266, 1978.
60. Liberson, WT: *Brief isometric exercise.* In Basmajian, JV (ed): *Therapeutic Exercise,* ed 3. Williams & Wilkins, Baltimore, 1978.
61. Licht, S: *Therapeutic Exercise,* ed 2. Waverly Press, Baltimore, 1965.
62. Lindh, M: *Increase of muscle strength from isometric quadriceps exercise at different knee angles.* Scand J Med 11:33,1979.
63. Lunnen, J: *Relationship between muscle length, muscle activity and torque of the hamstring muscles.* Phys Ther 61:190, 1981.
64. Malone, T, Blackburn, T, and Wallace, L: *Knee rehabilitation.* Phys Ther 60:1602, 1980.
65. McArdle, WD, Katch, FI, and Katch, VL: *Exercise Physiology: Energy, Nutrition and Human Performance.* Lea & Febiger, Philadelphia, 1981.
66. McGovern, RE and Luscombe, HB: *Useful modifications of programs and resistive exercise techniques.* Arch Phys Med Rehabil 34:475, 1953.
67. Moffroid, M, et al: *A study of isokinetic exercise.* Phys Ther 49:735, 1969.
68. Moffroid, M and Whipple, R: *Specificity of the speed of exercise.* Phys Ther 50:1693, 1970.
69. Moffroid, MT and Kusick, ET: *The power struggle: Definition and evaluation of power of muscular performance.* Phys Ther 55:1098, 1975.
70. Mortain, T and Devries, HA: *Neural factors vs. hypertrophy in the time course of muscle strength gain.* Am J Phys Med 58:115, 1979.
71. Muller, EA: *Influence of training and inactivity on muscle strength.* Arch Phys Med Rehabil 51:449, 1970.
72. Noland, R and Kuckhoff, F: *Adapted progressive resistance exercise device.* Phys Ther Rev 34:333, 1954.
73. Parry, CBW: *Vicarious motions (trick movements).* In Basmajian, JV (ed): *Therapeutic Exercise,* ed 3. Williams & Wilkins, Baltimore, 1978.
74. Petrofsky, JS: *Isometric Exercise and Its Clinical Implications.* Charles C Thomas, Springfield, IL, 1982.
75. Richard, G and Currier, D: *Back stabilization during knee strengthening exercise.* Phys Ther 57:1013, 1977.
76. Rose, DL: *Effect of brief maximal exercise on the strength of quadriceps femoris.* Arch Phys Med 38:157, 1957.
77. Rothstein, JM: *Muscle biology: Clinical considerations.* Phys Ther 62:1823, 1982.
78. Sanders, M and Sanders, B: *Mobility: active-resistive training.* In Gould, J and Davies, G (eds): *Orthopedic and Sports Physical Therapy.* CV Mosby, St Louis, 1985.
79. Sapega, AA and Drillings, G: *The definition and assessment of muscular power.* JOSPT 5(1):7, 1983.
80. Schram, DA: *Resistance exercise.* In Basmajian, JV (ed): *Therapeutic Exercise,* ed 3. Williams & Wilkins, Baltimore, 1978.
81. Sherman, WH, et al: *Isokinetic strength during rehabilitation following arthrotomy.* Athletic Train 16:138, 1981.
82. Smith, MJ and Melton, P: *Isokinetic vs. isotonic variable-resistance training.* Am J Sports Med 9:275, 1981.

83. Stephens, JA and Taylor, A: *Fatigue of maintained voluntary muscle contraction in man.* J Physiol (Lond) 220:1, 1972.
84. Talag, TS: *Residual muscular soreness as influenced by concentric eccentric and static contractions.* Res Q 44:458, 1973.
85. Thomeé, R, et al: *Slow or fast isokinetic training after knee ligament surgery.* J Orthop Sports Phys Ther 8:475, 1988.
86. Timm, KE: *Investigation of the physiological overflow effect from speed-specific isokinetic activity.* J Orthop Sports Phys Ther 9:106, 1987.
87. Vallbona, C: *Bodily responses to immobilization.* In Kottke, FJ, Stillwell, GK, and Lehmann, JF (eds): *Krusen's Handbook of Physical Medicine and Rehabilitation.* WB Saunders, Philadelphia, 1982.
88. Voss, DE, Ionta, MK, and Myers, BJ: *Proprioceptive Neuromuscular Facility,* ed 3. Harper & Row, New York, 1985.
89. Walsh, WM: *Anteromedial rotary instability of the knee.* Phys Ther 60:1633, 1980.
90. Waltrous, B, Armstrong, R, and Schwane, J: *The role of lactic acid in delayed onset muscular soreness.* Med Sci Sports Exerc 1:380, 1981.
91. Wilke, DV: *The relationship between force and velocity in human muscle.* J Physiol 110:249, 1950.
92. Williams, M and Stutzman, L: *Strength variations through the range of joint motion.* Phys Ther Rev 39:145, 1959.
93. Wolf, SL: *The morphological and functional basis of therapeutic exercise.* In Basmajian, JV (ed): *Therapeutic Exercise,* ed 3. Williams & Wilkins, Baltimore, 1978.
94. Zinowieff, AN: *Heavy resistance exercise: The Oxford technique.* Br J Phys Med 14:129, 1951.

CHAPTER ——————————— 4

Stretching

Mobility and flexibility of the soft tissues that surround a joint, that is, muscles, connective tissue, and skin, in conjunction with adequate joint mobility are necessary for normal range of motion. Conditions that may produce adaptive shortening of soft tissues around a joint and subsequent loss of range of motion include (1) prolonged immobilization, (2) restricted mobility, (3) connective tissue or neuromuscular diseases, (4) tissue pathology due to trauma, and (5) congenital and acquired bony deformities.

Prolonged immobilization can occur when a patient must wear a cast or a splint for an extended period of time after a fracture or surgery. An individual's mobility may be restricted because of prolonged bed rest or confinement to a wheelchair. This can lead to long-term static and often faulty positioning of joints and soft tissue. Neuromuscular diseases or trauma can lead to paralysis, spasticity, weakness, muscle imbalance, and pain, all of which make it difficult or impossible for a patient to move joints through a full range of motion. Connective tissue diseases (collagen diseases) such as scleroderma, dermatomyositis, and polymyositis as well as joint diseases such as rheumatoid arthritis and osteoarthritis can cause pain, muscle spasm, inflammation, and weakness and can alter the structure of soft tissues. Tissue pathology from trauma, inflammation, edema, ischemia, hemorrhage, surgical incision, laceration, and burns can lead to the production of dense fibrous tissue, which replaces normal soft tissue. These soft tissues then lose their normal elasticity and plasticity, resulting in loss of range of motion.

Muscle strength can also be altered when soft tissue adaptively shortens over time. As muscle loses its normal flexibility a change in the length-tension relationship of the muscle also occurs. As the muscle shortens, it no longer is capable of producing peak tension,[21] and *tight weakness* develops. Loss of flexibility, for whatever reason, can also cause pain arising from muscle, connective tissue, or periosteum. This, in turn, also decreases muscle strength.

Limitation of joint range of motion because of contracture (adaptive shortening) of soft tissue may be treated with passive stretching combined with relaxation procedures and active inhibition techniques. Each of these methods will be discussed in this chapter. Limitations of motion because of joint immobility are treated with joint mobilization and manipulation and will be dealt with in Chapter 5.

OBJECTIVES

After studying this chapter, the reader will be able to:
1. define specific terms related to stretching such as contracture, tightness, irreversible contracture, overstretching, and selective stretching.
2. identify the pathologic processes and clinical situations in which limitations of motion of soft tissues and joints can occur.
3. describe the properties of contractile and noncontractile soft tissue that affect the application and success of stretching procedures.
4. define and explain the different therapeutic techniques used to elongate muscle, including active inhibition and passive stretching.
5. describe the indications, goals, precautions, and contradictions to stretching.
6. discuss the correct procedures a therapist should follow when setting up and carrying out stretching exercises.
7. identify the general principles of relaxation exercises and apply them in preparation for stretching.
8. describe proper patient positioning, hand placement, and stabilization used when applying stretching techniques to the upper and lower extremities.
9. describe the appropriate application of active inhibition techniques.

I. DEFINITION OF TERMS RELATED TO STRETCHING

A. Stretching

A general term used to describe any therapeutic maneuver designed to lengthen (elongate) pathologically shortened soft-tissue structures and thereby to increase range of motion[1,3,5,31,52]

1. Passive stretching

While the patient is relaxed, an external force, applied either manually or mechanically, lengthens the shortened tissues.

2. Active inhibition

The patient participates in the stretching maneuver to inhibit tonus in a tight muscle.

B. Flexibility

Flexibility is a term sometimes used interchangeably with extensibility. It refers to the ability of muscle to relax and yield to a stretch force.[3,20] Flexibility exercises are stretching exercises designed to increase range of motion.

C. Selective Stretch

Selective stretch is a process whereby the overall function of a patient may be improved by applying stretching techniques selectively and allowing limitation of motion to develop in specific joints.
1. For example, in the patient with spinal cord injury, stability of the trunk is necessary for independence in sitting. With thoracic and cervical lesions, the patient will not have active control of the back extensors. If moderate tightness is allowed to develop in the extensors of the low back, the patient will be able to lean into the slightly tight structures and will have some trunk stability in sitting.

Note: The patient must also have adequate range for independence in dressing and transfers. Too much tightness in the low back can decrease function.
2. Allowing slight contractures to develop in the long flexors of the fingers will enable the patient with spinal cord injury, who lacks innervation of the intrinsic finger muscles, to develop grasp through a tenodesis action.

D. Overstretch[31]

Overstretch is a stretch well beyond the normal range of motion of a joint and the surrounding soft tissues, resulting in hypermobility.
1. Overstretching may be necessary for certain healthy individuals with normal strength and stability participating in sports such as gymnastics.
2. Overstretching becomes detrimental when the supporting structures of a joint and the strength of the muscles around a joint are insufficient and cannot hold a joint in a stable, functional position during activities.

E. Contracture

Contracture is defined as shortening of muscle or other tissues that cross a joint, which results in a limitation of joint motion.[13,28,29]
1. Contractures are described by identifying the tight muscle action. If a patient has tight elbow flexors and cannot fully extend the elbow, he is said to have an elbow flexion contracture. When a patient cannot fully abduct his leg because of tight adductors of the hip, he is said to have an adduction contracture of the hip.
2. The terms *contracture* and *contraction* (the process of tension developing in a muscle during shortening or lengthening)[3,26] are **not** synonymous and should not be used interchangeably.

F. Types of Contractures

Contractures can be more specifically defined and classified by the soft tissue structures involved.

1. Myostatic contracture[13]

a. There is no specific tissue pathology present. The musculotendinous unit has adaptively shortened and there is a significant loss of range of motion.
b. *Tightness*
Tightness is a nonspecific term referring to mild shortening of an otherwise healthy musculotendinous unit. The term *tightness* is sometimes used to describe a mild transient contracture. A muscle that is "tight" can be lengthened to all but the outer limits of its range. Normal individuals who do not regularly participate in a flexibility program can develop mild myostatic contractures or tightness, particularly in two-joint muscles such as the hamstrings, rectus femoris, or gastrocnemius.
c. Myostatic contractures can be resolved in a relatively short period of time with gentle stretching exercises.

2. Scar-tissue adhesions[13]

When scar tissue is laid down between otherwise normal tissues and ties down the motion of these tissues in relation to each other, an adhesion forms and limits motion and function. Contractures can develop from scar tissue adhesions in muscles, tendons, joint capsules, or skin. Most contractures resulting from scar tissue adhesions can be prevented or reduced with exercise.

3. Fibrotic adhesions[13]

Contractures can also develop as the result of a chronic inflammation and fibrotic changes of soft tissues. Fibrotic adhesions dramatically restrict motion. Contractures caused by fibrosis of tissues are very difficult to reduce.

4. Irreversible contracture

A permanent loss of extensibility of soft tissues that cannot be released by nonsurgical treatment occurs when normal soft tissue and organized connective tissue is replaced by an excessive amount of nonextensible tissue such as bone or fibrotic tissue.

5. Pseudomyostatic contracture[13]

Limitation of motion may also develop as the result of hypertonicity caused by a central nervous system lesion. The muscle appears to be in an inappropriate and constant state of contraction, resulting in an apparent limitation of motion.

II. PROPERTIES OF SOFT TISSUE THAT AFFECT ELONGATION

As mentioned earlier, the soft tissues that can restrict joint motion are muscles, connective tissue, and skin. Each has unique qualities that affect its extensibility, that is, its ability to elongate. When stretching procedures are applied to these soft tissues, the velocity, intensity, and duration of the stretch force will all affect the response of the different types of soft tissues. Mechanical characteristics of contractile and noncontractile tissue as well as the neurophysiologic properties of contractile tissue all affect soft tissue lengthening.

When soft tissue is stretched, either elastic or plastic changes occur. *Elasticity* is the ability of soft tissue to return to its resting length after passive stretch. *Plasticity* is the tendency of soft tissue to assume a new and greater length after the stretch force has been removed.[45] Both contractile and noncontractile tissues have elastic and plastic qualities.[3,31,45]

A. Mechanical Properties of Contractile Tissue

Muscle is primarily composed of contractile tissue but is interwoven with noncontractile tissue.

1. Contractile elements of muscle (Figure 4-1)

Individual muscles are composed of many *muscle fibers*. A single muscle fiber is made up of many *myofibrils*. A myofibril is composed of *sarcomeres*, which lie in series. The sarcomere is the contractile unit of the myofibril and is composed of overlapping cross-bridges of actin and myosin. The sarcomere gives a muscle its ability to contract and relax. When a muscle contracts, the actin-myosin filaments slide together and the muscle shortens. When a muscle relaxes, the cross-bridges slide apart slightly, and the muscle returns to its resting length (Figure 4-2).

2. Mechanical response of the contractile unit to stretch

a. When a muscle is passively stretched, initial lengthening occurs in the series elastic component and tension rises sharply. After a point there is

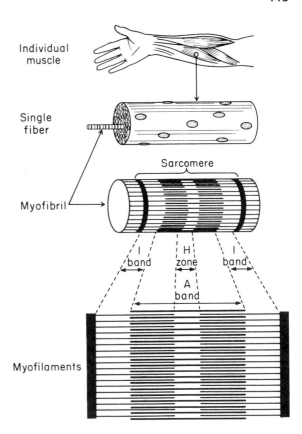

Individual muscle

Single fiber

Sarcomere

Myofibril

I band   H zone   I band

A band

Myofilaments

FIGURE 4–1. The structure of skeletal muscle.

a mechanical disruption of the cross-bridges as the filaments slide apart and an abrupt lengthening of the sarcomeres occurs (sarcomere give).[19] When the stretch force is released, the individual sarcomeres return to their resting length (Figure 4-2). The tendency of muscle to return to its resting length after short-term stretch is called *elasticity*.[45,49,51]

b. If a muscle is immobilized in a lengthened position over a prolonged period of time, the number of sarcomeres in series will increase, giving rise to a more permanent (plastic) form of muscle lengthening. A muscle will adjust its length over time to maintain the greatest functional overlap of actin-myosin.[49,51,59]

c. A muscle that has been immobilized in a shortened position produces increased amounts of connective tissue that serves to protect the muscle when it stretches. There is a reduction in the number of sarcomeres as the result of sarcomere absorption.[49,51,59]

d. The sarcomere adaptation to prolonged positions (either lengthened or shortened) is transient if the muscle is allowed to resume its normal length after immobilization.

B. Neurophysiologic Properties of Contractile Tissue

1. The muscle spindle (Figure 4-3)

The muscle spindle is the major sensory organ of muscle and is composed of microscopic intrafusal fibers that lie in parallel to the extrafusal fiber. The

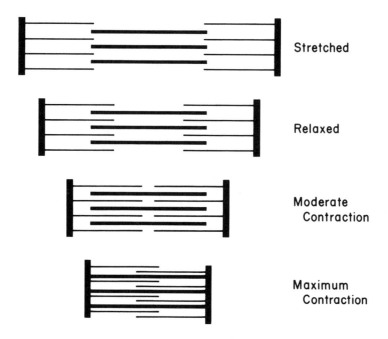

Stretched

Relaxed

Moderate
Contraction

Maximum
Contraction

FIGURE 4–2. Elongation and shortening of the sarcomere, the contractile unit of muscle.

muscle spindle monitors the velocity and duration of stretch. When a muscle is stretched the intrafusal and extrafusal fibers of that muscle are stretched. Fibers of the muscle spindle sense how quickly a muscle is stretched.

2. **The golgi tendon organ (GTO)**
   The GTO wraps around the ends of the extrafusal fibers of a muscle and is sensitive to the tension in a muscle caused by either passive stretch or active muscle contraction.
   a. The GTO is a protective mechanism that inhibits contraction of the muscle in which it lies. It has a very low threshold for firing (fires easily) after an active muscle contraction and has a high threshold for firing with passive stretch.
   b. When excessive tension develops in a muscle, the GTO fires and causes the muscle to relax.[3,15]

3. **The neurophysiologic response of muscle to stretch**[3,15]
   a. When a muscle is stretched very quickly, the muscle spindle contracts, which in turn stimulates the primary afferent fibers that causes the extrafusal fiber to fire, and tension increases in the muscle. This is called the *monosynaptic stretch reflex.* Stretching procedures that are performed at too high a velocity may actually increase the tension in a muscle that is to be lengthened.

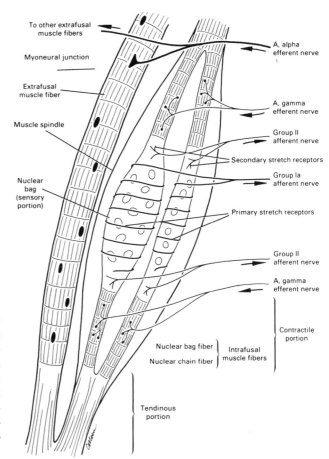

To other extrafusal
muscle fibers

Myoneural junction

Extrafusal
muscle fiber

Muscle spindle

Nuclear
bag
(sensory
portion)

A, alpha
efferent nerve

A, gamma
efferent nerve

Group II
afferent nerve

Secondary stretch receptors

Group Ia
afferent nerve

Primary stretch receptors

Group II
afferent nerve

A, gamma
efferent nerve

Contractile
portion

Nuclear bag fiber ⎱ Intrafusal
Nuclear chain fiber ⎰ muscle fibers

Tendinous
portion

FIGURE 4–3. The muscle spindle. Diagram shows intrafusal and extrafusal muscle fibers. The muscle spindle acts as a stretch receptor. (From Lehmkuhl, LD and Smith, LK: *Brunnstrom's Clinical Kinesiology,* ed 4. FA Davis, Philadelphia, 1983, p. 97 with permission.)

b. If a slow stretch force is applied to muscle, the GTO fires and inhibits the tension in the muscle, allowing the parallel elastic component (the sarcomere) of the muscle to lengthen.

C. Mechanical Characteristics of Noncontractile Soft Tissue

Noncontractile soft tissue permeates the entire body and is organized into various types of connective tissue to support the structures of the body. Ligaments, tendons, joint capsules, fascia, noncontractile tissue within muscles, and skin all have characteristics that will lead to the development of adhesions and contractures and thus affect the flexibility of the tissues crossing the joint. When these tissues restrict range of motion and require stretching, it is important to understand how they respond to various intensities and duration of stretch forces.

1. Material strength

The material strength of each tissue is related to its ability to resist a load or stress.[12,34]

a. *Stress* is force per unit area. Mechanical stress is the internal reaction or resistance to an external load. There are 3 kinds of stress.
   (1) *Tension:* a tensile force that is applied perpendicular to the cross-sectional area of the tissue in a direction away from the tissue. Tension stress is a stretching force.
   (2) *Compression:* a compressive force that is applied perpendicular to the cross-sectional area of the tissue in a direction toward the tissue. Compression stress occurs within joints, with muscle contraction and on weight bearing when a joint is loaded.
   (3) *Shear:* a force that is parallel to the cross-sectional area of the tissue.
b. *Strain* is the amount of deformation that occurs when a load (stress) is applied.
c. *Stress-strain curve (Figure 4-4)*
   (1) *Elastic range:* initially the strain is directly proportional to the ability of the material to resist the force. The tissue returns to its original size and shape when the load is released.
   (2) *Elastic limit:* the point beyond which the tissue will not return to its original shape and size.
   (3) *Plastic range:* the range beyond the elastic limit extending to the point of rupture. Tissue strained within this range will have permanent deformation.
   (4) *Yield strength:* the load beyond the elastic limit that produces permanent deformation within the tissue. Once the yield point is reached, there is sequential failure of the tissue with permanent deformation (remodeling), and the tissue passes into the plastic range of the stress-strain curve. The deformation may be from a single load or the summation of several subcritical loads.[12]
   (5) *Ultimate strength:* the greatest load the tissue can sustain. Once the maximum load is reached, there is increased strain (deformation) without an increase in stress.
   (6) *Necking:* the region where there is considerable weakening of the tissue; less force is needed for deformation, and failure rapidly approaches.
   (7) *Breaking strength:* the load at the time the tissue fails.
   (8) *Failure:* rupture of the integrity of the tissue.
d. Influences on the stress-strain curve
   (1) *Resilience:* the ability to absorb energy within the elastic range as work is accomplished. Energy is released when the load is removed and the tissue returns to its original shape.
   (2) *Toughness:* the ability to absorb energy within the plastic range without breaking (failing). If too much energy is absorbed with the stress, there will be rupture.
   (3) *Creep:* when a load is applied for an extended period of time, the tissue elongates, resulting in permanent deformation or failure. It is related to the viscosity of the tissue and is therefore time dependent. Deformation depends on the amount of force and the rate at which the force is applied. Creep occurs with low-magnitude load, usually in the elastic range, over a long period of time. The greater the load, the more rapid the rate of creep, but not in proportion to strain; therefore, a lesser load applied for a longer period of time will result in greater deformation. Increased temperature increases creep and therefore distensibility of the tissue.[32,56,57]

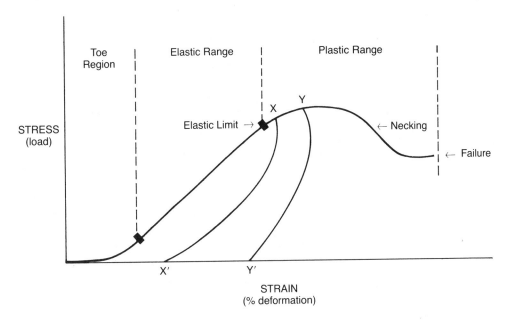

FIGURE 4–4. Stress–strain curve. When stressed, initially the wavy collagen fibers straighten (toe region). With additional stress, recoverable deformation occurs in the elastic range. Once the elastic limit is reached, sequential failure of the collagen fibers and tissue occurs in the plastic range, resulting in release of heat (hysteresis) and new length when the stress is released. The length from the stress point (X) results in a new length when released (X′); the heat released is represented by the area under the curve between these two points (hysteresis loop). (Y to Y′ represents additional length from additional stress with more heat released.) Necking is the region where there is considerable weakening of the tissue and less force is needed for deformation. Total failure quickly follows even under smaller loads.

(4) *Structural stiffness:* tissue with greater stiffness will have a higher slope in the elastic region of the curve, indicating there is less elastic deformation with greater stress. Contractures and scar tissue have greater stiffness, probably due to a greater degree of bonding between collagen fibers and their surrounding matrix.

(5) *Heat production:* energy is released as heat when stress is applied. It is depicted by the area under the curve (hysteresis loop) in the plastic range. As the tissue is heated, it more easily distends.

(6) *Fatigue:* cyclic loading of the tissue may cause failure below the yield point. The greater the applied load, the fewer number of cycles are needed for failure. A minimum load is required for this failure; below the minimum load an apparent infinite number of cycles will not cause failure. This is the *endurance limit*. Examples of fatigue are stress fractures and overuse syndromes. Biologic tissue has the ability to repair itself after cyclic loading if the load is not too great and time is allowed before the cyclic loading is again applied.

2. Composition of connective tissue

Connective tissue is composed of three types of fibers and nonfibrous ground substance.[12]

a. *Collagen fibers* resist tensile deformation and are responsible for the strength and stiffness of tissue. Collagen elongates quickly under light loads (wavy fibers straighten within the toe region); with increasing tension, the fibers continue to stiffen. They strongly resist the deforming force that begins to break the bonds between collagen fibrils and molecules. When a substantial number of bonds are broken, the fibers fail. Tissue with greater proportion of collagen provide greater stability. Collagen is five times as strong as elastin.

b. *Elastin fibers* provide extensibility. They show a great deal of elongation with small loads and fail abruptly without deformation at higher loads. Tissues with greater amounts of elastin have greater flexibility.

c. *Reticulin fibers* provide tissue with bulk.

d. *Ground substance,* mostly a gel containing water, reduces friction between fibers and may help prevent excessive cross-linking between fibers.[14]

3. Mechanical behavior of noncontractile tissue

The mechanical behavior of the various noncontractile tissues is determined by the proportion of collagen and elastin fibers and by the structural orientation of the fibers. Collagen is the structural element that absorbs most of the tensile stress.

a. In tendons, collagen fibers are parallel and can resist the greatest tensile load.

b. In skin, collagen fibers are random and weakest in resisting tension.

c. In ligaments, joint capsules, and fascia the collagen fibers vary between the two extremes. Ligaments that resist the major joint stresses have more parallel orientation of collagen fibers and a larger cross-sectional area.[43]

4. Interpreting the stress-strain curve[61]

a. Collagen fibers at rest are wavy, so initially they straighten as stress is applied. Little force is required for elongation in this range (toe region) where most functional activity normally occurs. Additionally, in the toe region stress removes any macroscopic slack in the 3-D matrix of collagenous tissues.

b. As the tissue is taken to the end of the full normal range of motion and a gentle stretch is applied, the tissue functions in the elastic portion (linear phase) of the curve. With this stress the collagen fibers line up with the applied force; the bonds between fibers and between the surrounding matrix are strained and some water may be displaced. There is complete recovery from this normal deformation.

c. If stress continues, the tissue reaches the yield point and sequential failure of the bonds between collagen fibrils and eventually of collagen fibers occurs. Heat is released and absorbed in the tissue and there is permanent deformation. Because collagen is crystalline, individual fibers do not stretch but respond to the forces by remodeling and rebonding over time in the lines of stress.

d. If maximum load and point of ultimate strength are reached, there is increased strain without an increase in stress. If necking is reached, the tissue rapidly fails. The therapist must be cognizant of the tissue feel when stretching because as the tissue begins necking and the stress is maintained, there will be complete failure (rupture). Experimentally, maximum tensile deformation of isolated collagen fibers prior to failure is 7 to 8%; whole ligaments may withstand strain of 20 to 40%.[43]

e. Using the principle of creep, low-magnitude loads over long periods of time increase the plastic deformation of noncontractile tissue, allowing a gradual rearrangement of collagen fibers and ground substance.[47] Increasing the temperature of the part will increase the creep.[32,57,58] Patient reaction dictates the time tolerated by a specific load. Fifteen to twenty minutes of low-intensity, sustained stretch, repeated on 5 consecutive days, has been documented to show change in the length of the hamstring muscles.[47]

f. Cyclic loading, or repetitive submaximal stress, increases the effects of the tissue adapting (remodeling) to a new length. Starring and coworkers[47] documented increased hamstring length using 10-second hold followed by an 8-second rest, repeated for 15 minutes on 5 consecutive days.

g. Tissue failure can occur as a single maximal event (acute tear from injury or manipulation that exceeds the failure point), or from repetitive submaximal stress (fatigue or stress failure from cyclic loading).

h. Healing and adaptive (remodeling) capabilities of biologic tissue allow tissue to respond to repetitive loads as long as time is allowed between bouts. This is important both for increasing flexibility as well as tensile strength of the tissue.

(1) If healing and remodeling time is not allowed, a breakdown of tissue (failure) will occur as in overuse syndromes and stress fractures.

(2) Intensive stretching is usually not done every day in order to allow time for healing.

(3) Greater precaution is required with aging because collagen looses its elasticity, and there is decreased capillary blood supply that reduces the healing capability.

5. **Changes in collagen affecting stress-strain response**

a. *Effects of immobilization*

There is weakening of the tissue seen as weakening of collagen, decrease in lubrication, and increase in adhesions.[14] Rate of return is slow. Following 8 weeks of immobilization the anterior cruciate ligament in monkeys failed at 61% of maximum load; after 5 months of reconditioning, failed at 79%; after 12 months of reconditioning, failed at 91%.[41,42] There was also a reduction in energy absorbed and an increase in compliance (decreased stiffness) prior to failure following immobilization. Partial- and near-complete recovery followed the same 5-month and 12-month pattern.[42]

b. *Effects of inactivity (decrease of normal activity)*

There is a decrease in size and amount of collagen fibers, resulting in weakening of the tissue; there is a proportional increase in the predominance of elastin fibers, resulting in an increased compliance. Recovery takes about 5 months of regular cyclic loading.

c. *Effects of age on collagen*

There is a decrease in the maximum tensile strength, a decrease in the elastic modulus, and the rate of adaptation to stress is slower.[43] There is an increased tendency for overuse syndromes, fatigue failures, and tears with stretching.[61]

d. *Effects of steroids*

There is a long-lasting deleterious effect on mechanical properties of collagen with a decrease in tensile strength.[61] There is fibrocyte death next to the injection site with delay in reappearance up to 15 weeks.[43]

An understanding of the qualities of contractile and noncontractile tissues and their responses to immobilization and stretch will assist the therapist in selecting the safest and most effective stretching procedures for patients.

III. THERAPEUTIC METHODS TO ELONGATE SOFT TISSUES

There are two basic methods to elongate contractile or noncontractile tissues: passive stretching and active inhibition of muscles.[5,10,20,26,31,52] All stretching procedures should be preceded by some low-intensity active exercise or therapeutic heat to warm up the tissues that are to be stretched. Soft tissue yields more easily to stretch if the muscle is warm when the stretch force is applied.

A. Passive Stretching

Passive stretching procedures are classified by the type of stretch force applied, the intensity of the stretch, and the duration of the stretch. Both contractile and noncontractile tissues can be elongated by passive stretching.

1. Manual passive stretching

a. The therapist applies the external force and controls the direction, speed, intensity, and duration of the stretch to the soft tissues that have caused the contracture and restriction of joint motion. The tissues are elongated beyond their resting length.

b. This technique should not be confused with passive range of motion exercises. Passive stretching takes the structures beyond the free range of motion. Passive range of motion is applied only within the unrestricted available range.

c. The patient must be as relaxed as possible during passive stretching.

d. The stretch force is usually applied for at least 15 to 30 seconds and repeated several times in an exercise session. Manual passive stretching is generally considered to be a short-duration stretch.[5,26]

   (1) No specific number of seconds has been determined to be the most effective duration for passive stretching.

   (2) In one study[23,27] passive stretching was applied to the hip abductors of healthy subjects for 15 seconds, 45 seconds, and 2 minutes at the same intensity. The 15-second stretch was just as effective as the 2-minute stretch.

e. The intensity and duration of the stretch are dependent on the patient's tolerance and the therapist's strength and endurance. A low-intensity manual stretch applied for as long as possible will be more comfortable and more readily tolerated by the patient.

f. Maintained versus ballistic stretch[44]

   (1) When manual passive stretching is appropriately applied, the stretch is very slow and gentle. The stretch force is *maintained,* as previously mentioned, for 15 seconds, 30 seconds, or longer. A slow, maintained stretch is less likely to facilitate the stretch reflex

and increase tension in the muscle being lengthened. This is some-times called a *static stretch*.

(2) Ballistic stretching is a high-intensity, very short-duration "bounc-ing" stretch. It is an inappropriate way to stretch muscle. A ballistic stretch quickly lengthens the muscle spindle and facilitates the stretch reflex, causing an increase in tension in the muscle that is being stretched. Muscles are more susceptible to microtrauma with ballistic stretching than with a maintained stretch.

(3) It has been shown that the tension created in a muscle during ballis-tic stretching is almost twice that created with low-intensity main-tained stretch.[55]

g. In comparison to long-duration mechanical stretching procedure, ap-plied for 20 minutes or more, manual passive stretching is a rather short-duration stretch. The gains achieved in range of motion are transient and are attributed to temporary sarcomere give (elastic changes in actin-myosin overlap).[22]

2. **Prolonged mechanical passive stretching**[32,45,47,48,56,57]

a. A low-intensity external force (5 to 15 lb) is applied to shortened tissues over a prolonged period of time with mechanical equipment.

b. The stretch force is applied through positioning of the patient, with weighted traction and pulley systems or with dynamic splints or serial casts.

c. The prolonged stretch may be maintained for 20 to 30 minutes or as long as several hours.

(1) Several studies have suggested that a period of 20 minutes or longer is necessary for a stretch to be effective and increase range of motion when low-intensity prolonged mechanical stretch is used.[31,45]

(2) Bohannon[8] evaluated the effectiveness of an 8-minute stretch of the hamstrings in comparison to a 20-minute or longer stretch using an overhead cable-pulley system (Elgin Exercise Unit). The 8-minute stretch resulted in only a small increase in hamstring flexibility, which was lost within 24 hours. It was suggested that a 20-minute or longer-duration stretch is necessary to effectively increase range of motion on a more permanent basis.

(3) Bohannon and Larkin[9] also used a regimen of tilt table–wedge board standing for 30 minutes daily to increase the range of ankle dorsi-flexion in patients with neurologic disorders.

(4) Prolonged, low-intensity stretch and an increase in range can also be accomplished with a dynamic splint[24] such as the Dynasplint (Fig-ure 4-5). The splint is applied for 8 to 10 hours. Units are available for the elbow, wrist, knee, and ankle.

d. Low-intensity prolonged stretch (5 to 12 lb stretch force applied 1 hour per day) has been shown to be significantly more effective than manual passive stretching over a 4-week period in patients with long-standing bilateral knee flexion contractures.[36] The patients also reported that the prolonged mechanical stretch was more comfortable than the manual stretching procedure.

e. Permanent lengthening (plastic changes) in contractile and noncontract-ile tissues has been reported as the result of long duration stretch.

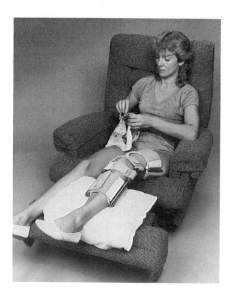

FIGURE 4–5. The Dynasplint Systems® Unit places a prolonged stretch on soft tissue to reduce a knee flexion contracture. (Courtesy of Dynasplint Systems, Inc., Baltimore, MD)

(1) When muscles are held in a lengthened position for several weeks, sarcomeres are added in series.[49,51,59]

(2) When noncontractile connective tissues are stretched with a low-intensity prolonged stretch force, plastic deformation occurs and the length of the tissue increases.[32,56,57]

Note: The term "permanent lengthening" means that length is maintained after the stretch force is removed. The increase in length will be "permanent" only if the new length is used regularly.

3. Cyclic mechanical stretching

Passive stretching using a mechanical device such as the Autorange (Valley City, ND) can also be done in a cyclic mode. Starring[47] reported significant increases in hamstring muscle flexibility using a 20-second, high-intensity (up to patient's pain tolerance) mechanical stretch. The intensity of the stretch, the length of each stretch cycle, and the number of stretch cycles per minute can all be adjusted on the mechanical stretching unit.

This type of stretching is similar in intensity and duration to manual passive stretching, but can be done independently by the patient. Cyclic mechanical stretching does improve range of motion and may be a useful alternative to manual passive stretching for some patients.

B. Active Inhibition[3,18,31,44,50,52,54]

Active inhibition refers to techniques in which the patient reflexively relaxes the muscle to be elongated prior to the stretching maneuver. When a muscle is inhibited (relaxed) there is minimal resistance to elongation of the muscle. Active inhibition techniques relax only the contractile structures within muscle, not connective tissues. This type of stretching is only possible if the muscle to be elongated is normally innervated and under voluntary control. It cannot be used in patients with severe muscle weakness, spasticity, or paralysis from neuromuscular dysfunction.

Therapists have used active inhibition techniques for many years as an adjunct or alternative to passive stretching. Inhibition techniques increase muscle length by stretching out elastic tissue. The assumption is that sarcomere give will occur more easily when the muscle is relaxed and there is less active resistance (tension) in the muscle as it is elongated. An advantage of inhibition techniques is that muscle elongation is a more comfortable form of stretching than traditional high-intensity, short-duration passive stretching. A disadvantage of active inhibition is that it is a high-intensity stretch that affects only the elastic structures of muscle and produces only temporary increases in muscle length.

There are 3 variations of active inhibition techniques that can be used to first relax and then elongate tight muscles. They are (1) contract-relax, (2) contract-relax-contract, and (3) agonist contraction.

1. Contract-relax (hold-relax)[11,18,44,54]

   a. This inhibition technique was originally associated with proprioceptive neuromuscular facilitation (PNF) but is now widely used in rehabilitation and training programs.
   b. The term *muscle energy* is also used by manual therapists to describe inhibition techniques used to elongate muscles and improve joint mobility in the spine or extremities.[18]
   c. In the contract-relax procedure, the patient performs an isometric contraction of the tight muscle before it is passively lengthened. The rationale behind this technique is that after a prestretch contraction of the tight muscle that same muscle will relax as the result of *autogenic inhibition* before it is passively lengthened. The Golgi tendon organ (GTO) may fire and inhibit tension in the muscle so that it can be more easily lengthened.
   d. Clinically therapists have assumed that the prestretch contraction causes a reflexive relaxation accompanied by a decrease in electromyographic (EMG) activity in the tight muscle. Some investigators[16,39] have refuted this assumption, whereas others have supported it. In two studies, a postcontraction sensory discharge (increased EMG activity) was identified in the muscle to be lengthened. This indicated that the muscle to be stretched was not effectively relaxed; but no postcontraction elevation in EMG activity was found in another study with the use of the contract-relax technique.[11]
   e. Obviously clinicians must evaluate the effectiveness of the contract-relax technique and determine its usefulness with individual patients.

2. Contract-relax-contract (hold-relax-contract)[11,17,18,39,54]

   a. A variation of the contract-relax technique is contraction of the tight muscle and relaxation of the tight muscle followed by a concentric contraction of the muscle opposite the tight muscle. As the muscle opposite the tight muscle shortens, the tight muscle lengthens. This technique combines *autogenic inhibition* and *reciprocal inhibition* to lengthen a tight muscle.
   b. In one study,[17] the contract-relax-contract technique produced a greater increase in ankle dorsiflexion range than the contract-relax technique. Both inhibition techniques produced a greater increase in range of ankle dorsiflexion than manual stretching. In another study, there was no sig-

nificant difference between contract-relax and contract-relax-contract techniques.[39]

3. Agonist contraction[3,10,11,18]

    a. Another inhibition technique is agonist contraction. This term has been used in several studies, but can be misunderstood. The "agonist" refers to the muscle opposite the tight muscle; and "antagonist," therefore, refers to the tight muscle. During this procedure, the patient dynamically contracts (shortens) the muscle *opposite the tight muscle* against resistance. This causes a *reciprocal inhibition* of the tight muscle, and the tight muscle lengthens more easily as the extremity moves.

    b. Therapists have found that this is an effective way to lengthen a tight muscle, particularly if the tight muscle is painful or in the early stages of healing. This method is least effective when a patient has close to normal range.

C. Self-stretching

Self-stretching is a type of flexibility exercise that the patient carries out himself. The patient may passively stretch out his own contractures by using his body weight as the stretch force. He may also actively inhibit a muscle to increase its length. The guidelines for the intensity and duration of the stretch that apply to self-stretching are the same as those for passive stretching carried out by a therapist or mechanical stretching procedures.

    Specific self-stretching procedures will not be discussed or illustrated in this chapter. Illustrations and explanation for many self-stretching exercises can be found in Chapters 7 through 12 and 14 through 17, which all deal with exercises for the upper and lower extremities and trunk.

IV. INDICATIONS AND GOALS OF STRETCHING[1,3,5,18,20,31,52]

A. Indications

1. when range of motion is limited as a result of contractures, adhesions, and scar tissue formation, leading to shortening of muscles, connective tissue and skin
2. when limitations might lead to structural (skeletal) deformities, otherwise preventable
3. when contractures interfere with everyday functional activities or nursing care
4. when there is muscle weakness and opposing tissue tightness. Tight muscles must be elongated before weak muscles can be effectively strengthened.

B. Goals

1. The overall goal of stretching is to regain or re-establish normal range of motion of joints and mobility of soft tissues that surround a joint.
2. Specific goals are to:
    a. prevent irreversible contractures.
    b. increase the general flexibility of a part of the body prior to vigorous strengthening exercises.
    c. prevent or minimize the risk of musculotendinous injuries related to specific physical activities and sports.

V. PROCEDURES FOR APPLYING PASSIVE STRETCHING[1,5,20,50]

A. Evaluation of the Patient Prior to Stretching

1. Determine if soft tissue or joint limitation is the cause of decreased motion and choose appropriate stretching or joint mobilization techniques or a combination of both to correct the limitation. Always evaluate the joint for adequate joint play. Before beginning a soft tissue stretching program, use joint mobilization techniques to re-establish joint play.
2. Assess the underlying strength of muscles where there is limitation of motion and realistically consider the value of stretching the limiting structures.

B. Prior to the Initiation of Stretching

1. Consider the best type of stretching or alternative to stretching to increase range.
2. Explain the goals of stretching to the patient.
3. Position the patient in a comfortable and stable position that will allow the best plane of motion in which the stretching procedure can be done. The direction of stretch will be exactly opposite the direction of tightness.
4. Explain the procedure to the patient and be certain he understands.
5. Free the area to be stretched of any restrictive clothing, bandages, or splints.
6. Explain to the patient that it is important that he be as relaxed as possible throughout the stretching period.
7. Employ relaxation techniques prior to stretching, if necessary. (See section VI of this chapter for more specific information.)
8. Apply heat to the soft tissues to be stretched. Warming tight structures increases their extensibility and decreases the possibility of injury.

C. When Applying the Stretch

1. Move the extremity slowly through the free range to the point of restriction.
2. Then grasp proximal and distal to the joint where motion is to occur. The grasp should be firm, but not uncomfortable to the patient. Use padding, if necessary, in areas where there is minimal subcutaneous tissue, over a bony surface, or where sensitivity is reduced. Use the broad surfaces of the hands to apply all forces.
3. Firmly stabilize the proximal segment (manually or with equipment) and move the distal segment.
   a. To stretch a multi-joint muscle, stabilize either the proximal or distal segment to which the tight muscle attaches.
   b. Stretch the muscle over one joint at a time, then over all joints simultaneously until optimum length of soft tissues is achieved.
   c. To minimize compressive forces in small joints, stretch the distal joints first and proceed proximally.
4. In order to avoid joint compression during the stretching procedure, apply very gentle (Grade I) traction to the moving joint.
5. Apply the stretch force in a gentle, slow, and sustained manner. Take the joint to the point of tightness and then move just beyond.
   a. The force must be enough to place tension on the soft-tissue structures, but not so great as to cause pain or injure the structures.
   b. Avoid ballistic stretching. Do not bounce the extremity at the end of the range. This will facilitate the stretch reflex and cause a reflex contraction

of the muscle being stretched. Ballistic stretching tends to cause the greatest amount of trauma and injury to tissues.

    c. In the stretched position, the patient should experience a sense of pulling or tightness of the structures being stretched, but not pain.

6. Hold the patient in the stretched position at least 15 to 30 seconds or longer.

    a. During this time the tension in the tissues should slowly decrease.

    b. When tension decreases, move the extremity or joint a little further.

7. Gradually release the stretch force.

8. Allow the patient and therapist to rest momentarily and then repeat the maneuver.

    Note: Do not attempt to gain full range in one or two treatment sessions. Increasing flexibility is a slow and gradual process. It may take several weeks of treatment to see significant results.

VI. RELAXATION AND INHIBITION IN PREPARATION FOR STRETCHING

Relaxation and inhibition procedures have been used for years by a variety of professionals to relieve pain, muscle tension, and associated physical and mental dysfunctions, including tension headaches, high blood pressure, and respiratory distress.[3,26,27,30,46,60]

Active inhibition techniques are reflex relaxation procedures that therapists use to inhibit muscle prior to lengthening. The background for these techniques has been discussed in section III B of this chapter. The procedures for application of active inhibition techniques will be outlined in this section.

A brief overview of other therapeutic modalities used to promote relaxation and extensibility of soft tissue will also be covered in this section.

A. Active Inhibition Techniques—Procedures For Application

    1. Contract-relax (hold relax)

        a. Procedure

            (1) Start with the tight muscle in a comfortably lengthened position.

            (2) Ask the patient to isometrically contract the tight muscle against substantial resistance for 5 to 10 seconds, until the muscle begins to fatigue.

            (3) Then have the patient voluntarily relax.

            (4) The therapist then lengthens the muscle by passively moving the extremity through the gained range.

            (5) Repeat the entire procedure after several seconds of rest.

        b. **Precautions**

            (1) The isometric contraction of the tight muscle should not be painful.

            (2) It is not necessary for the patient to perform a maximal isometric contraction of the tight muscle prior to stretch. A *submaximal* isometric contraction held for a longer period of time will adequately inhibit the tight muscle. Postcontraction sensory discharge (lingering tension in muscle after the prestretch contraction) may be a greater problem if a maximum contraction is performed. A submaximal, long-duration contraction will also be easier for the therapist to control if the patient is strong.

        c. Example: Tight ankle plantar flexors

            (1) Dorsiflex the ankle to a comfortable position to lengthen the tight muscles.

(2) Place your hand on the plantar surface of the patient's foot.
(3) Have the patient isometrically contract the plantar flexors against your resistance for 5 to 10 seconds.
(4) Tell the patient to relax and then passively dorsiflex the patient's ankle to lengthen the plantar flexors.

2. **Contract relax-contract (hold-relax-contract)**
   a. Procedure
      (1) Follow the same procedure as done for contract-relax.
      (2) After the patient relaxes the tight muscle, have the patient perform a concentric contraction of the muscle opposite the tight muscle. The patient actively moves his own extremity through the increased range.
   b. **Precautions:** same as for contract-relax
   c. Example: Tight ankle plantar flexors.
      (1) Follow the procedures described in contract-reflex.
      (2) After the patient relaxes the tight muscle, have him actively dorsiflex the foot.

3. **Agonist contraction**
   a. Procedure
      (1) Passively lengthen the tight muscle to a comfortable position.
      (2) Have the patient perform a dynamic (shortening) contraction of the muscle opposite the tight muscle.
      (3) Apply mild resistance to the contracting muscle, but allow joint movement to occur.
      (4) The tight muscle will relax as the result of reciprocal inhibition as joint movement occurs.
   b. **Precautions**
      (1) Do not apply excessive resistance to the contracting muscle. This may cause irradiation of tension to the tight muscle rather than relaxation and may restrict movement of the joint or cause pain.
      (2) Remember: This procedure is often used when muscle spasm restricts joint movement. This type of active inhibition is very useful if a patient cannot generate a strong pain-free contraction of the tight muscle, which must be done in the contract-relax procedure.
   c. Example: Pain and tight ankle plantar flexors
      (1) Place the patient's ankle in a comfortable position.
      (2) Apply mild resistance to the dorsum of the foot as the patient dynamically contracts the dorsiflexors. Allow joint movement (increased dorsiflexion) to occur.

B. Local Relaxation

1. **Heat**[18,20,45,56,57]

   Superficial or deep heat applied to soft tissue prior to stretching will increase the extensibility of the shortened tissue. Low-intensity active exercise done prior to stretching will increase circulation to soft tissue and warm the tissues to be stretched. Muscles that are warm relax and lengthen more easily, making stretching more comfortable for the patient. Connective tissue yields more easily to passive stretch if the tissue is warm.

2. Massage[4,30]

It is well documented that massage, particularly deep massage, can be used to increase local circulation and to decrease muscle spasm and stiffness. Massage is often preceded by the application of heat to further improve the extensibility of soft tissues.

3. Biofeedback[3,30]

A patient, if properly trained, can monitor and reduce the amount of tension in a muscle through biofeedback. Through visual or auditory feedback, a patient can begin to sense or feel what muscle relaxation is. Biofeedback is just one tool that can be useful in helping the patient learn and practice the process of relaxation. By reducing muscle tension, pain can be decreased and flexibility of muscle increased.

4. Joint traction or oscillation

a. Slight manual distraction of joint surfaces prior to or in conjunction with joint mobilization or stretching techniques can be used to decrease joint pain and spasm of muscles around a joint (see Chapter 5).

b. Pendular motions[26] of a joint, advocated by Codman, use the weight of the limb to distract the joint surfaces and thereby to relax and increase mobility of a limb. The joint may be further distracted by adding a 1- or 2-lb weight to the extremity.

C. General Relaxation[27,30,46]

1. General progressive relaxation techniques may also be a useful adjunct to a stretching program. A patient may learn to relax the total body or an extremity. Tension in muscles can be relieved by conscious effort and thought. Some techniques, such as autogenic relaxation advocated by Schultz,[46] suggest progressive conscious control and relaxation of muscle and body tension. Other techniques, such as Jacobson's progressive relaxation,[27] suggest a systematic distal to proximal progression of conscious contraction and relaxation of musculature.

2. Procedures for progressive relaxation training[3,7,27,30,46]

a. Place the patient in a quiet area and in a comfortable position, and be sure that he is free of restrictive clothing.

b. Have the patient breathe in a deep, relaxed manner.

c. Ask the patient to voluntarily contract the distal musculature in the hands or feet for a few seconds. Then have the patient consciously relax those muscles.

d. Suggest that the patient try to feel a sense of heaviness in his hands or feet.

e. Suggest to the patient that he feels a sense of warmth in the muscles he has just relaxed.

f. Progress to a more proximal area of the body. Have the patient actively contract and then actively relax more proximal musculature. Eventually have the patient isometrically contract and then consciously relax the entire extremity.

g. Suggest to the patient that he should feel a sense of heaviness and warmth throughout the entire limb and eventually throughout the whole body.

Note: Any combination of local and general relaxation may be used by the therapist to promote maximum muscle relaxation and therefore the potential for maximum muscle flexibility in a stretching program.

VII. PRECAUTIONS FOR AND CONTRAINDICATIONS TO STRETCHING

A. Precautions for Stretching[1,3,5,18,20,25,31]

1. Do not passively force a joint beyond its normal range of motion. Remember, normal range of motion varies among normal individuals.
2. Newly united fractures should be protected by stabilization between the fracture site and the joint where the motion takes place.
3. Use extra caution in patients with known or suspected osteoporosis due to disease, prolonged bed rest, age, and prolonged use of steroids.
4. Avoid vigorous stretching of muscles and connective tissues that have been immobilized over a long period of time. Connective tissues (tendons and ligaments) lose their tensile strength after prolonged immobilization.
   a. High-intensity, short-duration stretching procedures tend to cause more trauma and resulting weakness of soft tissues than low-intensity, long-duration stretch.
   b. Strengthening exercises should be added to a stretching program at some point so that a patient will be able to develop an appropriate balance between flexibility and strength.
5. If a patient experiences joint pain or muscle soreness lasting more than 24 hours, too much force has been used during stretching. Patients should experience no more residual discomfort than a transitory feeling of tenderness.
6. Avoid stretching edematous tissue, as it is more susceptible to injury than normal tissue. Continued irritation of edematous tissues usually causes increased pain and edema.
7. Avoid overstretching weak muscles, particularly those that support body structures in relation to gravity.

B. Contraindications to Stretching

1. when a bony block limits joint motion.
2. after a recent fracture.
3. whenever there is evidence of an acute inflammatory or infectious process (heat and swelling) in or around joints.
4. whenever there is sharp, acute pain with joint movement or muscle elongation.
5. when a hematoma or other indication of tissue trauma is observed.
6. when contractures or shortened soft tissues are providing increased joint stability in lieu of normal structural stability or muscle strength.
7. when contractures or shortened soft tissues are the basis for increased functional abilities, particularly in patients with paralysis or severe muscle weakness.

VIII. TECHNIQUES OF STRETCHING USING ANATOMIC PLANES OF MOTION

As with range of motion (ROM) exercises described in Chapter 2, the following techniques are described with the patient in a supine position. Alternate positions for patients are indicated for some motions and are noted when necessary.

Effective manual stretching techniques require adequate stabilization of the patient and sufficient strength and good body mechanics of the therapist. Depending on the size (height and weight) of the therapist and patient, variations in the position of the patient and suggested hand placements might have to be made by the therapist.

Each description of a stretching technique is identified by the plane of motion that is to be increased and followed by a notation of the muscle group being stretched. Each section contains a discussion of special considerations for each joint being stretched.

Prolonged passive stretching techniques using mechanical equipment are applied in the same positions and using the same points of stabilization as manual passive stretching. The stretch force is applied at a lower intensity and is applied over a much longer period of time than with manual passive stretching. The stretch force is provided by a weighted pulley system rather than the strength of a therapist. The patient is stabilized with belts, straps, or counterweights.

Self-stretching techniques of the extremities and trunk, which the patient can do without assistance from the therapist, will not be covered in this chapter. These techniques will be found for each joint of the extremities in Chapters 7 through 12. Stretching procedures for the musculature of the cervical, thoracic, and lumbar spine will be found in Chapters 14 through 17.

A. The Upper Extremity

1. The shoulder—Special considerations

Many muscles involved with shoulder motion attach to the scapula rather than the thorax. Therefore, when most muscles of the shoulder girdle are stretched, it is mandatory to stabilize the scapula. Without scapular stabilization the stretch force will be transmitted to those muscles that normally stabilize the scapula during movement of the arm. This subjects these muscles to possible overstretching and disguises the true range of motion of the glenohumeral joint.

Remember:

— When the scapula is stabilized and not allowed to abduct or upwardly rotate, only 120 degrees of shoulder flexion and abduction can occur at the glenohumeral joint.

— When scapular movement is stabilized, the humerus must be externally rotated to gain full range of motion.

— Muscles most apt to exhibit tightness are those that *prevent* full shoulder flexion, abduction, and rotation. It is rare to find tightness in structures that prevent shoulder adduction and extension to neutral.

a. **To increase flexion of the shoulder** (to stretch the shoulder extensors) (Figure 4-6A)

    (1) Hand placement

        Grasp the posterior aspect of the distal humerus, just above the elbow.

    (2) Stabilize the axillary border of the scapula.

    (3) Move the patient into full shoulder flexion to elongate the shoulder extensors.

b. **To increase hyperextension of the shoulder** (to stretch the shoulder flexors) (Figure 4-6B)

    (1) Alternate position

        Place the patient in a prone position.

    (2) Hand placement

        Support the forearm and grasp the distal humerus.

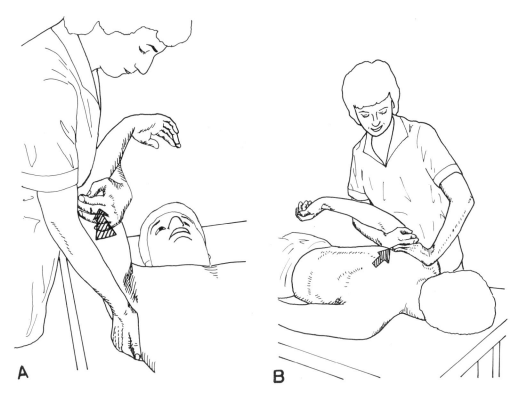

FIGURE 4–6. (*A*), Hand placement and stabilization of the scapula for stretching procedure to increase shoulder flexion. (*B*), Hand placement and stabilization of the scapula to increase hyperextension of the shoulder.

      (3) Stabilize the posterior aspect of the scapula to prevent substitute movements.

      (4) Move the patient's arm into full hyperextension of the shoulder to elongate the shoulder flexors.

  c. **To increase abduction of the shoulder** (to stretch the adductors) (Figure 4-7)

      (1) Hand placement
With the elbow flexed to 90 degrees, grasp the distal humerus.

      (2) Stabilize the axillary border of the scapula.

      (3) Move the patient into full shoulder abduction to lengthen the adductors of the shoulder.

  d. **To increase adduction of the shoulder** (to stretch the abductors)

      (1) It is rare that a patient will not be able to fully adduct the shoulder to 0 degrees (so the upper arm is at the patient's side).

      (2) Even if a patient has worn an abduction splint after a soft-tissue or joint injury of the shoulder, when the patient is upright, the constant pull of gravity will elongate the shoulder abductors so the patient can adduct to a neutral position.

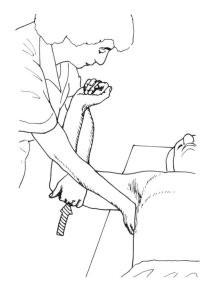

FIGURE 4–7. Hand placement and stabilization of the scapula for stretching procedure to increase shoulder abduction.

e. **To increase external rotation of the shoulder** (to stretch the internal rotators) (Figure 4-8)
   (1) Hand placement
       Abduct the shoulder to 90 degrees and flex the elbow to 90 degrees. Grasp the distal forearm.
   (2) Stabilization of the scapula will be provided by the table upon which the patient is lying.
   (3) Externally rotate the patient's shoulder by moving the patient's forearm closer to the table. This will fully lengthen the internal rotators.
   Note: It is necessary to apply the stretch forces across the intermediate elbow joint when elongating the internal and external rotators of the shoulder. Therefore, be sure the elbow joint is stable and pain free.
f. **To increase internal rotation of the shoulder** (to stretch the external rotators) (Figure 4-9)
   (1) Hand placement
       Same as when increasing external rotation of the shoulder
   (2) Stabilize the anterior aspect of the shoulder.
   (3) Move the patient into internal rotation to lengthen the external rotators of the shoulder.
g. **To increase horizontal abduction of the shoulder** (to stretch the pectoralis muscles)
   (1) Alternate position
       To reach full horizontal abduction in supine position, the patient's shoulder must be at the edge of the table. As with passive ROM (see Figure 2-5A), begin with the shoulder in 90 degrees of abduction; the patient's elbow may also be flexed.
   (2) Hand placement
       Grasp the anterior aspect of the distal humerus.
   (3) Stabilize the anterior aspect of the shoulder.
   (4) Move the patient's arm into full horizontal abduction to stretch the horizontal adductors.

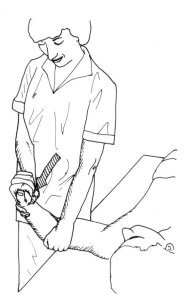

FIGURE 4–8. Hand placement and stabilization of the shoulder for stretching procedure to increase external rotation of the shoulder.

Note: The horizontal adductors are usually tight bilaterally. Stretching techniques can be applied bilaterally by the therapist, or a bilateral self-stretch can be done by the patient with doorframe exercises (see Chapter 14, Figures 14-5 and 14-6).

h. **Scapular Mobilization**
   (1) In order to have full shoulder motion, a patient must have normal scapular mobility.
   (2) See scapular mobilization techniques in Chapter 5.

2. **Elbow and forearm—Special considerations**

   Several muscles that cross the elbow, such as the biceps brachii and brachioradialis, also influence supination and pronation of the forearm. Therefore, when stretching the elbow flexors and extensors, the forearm should be pronated and supinated.

   Precaution: Vigorous stretching of the elbow flexors may cause internal trauma to these muscles. This may precipitate myositis ossificans, especially in children. Passive stretching should be done gently, or the use of active inhibition techniques should be considered.

   a. **To increase elbow flexion** (to stretch the elbow extensors) (see Figure 2-7).
      (1) Hand placement
          Grasp the distal forearm just proximal to the wrist.
      (2) Stabilize the humerus.
      (3) Flex the patient's elbow just past the point of tightness to lengthen the elbow extensors.

   b. **To increase elbow extension** (to stretch the elbow flexors) (Figure 4-10).
      (1) Hand placement
          Grasp the distal forearm.

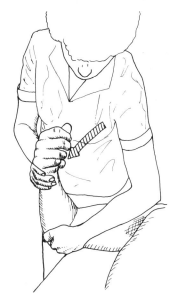

FIGURE 4–9. Hand placement and stabilization of the shoulder to increase internal rotation of the shoulder.

    (2) Stabilize the anterior aspect of the proximal humerus.
    (3) Extend the elbow as far as possible to lengthen the elbow flexors.
    Note: Be sure to do this with the forearm in supination, pronation, and a neutral position to stretch each of the elbow flexors.
  c. **To increase supination or pronation of the forearm** (see Figure 2-10)
    (1) Hand placement
        With the patient's humerus supported on the table and the elbow flexed to 90 degrees, grasp the distal forearm.
    (2) Stabilize the humerus.
    (3) Supinate or pronate the forearm just beyond the point of tightness as indicated. Be sure the force is applied to the radius rotating around the ulna. Do not twist the hand.
    (4) Repeat the procedure with the elbow extended. Be sure to stabilize the humerus to prevent internal or external rotation of the shoulder.

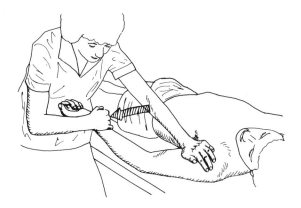

FIGURE 4–10. Hand placement and stabilization of the humerus for stretching procedure to increase elbow extension.

3. The wrist—Special considerations

The extrinsic muscles of the fingers cross the wrist joint and therefore may influence the range of motion of the wrist.

When stretching the musculature of the wrist, the stretch force should be applied proximal to the metacarpophalangeal (MCP) joints, and the fingers should be relaxed.

Alternate position

It may be easier to have the patient sitting in a chair adjacent to the therapist, with the forearm supported on the table, rather than lying supine.

a. **To increase wrist flexion** (see Figure 2-11)

  (1) Hand placement

    Supinate the forearm and grasp the patient at the dorsal aspect of the hand.

  (2) Stabilize the forearm.

  (3) To elongate the wrist extensors, flex the patient's wrist and allow the fingers to extend passively.

  (4) Alternate position

    The patient's forearm may also be in mid-position and supported along the ulna.

b. **To increase wrist extension** (Figure 4-11)

  (1) Hand placement

    Pronate the forearm and grasp the patient at the palmar aspect of the hand.

  (2) Stabilize the forearm.

  (3) To lengthen the wrist flexors, extend the patient's wrist, allowing the fingers to passively flex.

  (4) Alternate position

    Support the patient's forearm on the table but allow the hand to drop over the edge of the table. Then passively extend the wrist. This may be more comfortable for the therapist or necessary if the patient has a severe wrist flexion contracture.

  (5) Alternate position

    The patient's forearm may also be in mid-position and supported along the ulna.

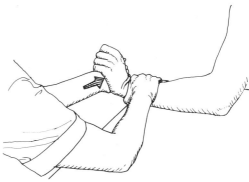

FIGURE 4–11. Hand placement and stabilization of the forearm for stretching procedure to increase extension of the wrist.

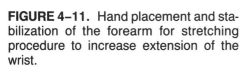

c. **To increase radial deviation**
   (1) Hand placement
      Grasp the ulnar aspect of the hand, along the fifth metacarpal. Hold the wrist in mid-position.
   (2) Stabilize the forearm.
   (3) Radially deviate the wrist to lengthen the ulnar deviators of the wrist.
d. **To increase ulnar deviation**
   (1) Hand placement
      Grasp the radial aspect of the hand along the second metacarpal, not the thumb.
   (2) Stabilize the forearm.
   (3) Ulnarly deviate the wrist to lengthen the radial deviators.

4. **The fingers—Special considerations**
   The complexity of joints and multi-joint muscles of the fingers requires careful evaluation of what is limiting motion and specifically where the motion is limited. Fingers should always be stretched individually, not grossly stretched.

   If an extrinsic muscle limits motion, lengthen it over one joint while stabilizing the other joints. Then lengthen it over two joints simultaneously, and so forth, until normal length is obtained. As noted in Chapter 2, begin the motion with the most distal joint in order to minimize joint compression of the small joints of the fingers.

   Do not produce hypermobility in one joint while stretching a tendon across two more joints simultaneously. This is particularly important at the MCP joints when stretching the flexor digitorum profundus.

   The web space between the first and second metacarpals is crucial for a functional hand. Stretch this area by applying force to the heads of the first and second metacarpals, not the phalanges.
   a. **To increase flexion and extension and abduction and adduction of the MCP joints** (see Figure 2-13A)
      (1) Hand placement
         Grasp the proximal phalanx with your thumb and index finger.
      (2) Stabilize the metacarpal with your other thumb and index finger. Keep the wrist in mid-position.
      (3) Move the MCP joint in the desired direction for stretch. Allow the PIP and DIP joints to passively flex or extend.
   b. **To increase flexion and extension of the PIP and DIP joints** (see Figure 2-13B)
      (1) Hand placement
         Grasp the middle or distal phalanx with your thumb and finger.
      (2) Stabilize the proximal or middle phalanx with your other thumb and finger.
      (3) Move the PIP or DIP joint in the desired direction for stretch.
   c. **Stretching specific extrinsic and intrinsic muscles of the fingers.**
      In Chapter 2 (section VI, A 13) elongation of extrinsic and intrinsic muscles of the hand was described. In order to stretch these muscles beyond their available range, the same hand placement and stabilization is used as with passive ROM. The only difference in technique is that the therapist moves the patient beyond the point of tightness.

B. The Lower Extremity

1. The hip—Special considerations

Since muscles of the hip attach to the pelvis or lumbar spine, the pelvis must always be stabilized when lengthening muscles about the hip. If the pelvis is not stabilized, the stretch force will be transferred to the lumbar spine where unwanted compensatory motion will occur.

a. **To increase flexion of the hip with the knee flexed** (to stretch the gluteus maximus) (see Figure 2-15B)

    (1) Hand placement

        Flex the hip and knee simultaneously.

    (2) Stabilize the opposite femur in extension to prevent a posterior tilt of the pelvis.

    (3) Move the patient's hip and knee into full flexion to lengthen the one-joint hip extensor.

b. **To increase flexion of the hip with the knee extended** (to stretch the hamstrings (Figure 4-12A)

    (1) Hand placement

        With the patient's knee fully extended, support the patient's lower leg with your arm or shoulder.

    (2) Stabilize the opposite extremity along the anterior aspect of the thigh with your other hand or a belt or with the assistance of another person.

    (3) With the knee in maximum extension, flex the hip as far as possible.

    (4) Alternate position (Figure 4-12B)

        (a) The therapist may kneel on the mat, place the patient's heel against her shoulder, and place both hands along the anterior aspect of the distal femur to keep the knee extended.

        (b) The opposite extremity is stabilized in extension by a belt or towel and held in place by the therapist's knee.

c. **To increase hip extension** (to stretch the iliopsoas) (Figure 4-13)

    (1) Stabilize the pelvis by flexing the opposite hip and knee to the pa-

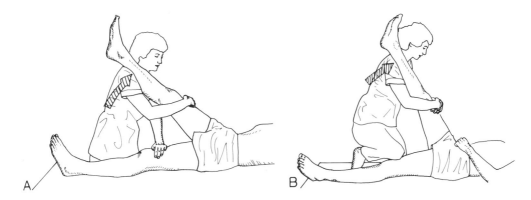

FIGURE 4–12. (*A* and *B*), Hand placement and stabilization of the pelvis and low back for stretching procedures to increase hip flexion with knee extension (stretch the hamstrings).

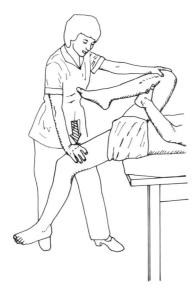

FIGURE 4–13. Hand placement and stabilization of the pelvis to increase hyperextension of the hip (stretch the iliopsoas) with the patient lying supine.

tient's chest. Maintain that position to prevent an anterior tilt of the pelvis during stretching.
(2) Hand placement and position of patient
    (a) Have the patient close to the edge of the bed so that the hip being stretched can be hyperextended.
    (b) While stabilizing the opposite hip and pelvis with one hand, move the hip to be stretched into extension or hyperextension by placing a downward pressure on the anterior aspect of the distal femur with your other hand.
(3) Alternate position
    Patient lying prone (Figure 4-14)
    (a) Hand placement
    Support and grasp the anterior aspect of the patient's distal femur.
    (b) Stabilize the patient's buttocks to prevent movement of the pelvis.
    (c) Hyperextend the patient's hip by lifting the femur off the table.
d. **To increase hip extension and knee flexion simultaneously** (to stretch the rectus femoris)
    (1) Position of patient (see Figure 4-13)
    Flex the opposite hip and knee to the patient's chest to stabilize the pelvis.
    (2) Hand placement
    With the hip to be stretched in full extension, place your hand on the distal tibia and gently flex the knee of that extremity as far as possible.
e. **To increase abduction of the hip** (to stretch the adductors) (Figure 4-15)
    (1) Hand placement
    Support the distal thigh with your arm and forearm.

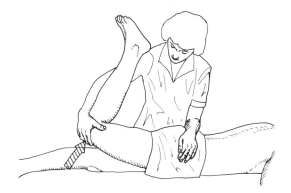

FIGURE 4–14. Hand placement and stabilization to increase hyperextension of the hip with the patient lying prone.

(2) Stabilize the pelvis by placing pressure on the opposite anterior iliac crest or by maintaining the opposite lower extremity in slight abduction.

(3) Abduct the hip as far as possible to stretch the adductors.

Note: You may apply your stretch force cautiously at the medial malleolus only if the knee is stable and pain free. This creates a great deal of stress to the medial supporting structures of the knee and is generally not recommended by us.

f. **To increase adduction of the hip** (to stretch the iliotibial band)

(1) Alternate position (Figure 4-16)

Place the patient in a side-lying position with the hip to be stretched uppermost. Flex the bottom hip and knee to stabilize the patient.

(2) Hand placement

Extend the patient's hip to neutral or into slight hyperextension, if possible. Place your hand on the lateral aspect of the distal femur.

(3) Stabilize the pelvis at the iliac crest with your other hand.

(4) Let the patient's hip adduct with gravity and apply the stretch force to the lateral aspect of the distal femur to further adduct the hip.

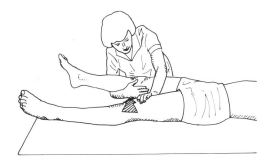

FIGURE 4–15. Hand placement and stabilization of the opposite extremity and pelvis for stretching procedure to increase abduction of the hip.

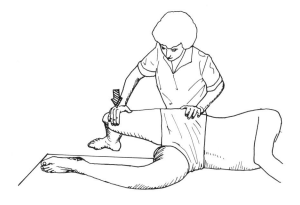

FIGURE 4–16. Patient positioned side-lying. Hand placement and procedure to stretch the iliotibial band.

g. **To increase external rotation of the hip** (to stretch the internal rotators)
   (1) Alternate position (Figure 4-17A)
       Place the patient in a prone position, hips extended and knee flexed to 90 degrees.
   (2) Hand placement
       Grasp the distal tibia of the extremity to be stretched.
   (3) Stabilize the pelvis by applying pressure with your other hand across the buttocks.
   (4) Apply pressure to the lateral malleolus and externally rotate the hip as far as possible.
   Note: You must apply your stretch force at the ankle, thus crossing the knee joint. If you stretch the hip rotators in this manner, the knee must be stable and pain free.
h. **To increase internal rotation of the hip** (to stretch the external rotators)
   (1) Alternate position and stabilization (Figure 4-17B)
       Same as when increasing external rotation described above.
   (2) Hand placement
       Apply pressure to the medial malleolus and internally rotate the hip as far as possible.

2. **The knee—Special considerations**
   The position of the hip during stretching will influence the flexibility of the flexors and extensors of the knee. The flexibility of the hamstrings and the rectus femoris must be evaluated separately from the one-joint muscles that affect knee motion.
   a. **To increase knee flexion** (to stretch the knee extensors)
      (1) Alternate position
          Patient lying prone (Figure 4-18)
          (a) Stabilize the pelvis by applying a downward pressure across the buttocks.
          (b) Hand placement
              Grasp the anterior aspect of the distal tibia and flex the patient's knee.

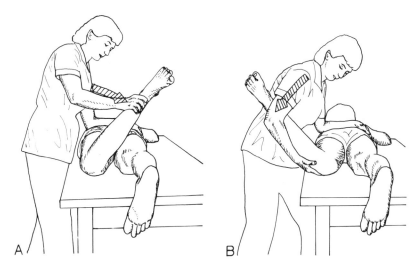

FIGURE 4–17. (*A* and *B*) Hand placement and stabilization to increase external and internal rotation of the hip with the patient prone.

Note: Place a rolled towel under the thigh just above the knee to prevent compression of the patella against the table during the stretch.

Precaution: Stretching the knee extensors too vigorously in the prone position can traumatize the knee joint and cause edema.

(2) Alternate position
  (a) Have the patient sit over the edge of a table (hips flexed to 90 degrees and knee flexed as far as possible).
  (b) Stabilize the anterior aspect of the proximal femur with one hand.
  (c) Apply the stretch force to the anterior aspect of the distal tibia and flex the patient's knee as far as possible.

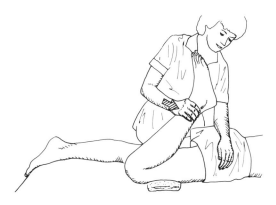

FIGURE 4–18. Hand placement and stabilization to increase knee flexion (stretch the rectus femoris and quadriceps) with the patient lying prone.

Note:
   i. This position is useful when working in the 0- to 100-degree range of knee flexion.
   ii. The prone position is best for increasing knee flexion from 90 to 135 degrees.
b. **To increase knee extension in the mid-range** (to stretch the knee flexors)
   (1) Alternate position (Figure 4-19)
       Place the patient in a prone position and put a small rolled towel under the patient's distal femur, just above the patella.
   (2) Hand placement and stabilization
       Grasp the distal tibia with one hand and stabilize the buttocks to prevent hip flexion with the other hand. Slowly extend the knee to stretch the knee flexors.
c. **To increase knee extension at the end of the range** (Figure 4-20)
   (1) Hand placement
       Grasp the distal tibia of the knee to be stretched.
   (2) Stabilize the hip by placing your hand or forearm across the anterior thigh. This will prevent hip flexion during stretching.
   (3) Apply the stretch force to the posterior aspect of the distal tibia and extend the patient's knee.

3. **The ankle—Special considerations**
   The ankle is composed of multiple joints. Consider the mobility of these joints (see Chapter 5) was well as the soft tissues around these joints when increasing range of motion of the ankle.
   a. **To increase dorsiflexion of the ankle with the knee extended** (to stretch the gastrocnemius muscle) (see Figure 2-20)
      (1) Hand placement
          Grasp the patient's heel (calcaneus) with one hand.
      (2) Stabilize the anterior aspect of the tibia with your other hand.
      (3) Pull the calcaneus downward with your thumb and fingers and gently push upward on the heads of the metatarsals.

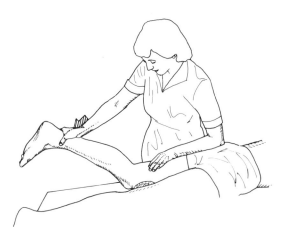

FIGURE 4–19. Hand placement and stabilization to increase mid-range knee extension with the patient lying prone.

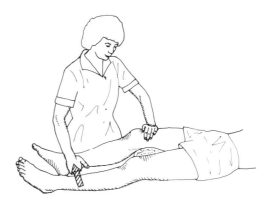

FIGURE 4–20. Hand placement and stabilization to increase knee extension at the end of the range.

 b. **To increase dorsiflexion of the ankle with the knee flexed** (to stretch the soleus muscle)
  (1) In order to eliminate the effect of the two-joint gastrocnemius muscle, the knee must be flexed.
  (2) Hand placement, stabilization, and stretch force are the same as when stretching the gastrocnemius.
   Precaution: Avoid placing too much pressure against the heads of the metatarsals and stretching the long arch of the foot. Overstretching the long arch of the foot can cause a rocker-bottom foot.
 c. **To increase plantarflexion of the ankle**
  (1) Hand placement:
   (a) Support the posterior aspect of the distal tibia with one hand.
   (b) Grasp the foot along the tarsal and metatarsal areas.
  (2) Apply the stretch force to the anterior aspect of the foot and plantarflex the foot as far as possible.
 d. **To increase inversion and eversion of the ankle**
  Inversion and eversion of the ankle occur at the subtalar joint. Mobility of the subtalar joint (with appropriate strength) is important for walking on uneven surfaces.
  (1) To increase motion in this joint, grasp the calcaneus and move it medially and laterally while stabilizing the talus (see Figure 2-21A and B)
  (2) To stretch the tibialis anterior (which inverts and dorsiflexes the ankle)
   (a) Grasp the anterior aspect of the foot.
   (b) Plantarflex and evert the ankle.
  (3) To stretch the tibialis posterior (which plantarflexes and inverts the foot)
   (a) Grasp the plantar surface of the foot.
   (b) Dorsiflex and evert the foot.
  (4) To stretch the peroneals (which evert the foot)
   (a) Grasp the tarsal region of the foot.
   (b) Invert the foot.
 e. **To increase flexion and extension of the toes** (see Figure 2-23).
 Note: It is best to individually stretch any tight musculature that effects

motion in the toes. With one hand stabilize the bone proximal to the tight joint, and with the other hand move the joint in the desired direction.

C. The Trunk

Stretching techniques to increase motion in the cervical, thoracic, and lumbar spine can be found in Chapters 14 through 17.

IX. SUMMARY

This chapter has provided an overview of background, principles, and procedures for the application of stretching techniques. Causes of soft tissue contractures related to immobilization, trauma, and disease and the changes that occur in muscle and connective tissue when immobilized were reviewed.

The mechanical and neurophysiologic properties of contractile and noncontractile tissues were described. The response of these tissues to stretching procedures were also discussed. Indications and goals for stretching as well as precautions and contraindications were reviewed.

Various methods of active inhibition and passive stretching were explained. Procedures and techniques of relaxation, active inhibition, and passive stretching were covered in detail. Emphasis was placed on positioning of patient, stabilization of joints, and placement of the therapist's hand. Finally, precautions for stretching were discussed.

REFERENCES

1. Agre, JC: *Static stretching for athletes.* Arch Phys Med Rehabil 59:561, 1978.
2. Astrand, PO and Rodahl, K: *Textbook of Work Physiology,* ed 2. McGraw-Hill, New York, 1977.
3. Basmajian, JV (ed): *Therapeutic Exercise,* ed 3. Williams & Wilkins, Baltimore, 1978.
4. Beard, G and Wood, E: *Massage: Principles and Techniques.* WB Saunders, Philadelphia, 1964.
5. Beaulieu, JA: *Developing a stretching program.* Physician Sports Med 9:59, 1981.
6. Becker, RO: *The electrical response of human skeletal muscle to passive stretch.* Surg Forum 10:828, 1960.
7. Benson, H, Beary, JF, and Carol, MP: *The relaxation response.* Psychiatry 37:37, 1974.
8. Bohannon, RW: *Effect of repeated eight minute muscle loading on the angle of straight leg raising.* Phys Ther 64:491, 1984.
9. Bohannon, RW and Larkin, PA: *Passive ankle dorsiflexion increases in patients after a regimen of tilt table–wedge board standing.* Phys Ther 65:1676, 1985.
10. Cherry, D: *Review of physical therapy alternatives for reducing muscle contracture.* Phys Ther 60:877, 1980.
11. Condon, SN and Hutton, RS: *Soleus muscle electromyographic activity and ankle dorsiflexion range of motion during four stretching procedures.* Phys Ther 67:24, 1987.
12. Cornwall, M: *Biomechanics of noncontractile tissue: A review.* Phys Ther 64:1869, 1984.
13. Cummings, GS, Crutchfeld, CA, and Barnes, MR: *Soft Tissue Changes in Contractures, Vol. 1.* Stokesville Publishing, Atlanta, 1983.
14. Donatelli, R and Owens-Burkhart, H: *Effects of immobilization on the extensibility of periarticular connective tissue.* J Orthop Sports Phys Ther 3:67, 1981.
15. Downey, J and Darling, R (eds): *Physiological Basis of Rehabilitation Medicine.* WB Saunders, Philadelphia, 1971.
16. Eldred, E, Hulton, RS, and Smith, JL: *Nature of persisting changes in afferent discharge from muscle following its contraction.* Prog Brain Res 44:157, 1976.
17. Etnyre, BR and Abraham, LD: *Gains in range of ankle dorsiflexion using three popular stretching techniques.* Am J Phys Med 65:189, 1986.
18. Evjenth, O and Hamberg, J: *Muscle Stretching in Manual Therapy—A Clinical Manual, Vol 1.* Alfta, Rehab, Alfta, Sweden, 1984.

19. Flitney, FW and Hirst, DG: *Cross bridge detachment and sarcomere "give" during stretch of active frog's muscle.* J Physiol 276:449, 1978.
20. Fox, E and Matthews, D: *The Physiological Basis of Physical Education and Athletics.* Saunders College Publishing, Philadelphia, 1981.
21. Gossman, M, Sahrmann, S, and Rose, S: *Review of length-associated changes in muscle.* Phys Ther 62:1799, 1982.
22. Griffiths, PJ, Goth, K, Kuhn, HJ, et al: *Cross bridge slippage in skinned frog muscle fibers.* Biophys Struct Mech 7:107, 1980.
23. Hallum, A and Medeiros, JM: *Effect of duration of passive stretch on hip abduction range of motion.* J Orthop Sports Phys Ther 18:409, 1987.
24. Hepburn, G and Crivelli, K: *Use of elbow Dynasplint for reduction of elbow flexion contracture: A case study.* J Orthop Sports Phys Ther 5:269, 1984.
25. Hlasney, J: *Effect of flexibility exercises on muscle strength.* Phys Ther Forum 7:3, 15, 1988.
26. Hollis, M: *Practical Exercise Therapy,* ed 2. Blackwell Scientific Publications, Oxford, 1982.
27. Jacobson, E: *Progressive Relaxation.* University of Chicago Press, Chicago, 1929.
28. Kendall, F and McCreary, E: *Muscles: Testing and Function,* ed 3. Williams & Wilkins, Baltimore, 1983.
29. Kendall, H and Kendall, F: *Posture and Pain.* Williams & Wilkins, Baltimore, 1952.
30. Kessler, R and Hertling, D: *Management of Common Musculoskeletal Disorders.* Harper & Row, Philadelphia, 1983.
31. Kottke, F: *Therapeutic exercise.* In Krusen, F, Kottke, F, and Ellwood, M: *Handbook of Physical Medicine and Rehabilitation,* ed 2. WB Saunders, Philadelphia, 1971.
32. Kottke, FJ, Pauley, DL, and Park, KA: *The rationale for prolonged stretching for correction of shortening of connective tissue.* Arch Phys Med Rehabil 47:345, 1966.
33. Lehmann, JF, Masock, AJ, et al: *The effect of therapeutic temperatures on tendon extensibility.* Arch Phys Med Rehabil 51:481, 1970.
34. Leveau, B: *Basic biomechanics in sports and orthopedic therapy.* In Gould, J and Davies, G: *Orthopedic and Sports Physical Therapy.* CV Mosby, St Louis, 1985.
35. Levine, HG, Kabat, H, Knott, M, et al: *Relaxation of spasticity by physiological techniques.* Arch Phys Med 45:214, 1964.
36. Light, KE, Nuzik, S, Personius, W, and Barstrom, A: *Low-load prolonged stretch vs. high-load brief stretch in treating knee contractures.* Phys Ther 64:330, 1984.
37. Madding, SW, Wong, JG, Hallum, A, and Medeiros, JM: *Effects of duration of passive stretch on hip abduction range of motion.* J Orthop Sports Phys Ther 8:409, 1987.
38. Medeiros, J, Smidt, G, Burmeister, L, et al: *The influence of isometric exercise and passive stretch on hip joint motion.* Phys Ther 57:510, 1977.
39. Moore, MA and Hutton, R: *Electromyographic investigation of muscle stretching techniques.* Med Sci Sports Exer 12:322, 1980.
40. Nicholas, JA: *Injuries to knee ligaments: relationships to looseness and tightness in football players.* JAMA 212:2236, 1970.
41. Noyes, FR, Tarvik, TJ, Hyde, WB, and DeLucas, JL: *Biomechanics of ligament failure.* J Bone Joint Surg 56A:1406, 1974.
42. Noyes, FR: *Functional properties of knee ligaments and alterations induced by immobilization.* Clin Orthop Rel Res 123:210, 1977.
43. Noyes, FR, Keller, CS, Grood, ES, and Butler, DL: *Advances in understanding of knee ligament injury, repair and rehabilitation.* Med Sci Sports Exerc 16:427, 1984.
44. Sady, SP, Wortman, M, and Blanke, D: *Flexibility training: ballistic, static or proprioceptive neuromuscular facilitation.* Arch Phys Med Rehabil 63:261, 1982.
45. Sapega, A, Quedenfeld, T, Moyer, R, et al: *Biophysical factors in range of motion exercises.* Physician Sports Med 9:57, 1981.
46. Schultz, JH and Luthe, W: *Autogenic Training: A Psychophysiologic Approach in Psychotherapy.* Grune & Stratton, New York, 1959.
47. Starring, DT, et al: *Comparison of cyclic and sustained passive stretching using a mechanical device to increase resting length of hamstring muscles.* Phys Ther 68:314, 1988.
48. Sussman, M and Cusick, B: *Preliminary report: The role of short-leg tone-reducing casts as an adjunct to physical therapy for patients with cerebral palsy.* Johns Hopkins Med J 145:112, 1979.

49. Tabary, JC, et al: *Physiological and structural changes in the cat soleus muscle due to immobilization at different lengths by plaster casts.* J Physiol (Lond) 224:231, 1972.
50. Tannigawa, M: *Comparison of the hold-relax procedure and passive mobilization on increasing muscle length.* Phys Ther 52:725, 1972.
51. Tardieu, C, et al: *Adaptation of connective tissue length to immobilization in the lengthened and shortened position in cat soleus muscle.* J Physiol (Paris) 78:214, 1982.
52. Trombly, CA: *Occupational Therapy for Physical Dysfunction,* ed 2. Williams & Wilkins, Baltimore, 1983.
53. Van Beveren, PS: *Effects of muscle stretching program on muscle strength.* Empire State Phys Ther 20:5, 1979.
54. Voss, DE, Ionla, MK, and Myers, BJ: *Proprioceptive Neuromuscular Facilitation,* ed 3. Harper & Row Publishers, Philadelphia, 1985.
55. Walker, SM: *Delay of twitch relaxation induced by stress and stress relaxation.* J Appl Physiol 16:801, 1961.
56. Warren, CG, Lehmann, JF, and Koblanski, JN: *Heat and stretch procedures: An evaluation using rat tail tendon.* Arch Phys Med Rehabil 57:122, 1976.
57. Warren, CG, Lehmann, JF, and Koblanski, JN: *Elongation of rat tail tendon: effect of load and temperature.* Arch Phys Med Rehabil 51:481, 1970.
58. Wessling, KC, Derane, DA, and Hylton, CR: *Effect of static stretch vs. static stretch and ultrasound combined on triceps surae muscle extensibility in healthy women.* Phys Ther 67:674, 1987.
59. Wiliams, PR and Goldspink, G: *Changes in sarcomere length and physiological properties in immobilized muscle.* J Anat 127:459, 1978.
60. Wolpe, J: *Psychotherapy by Reciprocal Inhibition.* Stanford University Press, Stanford, 1958.
61. Zarins, B: *Soft tissue injury and repair—biomechanical aspects.* Int J Sports Med 3:9, 1982.

CHAPTER ——————————— 5

Peripheral Joint Mobilization

Historically, when a patient has had limited range of motion, the therapeutic approach was to stretch the region with passive stretching techniques (see Chapter 4). Over the past 30 years, therapists have identified and learned techniques that deal more directly with stretching the *source* of the limitation, and thus they are managing dysfunctions better and with less trauma. Muscle elongation or active inhibition techniques are used to counteract loss of elasticity in contractile structures (see Chapter 4); cross-fiber massage techniques are used to increase mobility in selected ligaments and tendons; and joint mobilization and manipulation techniques are used to safely stretch or snap structures to restore normal joint mechanics with less trauma than passive stretching.

Joint mobilization refers to techniques that are used to treat joint dysfunction such as when there is stiffness, reversible joint hypomobility, or pain.[8] Currently there are several schools of thought and treatment techniques that are popular in the United States, and leading practitioners and educators are attempting to blend common points to yield more uniform treatment from the various approaches.[2,9]

In order to effectively use joint mobilization for treatment, the practitioner must know and be able to evaluate the anatomy, arthrokinematics, and pathology of the neuromusculoskeletal system[8] and to recognize when the techniques are indicated or when other stretching techniques would be more effective for regaining lost motion. Indiscriminate use of joint mobilization techniques when not indicated could lead to potential harm to the patient's joints.

The importance of evaluation skills and of the ability to identify the various structures that can cause decreased range of motion and pain underlies the presentation of material in this chapter. We assume that, prior to learning the joint mobilization techniques presented here, the student or therapist will have had (or will be concurrently taking) a course in orthopedic evaluation and therefore is able to choose appropriate, safe techniques for treating the patient's functional limitation. (See evaluation outline in Chapter 1 and guidelines in Chapter 6.) The reader is referred to several resources for additional study of evaluation procedures.[2,3,7,8,9,11,19,20]

When indicated, joint mobilization is a safe and effective means of restoring or maintaining joint play within a joint and can also be used for treating pain.[8,10,13]

OBJECTIVES

After studying this chapter, the reader will be able to:
1. define terminology of joint mobilization.
2. summarize basic concepts of joint motion.
3. identify indications and goals for joint mobilization.
4. identify limitations of joint mobilization.
5. identify contraindications for joint mobilization.
6. describe procedures for applying joint mobilization.
7. apply basic techniques of joint mobilization to the extremity joints.

I. DEFINITIONS OF JOINT MOBILIZATION

A. Mobilization

A passive movement performed by the therapist at a speed slow enough that the patient can stop the movement. The technique may be applied with an oscillatory motion or a sustained stretch intended to decrease pain or increase mobility. The techniques may use physiologic movements or accessory movements.[8,11]

1. Physiologic movements

Movements that the patient can do voluntarily; for example, the classic or traditional movements such as flexion, abduction, and rotation. The term *osteokinematics* is used when these motions of the bones are described.

2. Accessory movements

Movements within the joint and surrounding tissues that are necessary for normal range of motion but that cannot be performed by the patient.[13] Terms that relate to *accessory movements* are *component motions* and joint play.
a. *Component motions* are those motions that accompany active motion but are not under voluntary control; the term is often used synonymously with accessory movement.[9] Motions such as upward rotation of the scapula and clavicle, which occur with shoulder flexion, are component motions.
b. *Joint play* describes the motions that occur in the joint and describes the distensibility or "give" in the joint capsule, which allows the bones to move. The movements are necessary for normal joint functioning through the range of motion and can be demonstrated passively, but they cannot be performed actively by the patient.[13] The movements include distractions, sliding, compression, rolling, and spinning of the joint surfaces (see Section II).[9] The term *arthrokinematics* is used when these motions of the bone surfaces within the joint are described.
Note: Procedures to distract or slide the joint surfaces in order to decrease pain or restore joint play are the fundamental joint mobilization techniques described in this text.

B. Manipulation

A passive movement using physiologic or accessory motions, which may be applied with a thrust or when the patient is under anesthesia.

1. Thrust

A sudden movement performed with a high-velocity, short-amplitude motion such that the patient cannot prevent the motion.[11,13] The motion is performed at the end of the pathologic limit of the joint and is intended to alter positional relationships, to snap adhesions, or to stimulate joint receptors.[13] Pathologic limit means the end of the available range of motion when there is restriction. THRUST TECHNIQUES ARE BEYOND THE SCOPE OF THIS TEXT.

2. Manipulation under anesthesia

A medical procedure used to restore full range of movement by breaking adhesions around a joint while the patient is anesthetized. The technique may be a rapid thrust or a passive stretch using physiologic or accessory movements.

II. BASIC CONCEPTS OF JOINT MOTION

A. Joint Shapes

The type of motion occurring between bony partners within a joint is influenced by the shapes of the joint surfaces. The shapes may be described as *ovoid* or *sellar*.[14]

1. Ovoid

One surface is convex; the other is concave (Figure 5-1A)

2. Sellar (Saddle)

One surface is concave in one direction and convex in the other, with the opposing surface convex and concave, respectively; similar to a horseback rider being in complementary opposition to the shape of a saddle (Figure 5-1B).

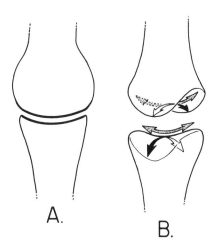

FIGURE 5–1. (*A*), With ovoid joints, one surface is convex and the other concave; (*B*), with sellar joints, one surface is concave in one direction and convex in the other, with the opposing surface convex and concave, respectively.

A.   B.

B. Types of Motion

As a bony lever moves about an axis of motion, there is also movement of the bone surface on the opposing bone surface within the joint.

1. The movement of the bony lever is called *swing* and is classically described as flexion, extension, abduction, adduction, and rotation. The amount of movement can be measured in degrees with a goniometer and is called range of motion.

2. Motion of the bone surfaces within the joint is a variable combination of *rolling, sliding,* or *spinning.*[8,9,12,15] These accessory motions allow for greater angulation of the bone as it swings. For the rolling, sliding, or spinning to occur, there must be adequate capsule laxity or joint play.

   a. *Roll*

   Characteristics of one bone rolling on another (Figure 5-2)

   (1) The surfaces are incongruent.

   (2) New points on one surface meet new points on the opposing surface.

   (3) Rolling results in angular motion of the bone.

   (4) Rolling is always in the same direction as the angulating bone motion (Figure 5-3A and B), whether the surface is convex or concave.

   (5) Rolling, if it occurs alone, causes compression of the surfaces on the side to which the bone is angulating and separation on the other side. Passive stretching using bone angulation alone may cause stressful compressive forces to portions of the joint surface, potentially leading to joint damage.

   (6) In normal functioning joints, pure rolling does not occur alone but in combination with joint sliding and spinning. Some muscles may function to cause the slide with normal active motion.

   b. *Slide*

   Characteristics of one bone sliding across another

   (1) For a pure slide, the surfaces must be congruent, either flat (Figure 5-4A) or curved (Figure 5-4B).

   (2) The same point on one surface comes into contact with new points on the opposing surface.

   (3) Pure sliding does not occur in joints, since the surfaces are not completely congruent.

   (4) The direction in which sliding occurs depends on whether the moving surface is concave or convex. Sliding is in the opposite direction of the angular movement of the bone if the moving joint surface is convex (Figure 5-5A). Sliding is in the same direction as the angular

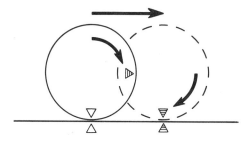

FIGURE 5–2. Diagrammatic representation of one surface rolling on another. New points on one surface meet new points on the opposing surface.

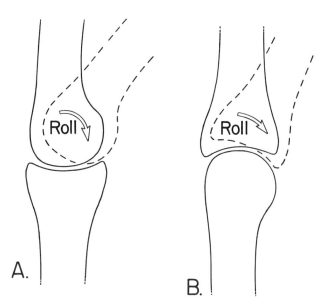

FIGURE 5–3. Rolling is always in the same direction as bone motion, whether the moving bone is convex (*A*) or concave (*B*).

movement of the bone if the moving surface is concave (Figure 5-5B).

Note: This mechanical relationship is known as the convex-concave rule and is the basis for determining the direction of the mobilizing force when joint mobilization gliding techniques are used.

c. *Combined roll-sliding in a joint*[8]
  (1) The more congruent the joint surfaces are, the more sliding there is of one bony partner on the other with movement.
  (2) The more incongruent the joint surfaces are, the more rolling there is of one bony partner on the other with movement.
  (3) For joint mobilization techniques, the sliding component of joint motion is used to restore joint play and reverse joint hypomobility. Rolling is not used since it causes joint compression.
  Note: When the therapist passively moves the articulating surface in the direction in which the slide normally occurs, the technique is

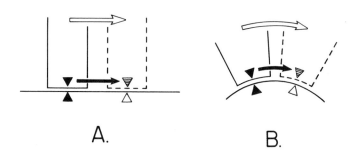

FIGURE 5–4. Diagrammatic representation of one surface sliding on another, whether flat (*A*) or curved (*B*). The same point on one surface comes into contact with new points on the opposing surface.

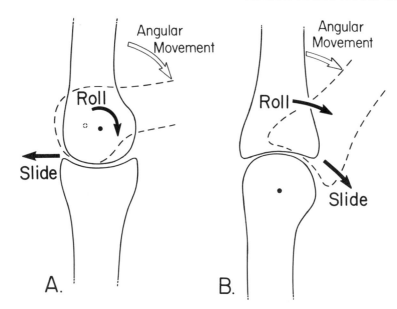

FIGURE 5–5. Diagrammatic representation of the concave-convex rule. (*A*), If the surface of the moving bone is convex, sliding is in the opposite direction of the angular movement of the bone. (*B*), If the surface of the moving bone is concave, sliding is in the same direction as the angular movement of the bone.

called translatoric glide, or glide.[8] It is used to control pain when applied gently or to stretch the capsule when applied with a stretch force.

   d. *Spin*

   Characteristics of one bone spinning on another

     (1) There is rotation of a segment about a stationary mechanical axis (Figure 5-6).

     (2) The same point on the moving surface creates an arc of a circle as the bone spins.

     (3) Spinning rarely occurs alone in joints but in combination with rolling and sliding.

     (4) Three examples of where spin occurs in joints of the body are the shoulder with flexion/extension, the hip with flexion/extension, and the radiohumeral joint with pronation/supination (Figure 5-7).

C. Arc Stretching Versus Joint Glide Stretching[10]

   1. Passive range of motion exercises, or arc stretching procedures, when the bony lever is used to stretch a tight joint capsule, may cause increased pain or joint trauma because

     a. the use of a lever significantly magnifies the force at the joint.

     b. the force causes excessive joint compression in the direction of the rolling bone (see Figure 5-3).

     c. the roll without a slide does not replicate normal joint mechanics.

   2. Joint mobilization stretching procedures, when the translatoric slide com-

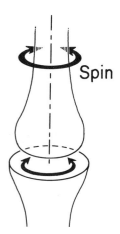

FIGURE 5–6. Diagrammatic representation of spinning. There is rotation of a segment about a stationary mechanical axis.

ponent of the bones is used to stretch a tight capsule, are safer and more selective because

 a. the force is applied close to the joint surface and controlled at an intensity compatible with the pathology.
 b. the direction of the force replicates the joint mechanics.
 c. the amplitude of the motion is small yet specific to the restricted portion of the capsule or ligaments, thus the forces are selectively applied to the desired tissue.

D. **Other Accessory Motions that Affect the Joint Include Compression and Traction**
   1. **Compression** is the decrease in the joint space between bony partners.
      a. Compression occurs in the lower extremity and spinal joints when weight bearing.

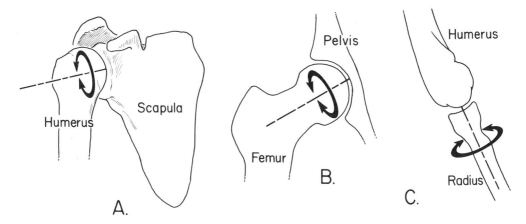

FIGURE 5–7. Examples of where joint spin occurs in the body: (*A*), humerus with flexion/extension; (*B*), femur with flexion/extension; and (*C*) head of the radius with pronation/supination.

     b. Some compression occurs as muscles contract; this provides stability to the joints.

     c. As one bone rolls on the other (see Figure 5-13) some compression also occurs on the side to which the bone is angulating.

     d. Normal intermittent compressive loads help move synovial fluid and thus help maintain cartilage health.

     e. Abnormally high compression loads may lead to articular cartilage changes and deterioration.[6]

  2. Traction is the distraction or separation of the joint surfaces.

     a. For distraction to occur within the joint, the surfaces must be pulled apart. The movement is not always the same as pulling on the long axis of one of the bony partners. For example, if traction is applied to the shaft of the humerus, it will result in a glide of the joint surface (Figure 5-8A). Distraction of the glenohumeral joint requires a pull at right angles to the glenoid fossa (Figure 5-8B).

     b. For clarity, whenever there is pulling on the long axis of a bone, the phrase *long-axis traction* will be used. Whenever the surfaces are to be pulled apart at right angles, the terms *distraction, joint traction,* or *joint separation* will be used.

     Note: For joint mobilization techniques, distraction is used to control or relieve pain when applied gently or to stretch the capsule when applied with a stretch force.

E. Effects of Joint Motion

  1. It stimulates biologic activity by moving synovial fluid, which brings nutrients to the avascular articular cartilage of the joint surfaces and intra-articular fibrocartilage of the menisci.[9] Atrophy of the articular cartilage begins soon after immobilization is imposed on joints.[1,4,5,6]

  2. It maintains extensibility and tensile strength of the articular and periarticular tissues. With immobilization there is fibrofatty proliferation, which causes intra-articular adhesions, as well as biochemical changes in tendon, ligament, and joint capsule tissue, which causes joint contractures and ligamentous weakening.[1]

  3. Afferent nerve impulses from joint receptors transmit information to the central nervous system and therefore provide for awareness of position and motion. With injury or degeneration of the capsule, there is a potential decrease in an important source of proprioceptive feedback. Joint motion

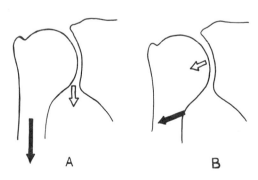

FIGURE 5–8. (*A*), Traction applied to the shaft of the humerus results in caudal gliding of the joint surface. (*B*), Distraction of the glenohumeral joint requires separation at right angles to the glenoid fossa.

provides sensory input relative to [16,17]

  a. static position and sense of speed of movement (type I receptors found in the superficial joint capsule).

  b. change of speed of movement (type II receptors found in deep layers of the joint capsule and articular fat pads).

  c. sense of direction of movement (type I and III receptors; type III found in joint ligaments).

  d. regulation of muscle tone (type I, II, and III receptors).

  e. nociceptive stimuli (type IV receptors found in the fibrous capsule, ligaments, articular fat pads, periosteum, and walls of blood vessels).

III. INDICATIONS FOR JOINT MOBILIZATION

A. Pain, Muscle Guarding, and Spasm

Painful joints, reflex muscle guarding, and muscle spasm can be treated with *gentle joint-play* techniques to stimulate neurophysiologic and mechanical effects.[6,9,11]

1. Neurophysiologic effects

Small-amplitude oscillatory movements are used to stimulate the mechanoreceptors that may inhibit the transmission of nociceptive stimuli at the spinal cord or brain stem levels.[9,13,15]

2. Mechanical effects

Small-amplitude distraction or gliding movements of the joint are used to cause synovial fluid motion, which is the vehicle for bringing nutrients to the avascular portions of the articular cartilage (and intra-articular fibrocartilage when present).[6,9] Gentle joint-play techniques help maintain nutrient exchange and thus prevent the painful and degenerating effects of stasis when a joint is swollen or painful and cannot move through a range of motion.

Note: The small-amplitude joint techniques used to treat pain, muscle guarding, or muscle spasm should not place a stretch on the reactive tissues (see Contraindications and Precautions under Section V).

B. Reversible Joint Hypomobility

Reversible joint hypomobility can be treated with *progressively vigorous joint-play stretching* techniques to elongate hypomobile structures. Sustained or oscillatory stretch forces are used to mechanically distend the shortened tissue.[8,9,11]

C. Progressive Limitation

Diseases that progressively limit movement can be treated with joint-play techniques to maintain available motion or retard progressive mechanical restrictions. The dosage of distraction or glide is dictated by the patient's response to treatment and the state of the disease.

D. Functional Immobility

When a patient cannot functionally move a joint for a period of time, the joint can be treated to maintain available joint play and prevent the degenerating and restricting effects of immobility. (See Section VI for descriptions of dosages.)

IV. LIMITATIONS OF JOINT MOBILIZATION TECHNIQUES

A. Mobilization techniques cannot change the disease process of disorders such as rheumatoid arthritis or the inflammatory process of injury. In these cases treatment is directed toward minimizing pain, maintaining available joint play, and reducing the effects of any mechanical limitations (see Chapter 6).

B. The skill of the therapist will affect the outcome. The techniques described in this text are relatively safe if directions are followed and precautions are heeded, but if these techniques are used indiscriminately on patients not properly evaluated and screened for such maneuvers, or if they are applied too vigorously for the condition, joint trauma or hypermobility may result.

V. CONTRAINDICATIONS AND PRECAUTIONS

A. The Only True Contraindications to Stretching Techniques are Hypermobility, Joint Effusion, and Inflammation[8]

1. **Hypermobility**
   a. Patients with potential necrosis of the ligaments or capsule should not be stretched.
   b. Patients with hypermobility may benefit from gentle joint play techniques (see Section III A) if kept within the limits of motion. Stretching is not done.

2. **Joint effusion**
   There may be joint swelling (effusion) from trauma or disease.
   a. Never stretch a swollen joint with mobilization or passive stretching techniques. The capsule is already on a stretch by being distended to accommodate the extra fluid. The limited motion is from the extra fluid and muscle response to pain, not from shortened fibers.
   b. Gentle oscillating motions that do not stress or stretch the capsule may help block the transmission of a pain stimulus so that it is not perceived and may also help improve fluid flow while maintaining available joint play (see Section III, A).
   c. If the patient's response to gentle techniques results in increased pain or joint irritability, the techniques were applied too vigorously or should not be done with the current state of pathology.

3. **Inflammation**
   Whenever inflammation is present, stretching will increase pain and muscle guarding and will result in greater tissue damage. See Chapter 6 for an appropriate approach to treatment when inflammation is present.

B. Conditions Requiring Special Precautions

In most cases, joint mobilization techniques are safer than passive angular stretching in which the bony lever is used to stretch tight tissue and joint compression results. Mobilization may be used with extreme care in the following conditions if signs and the patient's response are favorable.
1. Malignancy
2. Bone disease detectable on x-ray
3. Unhealed fracture (depends on the site of the fracture and stabilization provided)

4. Excessive pain (determine the cause of pain and modify treatment accordingly)
5. Hypermobility in associated joints (associated joints must be properly stabilized so the mobilization force is not transmitted to them)
6. Total joint replacements (the mechanism of the replacement is self-limiting, and therefore the mobilization gliding techniques may be inappropriate)

VI.   PROCEDURES FOR APPLYING JOINT MOBILIZATION TECHNIQUES

A. Evaluation and Assessment

If the patient has limited or painful motion, evaluate and assess what tissues are limiting function and the state of pathology (see Chapter 1). Determine whether treatment will be directed primarily toward relieving pain or stretching a joint or soft tissue limitation.[3,11]

1. The quality of pain helps determine the stage of recovery and the dosage of techniques used for treatment. (See Figures 6-2 and 6-3.)
   a. If pain is experienced before tissue limitation—such as the pain that occurs with muscle guarding following an acute injury or during the active stage of a disease—pain-inhibiting joint techniques may be used to relieve pain. The same techniques will also help maintain joint play. (See Section B, Grades or dosages of movement.) Stretching under these circumstances is contraindicated.
   b. If pain is experienced concurrently with tissue limitation—such as the pain and limitation that occur when damaged tissue begins to heal—the limitation is treated cautiously. Gentle stretching techniques specific to the tight structure are used in order to gradually improve movement yet not exacerbate the pain by reinjuring the tissue.
   c. If pain is experienced after tissue limitation is met because of stretching of tight capsular or periarticular tissue, the stiff joint can be aggressively stretched with joint-play techniques and the periarticular tissue with the stretching techniques described in Chapter 4.
2. The joint capsule is limiting motion and should respond to mobilization techniques if the following signs are present:
   a. The passive range of motion for that joint is limited in a capsular pattern. (These patterns are described for each peripheral joint under the respective sections on joint problems in Chapters 7 through 12).
   b. There is a firm capsular end feel when overpressure is applied to the tissues limiting the range.
   c. There is decreased joint play movement when mobility tests (articulations) are done.
3. An adhered or contracted ligament is limiting motion if there is decreased joint play and pain when the fibers of the ligament are stressed. Ligaments often respond to joint mobilization techniques if applied specific to their line of stress.
4. Subluxation or dislocation of one bony part on another and loose intra-articular structures that block normal motion may respond to joint manipulation or thrust techniques. Some of the simpler manipulations are described in appropriate sections in this text. Others require more advanced training and are beyond the scope of this book.

B. Grades or Dosages of Movement

Two systems of grading dosages for mobilization are used.

1. Graded oscillation techniques[11] (Figure 5-9)

a. Dosages

   (1) Grade I

   Small-amplitude rhythmic oscillations are performed at the beginning of the range.

   (2) Grade II

   Large-amplitude rhythmic oscillations are performed within the range, not reaching the limit.

   (3) Grade III

   Large-amplitude rhythmic oscillations are performed up to the limit of the available motion and stressed into the tissue resistance.

   (4) Grade IV

   Small-amplitude rhythmic oscillations are performed at the limit of the available motion and stressed into the tissue resistance.

   (5) Grade V

   A small-amplitude, high-velocity thrust technique is performed to snap adhesions at the limit of the available motion. Thrust techniques used for this purpose require advanced training and are beyond the scope of this book.

b. Uses

   (1) Grades I and II are primarily used for treating joints limited by pain. The oscillations may have an inhibitory effect on perception of painful stimuli by repetitively stimulating mechanoreceptors that block nociceptive pathways at the spinal cord or brain stem levels.[13,18] These nonstretch motions help move synovial fluid to improve nutrition to the cartilage.

   (2) Grades III and IV are primarily used as stretching maneuvers.

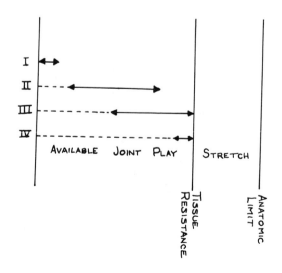

FIGURE 5–9. Diagrammatic representation of graded oscillation techniques. (Adapted from Maitland,[11] p. 29, with permission.)

c. Techniques

The oscillations may be done using physiologic (osteokinematic) motions or joint-play (arthrokinematic) techniques.

2. **Sustained translatory joint-play techniques[8] (Figure 5-10)**

a. Dosages

(1) Grade I (Loosen)

Small-amplitude distraction is applied where no stress is placed on the capsule. It equalizes cohesive forces, muscle tension, and atmospheric pressure acting on the joint.

(2) Grade II (Tighten)

Enough distraction or glide is applied to tighten the tissues around the joint. Kaltenborn[8] calls this "taking up the slack."

(3) Grade III (Stretch)

A distraction or glide is applied with an amplitude large enough to place a stretch on the joint capsule and on surrounding periarticular structures.

b. Uses

(1) Grade I distraction is used with all gliding motions and may be used for relief of pain.

(2) Grade II distraction is used for the initial treatment to determine how sensitive the joint is. Once joint reaction is known, the dosage of treatment is either increased or decreased accordingly.

(3) Grade III joint distraction or glides are used to stretch the joint structures and thus increase joint play.

c. Techniques

This grading system describes only joint-play techniques that separate (distract) or glide (slide) the joint surfaces.

3. **Comparison**

The only consistency between the dosages of the two grading systems is in Grade I in which no tension is placed on the joint capsule or surrounding tissue. Grade IV oscillation and Grade III sustained stretch techniques are

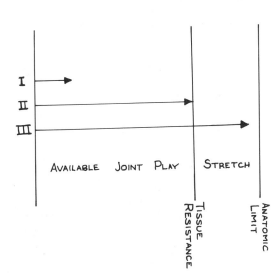

FIGURE 5–10. Diagrammatic representation of sustained translatory joint-play techniques. (Adapted from Kaltenborn, p. 25.[8])

similar in dosage in that they are applied with a stretch force at the limit of motion.

   a. For clarity and consistency, when referring to dosages in this text:

      (1) the notation *graded oscillations* means: use the dosages as described in the section on graded oscillation techniques.

      (2) the notation *sustained grade* means: use the dosages as described in the section on sustained translatory joint-play techniques.

   b. The choice of using oscillating or sustained techniques depends on the patient's response.

      (1) When dealing with pain management, oscillating techniques are recommended.

      (2) When dealing with loss of joint play and thus decreased functional range, sustained techniques are recommended.

      (3) When attempting to maintain available range by using joint-play techniques, either Grade II oscillating or sustained Grade II techniques can be used.

C. Patient Position

The patient and the extremity to be treated should be positioned so the patient can relax. Techniques of relaxation (see Chapter 4) may be appropriately used prior to or between stretching.

D. Joint Position

Evaluation of joint play and the first treatment are performed in the RESTING POSITION for that joint, that is, that position in which the capsule has greatest laxity. Maximum joint traction and joint play are available in that position (see Section H). In some cases, the position to use is the one in which the joint is least painful.

E. Stabilization

Firmly and comfortably stabilize one joint partner, usually the proximal bone. Stabilization may be provided by a belt, one of the therapist's hands, or an assistant holding the part.

F. Treatment Force

The treatment force (either gentle or strong) is applied as close to the opposing joint surface as possible. The larger the contact surface is, the more comfortable the procedure will be. For example, instead of forcing with your thumb, use the flat surface of your hand.

G. Direction of Movement

1. The direction of movement during treatment is either parallel to or perpendicular to the treatment plane. TREATMENT PLANE is described by Kaltenborn[8] as a plane perpendicular to a line running from the axis of rotation to the middle of the concave articular surface. The plane is in the concave partner so its position is determined by the position of the concave bone (Figure 5-11).

2. Joint traction techniques are applied perpendicular to the treatment plane. The entire bone is moved so that the joint surfaces are separated.

3. Gliding techniques are applied parallel to the treatment plane.

   a. Glide in the direction in which the slide would normally occur for the desired motion. Direction of sliding is easily determined by using the

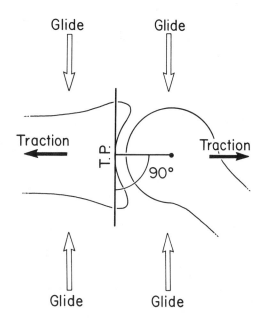

FIGURE 5–11. Treatment plane (T.P.) is at right angles to a line drawn from the axis of rotation to the center of the concave articulating surface and lies in the concave surface. Traction is applied perpendicular and glides are applied parallel to the treatment plane.

convex-concave rule (see Section II, B 2). If the surface of the moving bony partner is convex, the treatment glide should be opposite to the direction in which the bone swings. If the surface of the moving bony partner is concave, the treatment glide should be in the same direction (see Figure 5-5A and B).

    b. The entire bone is moved so that there is gliding of one joint surface on the other. There should be no arcing motion (swing) of the bone that would cause rolling and thus compression of the joint surfaces.

H. Initiation and Progression of Treatment (Table 5-1)

1. The initial treatment is the same whether treating for pain or increased joint play. The purpose is to determine joint reactivity before proceeding. Use a sustained Grade II distraction of the joint surfaces with the joint held in resting position or the position of greatest relaxation.[8] Note the immediate joint response relative to irritability and range.
2. The next day, evaluate joint response.
   a. If there is increased pain and sensitivity, reduce the amplitude of treatment to Grade I oscillations.
   b. If the joint is the same or better:
      (1) repeat the same maneuver if the goal of treatment is to maintain joint play
      (2) or progress the maneuver to sustained Grade III traction or glides if the goal of treatment is to increase joint play.
3. As the range plateaus, move the joint to the end of the available range of motion, then apply the sustained Grade III distraction or glide techniques. Advanced progressions include rotating the part at the end of the available range prior to applying Grade III distraction or glide techniques (not illustrated in this chapter).

TABLE 5–1. Initiation and Progression of Treatment

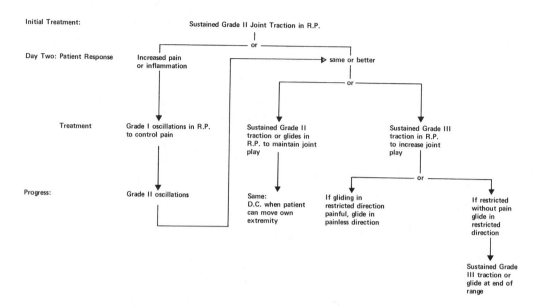

4. Hints[8]

a. Prepare the tissue around the joint prior to stretching with modalities, soft tissue mobilization, or muscle relaxation techniques.

b. When using sustained gliding techniques, a Grade I distraction should be used with it. A Grade II or III distraction should not be used with a Grade III glide in order to avoid excessive trauma to the joint.

c. If gliding in the restricted direction is too painful, begin gliding mobilizations in the painless direction. Progress to gliding in the restricted direction when mobility improves a little and it is not painful.

d. When applying stretching techniques, move the bony partner through the available range of joint play first, that is, "take up the slack;" when tissue resistance is felt, apply the stretch force against the restriction.

5. To maintain joint play by using gliding techniques when range of motion techniques are contraindicated or not possible for a period of time, use sustained Grade II or Grade II oscillation techniques.

I. Speed, Rhythm, and Duration of Movements

1. Oscillations[11]

a. Apply smooth, regular oscillations, at 2 or 3 per second, for 1 to 2 minutes.

b. Vary the speed of oscillations for different effects such as low-amplitude, high-speed to inhibit pain, or slow speed to relax muscle guarding.

2. Sustained[8]

a. For painful joints, apply intermittent distraction for 10 seconds with a few seconds of rest in between for several cycles. Note response and either repeat or discontinue.

b. For restricted joints apply a minimum of a 6-second stretch force, followed by partial release (to Grade I or II), then repeat at 3- to 4-second intervals.

J. Treatment Soreness

Stretching maneuvers usually cause soreness. Perform the maneuvers on alternate days in order to allow soreness to decrease and tissue healing to occur between stretching sessions. If there is increased pain after 24 hours, the dosage (amplitude) or duration of treatment was too vigorous. Decrease the dosage or duration until the pain is under control.

K. Reassessment

The patient's joint and range of motion should be reassessed after treatment and again before the next treatment. Alterations in treatment are dictated by the joint response.

L. Total Program

Mobilization techniques are one part of a total treatment for decreased function. Therapy should also include appropriate range of motion, strengthening, and functional techniques (see Chapters 7 through 12).

VII. PERIPHERAL JOINT MOBILIZATION TECHNIQUES

The following are suggested joint distraction and gliding techniques for use by entry level therapists and those attempting to gain a foundation in joint mobilization. A variety of adaptations can be made from these techniques. The distraction and glide techniques should be applied with respect to the dosage, frequency, progression, precautions, and procedures as described in the previous sections.

Note: Terms such as proximal hand, distal hand, or lateral hand, or other descriptive terms, indicate that the therapist should use the hand that is more proximal, distal, or lateral to the patient or the patient's extremity.

A. Shoulder Girdle Complex (Figure 5-12)

1. Glenohumeral joint. (concave glenoid fossa receives the convex humeral head)

RESTING POSITION

Shoulder abducted 55 degrees, horizontally adducted 30 degrees, and rotated so that the forearm is in the horizontal plane.

TREATMENT PLANE

In the glenoid fossa and moves with the scapula. (See definition in section VI G).

STABILIZATION

Fixate the scapula with a belt or have an assistant help.

a. **Joint traction** (distraction) (Figure 5-13)

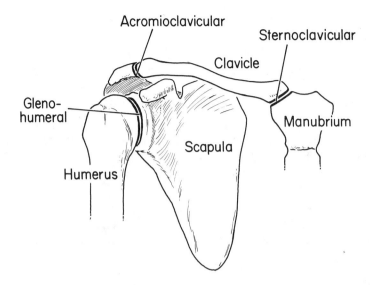

Acromioclavicular
Sternoclavicular
Clavicle
Gleno-
humeral
Manubrium
Scapula
Humerus

FIGURE 5–12. Bones and joints of the shoulder girdle complex.

INDICATIONS
Testing; initial treatment (sustained Grade II); pain control (Grade I or II oscillations); general mobility (sustained Grade III)

POSITION OF PATIENT
Supine, with arm in resting position; support the forearm between your trunk and elbow.

HAND PLACEMENT
Use the hand nearest the part being treated (for example right hand if treating the patient's right shoulder) and place it in the patient's axilla with your thumb just distal to the joint margin anteriorly and fingers posteriorly. Your other hand supports the humerus from the lateral surface.

MOBILIZING FORCE
With the hand in the axilla, move the humerus laterally.
Note: The entire arm moves in a translatoric motion away from the plane of the glenoid fossa. Distractions may be done with the humerus in any position (see Figures 5-16, 5-18, and 7-12). The therapist must be aware of the amount of scapular rotation and adjust the distraction force against the humerus so it is perpendicular to the plane of the glenoid fossa.

b. **Caudal glide** (Figure 5-14)

INDICATIONS
To increase abduction (sustained Grade III); to reposition humeral head if superiorly positioned.

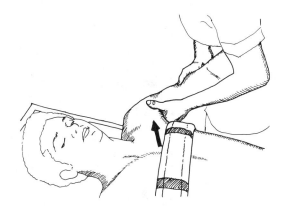

FIGURE 5–13. Joint traction; gleno-humeral joint.

PATIENT POSITION
Same as with distraction

HAND PLACEMENT
Place one hand in the patient's axilla (as in section a) to provide the Grade I distraction; the web space of your other hand is placed just distal to the acromion process.

MOBILIZING FORCE
With the superiorly placed hand, glide the humerus in an inferior direction.

c. **Caudal glide—alternate**

HAND PLACEMENT
Same as with distraction (see Figure 5-13)

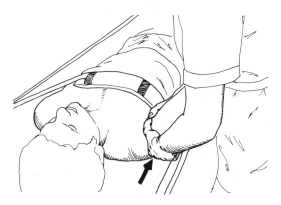

FIGURE 5–14. Caudal glide; gleno-humeral joint.

MOBILIZING FORCE
Comes from the hand around the arm, pulling caudally as you lean backward
Note: This glide is also called long-axis traction.

d. **Caudal glide progression** (Figure 5-15A)

INDICATION
To increase abduction when range approaches 90 degrees

POSITION OF PATIENT
Supine, with the arm abducted to the end of its available range. External rotation of the humerus should be added to the end range position as the arm approaches and goes beyond 90 degrees.

POSITION OF THERAPIST AND HAND PLACEMENT
Stand facing the patient's feet, and stabilize the patient's arm against your trunk with the hand farthest from the patient. A slight lateral motion of your trunk will provide the Grade I distraction. Place the web space of your other hand just distal to the acromion process on the proximal humerus.

MOBILIZING FORCE
With the hand on the proximal humerus, glide the humerus in an inferior direction.

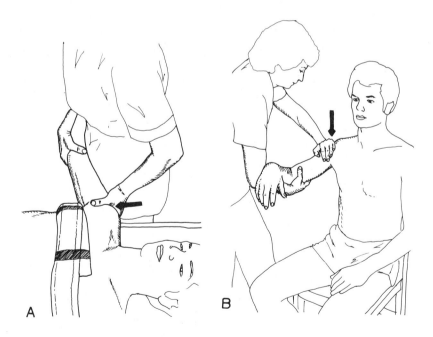

FIGURE 5–15. Caudal glide with the shoulder near 90 degrees, supine (*A*), and sitting (*B*).

ALTERNATE POSITION
Sitting (Figure 5-15B)

e. **Elevation progression** (Figure 5-16A)

INDICATION
To increase elevation beyond 90 degrees of abduction

POSITION OF PATIENT
Supine, with the arm abducted and elevated to the end of its available range. The humerus is then externally rotated to its limit.

POSITION OF THERAPIST AND HAND PLACEMENT
Same as caudal glide progression; the therapist adjusts his or her body position so that the hand applying the mobilizing force is aligned with the treatment plane.

MOBILIZING FORCE
With the hand on the proximal humerus, glide the humerus in a progressively anterior direction. The direction of force will depend on the amount of upward rotation and protraction of the scapula. The force directs the head of the humerus against the inferior folds of the capsule.

ALTERNATE POSITION
Sitting (Figure 5-16B)

f. **Posterior glide** (Figure 5-17)

INDICATIONS
To increase flexion; to increase internal rotation

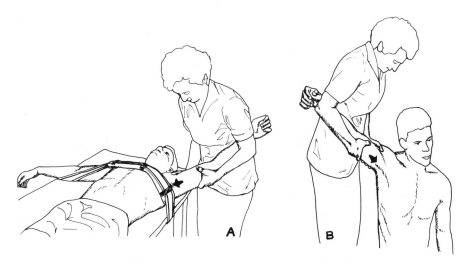

FIGURE 5–16. Elevation progression; glenohumeral joint supine (*A*) and sitting (*B*). Used when the range is greater than 90 degrees. Note the externally rotated position of the humerus.

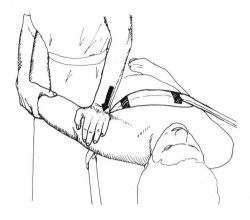

FIGURE 5-17. Posterior glide; glenohumeral joint.

POSITION OF PATIENT
Supine, with the arm in resting position.

POSITION OF THERAPIST AND HAND PLACEMENT
Stand with your back to the patient, between the patient's trunk and arm; support his arm against your trunk, grasping the distal humerus with your lateral hand. This position provides Grade I distraction to the joint. Place the lateral border of your top hand just distal to the anterior margin of the joint, with your fingers pointing superiorly. This hand gives the mobilizing force.

MOBILIZING FORCE
Glide the humeral head posteriorly by moving the entire arm as you bend your knees.

g. **Posterior glide progression** (Figure 5-18)

INDICATIONS
To increase posterior gliding when flexion approaches 90 degrees; to increase horizontal adduction

POSITION OF PATIENT
Supine, with arm flexed to 90 degrees, internally rotated, with elbow flexed. The arm may also be placed in horizontal adduction.

HAND PLACEMENT
Place padding under the scapula for stabilization. Place one hand across the proximal surface of the humerus to apply a Grade I distraction. Place your other hand over the patient's elbow.

MOBILIZING FORCE
Glide the humerus posteriorly by pushing down at the elbow through the long axis of the humerus.

h. **Anterior glide** (Figure 5-19)

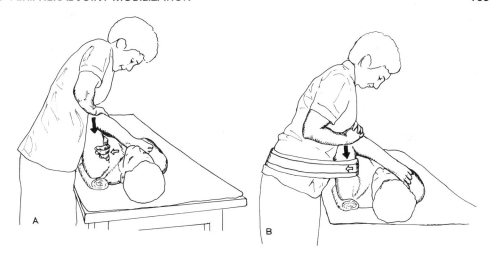

FIGURE 5–18. Posterior glide progression; glenohumeral joint; (*A*) using one hand or (*B*) using a belt to give a Grade I distraction force.

INDICATIONS
To increase extension; to increase external rotation

POSITION OF PATIENT
Prone, with arm in resting position over the edge of the treatment table, supported on your thigh. Stabilize the acromion with padding.

POSITION OF THERAPIST AND HAND PLACEMENT
Stand facing the top of the table with the leg closest to the table in a forward stride position. Support the patient's arm against your thigh with your outside hand. The weight of the patient's arm provides a Grade I distraction. Place the ulnar border of your other hand just distal to the posterior angle of the acromion process, with your fingers pointing superiorly. This hand gives the mobilizing force.

MOBILIZING FORCE
Apply in an anterior and slightly medial direction. Bend both knees so the entire arm moves anterior.
Precaution: Do not lift the arm at the elbow and thereby cause an angulation of the humerus; such angulation could lead to an anterior subluxation of the humeral head.

i. **Anterior glide progression**

INDICATIONS
To increase external rotation
Precaution: Do not place the shoulder in 90 degrees abduction and then progress to externally rotating the arm while applying an anterior glide. Such a technique may lead to anterior subluxation of the humeral head.

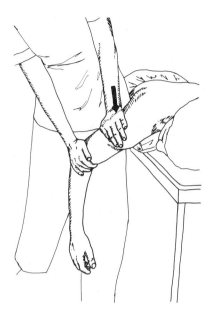

FIGURE 5–19. Anterior glide; glenohumeral joint.

TECHNIQUES
(1) Use elevation progression (see Figure 5-16) since external rotation is incorporated into that technique.
(2) Use a distraction progression of the humerus. Begin with the shoulder in resting position, externally rotate the humerus, then apply a Grade III distraction perpendicular to the plane of the glenoid fossa (see Figure 7-12).

Note: To gain full elevation of the humerus, the accessory and component motions of clavicular elevation and rotation, scapular rotation, and external rotation of the humerus as well as adequate joint play anteriorly and inferiorly are necessary. The clavicular and scapular mobilizations are described in the following sections.

2. Acromioclavicular joint. Anterior glide (Figure 5-20)

INDICATION
To increase mobility of the joint

STABILIZATION
Fixate the scapula at the acromion process.

POSITION OF PATIENT
Sitting or prone

HAND PLACEMENT
With the patient sitting, stand behind him and stabilize the acromion process with the fingers of your lateral hand. The thumb of your other hand is placed posteriorly on the clavicle, just medial to the joint space. With the patient prone, stabilize the acromion with a towel roll under the shoulder.

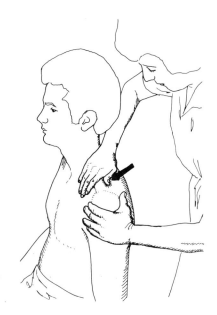

FIGURE 5–20. Anterior glide; acromioclavicular joint.

MOBILIZING FORCE
Your thumb pushes the clavicle anteriorly.

3. **Sternoclavicular joint. (The proximal articulating surface of the clavicle is convex superior/inferior and concave anterior/posterior.)**
POSITION OF PATIENT AND STABILIZATION
Supine. The thorax provides stability to the sternum.
a. **Posterior glide** (Figure 5-21)

INDICATION
To increase retraction

HAND PLACEMENT
Place your thumb on the anterior surface of the proximal end of the clavicle; flex your index finger and place the middle phalanx along the caudal surface of the clavicle to support the thumb.

MOBILIZING FORCE
Push with your thumb in a posterior direction.
b. **Anterior glide** (Figure 5-22A)

INDICATION
To increase protraction

HAND PLACEMENT
Your fingers are placed superiorly and thumb inferiorly around the clavicle.

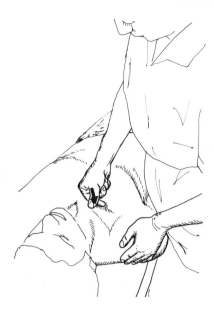

FIGURE 5–21. Posterior glide of the sternoclavicular joint; the same hand placement is used for superior glide.

MOBILIZING FORCE
The fingers and thumb lift the clavicle anteriorly.
c. **Inferior glide** (Figure 5-22B)

INDICATION
To increase elevation

HAND PLACEMENT
Your fingers are placed superior to the clavicle as in section b.

MOBILIZING FORCE
Your fingers pull the proximal clavicle caudally.
d. **Superior glide** (see Figure 5-21)

INDICATION
To increase depression

HAND PLACEMENT
Same as section a above

MOBILIZING FORCE
Your index finger forces in a superior direction.

4. **Scapulothoracic articulation. (This is not a true joint, but the soft tissue is stretched in order to obtain normal shoulder girdle mobility.) (Figure 5-23)**

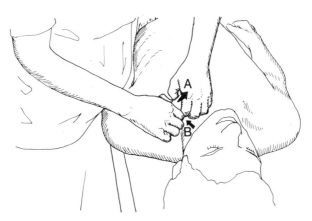

FIGURE 5-22. (A), Anterior glide of the sternoclavicular joint; (B), the same hand placement is used for inferior glide.

INDICATIONS
To increase scapular motions of elevation, depression, protraction, retraction, rotation, and winging. (Winging is an accessory motion that occurs when a person attempts to place the hand behind the back, accompanying shoulder internal rotation and scapular downward rotation.)

POSITION OF PATIENT
If there is little mobility, begin prone (see Figure 2-6), and progress to side-lying, with the patient facing you. The patient's arm is draped over your inferior arm and allowed to hang so that the muscles are relaxed.

HAND PLACEMENT
Your superior hand is placed across the acromion process to control the direction of motion. The fingers of your inferior hand scoop under the medial border and inferior angle of the scapula.

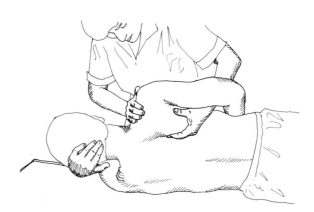

FIGURE 5-23. Scapulothoracic mobilization.

MOBILIZING FORCE
The scapula is moved in the desired direction by lifting from the inferior angle or by pushing on the acromion process.

B. The Elbow and Forearm Complex (Figure 5-24)

1. The humeroulnar articulation. (The convex trochlea articulates with the concave olecranon fossa.)

RESTING POSITION
Elbow flexed 70 degrees, forearm supinated 10 degrees

TREATMENT PLANE
In the olecranon fossa, angled approximately 45 degrees from the long axis of the ulna (Figure 5-25)

STABILIZATION
Fixate the humerus against the treatment table with a belt or use an assistant to hold it.

a. **Joint traction** (Figure 5-26A)

INDICATIONS
Testing; initial treatment (sustained Grade II); pain control (Grade I or II oscillation); to increase flexion or extension

POSITION OF PATIENT
Supine, elbow over the edge of the treatment table or supported with padding just proximal to the olecranon process. The wrist rests against the therapist's shoulder, allowing the elbow to be in resting position.

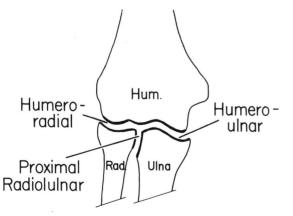

Humero-radial

Hum.

Humero-ulnar

Proximal Radiolulnar

Rad

Ulna

FIGURE 5–24. Bones and joints of the elbow complex.

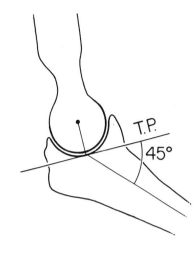

FIGURE 5–25. Lateral view of the humeroulnar joint, depicting the treatment plane (T.P.).

HAND PLACEMENT
Using your medial hand, place your fingers over the proximal ulna on the volar surface; reinforce it with your other hand.

MOBILIZING FORCE
Force against the proximal ulna at a 45-degree angle to the shaft

b. **Traction progression**

INDICATIONS
To increase flexion or extension

POSITION OF PATIENT
Same as in section a, except the elbow is positioned at the end of its available range of motion before applying the mobilizing force.

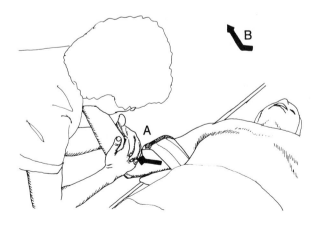

FIGURE 5–26. Joint traction: (*A*), humeroulnar articulation; (*B*), arrow indicating joint traction with distal glide.

HAND PLACEMENT
Adjust your position to best apply the mobilization force and stabilize the forearm.

MOBILIZING FORCE
Always force against the ulna at a 45-degree angle, no matter at what angle the elbow is.

c. **Distal glide** (Figure 5-26B)

INDICATION
To increase flexion

POSITION OF PATIENT AND HAND PLACEMENT
Same as in section a.

MOBILIZING FORCE
Use a scooping motion in which distraction is applied to the joint first as in section a, then pull along the long axis of the ulna (distal traction).

2. **The humeroradial articulation. (The convex capitulum articulates with the concave radial head.)**

RESTING POSITION
Elbow extended, forearm supinated

TREATMENT PLANE
In the concave radial head perpendicular to the long axis of the radius

STABILIZATION
Fixate the humerus with one of your hands.

a. **Joint traction** (Figure 5-27)

INDICATIONS
To increase mobility of the radius; to correct a pushed elbow (proximal displacement of the radius)

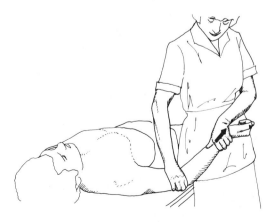

FIGURE 5–27. Joint traction; humeroradial articulation.

POSITION OF PATIENT
Supine; or sitting, with the arm resting on the treatment table.

POSITION OF THERAPIST AND HAND PLACEMENT
Position yourself on the ulnar side of the patient's forearm. Stabilize the patient's humerus with your superior hand; grasp around the distal radius with the fingers and thenar eminence of your inferior hand; be sure you are not grasping around the distal ulna.

MOBILIZING FORCE
Pull the radius distally (long-axis traction will cause joint traction).

b. **Dorsal or volar glide of the radius** (Figure 5-28)

INDICATIONS
Dorsal glide, to increase extension; volar glide, to increase flexion

POSITION OF PATIENT
Supine, or sitting with the elbow extended and supinated as far as possible.

HAND PLACEMENT
Stabilize the humerus from the medial side of the patient's arm. Place the palmar surface of your lateral hand on the volar aspect and your fingers on the dorsal aspect of the radial head.

MOBILIZING FORCE
Force the radial head dorsally with the palm of your hand or volarly with your fingers. If a stronger force is needed for the volar glide, turn the

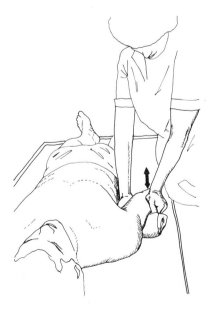

FIGURE 5–28. Dorsal and volar glide; humeroradial articulation.

forearm over, realign your body, and push with the base of your hand against the dorsal surface in a volar direction.

c. **Joint compression** (Figure 5-29)

INDICATION
To reduce a pulled elbow subluxation

POSITION OF PATIENT
May be sitting or supine

HAND PLACEMENT
Using the same hand as that of the patient, place your thenar eminence against the patient's thenar eminence (locking thumbs). Fixate the humerus and proximal ulna against a firm object (treatment table or your other hand).

MOBILIZING FORCE
Push along the long axis of the radius by putting pressure against the thenar eminence; simultaneously supinate the forearm.
Note: To replace an acute subluxation, a quick motion (manipulation) is used.

3. **Radioulnar articulations**
   a. **Proximal radioulnar joint** (Figure 5-30). (Convex rim of the radial head articulates with the concave radial notch on the ulna.)

RESTING POSITION
Elbow flexed 70 degrees, forearm supinated 35 degrees.

TREATMENT PLANE
In the radial notch of the ulna, parallel to the long axis of the ulna

STABILIZATION
Proximal ulna

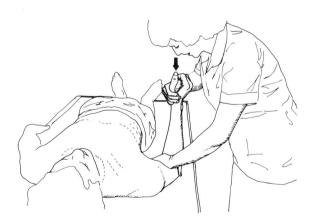

FIGURE 5–29. Joint compression; humeroradial articulation.

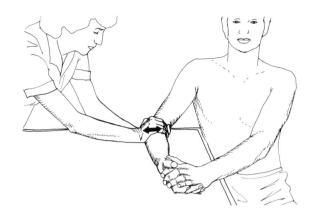

FIGURE 5–30. Dorsal-volar glide; proximal radioulnar joint.

INDICATIONS
Dorsal glide, to increase pronation; volar glide, to increase supination

Position of Patient
Sitting or supine, with the elbow and forearm in resting position.

HAND PLACEMENT
Fixate the ulna with your medial hand around the medial aspect of the forearm; place your other hand around the head of the radius with the fingers on the volar surface and the palm on the dorsal surface.

MOBILIZING FORCE
Force the radial head volarly by pushing with your palm, or dorsally by pulling with your fingers. If a stronger force is needed for the dorsal glide, move around to the other side of the patient, switch hands, and push from the volar surface with the base of your hand against the radial head.

b. **Distal radioulnar joint** (Figure 5-31). (The concave ulnar notch of the radius articulates with the convex head of the ulna.)

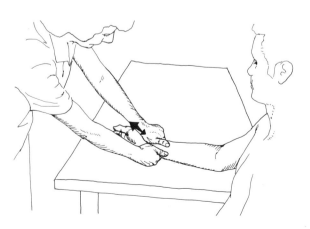

FIGURE 5–31. Dorsal-volar glide; distal radioulnar joint.

RESTING POSITION
Supinated 10 degrees.

TREATMENT PLANE
Articulating surface of the radius, parallel to the long axis of the radius

STABILIZATION
Distal ulna

INDICATIONS
Dorsal glide, to increase supination; volar glide, to increase pronation

POSITION OF PATIENT
Sitting, with arm on the treatment table; forearm in resting position

HAND PLACEMENT
Stabilize the distal ulna by placing the fingers of one hand on the dorsal surface, and the thenar eminence and thumb on the volar surface. Place your other hand in the same manner around the distal radius.

MOBILIZING FORCE
Glide the distal radius dorsally or volarly parallel to the ulna.

C. The Wrist Complex (Figure 5-32)

1. Radiocarpal joint. (Concave distal radius articulates with the convex proximal row of carpals which is composed of the scaphoid, lunate, and triquetrum.)

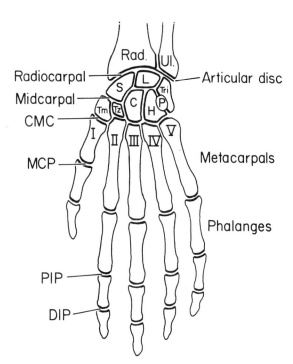

FIGURE 5–32. Bones and joints of the wrist and hand.

RESTING POSITION
Straight line through the radius and third metacarpal with slight ulnar deviation

TREATMENT PLANE
In the articulating surface of the radius perpendicular to the long axis of the radius

STABILIZATION
Distal radius and ulna
a. **Joint traction** (distraction) (Figure 5-33)

INDICATIONS
Testing; initial treatment; pain control; general mobility of the wrist

POSITION OF PATIENT
Sitting, with forearm supported on the treatment table, wrist over the edge of the table

HAND PLACEMENT
With the hand closest to the patient, grasp around the styloid processes and fixate the radius and ulna against the table. Your other hand grasps around the distal row of carpals.

MOBILIZING FORCE
Pull in a distal direction with respect to the arm.
b. **General glides**

INDICATIONS
Dorsal glide to increase flexion (Figure 5-34); volar glide to increase extension (Figure 5-35); radial glide to increase ulnar deviation; ulnar glide to increase radial deviation (Figure 5-36)

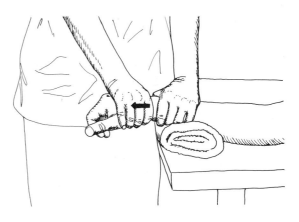

FIGURE 5–33. Joint traction; wrist joint.

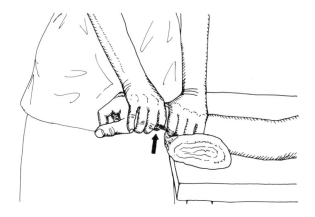

FIGURE 5-34. Dorsal glide; general mobilization of the wrist joint.

POSITION OF PATIENT AND HAND PLACEMENT
Same as in section a, except rotate the forearm when doing radial or ulnar glide for ease in doing the technique

MOBILIZING FORCE
Comes from the hand around the distal carpals

2. **Specific glides of the carpals in the proximal row with the radius and ulna**

POSITION OF PATIENT
Sitting, with the hand being held by the therapist so that the elbow hangs unsupported. The weight of the arm provides slight joint traction (Grade I) so the therapist then needs only to apply the glides.

HAND PLACEMENT
Place your index fingers on the volar surface of the bone to be stabilized (see stabilization); the thumbs on the dorsal surface of the bone to be mobilized.

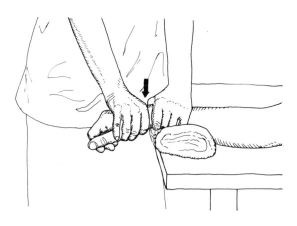

FIGURE 5-35. Volar glide; general mobilization of the wrist joint.

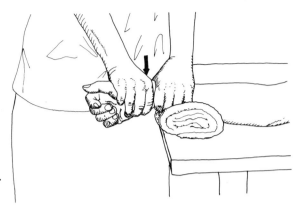

FIGURE 5–36. Ulnar glide; general mobilization of the wrist joint.

STABILIZATION
To increase flexion, the index fingers stabilize the distal bone (scaphoid or lunate) (Figure 5-37). To increase extension, the index fingers stabilize the proximal bone (radius) (Figure 5-38).

MOBILIZING FORCE
In each case, the force comes from the thumbs on the dorsal surface of the bone to be mobilized. By mobilizing from the dorsal surface, pressure against the nerves, blood vessels, and tendons in the carpal tunnel and Guyon's canal is minimized and a stronger mobilizing force can be used without pain.

a. **Scaphoid-radius** (Scaphoid convex, radius concave) and **lunate-radius** (lunate convex, radius concave)

INDICATIONS
To increase flexion, glide radius volarly on fixed scaphoid, or glide radius volarly on fixed lunate (see Figure 5-37). To increase extension,

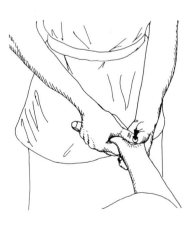

FIGURE 5–37. Stabilization of the distal bone; volar glide of the proximal bone; shown is stabilization of the scaphoid and lunate with volar glide to the radius.

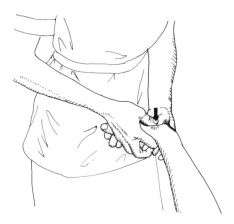

FIGURE 5-38. Stabilization of the proximal bone; volar glide of the distal bone; shown is stabilization of the radius with volar glide to the lunate.

glide scaphoid volarly on fixed radius, or glide lunate volarly on fixed radius (Figure 5-38).

b. **Ulnar-meniscal triquetral articulation**

INDICATIONS

To unlock the articular disk, which may block motions of the wrist or forearm glide ulna volarly on fixed triquetrum.

3. Specific glides of the intercarpal joints

POSITION OF PATIENT AND HAND PLACEMENT
Same as described in section 2.

STABILIZATION

In all cases the stabilization is applied with the index fingers overlapped on the volar surface.

MOBILIZATION FORCE

In all cases the force comes from the overlapped thumbs on the dorsal surface.

a. Glides to increase extension
Stabilize the bone that has the concave articulating surface, and apply the mobilizing force against the dorsal surface of the bone with the convex articulating surface. The force is in a volar direction.

EXAMPLES

(1) To increase extension and radial deviation at the trapezium-trapezoid/scaphoid articulation, glide the scaphoid volarly with your thumbs while stabilizing the trapezium-trapezoid unit with your index fingers.

(2) To increase extension at the capitate/lunate articulation, glide the capitate volarly with your thumbs while stabilizing the lunate with your index fingers.

b. Glides to increase flexion
Stabilize the bone that has the convex articulating surface and apply the mobilizing force against the dorsal surface of the bone with the concave articulating surface. The force is in a volar direction.

EXAMPLES
(1) To increase flexion at the trapezium-trapezoid/scaphoid articulation, glide the trapezium-trapezoid unit volarly with your thumbs while stabilizing the scaphoid with your index fingers.
(2) To increase flexion at the capitate/lunate articulation, glide the lunate volarly with your thumbs while stabilizing the capitate.

D. The Hand and Finger Joints

1. The carpometacarpal and intermetacarpal joints of digits II through V.

a. **Joint traction** (Figure 5-39)

INDICATION
To increase mobility of the hand

STABILIZATION AND HAND PLACEMENT
Stabilize the respective carpal with one hand, grasp with your thumb dorsal and index fingers volar. Your other hand grasps around the proximal portion of a metacarpal, thumb dorsal and fingers volar.

MOBILIZING FORCE
Apply long-axis traction to the metacarpal to separate the joint surfaces.

b. **Volar glide**

INDICATION
To increase mobility of the arch of the hand

STABILIZATION AND HAND PLACEMENT
Same as in section a

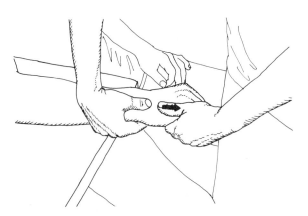

FIGURE 5–39. Joint traction; carpometacarpal joint.

MOBILIZING FORCE
The thumb on the dorsum of the metacarpal glides the proximal portion of the bone volarward.

c. See also the technique for cupping and flattening the arch of the hand described in Chapter 2.

2. The carpometacarpal joint of the thumb. (A saddle joint: The trapezium is concave, proximal metacarpal convex for abduction/adduction; the trapezium is convex, proximal metacarpal concave for flexion/extension.)

RESTING POSITION
Midway between flexion and extension, and between abduction and adduction.

STABILIZATION
Fixate the trapezium with the hand closest to the patient.

TREATMENT PLANE
In the trapezium for abduction-adduction; in the proximal metacarpal for flexion-extension.

a. **Joint traction**

INDICATIONS
Testing; initial treatment; pain control; general mobility

POSITION OF PATIENT
Forearm and hand resting on the treatment table

HAND PLACEMENT
Fixate the trapezium with the hand closest to the patient; grasp the patient's metacarpal by wrapping your fingers around it (similar to Figure 5-40A).

MOBILIZING FORCE
Apply long-axis traction to separate the joint surfaces.

b. **Glides** (Figure 5-40)

INDICATIONS
To increase flexion, ulnar glide; to increase extension, radial glide; to increase abduction, dorsal glide; to increase adduction, volar glide

POSITION OF PATIENT AND HAND PLACEMENT
Same as in section a. The volar surface of the hand around the metacarpal is placed opposite the direction of the glide. (In Figure 5-40, the surface of the hand is on the radial side of the metacarpal in order to cause an ulnar glide.)

MOBILIZING FORCE
Comes from the volar surface of the hand on the metacarpal, and glides the base of the metacarpal in the appropriate direction.

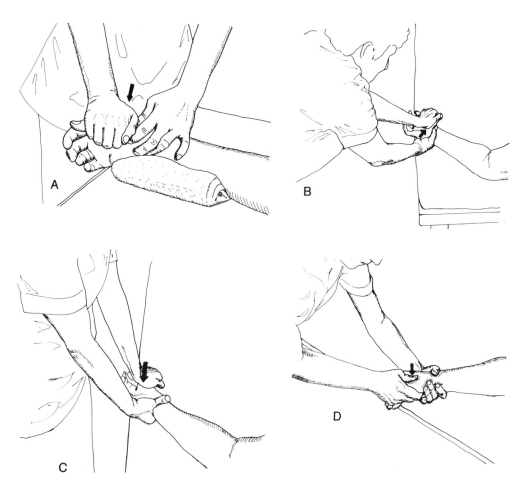

FIGURE 5–40. Carpometacarpal joint of the thumb; (*A*) ulnar glide to increase flexion, (*B*) radial glide to increase extension, (*C*) dorsal glide to increase abduction, (*D*) volar glide to increase adduction. Note the thumb of the therapist is placed in the web space between the index and thumb of the patient's hand in order to apply a volar glide.

3. **The metacarpophalangeal and interphalangeal joints of the fingers. (In all cases, the distal end of the proximal articulating surface is convex, and the proximal end of the distal articulating surface is concave.)**

   Note: Since all the articulating surfaces are the same for the digits, all techniques are applied in the same manner to each joint.

   RESTING POSITION
   Slight flexion in all joints

   TREATMENT PLANE
   In the distal articulating surface

STABILIZATION
Rest the forearm and hand on the treatment table; fixate the proximal articulating surface with the fingers of one of your hands.

a. **Joint traction** (Figure 5-41)

INDICATIONS
Testing; initial treatment; pain control; general mobility

HAND PLACEMENT
Use your proximal hand to stabilize the proximal bone; wrap the fingers and thumb of your other hand around the distal bone close to the joint.

MOBILIZING FORCE
Apply long-axis traction to separate the joint surface.

b. **Glides**

INDICATIONS
To increase flexion, volar glide (Figure 5-42); to increase extension, dorsal glide; to increase abduction or adduction, radial or ulnar glide (depending on finger)

MOBILIZING FORCE
The glide force is applied by the thumb against the proximal end of the bone to be moved.

c. **Rotations** (Figure 5-43)

INDICATIONS
To increase final degrees of motion

MOBILIZING FORCE
Initially, rotate the distal bone on the stabilized proximal bone, then apply a traction force.

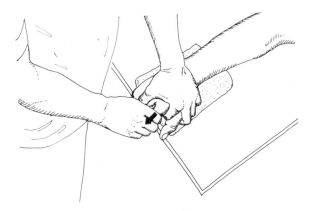

FIGURE 5–41. Joint traction of a metacarpophalangeal joint.

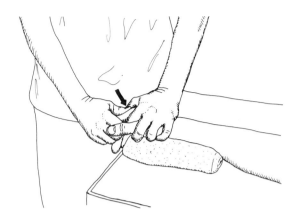

FIGURE 5–42. Volar glide of a metacarpophalangeal joint.

E. The Hip Joint.
(The Concave Acetabulum Receives The Convex Femoral Head.) (Figure 5-44)

RESTING POSITION
Hip flexion 30 degrees, abduction 30 degrees, and slight external rotation

STABILIZATION
Fixate the pelvis to the treatment table with belts.

1. Distraction of the weight-bearing surface—caudal glide (Figure 5-45)
   Note: Because of the deep configuration of this joint, when traction is applied perpendicular to the treatment plane, there is a lateral glide of the superior, weight-bearing surface. To get separation of the weight-bearing surface, a caudal glide is used.

   INDICATIONS
   Testing; initial treatment; pain control; general mobility

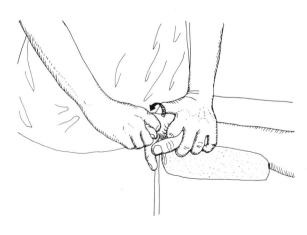

FIGURE 5–43. Rotation of a meta-carpophalangeal joint.

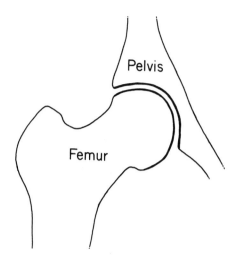

FIGURE 5–44. Bones of the hip joint.

POSITION OF PATIENT
Supine, with hip in resting position and the knee extended.
Caution: If there is knee dysfunction, this position should not be used; see alternate position under section 2.

POSITION OF THERAPIST AND HAND PLACEMENT
Stand at the end of the treatment table; place a belt around your trunk, then cross the belt over the patient's foot and around his ankle. Place your hands proximal to the malleoli, under the belt. The belt allows you to use your body weight to apply the mobilizing force.

MOBILIZING FORCE
A long-axis traction is applied by pulling on the leg as you lean backward.

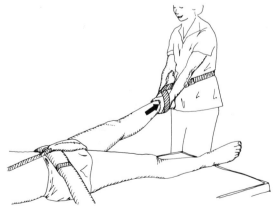

FIGURE 5–45. Distraction of the weight-bearing surface of the hip joint: caudal glide.

2. Alternate position for caudal glide

INDICATION
Same as in section 1, to apply distraction to the weight-bearing surface of the hip when there is knee dysfunction.

POSITION OF PATIENT
Supine, with the hip and knee flexed

POSITION OF THERAPIST AND HAND PLACEMENT
Crouch close to the patient's hip; have the patient's leg over your shoulder. Wrap both of your hands around the proximal thigh.

MOBILIZING FORCE
Comes from your hands and is applied in a caudal direction as you lean backward

3. Posterior glide (Figure 5-46)

INDICATIONS
To increase flexion; to increase internal rotation

POSITION OF PATIENT
Supine, with hips at the end of the table. The patient helps stabilize his pelvis by flexing the opposite hip and holding the thigh with his hands. The hip to be mobilized is in resting position.

POSITION OF THERAPIST AND HAND PLACEMENT
Stand on the medial side of the patient's thigh. Place a belt around your shoulder and under the patient's thigh to help hold the weight of the lower extremity. Place your most distal hand under the belt and distal thigh. Place your proximal hand on the anterior surface of the proximal thigh.

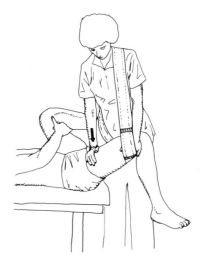

FIGURE 5–46. Posterior glide; hip joint.

MOBILIZING FORCE

Keep your elbows extended and flex your knees, and apply the force through your proximal hand in a posterior direction.

4. Anterior glide (Figure 5-47A)

INDICATIONS

To increase extension; to increase external rotation

POSITION OF PATIENT

Prone, with trunk resting on the table and hips over the edge. The opposite foot is on the floor.

POSITION OF THERAPIST AND HAND PLACEMENT

Stand on the medial side of the patient's thigh; place a belt around your shoulder and the patient's thigh to help support the weight of the leg. With your distal hand, hold the patient's leg. Place your proximal hand posteriorly on the proximal thigh, just below the buttock.

MOBILIZING FORCE

Keep your elbow extended and flex your knees, and apply the force through your proximal hand in an anterior direction.

ALTERNATE POSITION (Figure 5-47B)

Position patient side-lying with the thigh comfortably flexed and supported by pillows. Stand posterior to the patient, stabilize the pelvis across the anterior superior iliac spine with your cranial hand. Push against the posterior aspect of the greater trochanter in an anterior direction with your caudal hand.

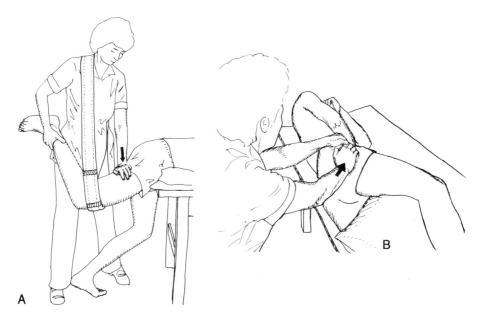

FIGURE 5–47. Anterior glide; hip joint prone (A), and side-lying (B).

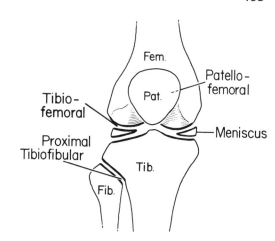

FIGURE 5–48. Bones and joints of the knee and leg.

F. The Knee and Leg (Figure 5-48)

1. The tibiofemoral articulation. (Concave tibial plateaus articulate on the convex femoral condyles.)

RESTING POSITION
Flexion 25 degrees

TREATMENT PLANE
Along the surface of the tibial plateaus. Therefore, it moves with the tibia as the knee angle changes.

STABILIZATION
In most cases, the femur is stabilized with a belt or by the table.

a. Joint traction—long-axis traction (Figure 5-49A, B, and C)

INDICATIONS
Testing; initial treatment; pain control; general mobility

POSITION OF PATIENT
Sitting, supine, or prone, beginning with the knee in resting position

HAND PLACEMENT
Grasp around the distal leg, proximal to the malleoli with both hands.

MOBILIZING FORCE
Pull on the long axis of the tibia to separate the joint surfaces.

b. Posterior glide—drawer test (Figure 5-50)

INDICATIONS
Testing; to increase flexion

POSITION OF PATIENT
Supine, with the foot resting on the table. The position for the drawer test can be used to mobilize the tibia either anteriorly or posteriorly, although no Grade I distraction can be applied with the glides.

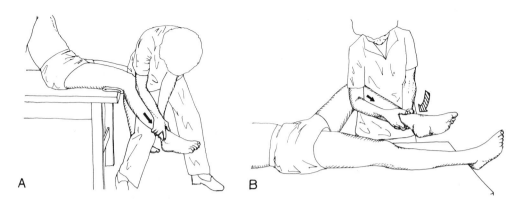

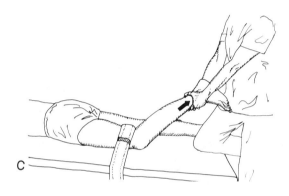

FIGURE 5–49. Traction of the knee joint sitting (*A*), supine (*B*), or prone (*C*).

POSITION OF THERAPIST AND HAND PLACEMENT
Sit on the table with your thigh fixating the patient's foot. With both hands, grasp around the tibia, fingers pointing posteriorly and thumbs anteriorly.

MOBILIZING FORCE
Extend your elbows and lean your body weight forward, and push the tibia posteriorly with your thumbs.

c. **Posterior glide, alternate position and progression** (Figure 5-51)

INDICATIONS
To increase flexion

POSITION OF PATIENT
Sitting, with the knee flexed over the edge of the treatment table, beginning in resting position (Figure 5-51A) and progressing to near 90 degrees (Figure 5-51B).

POSITION OF THERAPIST AND HAND PLACEMENT
When in resting position, stand on the medial side of the patient's leg.

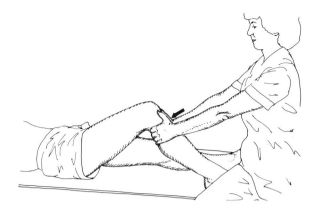

FIGURE 5–50. Posterior glide (drawer); knee joint.

Hold the distal leg with your distal hand and place the palm of your proximal hand along the anterior aspect of the tibia. When near 90 degrees, sit on a low stool; stabilize the leg between your knees and place one hand on the anterior aspect of the tibia.

MOBILIZING FORCE
Extend your elbow and lean your body weight onto the tibia, gliding it posteriorly.

d. **Anterior glide** (Figure 5-52)

INDICATIONS
To increase extension

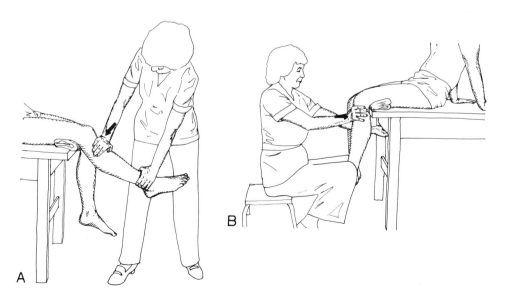

FIGURE 5–51. Posterior glide of the knee joint in resting position (*A*) and near 90 degrees (*B*).

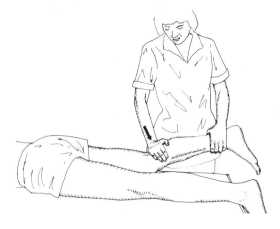

FIGURE 5-52. Anterior glide; knee joint.

POSITION OF PATIENT
Prone, with the knee in resting position. Place a small pad under the distal femur in order to prevent patellar compression.

HAND PLACEMENT
Grasp the distal tibia with the hand closest to it, and place the palm of the proximal hand on the posterior aspect of the proximal tibia.

MOBILIZING FORCE
Force with the hand on the proximal tibia in an anterior direction
Note: The drawer test position can also be used (see section a). The mobilizing force comes from the fingers on the posterior tibia as you lean backwards (see Figure 5-50).

2. **Patellofemoral joint**
   a. **Distal glide** (Figure 5-53)

   INDICATION
   To increase patellar mobility for knee flexion

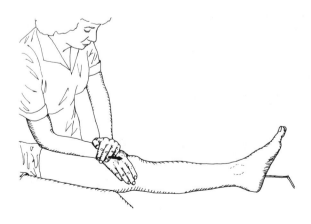

FIGURE 5-53. Distal glide; patellofemoral joint.

POSITION OF PATIENT
Supine, with knee extended

HAND PLACEMENT
Stand next to the patient's thigh, facing his feet. Place the web space of the hand closest to the thigh around the superior border of the patella. Use the other hand for reinforcement.

MOBILIZING FORCE
Glide the patella in a caudal direction, parallel to the femur.
Caution: Do not compress the patella into the femoral condyles while performing this technique.

b. **Medial-lateral glide** (Figure 5-54)

INDICATION
To increase patellar mobility

POSITION OF PATIENT
Supine, with knee extended

HAND PLACEMENT
Place your fingers medially and thumbs laterally around the medial and lateral borders of the patella, respectively.

MOBILIZING FORCE
Glide the patella in a medial or lateral direction, against the restriction

3. **Proximal tibiofibular articulation—Anterior (ventral) glide (Figure 5-55)**

INDICATIONS
To increase movement of the fibular head; to reposition a posteriorly positioned head

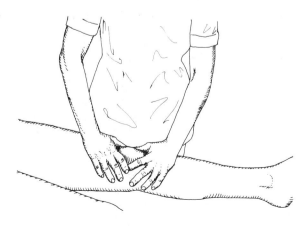

FIGURE 5–54. Medial-lateral glide of the patella.

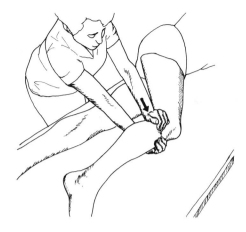

FIGURE 5–55. Anterior glide; fibular head.

POSITION OF PATIENT
Side-lying, with the trunk and hips rotated partially toward prone; the top leg is flexed forward so that the knee and lower leg are resting on the table.

POSITION OF THERAPIST AND HAND PLACEMENT
Stand behind the patient, placing your most distal hand under the tibia to stabilize it. Place the base of your proximal hand posterior to the head of the fibula, wrapping your fingers anteriorly.

MOBILIZING FORCE
Comes from the heel of your hand against the posterior aspect of the fibular head, in an anterior-lateral direction.

4. **Distal tibiofibular articulation—Anterior (ventral) or posterior (dorsal) glide (Figure 5-56)**

INDICATION
To increase mobility of the mortice when it is restricting ankle dorsiflexion

POSITION OF PATIENT
Supine or prone

HAND PLACEMENT
Working from the end of the table, place the fingers of the more medial hand under the tibia and the thumb over the tibia to stabilize it. Place the base of your other hand over the lateral malleolus, with the fingers underneath.

MOBILIZING FORCE
Against the fibula in an anterior direction when prone, and a posterior direction when supine

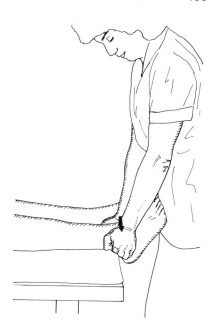

FIGURE 5–56. Posterior glide; distal tibiofibular articulation.

G. Ankle and Tarsal Joints (Figure 5-57)

1. Talocrural (upper ankle joint). (Convex talus articulates with the concave mortice made up of the tibia and fibula.)

RESTING POSITION
Plantarflexion 10 degrees

TREATMENT PLANE
In the mortice, going in an anterior-posterior direction with respect to the leg

STABILIZATION
Tibia strapped or held against the table

a. Joint traction (distraction) (Figure 5-58)

INDICATIONS
Testing; initial treatment; pain control; general mobility

POSITION OF PATIENT
Supine, with the lower extremity extended and the ankle in resting position

POSITION OF THERAPIST AND HAND PLACEMENT
Stand at the end of the table; wrap the fingers of both hands over the dorsum of the patient's foot, just distal to the mortice; place your thumbs on the plantar surface of the foot to hold it in resting position.

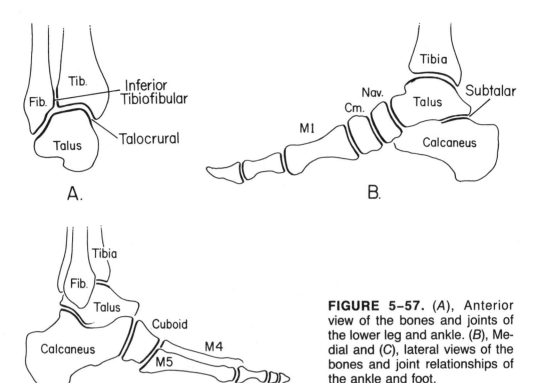

FIGURE 5–57. (*A*), Anterior view of the bones and joints of the lower leg and ankle. (*B*), Medial and (*C*), lateral views of the bones and joint relationships of the ankle and foot.

Mobilization Force
Pull the foot away from the long axis of the leg in a distal direction by leaning backward.

b. **Dorsal (posterior) glide** (Figure 5-59)

INDICATION
To increase dorsiflexion

POSITION OF PATIENT
Supine, with the leg supported on the table and the heel over the edge

POSITION OF THERAPIST AND HAND PLACEMENT
Stand to the side of the patient. Stabilize the leg with your cranial hand, or use a belt to secure the leg to the table. Place the palmar aspect of the web space of your other hand over the talus just distal to the mortise. Wrap your fingers and thumb around the foot to maintain the ankle in resting position. A Grade I distraction force is applied in a caudal direction.

MOBILIZING FORCE
Glide the talus posteriorly with respect to the tibia by pushing against the talus.

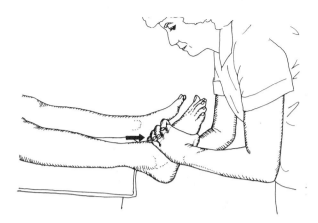

FIGURE 5–58. Joint traction; talocrural joint.

c. **Ventral (anterior) glide** (Figure 5-60)

INDICATION
To increase plantarflexion

POSITION OF PATIENT
Prone, with the foot over the edge of the table

POSITION OF THERAPIST AND HAND PLACEMENT
Working from the end of the table, place your lateral hand across the dorsum of the foot to apply a Grade I distraction. Place the web space of your other hand just distal to the mortice on the posterior aspect of the talus and calcaneus.

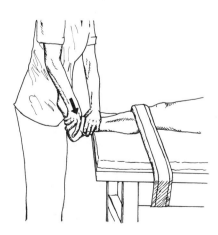

FIGURE 5–59. Posterior glide; talocrural joint.

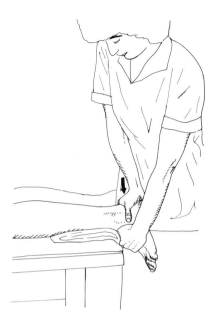

FIGURE 5–60. Anterior glide; talocrural joint.

MOBILIZING FORCE
Push against the calcaneus in an anterior direction (with respect to the tibia); this glides the talus anteriorly.

ALTERNATE POSITION
Patient is supine. Stabilize the distal leg anterior to the mortise with your proximal hand. The distal hand cups under the calcaneus. When you push against the calcaneus in an anterior direction, the talus glides anteriorly.

2. **Subtalar (talocalcaneal) joint, posterior compartment. (The calcaneus is convex, articulating with a concave talus in the posterior compartment.)**

RESTING POSITION
Midway between inversion and eversion

TREATMENT PLANE
In the talus, parallel to the sole of the foot
a. **Joint traction (distraction)** (Figure 5-61)

INDICATIONS
Testing; initial treatment; pain control; general mobility for inversion/ eversion

POSITION OF PATIENT
Supine, with the leg supported on the table and heel over the edge. The ankle is stabilized in dorsiflexion with pressure from the therapist's thigh.

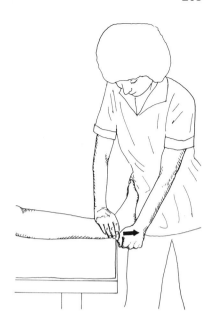

FIGURE 5–61. Joint traction; subtalar (talocalcaneal) joint.

HAND PLACEMENT
The distal hand grasps around the calcaneus from the posterior aspect of the foot. The other hand fixes the talus and malleoli against the table.

MOBILIZING FORCE
Pull the calcaneus distally with respect to the long axis of the leg.

b. **Medial glide or lateral glide** (Figure 5-62)

INDICATION
Medial glide to increase eversion; lateral glide to increase inversion

POSITION OF PATIENT
Patient is side-lying or prone, with the leg supported on the table or with a towel roll.

POSITION OF THERAPIST AND HAND PLACEMENT
Align your shoulder and arm parallel to the bottom of the foot. Stabilize the talus with your proximal hand. Place the base of the distal hand on the side of the calcaneus, medially to cause a lateral glide and laterally to cause a medial glide, and wrap the fingers around the plantar surface.

MOBILIZING FORCE
Apply a Grade I distraction force in a caudal direction, then push with the base of your hand against the side of the calcaneus parallel to the plantar surface of the heel.

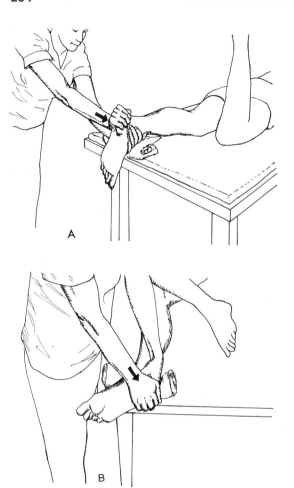

FIGURE 5–62. (*A*) Medial glide with patient prone to increase eversion, (*B*) lateral glide with patient side-lying to increase inversion; subtalar joint.

ALTERNATE POSITION
Same as in section a, moving the calcaneus in a medial direction with the fingers, or a lateral direction with the base of the hand.

3. **Intertarsal joints and tarsometatarsal joints. (When moving in a dorsal-plantar direction with respect to the foot, all of the articulating surfaces are concave and convex in the same direction; for example, the proximal articulating surface is convex and the distal articulating surface is concave. The technique for mobilizing each joint is the same; the hand placement is adjusted to stabilize the proximal bone partner so the distal bone partner can be moved.)**
   a. **Plantar glide** (Figure 5-63)

   INDICATION
   To increase plantarflexion accessory motions (for example, to increase the arch)

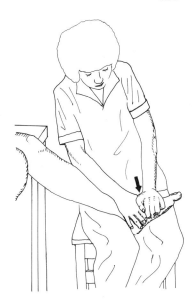

FIGURE 5–63. Plantar glide of a distal tarsal bone on a stabilized proximal bone; shown is the cuneiform bone on the navicular.

POSITION OF PATIENT
Supine, with hip and knee flexed; or sitting, with knee flexed over the edge of the table and heel resting in the therapist's lap

STABILIZATION
Fixate the more proximal bone with your index finger on the plantar surface of the bone.

HAND PLACEMENT
To mobilize the medial tarsal joints, place the stabilizing hand on the dorsum of the foot with the fingers pointing medially, so the index finger can be placed under the bone to be stabilized. Wrap the fingers of the other hand around the plantar surface of the tarsal joint to be moved and the base of the hand over the dorsal surface. To mobilize the lateral tarsal joints, position yourself medially and point your fingers laterally.

MOBILIZING FORCE
Push in a plantar direction from the dorsum of the foot
b. **Dorsal glide** (Figure 5-64)

INDICATION
To increase dorsal gliding accessory motion

POSITION OF PATIENT
Prone, with knee flexed

STABILIZATION
Fixate the more proximal bone.

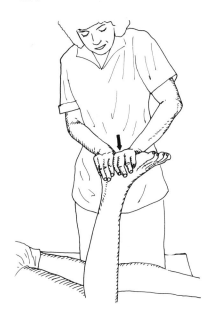

FIGURE 5–64. Dorsal gliding of a distal tarsal on a proximal tarsal; shown is the cuboid bone on the calcaneus.

HAND PLACEMENT
To mobilize the lateral tarsal joints (for example, cuboid on calcaneus), wrap your fingers around the lateral side of the foot (as in Figure 5-64). To mobilize the medial bones (for example, navicular on talus), wrap your fingers around the medial aspect of the foot. Place your second metacarpophalangeal joint against the bone to be moved.

MOBILIZING FORCE
Push from the plantar surface in a dorsal direction.

ALTERNATE TECHNIQUE
Same as position of patient in section a, except the distal bone is stabilized and the proximal bone is forced in a planter direction. This is a relative motion of the distal bone moving in a dorsal direction.

H. The Intermetatarsal, Metatarsophalangeal, and Interphalangeal Joints

The intermetatarsal, metatarsophalangeal, and interphalangeal joints of the toes are stabilized and mobilized in the same manner as the fingers. In each case, the articulating surface of the proximal bone is convex, and the articulating surface of the distal bone is concave. (See section D.)

VIII. SUMMARY

Basic concepts of joint mobilization were presented, including definitions of terminology, concepts of joint motion, and indications, limitations, and contraindications for the techniques. Basic procedures for applying the techniques were described, from which adaptations can be made and other techniques developed as the skill of the therapist progresses.

REFERENCES

1. Akeson, WH, et al: *Effects of immobilization on joints.* Clin Orthop Rel Res 219:28, 1987.
2. Cookson, JC and Kent, BE: *Orthopedic manual therapy an overview; Part I: The extremities.* Phys Ther 59:136, 1979.
3. Cyriax, J: *Textbook of Orthopaedic Medicine, Vol. I: The Diagnosis of Soft Tissue Lesions,* ed 8. Bailliere and Tindall, London, 1982.
4. Donatelli, R and Owens-Burkhart, H: *Effects of immobilization on the extensibility of periarticular connective tissue.* JOSPT 3:67, 1981.
5. Enneking, WF and Horowitz, M: *The intra-articular effects of immobilization on the human knee.* J Bone Joint Surg 54-A:973, 1972.
6. Grieve, G: *Manual mobilizing techniques in degenerative arthrosis of the hip.* Bulletin of the Orthopaedic Section, APTA 2/1:7, 1977.
7. Hoppenfeld, S: *Physical Examination of the Spine and Extremities.* Appleton-Century-Crofts, New York, 1976.
8. Kaltenborn, FM: *Mobilization of the Extremity Joints: Examination and Basic Treatment Techniques.* Olaf Norlis Bokhandel, Universitetsgaten, Oslo, 1980.
9. Kessler, R and Hertling, D: *Management of Common Musculoskeletal Disorders.* Harper & Row, Philadelphia, 1983.
10. Lehmkuhl, LD and Smith, LM: *Brunnstrom's Clinical Kinesiology,* ed 4. FA Davis, Philadelphia, 1983.
11. Maitland, GD: *Peripheral Manipulation,* ed 2. Butterworth, Boston, 1977.
12. Norkin, C and Levangie, P: *Joint Structure and Function: A Comprehensive Analysis.* FA Davis, Philadelphia, 1983.
13. Paris, SV: *Mobilization of the spine.* Phys Ther 59:988, 1979.
14. Svendsen, B, Moe, K, and Merritt, R: *Joint Mobilization Laboratory Manual: Extremity Joint Testing and Selected Treatment Techniques.* Bryn Mawr, CA, 1981.
15. Warwick, R and Williams, S (eds): *Arthrology.* In *Gray's Anatomy,* 35th British ed. WB Saunders, Philadelphia, 1973.
16. Wyke, B: *The neurology of joints.* Ann R Coll Surg 41:25, 1967.
17. Wyke, B: *Articular neurology—A review.* Physiotherapy March: 94, 1972.
18. Wyke, B: *Neurological Aspects of Pain for the Physical Therapy Clinician.* Physical Therapy Forum '82, Lecture, Columbus, 1982.
19. Magee, D: *Orthopedic Physical Assessment.* WB Saunders Co, Philadelphia, 1987.
20. Wadsworth, C: *Manual Examination of the Spine and Extremities.* Williams & Wilkins, Baltimore, 1988.

PART —————— 2

APPLICATION OF THERAPEUTIC EXERCISE TECHNIQUES TO REGIONS OF THE BODY

CHAPTER ——————— 6

Principles of Treating Soft-Tissue, Bony, and Postsurgical Problems

The proper use of therapeutic exercise in the treatment of musculoskeletal disorders depends on identifying the structure involved and recognizing its stage of recovery. Evaluation is an important prerequisite for identifying the anatomic structure or structures that are causing pain or limiting function and also for determining whether the tissue is in the acute, subacute, or chronic stage of recovery. Information summarizing an orthopedic evaluation and suggested references for study are included in Chapter 1. This chapter and subsequent chapters in this section have been written with the assumption that the reader has a background in evaluation and assessment.

OBJECTIVES

After studying this chapter, the reader will be able to:
1. identify examples of soft-tissue lesions.
2. identify characteristics of soft-tissue repair during the stages of inflammation, healing, and restoration of function.
3. identify special considerations, treatment goals, and plan of care for soft-tissue lesions during the inflammatory and healing stages of tissue repair and during the restoration of function.
4. identify special considerations, treatment goals, and a plan of care for specific joint disorders during exacerbation and remission of symptoms.
5. identify special considerations, treatment goals, and a plan of care for recovery following fractures.
6. identify special considerations, treatment goals, and a plan of care for presurgical and postsurgical management.

I. SOFT-TISSUE LESIONS

A. Examples of Soft-Tissue Lesions

1. **Strain**

   Overstretching, overexertion, overuse of soft tissue; tends to be less severe than a sprain. Occurs from slight trauma or unaccustomed repeated trauma of a minor degree.[4] This term is frequently used to refer specifically to some degree of disruption of the musculotendinous unit.[14]

2. **Sprain**

   Severe stress, stretch, or tear of soft tissues such as joint capsule, ligament, tendon, or muscle. This term is frequently used to refer specifically to injury of a ligament, and is graded as first- (mild), second- (moderate), or third- (severe) degree sprains.[14]

3. **Subluxation**

   An incomplete or partial dislocation that often involves secondary trauma to surrounding soft tissue

4. **Dislocation**

   Displacement of a part, usually the bony partners within a joint, leading to soft-tissue damage, inflammation, pain, and muscle spasm

5. **Muscle/tendon rupture or tear**

   If a rupture or tear is partial, pain is experienced in the region of the breach when the muscle is stretched or when it contracts against resistance. If a rupture or tear is complete, the muscle does not pull against the injury, so stretching or contraction of the muscle does not cause pain.[9]

6. **Tendinous lesions**[3,10]

   Tenosynovitis is an inflammation of the synovial sheath covering a tendon.
   Tendinitis is scarring or calcium deposits in a tendon.
   Tenovaginitis is a thickening of a tendon sheath.

7. **Synovitis**

   Inflammation of a synovial membrane; an excess of normal synovial fluid within a joint or tendon sheath from trauma or disease[29]

8. **Hemarthrosis**

   Bleeding into a joint, usually from severe trauma[29]

9. **Ganglia**

   A ballooning of the wall of a joint capsule or tendon sheath. Ganglia may arise following trauma; they sometimes occur with rheumatoid arthritis.

10. **Bursitis**

    Inflammation of a bursa

11. **Contusion**

    Bruising from a direct blow, resulting in capillary rupture, bleeding, edema, and an inflammatory response

12. **Overuse syndromes**

Repeated, submaximal overload and/or frictional wear to a muscle or tendon resulting in inflammation and pain

B. Clinical Conditions Resulting from Trauma or Pathology

In many conditions involving soft tissue, the primary pathology is difficult to define, or the tissue has healed with limitations, resulting in a secondary loss of function. The following are examples of clinical manifestations resulting from a variety of causes, including those listed under the previous section.

1. **Dysfunction**

Loss of normal function of a tissue or region. The dysfunction may be due to adaptive shortening of the soft tissues, adhesions, muscle weakness, or any condition resulting in loss of normal mobility.

2. **Joint dysfunction**

Mechanical loss of normal joint play in synovial joints; commonly causes loss of function and pain. Precipitating factors may be trauma, immobilization, disuse, aging, or a serious pathologic condition.[29]

3. **Contractures**

Shortening or tightening of skin, fascia, muscle, or joint capsule that prevents normal mobility or flexibility of that structure

4. **Adhesions**

Abnormal adherence of collagen fibers to surrounding structures during immobilization, following trauma, or as a complication of surgery, which restricts normal elasticity of the structures involved

5. **Reflex muscle guarding (see also intrinsic muscle spasm)**

The prolonged contraction of a muscle in response to a painful stimulus. The primary pain-causing lesion may be in nearby or underlying tissue or from a referred pain source. When not referred, the contracting muscle functionally splints the injured tissue against movement. Guarding ceases when the painful stimulus is relieved.

6. **Intrinsic muscle spasm**

The prolonged contraction of a muscle in response to the local circulatory and metabolic changes that occur when a muscle is in a continued state of contraction. Pain is a result of the altered circulatory and metabolic environment, so the muscle contraction becomes self-perpetuating regardless of whether the primary lesion that caused the initial guarding is still irritable (Figure 6-1). Spasm may also be a response of muscle to viral infection, cold, prolonged periods of immobilization, emotional tension, or direct trauma to muscle.[29]

7. **Muscle weakness**

A decrease in the strength of contraction of muscle. Muscle weakness may be the result of a systemic, chemical, or local lesion of a nerve of the central or peripheral nervous system or the myoneural junction. It may also be the result of a direct insult to the muscle or may simply be due to inactivity.

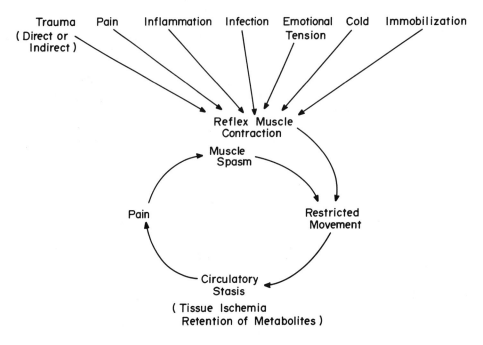

FIGURE 6-1. Schematic of the self-perpetuating cycle of muscle spasm.

C. Severity of Tissue Injury[14,15]

1. Grade 1 (first-degree)

Mild pain at the time of injury or within the first 24 hours; mild swelling, local tenderness, and pain occur when the tissue is stressed

2. Grade 2 (second-degree)

Moderate pain that requires stopping the activity. Stress and palpation of the tissue greatly increases the pain. When the injury is to ligaments, some of the fibers are torn, resulting in some increased joint mobility.

3. Grade 3 (third-degree)

Near-complete or complete tear or avulsion of the tissue (tendon or ligament) with severe pain. Stress to the tissue is usually painless; palpation may reveal the defect. A torn ligament results in instability of the joint.

II. STAGES OF INFLAMMATION AND REPAIR: GENERAL DESCRIPTIONS

Following any insult to connective tissue, whether it is from mechanical injury or chemical irritant, the body responses and stages of healing are similar (Figure 6-2). In the following outline, the number of days given for each stage is approximate, and the stages overlap. Differences in individual patients must also be taken into account. The response of the patient is the best guideline for determining when treatment should progress from one stage to the next.

PHYSICAL THERAPY	ACUTE STAGE Inflammatory-Reaction	SUBACUTE STAGE Repair and Healing	CHRONIC STAGE Maturation and Remodeling
CHARACTERISTICS	Vascular changes Exudation of cells and chemicals Clot formation Phagocytosis, neutralization of irritants Early fibroblastic activity	Removal of noxious stimuli Growth of capillary beds into area Collagen formation Granulation tissue Very fragile, easily injured tissue	Maturation of connective tissue Contracture of scar tissue Remodeling of scar Collagen aligns to stress
CLINICAL SIGNS	Inflammation Pain before tissue resistance	Decreasing inflammation Pain synchronous with tissue resistance	Absence of inflammation Pain after tissue resistance
TREATMENT APPROACH	Control effects of inflammation: Modalities Immobilization Cautious gentle movement	Prevent or minimize contracture and adhesion formation: Gentle active movement, gradually increasing in intensity and range	Restore function: Progressive stretching, strengthening, and functional exercises

FIGURE 6-2. Characteristics and clinical signs of the stages of inflammation, repair, and maturation of tissue.

A. Acute (Inflammatory-Reaction) Stage

1. Characteristics

This stage involves both cellular and humoral responses. During the first 48 hours following insult to soft tissue, vascular changes predominate. Exudation of cells and solutes from the blood vessels takes place, and clot formation occurs. Within this period, neutralization of the chemical irritants or noxious stimuli, phagocytosis (cleaning up of dead tissue), early fibroblastic activity, and formation of new capillary beds begin. These physiologic processes serve as a protective mechanism as well as a stimulus for subsequent healing and repair.[27,28] Usually this stage lasts 4 to 6 days unless the insult is perpetuated.

2. Clinical signs

The signs of inflammation are present: swelling, redness, heat, pain, and loss of function. When testing the range of motion (ROM), the patient will experience pain, and there may be muscle guarding before completion of the range (Figure 6-3A).

B. Subacute (Repair-Healing) Stage

As the inflammation decreases (during the 2nd to 4th day), resolution of the clot and repair of the injured site begins. This usually lasts an additional 10 to 17 days (14 to 21 days after the onset of injury), but may last up to 6 weeks.

1. Characteristics

This stage is characterized by the synthesis and deposition of collagen. Noxious stimuli are removed, and growth of capillary beds into the area takes place. Fibroblastic activity, collagen formation, and granulation tissue development increase. Fibroblasts are in tremendous number by the 4th day after injury and continue in large number until about the 21st day.[5] The fibroblasts produce new collagen. The immature collagen replaces the exudate that originally formed the clot. Wound closure in muscle and skin usually takes 5 to 8 days; in tendons and ligaments, 3 to 5 weeks. During this stage, immature connective tissue is produced that is thin and unorganized. It is very fragile and easily injured if overstressed, yet proper growth and alignment can be stimulated by appropriate tensile loading in the line of normal stresses for that tissue. At the same time, adherence to surrounding tissues can be minimized.[7]

2. Clinical signs

The signs of inflammation progressively decrease and eventually are absent. When testing ROM, the patient experiences pain synchronous with encountering tissue resistance at the end of the available ROM (Figure 6-3B).

C. Chronic (Maturation and Remodeling) Stage

1. The term *chronic* is used to describe:

a. that time during the late stages of tissue repair or recovery when there are no signs of inflammation, yet the patient has not gained full function (overlapping with the subacute stage around the 14th to 21st day after insult); or

b. a condition that is long-standing with recurring episodes of pain from

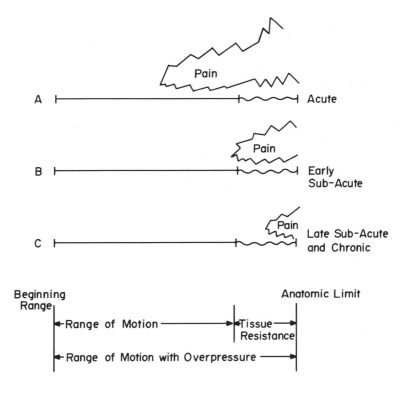

FIGURE 6-3. Pain experienced with range of motion when involved tissue is in the acute stage (*A*), early subacute stage (*B*), and late subacute or chronic stage (*C*).

chronic inflammation, or in which there are dysfunctions resulting from the healing process. (see Section D.)

2. Characteristics

There is maturation of the connective tissue as collagen fibers form from fibrils and scar tissue matures. Remodeling occurs as collagen fibers become thicker and reorient in response to stresses placed on the connective tissue. The scar begins to retract from activity of the myofibroblasts. The higher the density of the connective tissue, the longer the remodeling time.

a. Because of the way immature collagen molecules are held together (hydrogen bonding) and adhere to surrounding tissue, they can easily be remodeled with gentle and persistent treatment. This is possible for 8 to 10 weeks.[9] If not properly stressed, the fibers adhere to surrounding tissue and form a restricting scar.

b. As the structure of collagen changes (covalent bonding) and thickens, it becomes stronger and resistant to remodeling. At 14 weeks, the scar tissue is unresponsive to remodeling. An old scar has a poor response to stretch.[8] Treatment under these conditions requires adaptive lengthening in the tissue surrounding the scar or surgical release.

3. Clinical signs

There are no signs of inflammation. When testing ROM, the patient does not feel pain until after resistance from the tissue is met and overpressure is applied to shortened or weakened structures. The patient may have decreased strength, decreased range of motion, and some loss of function. Restoration of function begins in this stage (Figure 6-3C).

D. Chronic Inflammation

1. Characteristics[8]

If excessive stresses or irritants are applied to the developing and remodeling scar tissue, the inflammatory process is perpetuated at low levels of intensity. Proliferation of fibroblasts with increased collagen production and degradation of mature collagen leads to a predominance of new, immature collagen. This has an overall weakening effect on the tissue. The myofibroblastic activity continues, which may lead to progressive limitation of motion. Efforts to stretch the tissue perpetuate the irritation and progressive limitation.

2. Clinical signs[7,8]

There are increased pain, swelling, and muscle guarding that lasts more than several hours after activity. There are an increased feeling of stiffness after rest, loss of range of motion 24 hours after activity, and progressive increased stiffness of the tissue as long as the irritation persists.

III. THE ACUTE STAGE: GENERAL TREATMENT GUIDELINES

A. Clinical Considerations During the Acute (Inflammatory) Stage of Soft-Tissue Insult

1. During the inflammatory stage there are pain and impaired movement from:
    a. irritating chemicals.
       The altered chemical state from the tissue reaction irritates the nerve endings.
    b. edema.
       Increased interstitial fluid from the altered circulatory pattern causes increased tension in the connective tissue, which restricts movement and causes pain.
    c. muscle guarding and spasm.
       The body's way of immobilizing an injured or painful area is with reflex muscle contraction. The spasm may be the result of direct muscle trauma but is usually in response to tissue injury in structures underlying the muscle.
    d. joint swelling (effusion).
       This occurs if there is trauma to a joint or if there is an arthritic disease (see Sections VII and VIII). The increased effusion into the joint space distends the capsule and prevents normal movement of the bony partners. The joint assumes a position in which the capsule can distend to its maximum. This occurs only with joint trauma or joint disease.
2. In order to relieve the musculoskeletal pain and promote healing, RESTING the part affected by the inflammatory process is necessary during the first 24 hours, but complete immobilization can lead to the adherence of

developing fibrils to surrounding tissue,[9] weakening of connective tissue,[29] and changes in articular cartilage.[18]

3. The *ultimate goal of treatment* is the formation of a strong, mobile scar at the site of the lesion so that there is complete and painless restoration of function. Initially, the network of fibril formation is random. It acquires an organized arrangement according to the mechanical forces acting on the tissue. To influence the development of an organized scar, begin treatment during the acute stage, when tolerated, with PASSIVE MOVEMENTS.

   a. These movements should be specific to the structure involved in order to prevent abnormal adherence of the developing fibrils to surrounding tissue and thus avoid future disruption of the scar.

   b. The intensity (dosage) should be gentle enough so that the fibrils are not detached from the site of healing. Too much movement too soon will be painful and will re-injure the tissue. The dosage of passive movement depends on the severity of the lesion. Some patients tolerate no movement during the first 24 to 48 hours; others tolerate only a few degrees of gentle passive movement. Continuous passive movement (CPM; see Chapter 2) has been useful immediately following various types of surgery to joints; intra-articular, metaphyseal, and diaphyseal fractures; surgical release of extra-articular contractures and adhesions; as well as other selected conditions.[23] Any movement tolerated at this stage is beneficial, but it must NOT increase the inflammation or pain.

   c. Movement of structures in the same region should also be done in appropriate dosages to maintain functional integrity and mobility, but the movement should not be disruptive to the healing process of the involved tissue.

   d. Active movement is CONTRAINDICATED at the site of an active pathologic process.[29]

4. **Dosages and techniques specific to tissues** in a state of inflammation and to related structures in the same vicinity follow.

   Precaution: If the movement causes increased pain or an inflammatory response, it is either of too great a dosage or it should not be done. Extreme care must be used with movement at this stage.

   a. *Joint and ligamentous pathology*

      (1) Passive range of motion, within the limit of pain, to maintain movement without stress. This range will probably be very small initially.[29]

      (2) Gentle passive joint traction or glides within the limit of pain; do not stretch the capsule or ligaments. Grade I or II distraction, glides, or oscillations performed in a pain-free position can be attempted; note the joint response before proceeding[13,16] (see Chapter 5). Besides maintaining mobility in the capsule and supporting ligaments and moving the synovial fluid to enhance cartilage nutrition and diffusion of waste products, these techniques may help to block the transmission of nociceptive stimuli to relieve pain via neurologic mechanisms.

      (3) Gentle massage to the injured site may benefit circulation to decrease edema and decrease pain.[9]

      (4) Intermittent muscle setting benefits the related muscle and circulation without moving the joint.[29]

  b. *Muscle pathology*
   (1) Passive range of motion within the limit of pain to maintain movement without stress. Stretching at this stage is contraindicated.
   (2) Intermittent muscle setting, with the injured muscle in a relaxed or shortened position. This will cause the muscle to broaden and keep the developing scar mobile, yet will not cause separation of the healing breech.[9]
   (3) Electrical stimulation with the muscle in the shortened range will have the same benefit as muscle setting.
   (4) If tolerated, massage applied transverse to the healing fibers is advocated to keep the developing scar mobile.[5,9] The dosage should be gentle in this early stage and should be followed with gentle muscle setting contractions.
   (5) Gentle massage may benefit circulation to decrease edema and pain sensation.
   (6) Passive joint-play movements (Grade I or II) applied to related joints maintains normal motion while the muscle begins healing and cannot be moved through its full range of motion.[29]
  c. *Tendinous lesions*
   (1) Gentle dosage of massage applied transverse to the injured fibers is advocated to smooth roughened surfaces of a tendon. The tendon is kept taut during the massage.[9]
   (2) Passive ROM within the limit of pain and joint-play movements (Grade I or II) maintain joint range without stressing the injured tissue.
  d. *Other connective tissue*
   (1) Passive range of motion within the limit of pain to maintain movement without stress. Stretching is contraindicated at this stage.
   (2) Muscle-setting exercises to assist with circulation and muscle function.
   (3) Passive joint-play movements (Grade I or II) to maintain joint integrity.
   (4) Gentle massage to maintain mobility of the connective tissue and to assist lymphatic flow and circulation.
 5. Maintain as normal a physiologic state as possible in related areas of the body. Include techniques to maintain or improve
  a. range of motion. These may be done actively or passively, depending on the proximity to and the effect on the injured tissue.
  b. muscle strength. Resistance may be applied at an appropriate dosage to muscles not directly related to the injured tissue to prepare the patient for use of assistive devices such as crutches or walkers and to improve functional activities.
  c. functional activities. Supportive or adaptive devices may be necessary depending on area of injury and necessary functional activities.
  d. circulation. It will be helped by doing the above activities as well as by using supportive elastic wraps, by elevating the part, and by using muscle-setting techniques.

B. Treatment Considerations: Acute Stage (0 to 4 Days)
 1. Problems summarized
  a. Inflammation, pain, edema, muscle spasm
  b. Impaired movement

      c. Joint effusion (if the joint is injured or if there is arthritis)

      d. Decreased use of associated areas

  2. General treatment goals and plan of care

Goals	*Plan of Care*
a. Control pain, edema, spasm	a. Cold, compression, elevation (48 hours) Immobilize the part (rest, splint, tape, cast) Avoid positions of stress to the part Gentle (Grade I) joint oscillations with joint in pain-free position
b. Maintain soft-tissue and joint integrity and mobility	b. Appropriate dosage of passive movements within limit of pain, specific to structure involved Appropriate dosage of intermittent muscle setting or electrical stimulation
c. Reduce joint swelling if symptoms are present	c. May require medical intervention if swelling is rapid (blood) Provide protection (splint, cast)
d. Maintain integrity and function of associated areas	d. Active-assistive, free, or resistive exercises, depending on proximity to and effect on the primary lesion Adaptive or assistive devices as needed to protect the part during functional activities

Precautions: The proper dosage of rest and movement must be used during the inflammatory stage. Signs of too much movement are increased pain or increased inflammation.

Contraindication: Stretching activities and resistance exercises are contraindicated when there are signs of inflammation.[29]

IV. THE SUBACUTE STAGE: GENERAL TREATMENT GUIDELINES

A. Clinical Considerations During the Subacute Stage of Healing Following Soft-Tissue Insult

  1. Pain and inflammation decrease as healing progresses. The new tissue being developed is fragile and easily interrupted. The patient often feels good and returns to normal activity too soon.

    a. Exercises progressed too vigorously or functional activities begun too early can be injurious to the fragile, newly developing tissue and therefore may delay recovery by perpetuating the inflammatory response.[28,29]

    b. If movement is not progressed, the new tissue adheres to surrounding structures and will become a source of pain and limited tissue mobility.[9]

  2. Because of the restricted use of the injured region, some muscle weak-

ness occurs even in the absence of muscle pathology. Muscle strengthening exercises can begin during the subacute stage but must be kept within the tolerance of the healing tissues. In the early stages, submaximal isometric exercises should be used to provide resistance to the muscle; low-intensity isometric exercises will not interrupt the developing collagen network as isotonic exercises would.

3. This is a transition period during which active movement can begin and progress with care. If activity is kept within a safe dosage and frequency, symptoms of pain and swelling will progressively decrease each day. Patient response is the best guide to how quickly or vigorously the progression can be. If signs of inflammation increase or the range of motion decreases then the intensity of exercise and activity must decrease.[29]

4. Progression of dosage (intensity) of exercise should be specific to the tissue involved and related structures.

   a. *Joint and ligamentous pathology*
      (1) Progress from passive, to active-assistive, to active ROM, within the limits of pain.
      (2) Passive joint-play movements are continued within the limits of pain.
          —If there is limited range with joint effusion, stretching of the capsule is contraindicated; continue use of Grade I or II sustained or oscillating techniques.
          —If there is limited range and decreased joint play with no joint effusion, stretching techniques to the capsule can begin; use sustained Grade II techniques and note the joint response before proceeding (see Chapter 5).
      (3) Increase the intensity of cross-fiber massage or soft-tissue massage to keep the ligaments and surrounding soft tissue moving freely across the joint.
      (4) Continue to maintain associated muscle integrity by progressing isometric exercises as tolerated.

   b. *Muscle pathology*
      (1) Progress from passive, to active-assistive, to active ROM, within the limits of pain.
      (2) Progress lengthening of the muscle with gentle contract-relax techniques or electrical stimulation. Begin with the muscle in the shortened position; have the muscle contract isometrically against *minimal* resistance, then relax, then elongate it a short distance. Repeat with each new length. Do not elongate beyond the limit of pain; continue just to the point of discomfort.
      (3) Progress the intensity of the cross-fiber massage within the patient's tolerance. The muscle is kept in the shortened position while applying the massage.
      (4) Continue to maintain joint-play movements in associated joints until the muscle has regained full range of motion. Use sustained Grade II glides.

   c. *Tendinous lesions*
      (1) Increase the intensity of the cross-fiber massage.
      (2) Progress from passive to active ROM within the limits of pain.
      (3) Maintain joint play with sustained Grade II traction or glide techniques.

    d. *Other connective tissue*
      (1) Progress from passive, to active-assistive, to active ROM within the limit of pain.
      (2) Cross-fiber friction or soft-tissue massage can be applied to specific sites that have been injured. Begin gently and progress as the patient tolerates the massage.
      (3) Progress isometric exercises to maintain muscle and circulatory integrity.
      (4) Continue to maintain joint-play movements (sustained Grade II) in associated joints until soft tissue flexibility has been restored.
  5. Continue to maintain as normal a physiologic and functional state as possible in related areas of the body.

B. Treatment Considerations: Subacute Stage (Day 4 to Day 14 or 21)

1. Problems summarized
  a. Pain when end of available range of motion is reached
  b. Decreasing soft-tissue edema
  c. Decreasing joint effusion (if joints are involved)
  d. Developing soft tissue, muscle, and/or joint contractures
  e. Developing muscle weakness from reduced usage
  f. Decreased functional use of the part and associated areas

2. General treatment goals and plan of care

Goals	*Plan of Care*
a. Control pain, edema, and joint swelling	a. Monitor response of tissue to exercise progression, decrease intensity if inflammation increases Protect healing tissue with assistive devices, splints, tape, or wrap; gradually increase amount of time the joint is free to move each day
b. Progressively increase soft tissue, muscle, and/or joint mobility	b. Progress from passive to active-assistive to active ROM within limits of pain Gradually increase mobility of scar, specific to structure involved (see section IV A 4 above) Progressively increase mobility of related structures if they are tight; use techniques specific to tight structure
c. Strengthen supporting and related muscles	c. Initially, progress isometric exercises within patient's tolerance; begin cautiously with mild resistance As range of motion, joint play, and healing improve, prog-

d. Maintain integrity and function of associated areas

ress to isotonic exercises with resistance progressing as tolerated (see section V A 4)

d. Apply progressive strengthening exercises, depending on proximity to and effect on the primary lesion

Gradually decrease the amount of support from assistive devices as strength increases

Precautions: The signs of inflammation or joint swelling normally decrease early in this stage. Some discomfort will occur as the activity level is progressed, but it should not last longer than a couple of hours. Signs of too much motion or activity are resting pain, fatigue, increased weakness, and spasm.[29]

V. THE CHRONIC STAGE: GENERAL TREATMENT GUIDELINES

A. Clinical Considerations During the Chronic-Remodeling Stage

1. The primary differences between the late subacute and chronic stages are the improvement in quality (orientation and tensile strength) of the collagen and the reduction in size of the wound during the chronic stages.[7,8,15] The quantity of collagen stabilizes; there is a balance between the synthesis and degradation. Because remodeling of the maturing collagen occurs in response to the stresses placed on it, it is important to use controlled forces that duplicate normal stresses on the tissue. Maximal strength of the collagen will develop in the direction of the imposed forces. Excessive or abnormal stresses will lead to re-injury and chronic inflammation, which can be detrimental to the return of function.

2. If mobility has been maintained in the injured tissue as well as the related structures, progression of activity and function continues as already outlined (see Section IV B 2) but with greater intensity.

3. Pain that the patient now experiences arises only when stress is placed on contractures or adhesions beyond the available range of motion. Usually no pain is felt within the available range. To avoid chronic or recurring pain, the contractures need to be stretched or the adhesions need to be broken up. Stretching of the tissues should be selective, using techniques appropriate to the tissue involved (see Chapters 4 and 5; also B 2 b in this section).

4. For progression of the patient to independent functional activities, two considerations are important[29]

   a. Free joint play within a useful (or functional) range of motion is necessary to avoid joint trauma. If joint play is restricted, joint mobilizing techniques should be used. These stretching techniques can be vigorous as long as no signs of increased irritation result.

   b. Joint motion without adequate muscle support will cause trauma to that joint as functional activities are attempted. Zohn and Mennell[29] recommend that the criterion for strength be a muscle test grade of Good in lower extremity musculature before discontinuing use of supportive or assistive devices for ambulation.

(1) To increase strength when there is a loss of joint play, isometric exercises are recommended.

(2) Once joint play within the available ROM is restored, resistive isotonic exercises are recommended for that available range. This does not imply that normal ROM needs to be present before initiating isotonic exercises but that joint play, within the available range, be present (see Chapter 5 for information on joint play).

c. In summary, both joint dynamics and muscle strength and flexibility should be balanced as the injured part is restored to functional usage.

5. Any adhesions in the fascia, skin, or other soft tissue such as ligaments will restrict motion and should be mobilized with soft-tissue stretching techniques specific to the tissue.

6. Depending on the size of the structure or degree of injury or pathology, healing will continue for 12 to 18 months. The principles of treatment that follow should be continued until the part is pain free with normal range of motion and good strength.

7. To return to greater-than-normal activities (such as required in sports participation and heavy-work settings) prior to regaining normal pain-free range of motion and normal strength will probably result in recurring pain. Therefore, it is important that these goals be met under such circumstances.

B. TREATMENT CONSIDERATIONS

Chronic stage. (Begins between day 14 to 21 and lasts until there is pain-free functional use of the part.)

1. Problems summarized

(all, some, or none of the problems are present)

a. Pain is experienced only when stress is applied to structures in dysfunction (pain after tissue resistance is met).

b. Soft-tissue, muscle, and/or joint contractures or adhesions limit normal range of motion or joint play.

c. Muscle weakness.

d. Decreased functional usage of the involved part.

2. General treatment goals and plan of care

Goals	*Plan of Care*
a. Decrease pain from stress on contractures or adhesions	a. Modalities Stretching of limiting structures
b. Increase soft-tissue, muscle, and/or joint mobility	b. Select stretching techniques specific to the tight tissue: soft tissue: passive stretch and massage joints, capsules, and selected ligaments: joint mobilization ligaments, tendons, and soft-tissue adhesions: cross-fiber massage muscles: active inhibition or flexibility techniques

c. Strengthen supporting and related muscles

c. With limited range and joint play: isometric exercises at various angles of the range.
   When joint play is good: dynamic resistive exercise (isotonic or isokinetic)

d. Progress functional independence

d. Continue using supportive and/or assistive devices until the range of motion is functional with good joint play, and the results of supporting muscle strength tests are Good (see section V A 4)
   Progress functional training in ambulation, stair climbing, or other appropriate activities.
   Continue progressive strengthening exercises and training activities until the muscles are strong enough for the individual's functional level.

Precautions: There should be no signs of inflammation. Some discomfort will occur as the activity level is progressed, but it should not last longer than a couple of hours. Signs that activities are progressing too quickly or with too great a dosage are joint swelling, pain that lasts longer than 4 hours or that requires medication for relief, a decrease in strength, or fatiguing more easily.[29]

VI. CHRONIC RECURRING PAIN: GENERAL TREATMENT GUIDELINES

A. Pain that Recurs from an Old Injury May Be the Result of

1. too early return to function, before proper healing has occurred, resulting in re-injury, e.g., chronic inflammation.
2. tearing of scar tissue that had adhered to surrounding tissues and thus had poor mobility. This may be from scar tissue that was not properly aligned to stress while healing.[9]
3. contractures or poor mobility in structures that then become stressed with repeated or vigorous activity.

B. Treatment Approaches Include

1. treating chronic inflammation or a re-injury as an acute injury, following the principles and program as previously outlined. It is critical to decrease the inflammatory response as well as to eliminate the mechanism of chronic irritation. Evaluate for faulty mechanics or faulty habits that may be sustaining the problem and develop a program to correct them.
2. stretching any contractures as outlined in section V, with reference to Chapters 4 and 5. This should be done after the inflammation is gone. With unyielding scar tissue, stretching of the soft tissue surrounding the scar using techniques that are specific to that tissue may be necessary to increase the mobility of the region.

3. rupturing an adhesion (with cross-fiber massage or manipulation) and treating it as an acute condition, following the principles and progression as previously outlined.

VII. RHEUMATOID ARTHRITIS: GENERAL TREATMENT GUIDELINES

A. Characteristics of Rheumatoid Arthritis (RA)[3]

1. RA is a connective tissue disease. The onset and progression vary from mild joint symptoms with aching and stiffness to abrupt swelling, stiffness, and progressive deformity. There are usually periods of exacerbation (flare) and remission.
2. Joints are characteristically involved with early inflammatory changes in the synovial membrane, peripheral portions of the articular cartilage, and subchondral marrow spaces. In response, granulation tissue (pannus) forms, covers, and erodes the articular cartilage. Adhesions may form, restricting joint mobility. With progression of the disease, cancellous bone becomes exposed. Fibrosis or ossific ankylosis may eventually result, causing deformity and disability.
3. Inflammatory changes may also occur in tendon sheaths (tenosynovitis), and if subjected to a lot of friction, they may fray or rupture.
4. Extra-articular pathologic changes sometimes occur; these include rheumatoid nodules, atrophy, and fibrosis of muscles and mild cardiac changes.

B. Clinical Considerations

1. With synovial inflammation, there is effusion and swelling of the joints, which causes aching and limited motion. Usually there is pain on motion, and a slight increase in temperature can be detected over the joints.
2. Onset is usually in the smaller joints of the hands and feet, most commonly in the proximal interphalangeal joints. Usually symptoms are bilateral.
3. With progression, the joints become deformed and may ankylose or sublux.
4. Pain is often felt in adjoining muscles; eventually muscle atrophy and weakness occur. Asymmetry in muscle pull adds to the deforming forces.
5. The person fatigues easily and requires additional rest during periods of flare up in order not to stress the joints.
6. Therapeutic exercises cannot positively alter the pathologic process of rheumatoid arthritis, but if administered carefully, they can help prevent, retard, or correct the mechanical limitations that occur (see precautions and contraindications in section C below).

C. Treatment Considerations During the Active Disease Period

1. **Problems summarized**
   a. Tenderness and warmth over the involved joints with joint swelling
   b. Muscle guarding and pain on motion
   c. Joint stiffness and limited motion
   d. Muscle weakness and atrophy
   e. Potential deformity and ankylosis from the degenerative process and asymmetric muscle pull

2. General treatment goals and plan of care

Goals	Plan of Care
a. Relieve pain and muscle guarding and promote relaxation	a. Modalities Gentle massage Immobilize in splint Relaxation techniques
b. Minimize joint stiffness and maintain available motion	b. Passive or active-assistive ROM within limits of pain, gradual progression as tolerated Gentle joint techniques using Grade I or II oscillations (Chapter 5)
c. Minimize muscle atrophy	c. Gentle muscle setting
d. Prevent deformity and protect the joint structures	d. Use of supportive and assistive equipment for all pathologically active joints Good bed positioning while resting Avoidance of activities that stress the joints Patient education

Precautions during the active inflammatory period:
  The patient fatigues easily and therefore requires more rest than usual. He should be cautioned to avoid stress and fatigue and should be taught methods of energy conservation during daily activities.
  Secondary effects of medications and steroids may include osteoporosis and ligamentous laxity, so exercises should not cause stress to bones or joints.
  If medication controls the swelling and secondary pain, exercise can be progressed carefully.

Contraindications during the active inflammatory period:
  Maximum resistive exercise should not be done. Even though muscles tend to weaken, vigorous strengthening exercises will cause joint compression and increase the irritability of the joint, potentially increasing damage to the joint surfaces.
  Stretching techniques should not be done. The limited motion in a swollen joint is caused by excessive fluid in the joint space, not from adhesions. To force motion on the distended capsule will overstretch it with subsequent hypermobility (or subluxation) when the swelling abates. It may also increase the irritability of the joint and prolong the joint reaction.

D. Treatment Considerations During the Remission Period

1. Potential problems summarized

a. Pain when stress is applied to mechanical restrictions
b. Limited range of motion and joint play from soft-tissue, muscle, and/or joint contractures or adhesions
c. Secondary muscle weakness
d. Postural changes or joint deformities
e. Decreased functional usage of the part and related regions

2. Goals and plan of care are the same as with any subacute and chronic musculoskeletal disorder, except appropriate precautions must be taken because the pathologic changes from the disease process make the parts more susceptible to damage.

   Precautions: The joint capsule, ligaments, and tendons may be structurally weakened by the rheumatic process (also as a result of using steroids), so the dosage of stretching techniques used to counter any contractures or adhesions must be carefully graded.

   Contraindications: Vigorous stretching or manipulative techniques.[16,17]

VIII. OSTEOARTHRITIS: GENERAL TREATMENT GUIDELINES

A. Characteristics of Osteoarthritis or Degenerative Joint Disease (DJD)[3,24,26]

1. DJD is a chronic degenerative disorder primarily affecting the articular cartilage of synovial joints, with eventual bony remodeling and overgrowth at the margins of the joints (spurs and lipping). There is also a progression of synovial and capsular thickening and joint effusion. With degeneration, there may be capsular laxity as a result of bone remodeling and capsule distention, resulting in hypermobility or instability in some ranges. With pain and decreased willingness to move, contractures eventually develop in portions of the capsule and overlying muscle, so that as the disease progresses, motion becomes more limited.[26]

2. Causes may be due to mechanical injury, from either a major stress or repeated minor stresses, or due to poor movement of synovial fluid when the joint is immobilized.[24] Rapid destruction of articular cartilage occurs with immobilization, because the cartilage is not being bathed by moving synovial fluid and is thus deprived of its nutritional supply.

3. The cartilage loses its ability to withstand stress; it splits and thins out. Eventually the bone becomes exposed. There is increased density of the bone along the joint line, with cystic bone loss and osteoporosis in the adjacent metaphysis. In the early stages, the joint is usually asymptomatic since the cartilage is avascular and aneural.

B. Clinical Considerations

1. Pain usually occurs because of compressive stresses on or excessive activity of the involved joint and is relieved with rest. In the late stages of the disease, pain is often present at rest. The pain is probably from secondary involvement of subchondral bone, synovium, and the joint capsule. In the spine, if bony growth encroaches on the nerve root, there may be radicular pain.

2. Usually there are brief periods of stiffness in the morning or following periods of rest. Movement relieves the stiffness.

3. Affected joints may become enlarged. Heberden's nodes (enlargement of the distal interphalangeal joint of the fingers) are common.

4. Most commonly involved are weight-bearing joints (hips and knees), the cervical and lumbar spine, and the distal interphalangeal joints of the fingers and carpometacarpal joint of the thumb.

5. Crepitation or loose bodies may occur within the joint.

6. Stiffness occurs with inactivity, but increased pain occurs with excessive mechanical stress or activity. Therefore, moderation of activity and correc-

tion of the biomechanical stresses can prevent, retard, or correct the mechanical limitations.
7. With progression of the disease, the bony remodeling, swelling, and contractures alter the transmission of forces through the joint, which further perpetuates the deforming forces and creates joint deformity.
8. Progressive weakening in the muscle occurs either from inactivity or from inhibition of the neuronal pools.
9. Impairment of joint position sense may occur.

C. Treatment Considerations for Osteoarthritis

1. Problems summarized

a. Stiffness following inactivity
b. Pain with mechanical stress or excessive activity
c. Limitation of motion (as the condition progresses)
d. Pain at rest (in the advanced stages)
e. Potential deformity

2. General treatment goals and plan of care

Goals	Plan of Care
a. Decrease effects of stiffness from inactivity	a. Patient education Active range of motion Joint-play techniques
b. Decrease pain from mechanical stress	b. Supportive and/or assistive equipment to minimize stress or to correct faulty biomechanics Increase strength in supporting muscles Alternate activity with periods of rest.
c. Increase range of motion	c. Stretch muscle, joint, or soft-tissue restrictions with specific techniques
d. Decrease pain at rest if present	d. Modalities Grade I or II joint oscillations
e. Prevent deformities	e. Patient education in the above plan of care Splinting

Precautions: When strengthening supporting muscles, increased pain in the joint during or following resistive exercises probably means that too great a weight is being used or stress is being placed at an inappropriate part of the range of motion. Analyze the joint mechanics and at what point during the range the greatest compressive forces are occurring. Maximum resistance exercise should not be done through that range of the motion.

IX. FRACTURES: GENERAL TREATMENT GUIDELINES

Reduction, alignment, and immobilization for healing of a fracture are medical procedures and will not be discussed in this text.

A. Clinical Considerations During the Period of Immobilization

1. With immobilization, there is connective tissue weakening, articular cartilage degeneration, muscle atrophy, and contracture development as well as sluggish circulation.[18] Structures in the related area should be kept in a state as near to normal as possible by using appropriate exercises without jeopardizing alignment of the fracture site.

2. If bed rest or immobilization in bed is required, as with skeletal traction, secondary physiologic changes will occur systematically throughout the body. General exercises for the uninvolved portions of the body can minimize these problems.

3. If there is a lower extremity fracture, alternate modes of ambulation need to be taught to the patient who is allowed out of bed, such as use of crutches or walker. The choice of device and gait pattern will depend on the fracture site, the type of immobilization, and the functional capabilities of the patient.

B. Treatment Considerations During the Period of Immobilization

1. Problems summarized

a. Initially, inflammation and swelling
b. In the immobilized area, progressive muscle atrophy, contracture formation, cartilage degeneration, and decreased circulation
c. Potential overall body weakening if on bed rest
d. Functional limitations imposed by the fracture site and method of immobilization used

2. General treatment goals and plan of care

Goals	Plan of Care
a. Decrease effects of inflammation during acute period	a. Ice, elevation Intermittent muscle setting
b. Decrease effects of immobilization	b. Intermittent muscle setting Active ROM to joints above and below immobilized region
c. If patient is confined to bed, maintain strength and ROM in major muscle groups	c. Resistive ROM to major muscle groups not immobilized, especially in preparation for future ambulation
d. Teach functional adaptations	d. Use of assistive or supportive devices for ambulation or bed mobility

C. Clinical Considerations After the Period of Immobilization

1. There will be decreased ROM, muscle atrophy, and joint pain in the structures that have been immobilized. Activities should be initiated carefully in order not to traumatize the weakened structures (muscle, cartilage, and connective tissue).

2. Initially, the patient will experience pain as movement begins, but it should progressively decrease as joint movement, muscle strength, and range of motion progressively improve.

3. If there was soft-tissue damage at the time of fracture, an inelastic scar will form, leading to decreased ROM or pain when stretch is placed on the scar. The scar tissue will have to be mobilized to gain pain-free movement.

Choice of technique will depend on the tissue involved.

4. To determine if there is clinical or radiologic healing, consult with the referring physician. Until the fracture site is radiologically healed, use care any time stress is placed distal to the fracture site (for example, resistance, stretch force, or weight bearing). Once radiologically healed, the bone has normal structural integrity and can withstand normal stress.

5. Evaluate to determine the degree and ranges of motion lost, the strength available, and the tissues that are in dysfunction. When progressing stretching and strengthening exercises and functional activities, use the guidelines, goals, and plans of care presented in the sections in this chapter on subacute and chronic stages (see Sections IV and V).

X. SURGERY

Many disorders of the musculoskeletal system that affect muscles, tendons, ligaments, cartilage, joints, capsules, or bones of the upper and lower extremities are treated successfully through surgical intervention. A well-planned, individualized therapeutic exercise program is an integral part of the preoperative and postoperative care of the surgical patient and significantly contributes to the success of the surgical procedure.

Acute, traumatic, soft-tissue injuries, such as ruptures of muscles and tendons and severe lesions of cartilage and ligaments, often must be repaired surgically. Severe chronic joint dysfunction due to rheumatoid arthritis, osteoarthritis, or traumatic arthritis may also require surgical intervention. In order to effectively establish an exercise program for a patient, the therapist must understand the indications and rationale for surgery, must become familiar with the procedure itself, and must be aware of the overall postoperative management of the patient.[10,19] An overview of specific surgical procedures for the upper and lower extremities and guidelines for postoperative care are found in Chapters 7 through 12.

A. Indications for Surgery[3,21]

1. Severe pain due to trauma to soft tissue or deterioration of articular surfaces
2. Chronic joint swelling
3. Marked limitation of active or passive joint motion
4. Gross instability of a joint or bony segment that leads to limitation of function
5. Joint deformity and abnormal joint alignment
6. Overall decrease or loss of function to maintain daily activities and personal care

B. Complications of Surgery

1. Postoperative infection or poor wound healing
2. Postoperative vascular disorders, such as thrombophlebitis and pulmonary embolism
3. Delayed healing of soft tissue or bone
4. Adhesions and contractures of soft tissue and joints
5. Loosening of prosthetic implants leading to instability and pain
6. Biomechanical breakdown of implants
7. Increased pulmonary secretions and risk of pneumonia and atelectasis

C. General Considerations for Preoperative Therapeutic Management

Whenever possible, preoperative contact with the patient can be extremely valuable for the patient and the therapist. A specific evaluation of the patient's status should be done prior to elective surgery. This evaluation of the patient will help to determine the likelihood or extent of success of the proposed surgical procedure.[10] Patient education can also be initiated more easily before surgery.

1. Evaluation procedures
   a. Determine the amount and type of joint pain, swelling, or crepitation the patient is experiencing.
   b. Measure the active and passive range of motion of the involved joint or extremity.
   c. Check the range of motion of all other joints.
   d. Grade the strength of the affected extremity.
   e. Estimate the strength of the unaffected joints or extremities as a basis for postoperative ambulation, transfers, and activities of daily living (ADL).
   f. Determine the level of functional independence that the patient had preoperatively and the level that he expects postoperatively.
   g. Evaluate the gait characteristics, type of assistive devices, and degree of weight bearing used during ambulation. Note any inequalities in leg lengths.

2. Early patient education
   a. Explain the general plan of care the patient can expect during the postoperative period.
   b. Advise the patient of any precautions or contraindications to movement or weight bearing that must be followed postoperatively.
   c. Teach the patient any exercises that will be started in the very early postoperative period. These often include
      (1) deep-breathing exercises.
      (2) active ankle exercises, if possible, to prevent venous stasis.
      (3) gentle muscle-setting exercises of immobilized joints.
   d. Teach the patient basic bed mobility.
   e. Teach the patient how to use any assistive devices, such as crutches or canes, which he may need after surgery.

D. Postoperative Goals and Guidelines for Exercise
1. Problems summarized
   a. Postoperative pain because of disruption of soft tissue
   b. Postoperative edema
   c. Postoperative circulatory and pulmonary complications
   d. Joint stiffness or limitation of motion because of injury to soft tissue and necessary postoperative immobilization
   e. Muscle atrophy because of immobilization
   f. Loss of strength for functional activities
   g. Limitation of weight bearing
   h. Potential loss of strength and mobility in unoperated joints

2. General postoperative treatment goals and plan of care

Goals	Plan of Care
a. Decrease postoperative pain	a. Relaxation exercises
	a. Use of modalities such as transcutaneous nerve stimulation (TNS), cold or heat. Continuous passive otion (CPM) during the early postoperative period
b. Decrease or minimize postoperative edema	b. Elevation of the operated extremity Active pumping exercises at the distal joints
c. Prevent circulatory and pulmonary complications such as thrombophlebitis, pulmonary embolus, or pneumonia	c. Active exercises to distal musculature Deep-breathing exercises
d. Prevent unnecessary, residual joint stiffness and improve functional range of motion	d. CPM initiated in the immediate postoperative period Progress to early active-assistive and active joint motion, when possible, to maintain normal length and mobility of muscle and soft tissue
e. Decrease muscle atrophy across immobilized joints	e. Muscle-setting exercises begun immediately after surgery
f. Restore adequate strength necessary for daily functional activities when soft tissue and bony healing allows.	f. Graded resistance exercises
g. Provide the patient with a safe and efficient means of ambulation when weight bearing is restricted.	g. Gait training with appropriate assistive devices
h. Maintain or improve strength and mobility of unoperated joints	h. Graded resistance exercise

3. General precautions

a. Avoid specific joint motions or weight bearing consistent with the surgical procedure.

b. Progress exercise gradually during the early postoperative period. Soft tissues, which were disturbed during surgery, will be inflamed. Allow adequate time for healing to occur.

c. Avoid any stretching or resistance exercise to muscles or tendons that have been incised and reattached during surgery for at least 6 weeks to ensure adequate healing and stability.

d. Continually note the level of swelling, pain, and wound drainage. If a marked increase is noted, report immediately and discontinue exercise to that area until further notice.

E. **Overview of Common Orthopedic Surgical Procedures and Guidelines for Postoperative Care**

Note: The length of immobilization and the initiation, progression, and intensity of exercise may vary according to differences in surgical techniques and the philosophy of the surgeon.

1. **Repair of soft-tissue lesions**

In general, at least 6 weeks are needed for soft tissues to heal after surgical repair.

a. **Complete rupture of a muscle**[12]

(1) This is not common, but it may occur when a muscle that is already contracted takes a direct blow or is forcibly stretched.

(2) Procedure

The muscle is surgically resutured and immobilized so the muscle is in a shortened position for 10 to 21 days.

(3) Exercise

(a) Muscle-setting exercise to the sutured muscle may be started immediately after surgery.

(b) At 10 to 14 days postoperatively, the cast is removed and active exercise may be started to regain joint motion.

(c) Weight bearing is restricted until the patient achieves normal strength and mobility.

(d) Stretching and heavy resistance exercise are contraindicated until soft-tissue healing is complete—as long as 6 to 8 weeks postoperatively.

b. **Rupture of a tendon**[3,12]

(1) A tendon usually ruptures from severe trauma in a young person or with a sudden, unusual motion in an elderly person. It is most often seen in the bicipital tendon at the shoulder or the Achilles tendon.

(2) Procedure

The tendon is sutured, and the muscle and tendon are put in a shortened position, as with complete tears of a muscle. A longer immobilization period is required (usually 3 to 4 weeks) for a repaired tendon than for a repaired muscle, because the vascular supply to tendons is poor.

(3) Exercise

(a) Muscle-setting is begun immediately after surgery to prevent adhesions of the tendon to the sheath.

(b) Gentle active ROM exercise is allowed after approximately 4 weeks when the immobilization device can be safely removed.

(c) In a lower extremity repair, weight bearing is usually restricted for 6 to 8 weeks.

(d) Vigorous resistance exercise may be initiated after about 8 weeks, when complete healing of the tendon has occurred.

c. **Ligamentous tears**

(1) When ligaments cannot be approximated for healing through closed reduction, surgical repair is indicated. The knee and ankle joints are commonly affected.

(2) Procedure

The torn ligament is repaired, and the joint is immobilized in a position of least stretch to the sutured ligament. Immobilization is required for at least 10 to 21 days, and in many cases a much longer period of time.

(3) Exercise

The same procedure may be followed as with repaired tendons. Support should be worn, and weight bearing should be restricted when the repair is at a potentially unstable joint, such as the knee, until muscle power can adequately protect the joint.

2. Soft-tissue releases—Tenotomy, myotomy, and lengthening[3,21]

a. In order to improve range of motion in joints where severe contractures exist, surgical release of soft tissue may be indicated. This may be done in young patients with severe arthritis in whom joint replacement is not advisable or as a preliminary procedure in adults prior to joint replacement. Releases are also done in patients with myopathic and neuropathic diseases such as cerebral palsy and muscular dystrophy. Some form of splinting or bracing in the corrected position in conjunction with exercise is always used postoperatively to maintain the gained range of motion.

b. Procedure

The muscle or tendon is surgically sectioned and any fibrous contractures of all involved periarticular structures are released.

c. Exercise

(1) Active-assistive motion may be initiated within 3 to 4 days after surgery. This is followed by active exercise through the gained range as soft-tissue healing progresses.

(2) Strengthening to the antagonists of the released muscle should also be started early to maintain active joint motion.

3. Synovectomy

a. Procedure

Removal of the synovium (lining of the joint) in patients with chronic joint swelling. It is occasionally done in patients with rheumatoid arthritis with chronic proliferative synovitis but with minimal articular changes. The most common joints on which synovectomy is performed are the knee, wrist, elbow, and metacarpophalangeal joints.[10,21]

b. Postoperative care

(1) Immobilization

A soft, bulky compression dressing is applied at the time of surgery and worn for several days.

(2) Elevation

The operated extremity is elevated to reduce edema.

(3) Exercise

(a) During the period of immobilization the patient may begin gentle setting exercises to the muscles around the affected joint.

(b) CPM, active-assistive and active exercises are begun as soon as the dressing is removed. These exercises are gradually progressed to mild resistance exercise over 6 to 12 weeks.

c. Weight bearing or lifting heavy objects is restricted for 6 to 8 weeks.

4. Osteotomy

a. Procedure

Osteotomy is the surgical cutting and realignment of bone, done in cases of severe arthritis to correct joint deformity and reduce pain. It is most often done in osteoarthritis of the knee or hip.[1,3] An osteotomy is primarily done to reduce pain by realignment and modification of the loads placed on joint surfaces before significant deterioration of the joint occurs. Osteotomy of the hip is done in young patients with severe hip pain secondary to hip problems such as Legg-Calvé-Perthes disease or congenital dislocation of the hip.

  b. Postoperative care
    (1) Immobilization
        The osteotomy site is either immobilized with internal fixation, which allows early joint motion and protected weight bearing, or the involved joint is placed in a cast until bony healing occurs, which may take as long as 8 to 12 weeks.[1,3]
    (2) Exercise
        (a) During immobilization in a cast the patient should be encouraged to actively move the joints above and below the site of the osteotomy to prevent joint stiffness and undue weakness.
        (b) When motion and weight bearing are allowed or when the cast is removed, active-assistive, active, and mild-resistive exercise may be started to restore joint range of motion and strength. (See discussion of the chronic stage of soft-tissue lesions earlier in this chapter.)
        (c) If chronic stiffness persists because of the long-term immobilization, joint mobilization and soft-tissue stretching may also be necessary.

5. Arthrodesis
  a. Procedure
    Fusion of bony surfaces of a joint with internal fixation such as pins, nails, plates, and bone grafts. This is usually done in cases of severe joint pain and instability in which mobility of the joint is a lesser concern. It is commonly done at the wrist, thumb, and ankle. Arthrodesis may be the only salvage procedure left for a patient with a failed joint arthroplasty.[1,3]
  b. Postoperative care
    (1) Immobilization
        The joint is immobilized in a cast in the desired position for maximum function for 8 to 12 weeks to ensure bony fusion.
    (2) Exercise
        Since no movement will be possible in the fused joint, range of motion and strength must be maintained above and below the operated joint.
    (3) Weight bearing is restricted until x-ray studies show evidence of bony healing.
  c. Optimum positions for arthrodesis[1]
    (1) Shoulder: in a position so that the hand can reach the mouth
    (2) Wrist: in slight extension. If the patient has bilateral wrist joint disease, one joint may be fused and the other replaced.
    (3) Thumb: MCP joint is usually fused in 20 degrees of flexion
    (4) Hip: in 15 to 20 degrees of flexion to allow ambulation and comfortable sitting
    (5) Ankle: in neutral position (90 degrees) or slight equinus for women

who wear low heels. The subtalar joint is fused in neutral so there is no varus or valgus.

6. Arthroplasty

a. General definition

Any reconstructive joint procedure, with or without joint implant, designed to relieve pain and/or restore joint motion.

b. Types of procedures[2,3,10,21]

(1) Excision arthroplasty

Removal of periarticular bone from one or both articular surfaces. A space is left where fibrotic (scar) tissue is allowed to be laid down during the healing process. This is sometimes called resectional arthroplasty. This procedure may be done in a variety of joints such as the hip, elbow, wrist, and foot to reduce pain and increase joint motion. Disadvantages of these procedures are

(a) possible joint instability.

(b) a poor cosmetic result because of shortening of the operated extremity.

(c) persistent muscular imbalance and weakness.

Excision arthroplasty, although an old procedure, is still appropriate in selected cases.

(2) Excision arthroplasty with implant

After removal of the articular surface, an artificial implant is fixed in place to help in the remodeling of a new joint. This is sometimes called implant resection arthroplasty. The implant usually is made of a flexible silicone material and becomes encapsulated by fibrous tissue as the joint re-forms.[25]

(3) Interpositional arthroplasty[25]

Débridement of the joint is done initially, and a foreign material is placed between (interposed) the two joint surfaces. A variety of materials may be used to cover the joint surface such as fascia, Silastic material, or metal.

Some examples of interpositional arthroplasties are Smith-Petersen cup arthroplasty of the hip (rarely done now, with the advent of the total hip replacement), condylar replacement of the knee, and humeral replacement of the shoulder.

(4) Total joint replacement arthroplasty

Removal of both affected joint surfaces and replacement with an artificial joint. Implants can be held in place with an acrylic cement (methyl methacrylate); may be stabilized with bolts, pins, screws, or nails;[6,20,21] or most recently may be secured without cement using either a press-fit (a very tight fit between bone and implant) or biologic fixation (microscopic in growth of bone into a porous-coated prosthesis). A great amount of research is currently being done on cementless joint replacements.[20] The bone-cement interface is the portion of the joint replacement where loosening occurs and is the primary source of mechanical failure of total joint replacements.[20,22]

Prosthetic replacements for almost every joint of the extremities have been developed and refined. A more complete description of those implants will be reviewed joint by joint in Chapters 7 through 12. Overall, total joint replacement arthroplasty has been most successful in the large joints, such as the hip and knee, rather than in the smaller joints of the foot and hand.[7] Total joint implants generally require less postoperative immobilization and less supervised graded exercise than excision arthroplasty (with or without implant) or interpositional arthroplasty, because the success of the procedure is less dependent on the encapsulation process.

c. Types of materials used in arthroplasty[20,21]

Many different materials have been used in the developing years in reconstructive surgery. Materials used today may be classified into three broad areas

(1) rigid

inert metal, usually a cobalt-chrome alloy, stainless steel, or ceramic materials.

(2) semi-rigid

plastic, high-density polymers such as polyethylene.

(3) flexible

elastic polymers such as Silastic or silicone implants.

In general, flexible implants are used in conjunction with excision arthroplasty, and semi-rigid plastics and rigid metals or ceramics are used in total joint replacements.

d. Postoperative care

A detailed description of postoperative management and exercises for specific total joint replacements will be covered in Chapters 7 through 12.

XI. SUMMARY

Chapter 6 provided background information necessary to design therapeutic exercise programs based on a patient's level of orthopedic involvement during the acute, subacute, or chronic stage of soft-tissue and joint healing. This approach was used whether the problem involved injury from trauma, insult from overuse, disease, or surgical intervention.

Soft-tissue lesions and clinical conditions were defined; the stages of inflammation and repair were described with emphasis on how to manage soft tissues and joints with therapeutic exercise during each stage. Special considerations and therapeutic exercise management for rheumatoid arthritis, osteoarthritis, postfracture dysfunctions and postsurgical conditions were also described.

A problem list with goals and plan of care was outlined to summarize each clinical situation. A list of clinical problems will be used as the foundation for designing exercise programs for each region of the body as described in Chapters 7 through 12.

REFERENCES

1. Benke, GJ: *Osteotomy, arthrodesis and girdlestone arthroplasty.* In Downie, PA (ed): *Cash's Textbook of Orthopedics and Rheumatology for Physiotherapists.* JB Lippincott, Philadelphia, 1984.
2. Bentley, JA: *Physiotherapy following joint replacement.* In Downie, PA (ed): *Cash's Textbook of Orthopedics and Rheumatology for Physiotherapists.* JB Lippincott, Philadelphia, 1984.
3. Braschear, R and Raney, RB (eds): *Shands' Handbook of Orthopaedic Surgery,* ed 9. CV Mosby, St Louis, 1978.
4. Cailliet, R: *Soft Tissue Pain and Disability.* FA Davis, Philadelphia, 1977.
5. Chamberlain, G: *Cyriax's friction massage: A review.* JOSPT 4:16, 1982.
6. Cofield, R, Morrey, B, and Bryan, R: *Total shoulder and total elbow arthroplasties: The current state of development—Part I.* JCE Orthopedics 6:14, 1978.

7. Cummings, G, Crutchfield, C, and Barnes, MR: *Soft-Tissue Changes in Contractures.* Orthopedic Physical Therapy Series, Vol 1. Stokesville Pub, Atlanta, 1983.

8. Cummings, G: *Soft-Tissue Contractures,* lecture notes. Ohio Chapter APTA Conference, Columbus, 1987.

9. Cyriax, J: *Textbook of Orthopaedic Medicine, Vol 1. Diagnosis of Soft Tissue Lesions,* ed 8. Bailliere and Tindall, London, 1982.

10. Hyde, SA: *Physiotherapy in Rheumatology.* Blackwell Scientific Publications, Oxford, 1980.

11. Inglis, AE (ed): *Symposium on Total Joint Replacement of the Upper Extremity* (1979). American Academy of Orthopaedic Surgeons, CV Mosby, St Louis, 1982.

12. Iversen, LD, and Clawson, DK: *Manual of Acute Orthopedic Therapeutics,* ed 2. Little, Brown & Company, Boston, 1982.

13. Kaltenborn, F: *Mobilization of the Extremity Joints: Examination and Basic Treatment Techniques,* ed 3. Norway, 1980.

14. Keene, J: *Ligament and muscle-tendon unit injuries.* In Gould, J and Davies, GJ (eds): *Orthopaedic and Sports Physical Therapy.* CV Mosby, St Louis, 1985.

15. Kellett, J: *Acute soft-tissue injuries—a review of the literature.* Med Sci Sports Exerc 18:489, 1986.

16. Maitland, GD: *Peripheral Manipulation,* ed 2. Butterworth, Boston, 1977.

17. Maitland, GD: *Vertebral Manipulation,* ed 4. Butterworth, Boston, 1977.

18. McDonough, A: *Effect of immobilization and exercise on articular cartilage—A review of literature.* JOSPT 3:2, 1981.

19. Melvin, J: *Rheumatic Disease: Occupational Therapy and Rehabilitation,* ed 2. FA Davis, Philadelphia, 1982.

20. Morrey, BF and Kavanaugh, BF: *Cementless joint replacement: current status and future.* Bull Rheum Dis 37:1, 1987.

21. Nickel, VL (ed): *Orthopedic Rehabilitation.* Churchhill-Livingstone, New York, 1982.

22. Rand, JA, et al: *A comparison of cemented vs cementless porous-coated anatomic total knee arthroplasty.* In Rand, JA (ed): *Total Arthroplasty of the Knee.* Aspen Pub, Rockville, MD, 1987.

23. Salter, RB et al: *Clinical application of basic research on continuous passive motion for disorders and injuries of synovial joints: A preliminary report of a feasibility study.* J Orthop Res 1:325, 1984.

24. Schrier, RW (ed): *Clinical Internal Medicine in the Aged.* WB Saunders, Philadelphia, 1982.

25. Swanson, AB: *Flexible Implant Resection Arthroplasty in the Hand and Extremities.* CV Mosby, St Louis, 1973.

26. Threlkeld, JA and Currier, DP: *Osteoarthritis: effects on synovial joint tissues.* Phys Ther 68:346, 1988.

27. van der Meulen, JCH: *Present state of knowledge on processes of healing in collagen structures.* Int J Sports Med 3:4, 1982.

28. Wilhelm, DL: *Inflammation and healing.* In Anderson, WAD (ed): *Pathology.* CV Mosby, St Louis, 1971.

29. Zohn, D and Mennell, J: *Musculoskeletal Pain: Principles of Physical Diagnosis and Physical Treatment.* Little, Brown & Company, Boston, 1976.

CHAPTER —————————————— 7

The Shoulder and Shoulder Girdle

The design of the shoulder girdle allows for mobility of the upper extemity. As a result, the hand can be placed almost anywhere within a sphere of movement, being limited primarily by the length of the arm and the space taken up by the body. The combined mechanics of its joints and muscles provides for and controls the mobility. When establishing a therapeutic exercise program for problems in the shoulder region, as with any other region of the body, the unique anatomic and kinesiologic features must be taken into consideration as well as the state of pathology and functional limitations imposed by the problems. The first section of this chapter briefly reviews anatomic and kinesiologic information on the shoulder complex; the reader is referred to several textbooks for in-depth study of the material.[6,9,19,22,24,32] The reader is also referred to Chapter 6 for review of principles of management.

OBJECTIVES

After studying this chapter, the reader will be able to:
1. identify important aspects of shoulder girdle structure and function for review.
2. establish a therapeutic exercise program to manage soft tissue and joint lesions in the shoulder girdle region related to stages of recovery following an inflammatory insult to the tissues.
3. establish a therapeutic exercise program to manage common musculoskeletal lesions, recognizing unique circumstances for their management.
4. establish a therapeutic exercise program to manage patients following common surgical procedures.

I. REVIEW OF THE STRUCTURE AND FUNCTION OF THE SHOULDER AND SHOULDER GIRDLE

   A. Bony Parts Include the Proximal Humerus, Scapula, and Clavicle and Its Attachment to the Sternum (see Figure 5-12).

241

B. Synovial Joints

1. Glenohumeral (GH) joint

a. Characteristics

An incongruous, ball-and-socket (spheroidal) triaxial joint with a lax joint capsule. It is supported by the tendons of the rotator cuff and the glenohumeral (superior, middle, and inferior) and coracohumeral ligaments.

b. The concave bony partner, the glenoid fossa, is located on the superior-lateral margin of the scapula. It faces anteriorly, laterally, and upward, which provides some stability to the joint. A fibrocartilage lip, the glenoid labrum, deepens the fossa for greater congruity.

c. The convex bony partner is the head of the humerus. Only a small portion of the head comes in contact with the fossa at any one time.

d. With motions of the humerus (physiologic motions), the convex head slides in the opposite direction of the humerus.

Physiologic Motions of the Humerus	Direction of Slide of Humeral Head
Flexion	Posterior
Extension	Anterior
Abduction	Inferior
Adduction	Superior
Internal rotation	Posterior
External rotation	Anterior
Horizontal abduction	Anterior
Horizontal adduction	Posterior

e. If the humerus is stabilized and the scapula moves, the concave glenoid fossa slides in the same direction that the scapula moves.

2. Acromioclavicular (AC) joint

a. Characteristics

A plane, gliding triaxial joint, which may or may not have a disk. The weak capsule is reinforced by the superior and inferior acromioclavicular ligaments. Stability is primarily provided by the coracoclavicular ligament.

b. The convex bony partner is a facet on the lateral end of the clavicle.

c. The concave bony partner is a facet on the acromion of the scapula.

d. With motions of the scapula, the acromial surface slides in the same direction in which the scapula moves, since the surface is concave. Motions affecting this joint include upward rotation (the scapula turns so that the glenoid fossa rotates upward), downward rotation, winging of the vertebral border, and tipping of the inferior angle.

3. Sternoclavicular (SC) joint

a. Characteristics

An incongruent, triaxial, saddle-shaped joint with a disk. The joint is supported by the anterior and posterior sternoclavicular ligaments and the interclavicular and costoclavicular ligaments.

b. The medial end of the clavicle is convex superior to inferior and concave anterior to posterior. The joint disk attaches to the upper end.

    c. The superior-lateral portion of the manubrium and first costal cartilage is concave superior to inferior and convex anterior to posterior.

    d. With anterior-posterior motions of the clavicle, the articulating surface slides in the same direction. With superior-inferior motions of the clavicle, the articulating surface slides opposite.

Physiologic Motions of the Clavicle	Direction of Slide of the Clavicle
Elevation	Inferior
Depression	Superior
Protraction	Anterior
Retraction	Posterior
Rotation	Spin

    e. The motions of the clavicle occur as a result of the scapular motions of elevation, depression, protraction (abduction), and retraction (adduction), respectively. Rotation of the clavicle occurs as an accessory motion when the humerus is elevated above the horizontal and the scapula upwardly rotates; it cannot occur as an isolated voluntary motion.

C. Functional Articulations

1. Scapulothoracic

    a. Motions of the scapula require sliding of the scapula along the thorax. Normally there is considerable soft-tissue flexibility, allowing the scapula to participate in all upper extremity motions.

    b. Motions of the scapula are

        (1) elevation, depression, protraction (abduction), and retraction (adduction), seen with clavicular motions at the SC joint.

        (2) upward and downward rotation, seen with clavicular motions at the SC joint and rotation at the AC joint, concurrently with motions of the humerus. Upward rotation of the scapula is a necessary component motion for full range of motion of flexion and abduction of the humerus.

        (3) winging of the medial border and tipping of the inferior angle, seen with motion at the AC joint concurrently with motions of the humerus. Tipping of the scapula is necessary to reach the hand behind the back in conjunction with internal rotation and extension of the humerus. Winging is an accessory motion with horizontal adduction of the humerus.

2. Suprahumeral

    a. Coracoacromial arch, composed of the acromion and coracoacromial ligament, overlies the subacromial/subdeltoid bursa.[32] The bursa lies over the supraspinatus tendon and a portion of the muscle.

    b. These structures allow for and participate in normal shoulder function. Compromise of this space, faulty mechanics, or injury to the soft tissue in this region leads to impingement syndromes.[5,6,38]

D. Shoulder Girdle Function[24,32]

1. Scapulohumeral rhythm

    a. Motion of the scapula, synchronous with motions of the humerus, allows for 150 to 180 degrees of shoulder range of motion into flexion or abduction with elevation. The ratio has considerable variation among individuals but is commonly accepted to be 2:1 (two degrees of gleno-humeral motion to one degree of scapular rotation).

b. The synchronous motion of the scapula allows the muscles moving the humerus to maintain a good length-tension relationship throughout the activity.

c. Muscles causing the upward rotation of the scapula are the upper and lower trapezius and serratus anterior. Weakness or complete paralysis of these muscles results in the scapula being rotated downward by the contracting deltoid and supraspinatus as abduction or flexion is attempted. These two muscles then reach active insufficiency, and functional elevation of the arm cannot be reached, even though there may be normal passive ROM and normal strength in the shoulder abductor and flexor muscles.

d. Weakness or poor synchronization of the upward rotating muscles may alter the relationship of the humerus in the suprahumeral space as the arm is abducted, leading to microtrauma within the joint or impingement syndromes in the soft tissue of the suprahumeral space.

2. **Clavicular elevation and rotation with humeral motion**

a. Initially, with upward rotation of the scapula, 30 degrees of elevation of the clavicle occurs at the SC joint. Then, as the coracoclavicular ligament becomes taut, the clavicle rotates 38 to 50 degrees about its longitudinal axis, which elevates its acromial end (because it is crank shaped). The scapula then rotates an additional 30 degrees at the AC joint.

b. Loss of any of these functional components will decrease the amount of scapular rotation and thus the range of motion of the upper extremity.

3. **External rotation of the humerus with full elevation through abduction**

a. For the greater tubercle of the humerus to clear the coracoacromial arch, the humerus must externally rotate as it is elevated above the horizontal.

b. Weak or inadequate external rotation will result in impingement of the soft tissues in the suprahumeral space, causing pain, inflammation, and eventually loss of function.

4. **Internal rotation of the humerus with full elevation through flexion**[3,4,34]

a. Medial rotation begins around 50 degrees of passive shoulder flexion when all structures are intact.[34] With full range of shoulder flexion and elevation, the humerus medially rotates 90 degrees.[34]

b. Most of the shoulder flexor muscles are also medial rotators of the humerus.[24]

c. As the arm elevates above the horizontal in the sagittal plane, the anterior capsule and ligaments become taut, causing the humerus to medially rotate.

d. The bony configuration of the posterior aspect of the glenoid fossa contributes to the inward rotation motion of the humerus as the shoulder flexes.[34]

5. Deltoid—Short rotator cuff and supraspinatus mechanisms

a. The majority of the force of the deltoid muscle causes upward translation of the humerus; if unopposed, it leads to impingement of the soft tissues within the suprahumeral space between the humeral head and the coracoacromial arch.

b. The combined effect of the short rotator muscles (infraspinatus, teres minor, and subscapularis) causes compression and a downward translation of the humerus.

c. The actions of the deltoid and short rotators result in a force couple which is necessary for abduction of the humerus.

d. The supraspinatus muscle has a compressive and slight upward translation effect on the humerus; these effects, combined with the effect of gravity, lead to abduction of the arm.

e. Interruption or poor coordination of any of these muscles can lead to microtrauma and eventual dysfunction in the shoulder region.

II. GUIDELINES AND THERAPEUTIC EXERCISES FOR MANAGEMENT OF COMMON MUSCULOSKELETAL PROBLEMS IN THE SHOULDER AND SHOULDER GIRDLE

Chapter 6 provides background information on the stages of inflammation and repair and outlines a management approach by identifying typical problems and suggested goals and plan of care for each stage. This section describes techniques that may be useful in the management of clinical problems in the shoulder. In some cases, the reader is referred to techniques described in Chapters 2 through 5. Not all procedures and techniques described are appropriate for all patients; procedures and techniques should be used only when the patient's condition and responses are appropriate.

A. Joint Problems—Glenohumeral Joint

1. Acute joint lesions

a. Causes
Rheumatoid arthritis or osteoarthritis, trauma, diabetes mellitus, microtrauma from poor postural alignment and faulty mechanics, immobilization, or secondary effects from conditions such as ischemic heart disease or stroke.

b. Clinical picture
Pain and muscle guarding limit motion, usually preventing external rotation and abduction. Pain is experienced radiating below the elbow and may disturb sleep.

2. Management of acute joint lesions

a. See guidelines for management in Chapter 6, section III.

b. To control the pain, edema, and muscle guarding
  (1) immobilization in a sling provides rest to the part, but complete immobilization can lead to contractures and limited motion.
  (2) gentle joint oscillation techniques of small amplitude (Grade I) may be used with the joint in a pain-free position (see Chapter 5).
  Precaution: During the first two days following trauma, this technique may not be tolerated by some people. Use with extreme care and use only if it decreases the pain.

c. To maintain soft tissue and joint integrity and mobility

(1) passive range of motion (ROM) to all ranges of pain-free motion (see Chapter 2). As pain decreases, the patient should be able to progress to active ROM with or without assistance, depending on severity of the injury.

(2) passive joint traction and glides, with the joint placed in a pain-free position as it is treated (see Chapter 5). Begin with Grade I; progress to Grade II as symptoms improve.

Precaution: If there is increased pain or irritability in the joint following use of these techniques, either the dosage was too strong, or the techniques should not be used at this time.

Contraindication: Stretching (Grade III) techniques. If there are mechanical restrictions causing limited motion, appropriate stretching can be initiated AFTER the inflammation subsides.

(3) gentle muscle setting (see Chapter 3) to all muscle groups of the shoulder. Also include scapular and elbow muscles because of their close association with the shoulder. Instruct the patient to gently contract a group of muscles while you apply slight resistance—just enough to stimulate a muscle contraction. It should not provoke pain. The emphasis is on rhythmic contracting and relaxing of the muscles to help stimulate blood flow and prevent circulatory stasis.

d. To maintain integrity and function of associated areas

(1) Either the therapist or the patient should perform ROM to the elbow, forearm, wrist, and fingers several times each day while the shoulder is immobilized. If tolerated, active or gentle resistive ROM is preferred to passive for a greater effect on circulation and muscle integrity.

(2) Shoulder-hand syndrome is a potential complication following shoulder injury or immobility; special attention should be given to the hand with additional exercises, such as repetitively squeezing a ball or other soft object (see section II F).

(3) If edema is noted in the hand, the hand should be elevated, whenever possible, above the level of the heart.

(4) Instruct the patient in the importance of keeping the joints distal to the injured site as active and mobile as possible.

3. Subacute and chronic joint problems

a. Clinical picture: subacute

If the patient can be treated as the acute condition begins to subside by gradually increasing the shoulder motion and activity, the complication of joint and soft-tissue contractures can usually be avoided.

b. Clinical picture: chronic

If motion becomes restricted, or if the patient is not treated until there is limited motion, capsular tightness develops, with pain felt as the capsule is stretched. Often, because of the pain, the person does not use the arm normally, and the joint progressively becomes more limited. Usually, external rotation and abduction are most limited, and internal rotation least limited. There may be aching, localized to the deltoid region.

c. Clinical picture: *idiopathic frozen shoulder*

Frozen shoulder is also called adhesive capsulitis and periarthritis.[37,42] The insidious onset usually occurs between the ages of 40 and 60, without a known cause, although problems already mentioned such as rheumatoid arthritis or osteoarthritis, trauma, or immobilization may lead to a frozen shoulder. This clinical entity follows a classic pattern of

—"freezing"—characterized by intense pain even at rest and limitation of motion by 2 to 3 weeks following onset

—"frozen"—characterized by pain only with movement, substitute motions with the scapula, and atrophy of the deltoid, rotator cuff, biceps, and triceps brachii muscles

—"thawing"—characterized by no pain but significant capsular restrictions

Spontaneous recovery occurs on the average of 2 years from onset.[14] Inappropriately aggressive therapy at the wrong time may prolong the symptoms.[2] Treatment guidelines are the same as acute for the "freezing" stage, and subacute and chronic for the "frozen" and "thawing" stages.

4. **Management of subacute and chronic joint limitations**
   a. Follow the guidelines as described in Chapter 6, sections IV and V, emphasizing joint mobility.
   b. To control pain, edema, and joint effusion, carefully monitor increasing activities. If the joint was splinted, gradually increase the amount of time that the shoulder is free to move each day.
   c. To decrease the effect of contracture formation and progressively increase soft tissue and/or joint mobility
      (1) *Passive joint mobilization techniques* (see Chapter 5)
         Note: A Grade I distraction is used with all gliding techniques.
         Begin with sustained Grade II traction and gliding techniques with the joint placed in a pain-free position; as the joint responds, gradually progress to Grade III.
         If the joint is highly irritable and gliding in the direction of restriction is not tolerated, glide in the opposite direction. As the pain and irritability decrease, begin to glide in the direction of restriction.
         (a) To increase abduction, caudal glide humeral head (see Figures 5-14–5-16).
         (b) To increase flexion or internal rotation, posterior glide humeral head (see Figures 5-16–5-18).
         (c) To increase extension or external rotation, anterior glide humeral head (see Figure 5-19).
         (d) As joint pain decreases and the available range reaches a plateau, progress by taking the shoulder to the limits of its motion and apply the appropriate glide.
         Precaution: Vigorous stretching should not be done until the chronic stage.
         Note: For normal joint mechanics, there must be good scapular mobility and the humerus must be able to externally rotate. Increasing abduction beyond 90 degrees should not occur until adequate external rotation is available and the scapula has unrestricted motion. With a traumatic injury also involving the AC or SC joints, these joints tend to become hypermobile. Care should be taken not to stretch them when mobilizing the glenohumeral joint by providing good stabilization to the scapula.

(2) *Early joint mobility exercises; pendulum (Codman's) exercises*[7]

These are self-mobilization techniques that use the effects of gravity to distract the humerus from the glenoid fossa.[6,7] They help relieve pain through gentle traction and oscillating movements and provide early motion of joint structures and synovial fluid.

POSITION OF PATIENT

Standing, with the trunk flexed at the hips about 90 degrees, or prone on a treatment table, with the involved shoulder over the edge. The arm hangs loosely downward in a position of about 90 degrees flexion.

TECHNIQUE

A pendulum or swinging motion of the arm is initiated by having the patient move his trunk slightly back and forth. Motions of flexion, extension, and horizontal abduction, adduction, and circumduction can be done (Figure 7-1 done without the weight in the patient's hand). Increase the arc of motion as tolerated. This technique should not cause pain.

Precautions: Some patients may get dizzy when standing upright after being bent over; if so, have them sit and rest.

If a patient cannot balance himself leaning over, have him hold on to a solid object or use the prone position.

If the patient experiences back pain from bending over, use the prone position.

Adding a weight to the hand or using wrist cuffs causes a greater distraction force on the glenohumeral joint (Figure 7-1). This should only be done when joint stretching maneuvers are indicated late in the subacute and chronic stages—and then, only if the scapula is stabilized by the therapist so the stretch force is directed to the joint, not the soft tissue of the scapulothoracic region.

If there is increased pain or decreased ROM, the technique may be an inappropriate choice.

(3) *Range of Motion*

(a) Begin with active ROM up to the point of pain, including all shoulder and scapular motions (see Chapter 2).

(b) Use self-assistive ROM techniques, such as the shoulder wheel, overhead pulleys, or wand exercises (see Chapter 2).

(c) When the patient can tolerate stretching, the patient takes the extremity to the limit of the range and holds it 10 to 15 seconds or longer if tolerated, relaxes; then repeats.

Precaution: If there is increased pain or decreased motion, the activity may be too intense or the patient may be using faulty mechanics. Re-assess the technique and discontinue it if faulty joint mechanics exist.

(4) *Control of muscle spasm*

Muscle spasm may lead to a faulty deltoid-rotator cuff mechanism when the patient attempts abduction. The head of the humerus may be held in a cranial position within the joint, making it difficult and/or painful to abduct the shoulder because the greater tuberosity impinges on the coracoacromial arch. In this case, repositioning the head of the humerus with a caudal glide is necessary before proceeding with any other form of shoulder exercise.

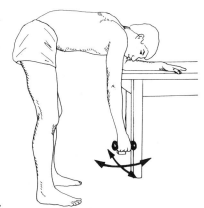

FIGURE 7-1. Pendulum exercises.

(a) Gentle oscillations will help decrease the muscle spasm (Grade I or II).
(b) Sustained caudal glides will help reposition the humeral head in the glenoid fossa.
(c) Training the external rotators of the shoulder will help to depress the humeral head as the arm abducts. This needs to be done if the patient tends to hike his shoulder while abducting, thus elevating rather than depressing the humeral head (Figure 7-2).

—Begin with active external rotation until the motion is pain free, then gradually add resistance.

—Elastic resistance: patient holds an elastic material in both hands, elbows flexed and held at the side, then moves his hands laterally, pulling against the resistance (Figure 7-3A).

—Wrist or hand weights: patient prone on a treatment table, shoulder at 90 degrees if possible, elbow flexed over the edge of the table. Lift the weight as far as possible by rotating the shoulder, not extending the elbow (Figure 7-3B).

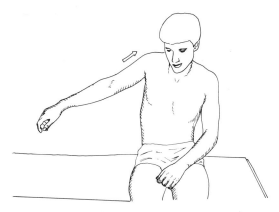

FIGURE 7-2. Patient hiking his shoulder while trying to abduct his shoulder, thus elevating rather than depressing the humeral head.

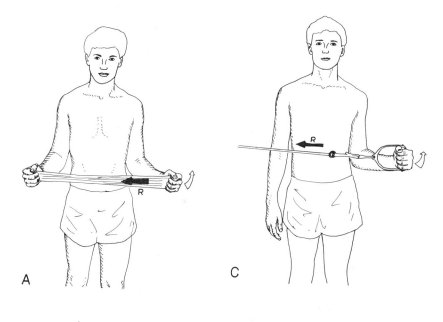

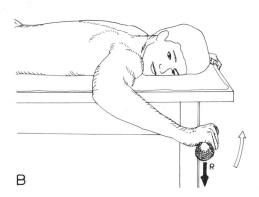

FIGURE 7-3. Resisting shoulder external rotation using elasticized material (*A*), hand-held weight (*B*), and wall pulley (*C*).

—Wall pulleys: the patient is positioned so that when his elbow is flexed 90 degrees and held at his side, his hand is at the level of the pulley. He then grasps the handle and rotates his arm outward (Figure 7-3C).

—Teach voluntary humeral depression. Have the patient attempt to push his arm caudally; provide slight resistance against his elbow for proprioceptive feedback (there will also be some scapular depression). Give verbal reinforcement any time the patient causes caudal glide of the humerus (Figure 7-4).

—Progress by having the patient attempt active abduction while maintaining the caudal glide.

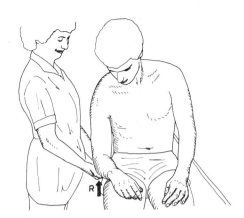

FIGURE 7-4. Resisting humeral depression.

(5) *Self-stretching exercises*[12,22]

As the joint reaction becomes predictable and the patient begins to tolerate stretching, he can be taught to stretch himself. His body is moved in relation to the stabilized arm. This technique uses the principle of moving the concave surface of the joint partner (the glenoid fossa) against the convex surface (the head of the humerus). When doing this, the concave surface slides in the same direction as the overall bone motion, which is the normal arthrokinematic relationship. Conversely, passive stretching by moving the humerus would cause the joint surface of the humeral head to roll in the same direction as the bone movement without the slide in the opposite direction. (The convex head needs to slide opposite the bone motion for normal joint mechanics. In active motion, the sliding of the head of the humerus is caused by the rotator cuff muscles. Passive stretching of the humerus in relation to the scapula does not result in correct joint mechanics unless the therapist simultaneously glides the head opposite the bone motion.) Moving the body in relation to the humerus is safer for the joint and less painful for the patient to do on himself.[21,22]

Instructions: Early in the subacute state, emphasize to the patient that he must begin gently with these activities and gradually progress the movement as tolerated. Too much stretching too soon will result in increased pain and decreased ROM. Once in the chronic stage, more intense stretching can be done. He is to move his body in relation to the arm, to the end of the available range; hold that position as long as comfortable for a low-grade, prolonged stretch, relax, then repeat.

(a) To increase flexion and elevation of the arm

The patient sits with his side next to the table, his forearm resting along the table edge with his elbow slightly flexed (Figure 7-5A). He then slides his forearm forward along the table as he bends from the waist. Eventually his head should be level with the shoulder (Figure 7-5B).

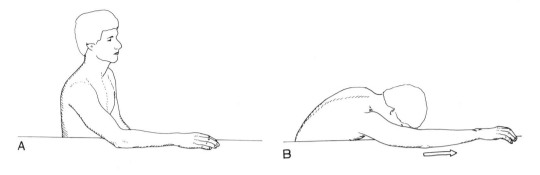

FIGURE 7-5. Beginning (*A*) and end (*B*) positions for self-stretching to increase shoulder flexion with elevation.

(b) To increase external (lateral) rotation
The patient sits as with flexion (Figure 7-5A). He then bends forward from the waist, bringing his head and shoulder level with the table (Figure 7-6).

(c) Alternate position for external rotation
The patient stands, facing the edge of a door frame with the palm of his hand against the frame and his elbow flexed 90 degrees. While keeping his arm against his side, the patient turns away from the fixed hand.

(d) To increase abduction and elevation of the arm
The patient sits with his side next to the table, his forearm resting with palm up on the table and pointing toward the opposite side of the table (Figure 7-7A). He then brings his head down toward his arm as he moves his thorax away from the table (Figure 7-7B).

(e) To increase extension
The patient stands with his back to the table, both hands grasping the edge with the fingers facing forward (Figure 7-8A). He then begins to squat while letting the elbows flex (Figure 7-8B).
Precaution: If a patient is prone to anterior subluxation or dislocation, this activity should not be done.

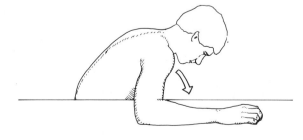

FIGURE 7-6. End position for self-stretching to increase shoulder external rotation.

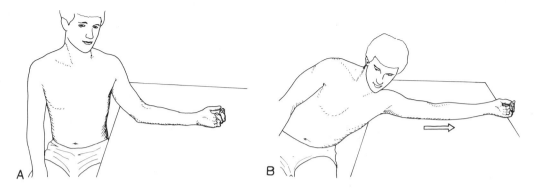

FIGURE 7-7. Beginning (*A*) and end (*B*) positions for self-stretching to increase shoulder abduction with elevation.

(6) *Self-mobilization techniques for a home program*
   (a) Caudal glide
      The patient sits on a firm surface and grasps his fingers under the edge. He then leans his trunk away from the stabilized arm (Figure 7-9).
   (b) Anterior glide
      The patient sits and places both arms behind him, fixing both hands on a solid surface. He then leans his body weight between his arms (Figure 7-10).

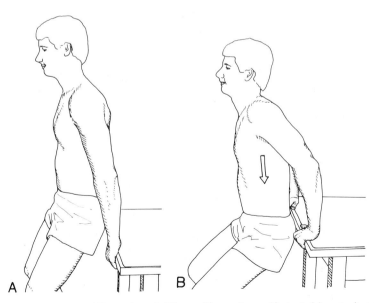

FIGURE 7-8. Beginning (*A*) and end (*B*) positions for self-stretching to increase shoulder extension.

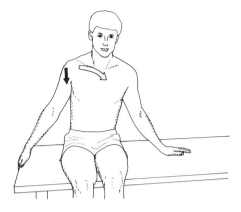

FIGURE 7-9. Self-mobilization; caudal glide of the humerus occurs as the person leans away from the fixed arm.

       (c) Posterior glide
           The patient lies prone and props himself up on both elbows. His body weight shifts downward between his arms (Figure 7-11).
    d. Determine if there are any faulty mechanics in the shoulder girdle or faulty posture. Stretch the tight and strengthen the weak components, then retrain the muscles to function within normal patterns of movement. If the patient returns to normal functional activities before normal mechanics are restored, the problem may be perpetuated. Frequent problems are
       (1) faulty deltoid rotator cuff mechanism.
       (2) faulty thoracic kyphosis posture (see Chapter 14).
       (3) poor scapular mobility.
       (4) muscle flexibility and strength imbalance.
    e. Once proper mechanics are restored, the patient should do active ROM of all shoulder motions daily and return to functional activities as much as tolerated.
    f. Occasionally, no progress is made, and the physician chooses to perform manipulation under anesthesia. Following this procedure, there is an inflammatory reaction and the joint is treated as though there were an acute lesion. Begin joint play and passive ROM techniques while the patient is still in the recovery room.

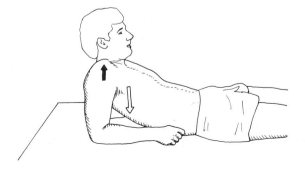

FIGURE 7-10. Self-mobilization; anterior glide of the humerus occurs as the person leans between the fixed arms.

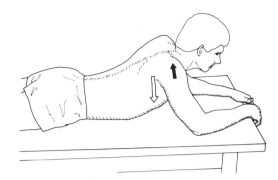

FIGURE 7-11. Self-mobilization; posterior glide of the humerus occurs as the person shifts his body weight downward between the fixed arms.

B. Joint Problems—Acromioclavicular (AC) and Sternoclavicular (SC) Joints

1. **Following trauma with overstretching of either the AC or SC joints, ligament or capsule hypermobility is permanent because there is no muscle support to restrict movement.**

2. **Clinical picture**
   a. Pain is localized to the joint or ligament.
   b. As the shoulder moves, there may be some pain in the injured joint either during the arc of movement or at the extremes of shoulder movement.

3. **Management if hypermobile**
   a. Rest the joint by putting the arm in a sling to support the weight of the arm.
   b. Cross-fiber massage to the capsule or ligaments
   c. ROM to the shoulder and Grade II traction and glides to the glenohumeral joint to prevent glenohumeral restriction.
   d. Teach the patient how to apply cross-fiber massage to himself if joint symptoms occur following excessive activity.

4. **Management if hypomobile**
   a. Sternoclavicular joint
      To increase elevation, caudal glide proximal clavicle (see Figure 5-22B).
      To increase depression, superior glide proximal clavicle (see Figure 5-21).
      To increase protraction, anterior glide proximal clavicle (see Figure 5-22A).
      To increase retraction, posterior glide proximal clavicle (see Figure 5-21).
   b. Acromioclavicular joint
      To increase motion, anterior glide distal clavicle (see Figure 5-20).

C. Anterior Shoulder Dislocation

1. Cause and clinical picture

The cause is usually trauma to the shoulder where there is excessive external rotation with abduction. The head of the humerus rests in the subcoracoid region rather than below the acromion process. This generally results in damage to the anterior portion of the capsule and subscapularis muscle.

2. Management

a. Following closed reduction (this should be undertaken only by someone specially trained), the part is immobilized for 3 to 4 weeks in a sling being removed only for exercise.

b. Exercises may be initiated early, using caution not to increase the inflammation or disrupt healing of the capsule and subscapularis muscle. The principles described in Section II A should be followed with the following *precautions* and treatment guidelines:

    (1) Protection

    While the soft tissues are healing, avoid full range of external rotation with abduction or hyperextension of the shoulder. Do external rotation motions during treatment with the elbow at the patient's side, progress to external rotation with the shoulder flexed in the sagittal plane and with the shoulder in resting position (abducted 55 degrees and horizontally adducted 30 degrees). Limit the range of external rotation to 50 degrees while healing. After 3 weeks of wearing the sling, the patient gradually increases the time the sling is off; the sling is used when the shoulder is tired or protection is needed.

    (2) Maintain joint play

    To maintain joint play, do sustained Grade II distraction or gentle Grade II oscillations with the glenohumeral joint at the side or in the resting position (see Figure 5-13).

    (3) Decrease joint contractures

    As healing occurs, if joint contractures develop, begin mobilization techniques using all appropriate glides to stretch the contractures, except the anterior glide. Anterior glide is *contraindicated* even though external rotation is necessary for functional elevation of the humerus. To safely stretch for external rotation, place the shoulder in resting position (abducted 55 degrees and horizontally adducted 30 degrees), then externally rotate it to the limit of its range, and then apply a Grade III distraction force (Figure 7-12).

    (4) Strengthening

    To maintain normal shoulder mechanics, both the internal and external rotators need to be strengthened as healing occurs. The internal rotators and adductors must be strong to support the anterior capsule; the external rotators must be strong to cause humeral depression and external rotation when elevating the humerus full range.

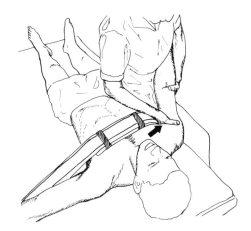

FIGURE 7-12. Mobilizing to increase external rotation when an anterior glide is contraindicated. Place the shoulder in resting position, externally rotate it, then apply a Grade III distraction force.

—Begin with **isometric resistance exercises** with the joint positioned at the side and progress to various pain-free positions within the available ranges.

—Progress to **isotonic resistance,** limiting external rotation to 50 degrees and avoiding the position of dislocation. Use elastic resistance for internal and external rotation with the arm at the side and elbow at 90 degrees. (see Figure 7–3A for external rotation.) For internal rotation, secure the elastic to a solid structure on the outside of the arm, and have the patient pull the hand in toward his waistline. Elastic resistance to adduction can be safely initiated by starting with the arm at the patient's side, elbow extended, the elastic secured lateral to the patient's hand. The patient pulls against the elastic by moving his hand across the front of his pelvis toward the opposite hip.

—At 3 weeks, begin supervised **isokinetic resistance** for internal rotation and adduction.[1] Position the patient standing with his arm at his side and elbow flexed 90 degrees. The patient does external rotation from the fully internal rotated position to the zero position. Progress to positioning the shoulder at 90 degrees flexion, then perform the rotations. Do not position in 90 degrees abduction.

—By 5 weeks, all shoulder motions are incorporated on isokinetic or other mechanical equipment—*except* the position of 90 degrees abduction with external rotation.

(5) Normal activities

The patient can return to normal activities when there is no weakness or muscle imbalance, and when the apprehension test result is negative. Full rehabilitation takes 2½ to 4 months.[1]

3. Management of recurrent dislocation

Recurrent dislocation is usually the result of severe ligamentous and capsule laxity. It may occur with any movement involving abduction of the shoulder. If anterior dislocation of the shoulder recurs on a regular basis and cannot be resolved with conservative management, surgical reconstruction is usually indicated. A brief explanation of several corrective procedures and postoperative rehabilitation is given in section III of this chapter.

D. Tendinitis

1. **Common sites of tendinous lesions at the shoulder include the tendon of the long head of the biceps brachii muscle in the bicipital groove (bicipital tendinitis), the infraspinatus tendon, and the supraspinatus tendon.**

2. **Causes**
   a. In young people, excessive activities.
      Overuse syndromes occur in the infraspinatus and long head of the biceps brachii tendon following a change or increase in exercise or training routine. Other musculotendinous units such as the pectoralis minor, short head of the biceps, and coracobrachialis are also subjected to microtraumas from excessive strain or overuse.
   b. In old people, degenerative lesions.
      The distal portion of the supraspinatus tendon is particularly vulnerable to impingement or overuse leading to degenerative changes, calcification, and eventual rupture.[38] Chronic ischemia caused by tension of the tendon, and decreased healing in the elderly are possible explanations.[22,38]

3. **Clinical picture**
   a. The onset may be acute, with pain intense enough to disturb sleep, or chronic, with low-grade irritation occurring with certain movements.[5,38]
   b. Referred pain occurs in the C-5 and C-6 dermatome reference zones.
   c. There may be a painful arc with ROM, and pain is experienced when isometric resistance is applied to the involved muscle, and when the muscle is stretched.
   d. Muscle contraction is strong unless there is a tear.
   e. Tenderness is experienced over the involved tendon when palpated.

4. **Management**
   a. See guidelines in Chapter 6, sections III and IV, with emphasis on modalities to decrease the inflammation during the acute stage and cross-fiber massage to the site of the lesion to produce a mobile scar and increase circulation.[10,22]
   b. Instruct the patient to avoid activities that cause the pain while the lesion is healing, so as not to continually irritate the structure.
   c. Progress strengthening of the involved muscle. Begin with isometric resistance with the muscle in the shortened position, then at various points through the range, until eventually in the stretched position. Progress to dynamic resistance exercises.
   d. Evaluate for muscle flexibility or strength imbalances throughout the

shoulder girdle. The exercise program should have a special emphasis on strengthening scapular retractors and the external rotators of the rotator cuff. If indicated, stretch and strengthen other muscles for good balance of length and strength.

e. Retrain for proper coordination of activities.

E. Bursitis

1. Clinical picture

Inflammation of the subdeltoid or subacromial bursa gives a clinical picture similar to tendinitis in the acute stage.

2. Management—Acute

a. See guidelines in Chapter 6, Section III B, with emphasis on splinting to prevent continued irritation of the bursa.

b. Intermittent periods of controlled motion to maintain range and inhibit pain

  (1) Use gentle (Grade I or II) joint techniques to the glenohumeral joint.

  (2) Pendulum exercises (see Figure 7-1, but the weight should not be used).

3. Management—Subacute

a. Regain function without irritating the bursa.

b. Analyze and eliminate faulty mechanics that perpetuate the problem by training and strengthening activities.

F. Shoulder-Hand Syndrome (Reflex Sympathetic Dystrophy)

1. Clinical picture[6,11,15]

a. Shoulder-hand syndrome is a reflex neurovascular disorder, often called reflex sympathetic dystrophy, which is characterized by

  (1) pain or hyperesthesia at the shoulder, wrist, or hand

  (2) limitation of motion of the

    (a) shoulder, with most restriction in lateral flexion and abduction

    (b) wrist, with most restriction in wrist extension

    (c) hand, with most restriction in metacarpophalangeal and proximal interphalangeal flexion secondary to shortened collateral ligaments

  (3) edema of the hand and wrist secondary to circulatory impairment of the venous and lymphatic systems, which in turn precipitates stiffness in the hand.

  (4) vasomotor instability

  (5) trophic changes in the skin

b. As the condition progresses

  (1) pain subsides but limitation of motion persists

  (2) the skin becomes cyanotic and shiny

  (3) intrinsic muscles of the hand atrophy

  (4) subcutaneous tissue in the fingers and palmar fascia thicken

  (5) nail changes occur

c. Shoulder-hand syndrome can develop in association with a cardiovascular accident, myocardial infarction, or cervical osteoarthritis or after trauma such as a fracture of the humerus or catheterization.

d. This condition can last for months or years, but spontaneous recovery often occurs in 18 to 24 months.

2. Management

This is a progressive disorder unless vigorous intervention is used.

a. Increase ROM of the shoulder and hand if limited, using techniques specific to the limiting structures and working within the pain-free range.
   (1) joint mobilization
   (2) muscle inhibition
   (3) soft-tissue stretching
b. Facilitate active muscle contractions with both isotonic and isometric exercise and light weight-bearing activities.
c. Relieve pain and increase sensory input with transcutaneous electrical nerve stimulation (TENS) or ice.
d. Apply intermittent pneumatic compression if there is edema. Elevate and use elastic compression when not receiving the pneumatic compression treatment.
e. Educate the patient on the importance of following the program of increased activity.
f. The physician may choose to perform a stellate block or use oral steroids or intramuscular medication in conjunction with therapeutic exercise.
g. Prevention is the best therapy. Whenever there is shoulder involvement or referred pain to the shoulder, the entire upper extremity should be moved as soon as allowed at an intensity safe for the condition.

G. Muscle Strength and Flexibility Imbalances

Whether the cause is nerve injury, disuse, or faulty posture or whether it is the result of some traumatic insult, muscle imbalance and faulty shoulder mechanics may precipitate or perpetuate painful syndromes. Restoring the balance of muscle strength, flexibility, and coordination is necessary for full recovery. (See also Chapter 14 for correction of cervical and thoracic postural problems that might underlie faulty shoulder girdle mechanics.)

1. Common problems and results

a. Weak external rotator muscles (infraspinatus and teres minor) will result in
   (1) abnormal deltoid-short rotator cuff mechanism.
   (2) incomplete external rotation when full humeral elevation is attempted in abduction.
   (3) the greater tubercle impinging on the coracoacromial arch when abduction is attempted, causing pain or impingement syndromes.
   (4) tightness in the antagonistic muscles and soft tissue (pectoralis major, teres major, subscapularis).
b. Weak upward rotator muscles of the scapula (upper and lower trapezius and serratus anterior) will cause
   (1) abnormal scapulohumeral rhythm when abduction or flexion of the shoulder is attempted.
   (2) decreased functional ROM of the shoulder girdle, because the scapula will not rotate upward through its full range or may rotate downward unopposed from the pull of the deltoid and supraspinatus muscles.
   (3) tightness in antagonistic muscles (levator scapulae and rhomboids, pectoralis minor) and soft tissue.

(4) postural abnormalities such as winging or tipping of the scapula.

  c. Weak postural muscles with tight antagonists will cause (see Chapter 14, section III B and C)

    (1) faulty alignment and mechanics of the shoulder girdle.[22]

    (2) postural pain syndromes.

2. Techniques to relax and progressively lengthen tight muscles if muscle is restricting motion

  a. Painful or restricting muscle guarding and spasm are the body's response to prevent motion when some underlying tissue has been damaged. Often there is no damage to the muscle itself. Since the cause of muscle guarding and spasm varies, different techniques have been found useful in gaining muscle relaxation. Whichever technique is most effective in relieving the spasm for a particular patient, its use should be continued until the spasm is under control. Besides use of modalities and massage, suggestions include techniques previously described

    (1) joint oscillations; see Section II A 2 b

    (2) gentle muscle setting; see Section II A 2 c

    (3) pendulum exercises; see Section II A 4 c (2)

    (4) caudal glide repositioning; see Section II A 4 c (4)

  b. Tight muscles can be effectively lengthened using inhibition techniques. Refer to Chapter 4 for principles, procedures, and techniques.

    (1) If there was an inflammatory reaction and the region now is in the early subacute stage of healing, the contraction of the muscle should be submaximal and not cause increased pain. As healing continues and the response of the tissue becomes predictable, the intensity of contraction can be progressively increased until maximum effort is used.

    (2) Conclude the lengthening procedure with active ROM through the available range.

  c. Self-stretching techniques such as those described in section IIA and illustrated in Figures 7-5 through 7-8 can be taught to the patient as well as end-range stretching using devices such as a wand, overhead pulleys, and finger ladder or wall climbing. Self-stretching with these devices requires careful instructions to avoid faulty mechanics or substitute motions (see Chapter 2). In addition, the patient should be cautioned in proper intensity of self-stretching (low-intensity, prolonged stretch).

  d. Following relaxation of muscle guarding and stretching of tight muscles or soft tissue, retrain or strengthen the antagonistic muscles for proper balance of strength and alignment.

3. Techniques to progressively strengthen muscles

Note: Chapter 3 presents principles and techniques of resistive exercises, and Chapter 6 presents procedures for exercising muscles at various stages of inflammation and repair. Refer to these chapters for guidelines and precautions.

  a. Isometric exercises

    (1) Initially use submaximal resistance; gradually increase the force at subsequent treatments if the patient responds favorably. Place the extremity in various positions in the pain-free range in order to

strengthen the muscle at different lengths. If pain from joint compression occurs, use manual resistance and apply a slight traction to the joint as resistance is given.

    (2) Examples of ways to teach the patient to do isometric exercises
        (a) The patient uses a wall or other solid structure and pushes against it for flexion (Figure 7-13A), abduction (Figure 7-13B), rotation (Figure 7-13C), or other variations.
        (b) The patient uses his contralateral extremity and resists against his humerus in the direction opposite the motion of the muscle for flexion (Figure 7-14A), abduction (Figure 7-14B), adduction, and extension; and resists against his forearm with the elbow flexed 90 degrees for rotation (Figure 7-14C).

  b. Progress to manual resistive exercises in the available range of motion. Use anatomic ranges of motion, isolated muscle function, or combined patterns of motion according to the defined needs and goals for the patient. Develop a plan that will improve the balance of muscle forces between the scapular and shoulder muscles.

  c. Progress to mechanical resistance when the patient's response to resistive exercise is predictable. Usually it is appropriate late in the subacute or chronic stage. Various types of resistance are available. Determine which piece of equipment best meets the treatment goals and ease of application. Some suggestions and examples are
    (1) wand exercises with weights added to the wand (see Figures 2-35, 2-36).
    (2) elasticized material that can be anchored with the opposite extremity or tied around a solid object (see Figure 7-3A).
    (3) wall pulleys (see Figure 7-3C).
    (4) Velcro weights and free hand-held weights (see Figures 3-30, 3-31, 7-3B, 7-15).

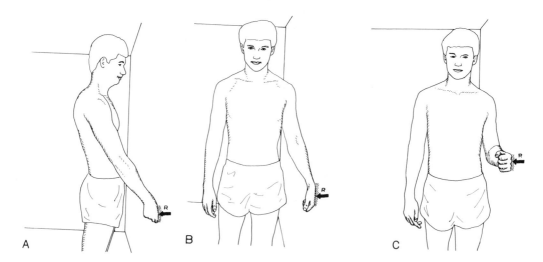

FIGURE 7-13. Using a wall to provide resistance for isometric shoulder flexion (*A*), abduction (*B*), or rotation (*C*).

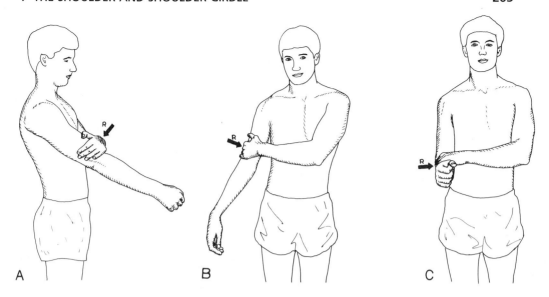

A   B   C

FIGURE 7-14. Self-resistance for isometric shoulder flexion (*A*), abduction (*B*), and rotation (*C*).

    (5) shoulder wheel with resistance added to the axis as the wheel turns (see Figures 2-40, 2-41).
    (6) variable resistance and isokinetic exercise equipment.

4. Functional usage of the shoulder

In preparation for activities, progressively increase the effort, repetitions, and speed using the desired functional pattern until functional ability is at a level where activity can be done safely without stress to the shoulder.

H. Referred Pain

1. Common sources referring pain into the shoulder region
  a. Cervical spine
    (1) vertebral joints between C-3 and C-4 or between C-4 and C-5
    (2) C-4 or C-5 nerve roots
  b. Dermatomal references from related tissues
    (1) C-4 dermatome is over the trapezius to the tip of the shoulder
    (2) C-5 dermatome is over the deltoid region and lateral arm
  c. Diaphragm: upper trapezius region
  d. Heart: axilla and left pectoral region
  e. Gallbladder irritation: tip of shoulder and posterior scapular region
  f. Myofascial pain patterns in the supraspinatus, infraspinatus, and trapezius.[41]

III. THERAPEUTIC EXERCISE FOR MANAGEMENT OF COMMON SURGICAL PROCEDURES OF THE SHOULDER

Severe trauma to musculoskeletal structures of the shoulder or progressive deterioration of the glenohumeral joint due to arthritis can cause pain, loss of mobility or stability of the

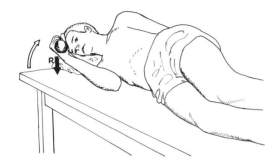

FIGURE 7-15. Resisted internal rotation of the shoulder using a hand-held weight. To resist external rotation, place the weight in the patient's upper hand.

shoulder, and complete loss of function of the upper extremity. When dysfunction is so pronounced, surgery is usually indicated.

The overall goal of all surgical procedures and postoperative rehabilitation of the shoulder is to regain functional use of the upper extremity. Specific goals include

1. relief of pain.
2. functional range of motion of the shoulder.
3. adequate strength and stability of the shoulder joint and upper extremity.
4. normal function of all unoperated joints in the upper extremity.

A. Repair of Rotator Cuff Tears

1. Indications for surgery

Rotator cuff tears can be classified as acute, chronic, degenerative, partial- or full-thickness tears. Rotator cuff tears occur most often in elderly individuals or as the result of a fall but can also occur in young athletes. Tears to the rotator cuff are associated with shoulder pain and limited upper extremity function. Weakness of shoulder abduction and external rotation is most common. Most rotator cuff tears are managed conservatively. Full-thickness rotator cuff tears usually require surgical repair to decrease pain and improve upper extremity function.[6,11,16,17,35,40]

2. Procedure[11,16,35,40]

a. Several surgical procedures can be used to repair rotator cuff tears. Most involve
   (1) approximation and reattachment with direct sutures of the torn tendons to the head of the humerus. The deltoid muscle must also be reflected and then reattached during the procedure.
   (2) decompression of the subacromial arch.
   (3) anterior acromioplasty and removal of the coracoacromial ligament if an impingement syndrome is present.
b. The shoulder is immobilized in a sling with the arm held at the side, or in an abduction splint to minimize tension on the repaired tendons for up to 6 weeks. The patient is only allowed out of the immobilization device for passive exercise.

3. Postoperative management[6,16,23,26,31,35,40]

a. Begin active exercise of the hand and wrist immediately after surgery to maintain range of motion.

b. As early as the first or by the fourth to sixth postoperative day, the sling can be temporarily removed for exercise.
  (1) Begin *passive* ROM exercises in the pain-free range, emphasizing forward flexion, abduction, and external rotation.
  (2) Add Codman's pendulum exercises during this early stage of healing.
  (3) Passive ROM helps the patient maintain movement while the reattached tendons are healing.

c. At 4 to 6 weeks postoperatively, begin *active* exercise of the shoulder, with emphasis on antigravity abduction in a protected position.[31]
  (1) While the patient is seated, the upper arm is held in 90 degrees of abduction by the therapist. The elbow is flexed to 90 degrees.
  (2) The patient attempts to lift the upper arm off the therapist's supporting hand.
  (3) This is done with the hand both pointing forward and toward the ceiling.

d. Start antigravity abduction from 0 degrees only after the patient can abduct the arm from the 90-degree position.

e. Begin gentle manual resistive exercise only after the patient can actively abduct the arm against gravity. This may be as long as 12 weeks after surgery. Increase resistance very gradually and conservatively. Resistance exercises can be done using elastic tubing, free weights, variable resistance, or isokinetic equipment.

f. At 3 months postoperatively, if the patient does not have near-normal ROM, begin stretching procedures.

B. Recurrent Dislocation of the Shoulder

Although recurrent anterior dislocation of the glenohumeral joint is the most common type of shoulder dislocation requiring surgical intervention, recurrent posterior dislocation can also be managed surgically when nonoperative, conservative treatment fails.

1. Reconstruction for recurrent anterior dislocation of the shoulder[23]

a. **Indications for surgery**
  (1) Recurrent dislocation requiring reduction
  (2) Recurrent subluxation that does not have to be reduced by someone else
  (3) Significant compromise of functional activities as the result of fear or putting the arm in positions that will cause dislocation

b. **Procedures**
  (1) Several reconstruction procedures may be done to improve anterior stability. They may include
    (a) transfer of the subscapularis muscle from the lesser tuberosity to the greater tuberosity.
    (b) transfer of the tip of the coracoid process with the short head of the biceps and coracobrachialis still attached to the anterior glenoid rim.
    (c) capsulorrhaphies (replacement of the torn shoulder capsule to the glenoid rim) with sutures or staples.
  (2) These procedures generally limit external rotation but support and tighten the anterior capsule.

(3) The upper extremity is immobilized, usually in a sling, for a few days to several weeks before exercises are begun.

c. **Postoperative management**
(1) After a period of immobilization, the sling is temporarily removed so that passive, active-assistive, and pendulum exercises can be carried out in the pain-free ROM. The repaired tissues of the shoulder region are treated as acute lesions. The sling is worn for about 1 month, except during exercise sessions.
(2) Begin active-free exercise at 4 to 6 weeks postoperatively.
(3) Add resistance during exercise at 10 to 12 weeks (see Figures 7-3A, 7-3C, and 7-15). Additional strengthening exercises may include those previously described in this chapter under management of anterior shoulder dislocation in Section IIC.
Precaution: Avoid the use of resistance equipment or activities that place the patient's involved upper extremity in the limits of external rotation, abduction, or hyperextension (see Figure 7-3B). Avoid functional or sports activities that require full range of shoulder external rotation or hyperextension if instability persists.

2. **Reconstruction for recurrent posterior dislocation of the shoulder**[16,18,23]

a. **Indications for surgery**
(1) Recurrent and painful subluxation or dislocation of the glenohumeral joint, particularly during activities that require full flexion or internal rotation.
(2) Upper extremity dysfunction as the result of recurrent dislocation.

b. **Procedures**
(1) Reconstruction is done to provide stability to the posterior portion of the capsule and will usually limit full internal rotation and forward flexion. The operative procedure may involve
(a) capsular plication and infraspinatus advancement.
(b) biceps tendon transfer and staple capsulorrhapy.
(c) posterior glenoid osteotomy.
(2) The shoulder is immobilized in external rotation in a reverse sling or spica cast for several days to several weeks.

c. **Postoperative management**
(1) As with reconstruction for anterior dislocation, passive ROM and pendulum exercises are begun after several days of complete immobilization. *Precaution:* During passive ROM, excessive forward flexion and internal rotation should be avoided.
(2) Active and resistive exercises are begun at a similar time in the postoperative period as with anterior reconstruction surgeries.
(a) A key muscle to strengthen is the supraspinatus.
(b) When strengthening the external rotators using weights or elastic resistance materials, do not begin in full internal rotation.
Precaution: as upper extremity function improves, educate the patient to avoid activities that might place the shoulder in the limits of shoulder flexion, internal rotation, or horizontal adduction and potentially cause recurrence of the posterior dislocation.

C. Glenohumeral (Total Shoulder) Joint Replacement

1. Indications for surgery[8,30]

a. Severe glenohumeral joint pain from osteoarthritis or traumatic or rheumatoid arthritis.

b. Decreased range of motion.

c. Loss of upper extremity strength and function.

2. Procedures[8,13,25,30,36,39]

Several types of glenohumeral joint replacements have been developed with varying amounts of shoulder stability built into the design. In general, the head of the humerus is removed and replaced with a stainless steel humeral stem prosthesis. The glenoid fossa is replaced with a high density polyethylene (plastic) component.

a. The most common procedure was developed by Neer[20,30] and is referred to as an unconstrained or resurfacing design. This is indicated when the rotator cuff is intact and functioning to give stability to the glenohumeral joint.

b. Partially constrained and constrained replacements have been designed to provide additional joint stability in patients with dysfunction of the rotator cuff and subsequent instability of the glenohumeral joint or more advanced deterioration of the joint surfaces.[8,11,36]

3. Postoperative management[20,31,33,39]

a. Immobilization of the operated shoulder is maintained for 4 to 5 days or longer depending on the type of procedure and the philosophy of the surgeon.

   (1) Immobilization is necessary after any type of total shoulder replacement. It is done to protect the anterior incision and capsule and the reattached rotator cuff and deltoid musculature.

   (2) The upper extremity is usually immobilized in a sling and swarthe or Velpeau dressing at the time of surgery, but a shoulder spica cast or splint may be used.

   (3) The shoulder is positioned in adduction, internal rotation, and slight forward flexion. The elbow is flexed, and the arm is supported by a sling.

   (4) When the patient is lying supine, the arm stays in the Velpeau dressing and a pillow is placed under the patient's arm to maintain the shoulder in 10 to 20 degrees of forward flexion. This is a comfortable position that protects the soft tissues repaired during surgery.

   (5) If the patient has a previous history of rotator cuff dysfunction and poor shoulder stability, immobilization may be required for several weeks before exercise may be initiated.

b. Exercise

The progression and type of exercise will vary with the type of surgical procedure chosen and the philosophy of the surgeon.

   (1) During the period of immobilization

      (a) encourage the patient to keep the shoulder, neck, and upper trunk musculature as relaxed as possible.

      (b) begin active exercises of the hand and wrist to maintain normal range of motion.

       (2) At 4 to 5 days postoperatively, the dressing is removed and re-placed with a supportive arm sling. The sling is removed only for exercise that includes
          (a) passive flexion of the shoulder with the elbow flexed.
          (b) passive abduction of the shoulder with the arm internally ro-tated.
          (c) passive external rotation only to neutral with the arm adducted (held at the patient's side).
          (d) active flexion and extension of the elbow.
          (e) active supination and pronation of the forearm.
          (f) active hand and wrist movements.
       (3) At 1 week begin
          (a) pendulum exercises with the arm held in internal rotation.
          (b) active-assistive forward flexion.
          (c) active-assistive abduction with the arm internally rotated.
       (4) At 1 to 2 weeks, progress to
          (a) active-assistive internal rotation.
          (b) active-assistive external rotation only to 20 degrees with the arm still adducted.
       (5) At 3 to 6 weeks, begin isometric exercise against gentle manual resistance to the shoulder flexors, abductors, and internal and ex-ternal rotators with the patient's arm adducted.
       (6) Active free exercise through the available range of motion should not be initiated before 6 weeks. During that time the patient should avoid leaning on the operated arm during activities of daily living.
       (7) By 8 weeks after surgery, the patient should use the operated arm in all activity except heavy lifting.
       (8) Strengthening exercises against light resistance with emphasis on the rotator cuff and deltoid muscles may be necessary for at least 1 year postoperatively for the patient to regain maximal function.
       (9) Gentle stretching exercises may also be required over a long-term period to gradually improve or maintain functional ROM.

    4. Long-term results[8,20,30,39]
      a. Almost all patients report total relief or a substantial decrease in shoul-der pain and therefore an improvement in function.
      b. Active range of motion and strength may be partially limited on a per-manent basis or for an extended period of time.
      c. If the rotator cuff and deltoid musculature is functioning well, a patient can expect to regain 70 percent normal strength and motion by 1 year after surgery.
      d. In one follow-up study the average active shoulder flexion 1 year after surgery was 115 degrees.[20]

D. Hemireplacement of the Shoulder (Humeral Head Replacement)[20,27–29,33,39]

  1. Indications for surgery
    a. Fracture dislocations of the proximal humerus
    b. Severe pain due to traumatic arthritis of the head of the humerus

  2. Procedure
    a. The head of the humerus is surgically excised and replaced with a

stainless steel intramedullary-stemmed prosthesis.

b. The prosthesis is held in place with methyl methacrylate, an acrylic cement.

c. The rotator cuff mechanism is repaired if indicated.

d. The patient is immobilized in an abduction splint for 2 to 4 weeks if a rotator cuff repair has been done. If no cuff repair was necessary, the patient's arm is immobilized and supported at his side in a Velpeau dressing.

3. Postoperative management[33]

a. If a surgical repair of the rotator cuff was done, follow the exercise plan discussed in the previous section of this chapter on complete rotator cuff tears.

b. If no cuff repair was necessary, the following exercise sequence is indicated.

   (1) During the period of immobilization (2 to 4 weeks), begin active range of motion exercises of the wrist and hand.

   (2) When the immobilization device is removed, begin

      (a) pendulum exercises with the arm internally rotated.

      (b) active-assistive flexion and abduction of the shoulder with the arm internally rotated.

      (c) active-assistive external rotation to neutral with the arm abducted or adducted (depending on the philosophy of the surgeon).

      (d) active flexion and extension of the elbow and supination and pronation of the forearm.

   (3) At 4 to 6 weeks isometric exercises of shoulder muscles against mild resistance may be started with the patient's arm kept at his side.

   (4) Active-resistive isotonic shoulder exercise should not be done for at least 6 more weeks.

E. Arthrodesis of the Shoulder[11,33]

1. Indications for surgery

a. Severe pain

b. Gross instability of the glenohumeral joint

c. Complete paralysis of the deltoid and rotator cuff muscles

d. Good compensatory scapular motion and strength of the serratus anterior and trapezius muscles

2. Procedure

a. The glenohumeral joint is fused with pins and bone grafts in a position of 15 to 20 degrees of flexion, 20 to 40 degrees of abduction, and neutral to internal rotation.

b. The shoulder is immobilized in a shoulder spica cast or brace that extends across the elbow joint for approximately 3 to 5 months.

3. Postoperative management[33]

a. While the shoulder is immobilized, the patient should be encouraged to maintain mobility in the wrist and hand.

b. If a brace with a hinged elbow is used, active elbow flexion and extension through the full range may be initiated the day after surgery.

    c. After the brace or cast has been removed, active and active-resistive scapulothoracic motion may be started.

  4. Long-term results[11,23]

    a. A patient may expect to achieve approximately 90 degrees of active elevation of the arm because of scapulothoracic motion.

    b. The shoulder will be stable and pain free for all activities that require strength or weight bearing at the shoulder. The patient will be able to bring his hand to his mouth and touch his hand behind his head.

IV. SUMMARY

Treatment of common orthopedic conditions in the shoulder girdle using appropriate therapeutic exercise techniques was described in Chapter 7, following a brief review of anatomy and kinesiology of the region.

Rather than using a cookbook protocol, the reader was provided with guidelines and suggestions for treatment. Section II of this chapter expanded the goals and plan of care described in Chapter 6, with reference to specific techniques that can be used to meet the goals.

The final section of Chapter 7 provided indications for and descriptions of common surgical procedures. The use and progression of therapeutic exercise for postoperative rehabilitation were also described.

REFERENCES

1. Aronen, JG and Regan, K: *Decreasing the incidence of recurrence of first-time anterior dislocations with rehabilitation.* Am J Sports Med 12:283, 1984.
2. Binder, AI, et al: *Frozen shoulder: a long-term prospective study.* Ann Rheum Dis 43:361, 1984.
3. Blakely, RL and Palmer, ML: *Analysis of rotation accompanying shoulder flexion.* Phys Ther 64:1214, 1984.
4. Blakely, RL and Palmer, ML: *Analysis of shoulder rotation accompanying a proprioceptive neuromuscular facilitation approach.* Phys Ther 66:1224, 1986.
5. Brunet, ME, Haddad, RJ, and Porche, EF: *Rotator cuff impingement syndrome in sports.* The Physician and Sports Medicine 10:87, 1982.
6. Cailliet, R: *Shoulder Pain,* ed 2. FA Davis, Philadelphia, 1981.
7. Codman, EA: *The Shoulder.* Thomas Todd Company, Boston, 1934.
8. Cofield, R, Morrey, B, and Bryan, R: *Total shoulder and total elbow arthroplasties: The current state of development—Part I.* JCE Orthopedics 6:14, 1978.
9. Cyriax, J: *Textbook of Orthopaedic Medicine, Volume One. Diagnosis of Soft Tissue Lesions,* ed 8. Baillière Tendall, London, 1982.
10. Cyriax, J: *Textbook of Orthopaedic Medicine, Volume Two. Treatment by Manipulation, Massage and Injection,* ed 10. Baillière Tendall, London, 1980.
11. DePalma, AF: *Surgery of the Shoulder,* ed 3. JB Lippincott, Philadelphia, 1983.
12. Dontigny, R: *Passive shoulder exercises.* Phys Ther 50:1707, 1970.
13. Fenlin, JM: *Total glenohumeral joint replacement.* Orthop Clin North Am 6:565, 1975.
14. Grey, RG: *The natural history of idiopathic frozen shoulder.* J Bone Joint Surg 60A:564, 1978.
15. Griffin, JW: *Hemiplegic shoulder pain.* Phys Ther 66:1884, 1986.
16. Hawkins, RJ, Koppert, G, and Johnston, G: *Recurrent posterior instability (subluxation) of the shoulder.* J Bone Joint Surg 66A:169, 1984.
17. Hawkins, RJ, Misamore, GW, and Hobeika, PE: *Surgery for full-thickness rotator cuff tears.* J Bone Joint Surg 67A:1349, 1985.
18. Hernandez, A and Drez, D: *Operative treatment of posterior shoulder dislocation by posterior glenoidplasty, capsulorrhapy and infraspinatus advancement.* Am J Sports Med 14:187, 1986.

19. Hoppenfeld, S: *Physical Examination of the Spine and Extremities.* Appleton-Century-Crofts, New York, 1976.
20. Hughes, M: *Glenohumeral joint replacement and post-operative rehabilitation.* Phys Ther 55:880, 1975.
21. Kaltenborn, F: *Course Notes.* Kent, Ohio, April, 1981.
22. Kessler, R and Hertling, D: *Management of Common Musculoskeletal Disorders.* Harper & Row, Philadelphia, 1983.
23. Kuland, DN: *The Injured Athlete,* ed 2. JB Lippincott, Philadelphia, 1988.
24. Lehmkuhl, LD and Smith, LK: *Brunnstrom's Clinical Kinesiology,* ed 4. FA Davis, Philadelphia, 1982.
25. Lettin, AWF and Scales, JT: *Total replacement of the shoulder joint (2 cases).* Proc Roy Soc Med 65:373, 1972.
26. Neer, CS: *Anterior acromioplasty for the chronic impingement syndrome in the shoulder. A preliminary report.* J Bone Joint Surg 54A:41, 1972.
27. Neer, CS: *Articular replacement of the humeral head.* J Bone Joint Surg 37A:215, 1955.
28. Neer, CS: *Displaced proximal humeral fractures.* J Bone Joint Surg 52A:1077, 1970.
29. Neer, CS: *Prosthetic replacement of the humeral head: Indications and operative technique.* Surg Clin North Am 43:158, 1963.
30. Neer, CS: *Replacement arthroplasty for glenohumeral osteoarthritis.* J Bone Joint Surg 56A:1, 1974.
31. Neviaser, RJ: *The painful shoulder.* In Nickel, VL (ed): *Orthopedic Rehabilitation.* Churchill-Livingstone, New York, 1982.
32. Norkin, C and Levangie, P: *Joint Structure and Function: A Comprehensive Analysis.* FA Davis, Philadelphia, 1983.
33. Occupational Therapy Staff: *Upper Extremity Surgeries for Patients with Arthritis—A Pre and Post-operative Occupational Therapy Treatment Guide.* Rancho Los Amigos Hospital, California, 1979.
34. Palmer, ML and Blakely, RL: *Documentation of medial rotation accompanying shoulder flexion: A case report.* Phys Ther 66:55, 1986.
35. Penny, JW and Welsh, MB: *Shoulder impingement syndromes in athletes and their surgical management.* Am J Sports Med 9:11, 1981.
36. Post, M, Haskel, S, and Finder, J: *Total shoulder replacement.* J Bone Joint Surg 57A:1171, 1975.
37. Rose, BS: *Frozen shoulder.* N Z Med J 98(792):1039, 1985.
38. Simkin, PA: *Tendinitis and bursitis of the shoulder, anatomy and therapy.* Postgrad Med 73:177, 1983.
39. Swanson, AB, et al: *Upper limb joint replacement.* In Nickel, VL (ed): *Orthopedic Rehabilitation.* Churchill-Livingstone, New York, 1982.
40. Tibone, JE, et al: *Surgical treatment of tears of the rotator cuff in athletes.* J Bone Joint Surg 68A:887, 1986.
41. Travell, JG and Rinzler, SH: *Myofascial genesis of pain.* Postgrad Med 11:425, 1952.
42. Wadsworth, CT: *Frozen shoulder.* Phys Ther 66:1878, 1986.

CHAPTER ——————————— 8

The Elbow and Forearm Complex

The design of the elbow and forearm adds to the mobility of the hand in space by shortening and lengthening the upper extremity and by rotating the forearm. The muscles provide control and stability to the region as the hand is used for various activities from eating, pushing, and pulling to coordinated use of tools and machines.[20]

The anatomic and kinesiologic relationships of the elbow and forearm are outlined in the first section of this chapter; the reader is also referred to several textbooks for in-depth study of the background material.[2,4,7,10,11,14] Chapter 6 presents information on principles of management; the reader should be familiar with that material before proceeding with establishing a therapeutic exercise program for the elbow and forearm.

OBJECTIVES

After studying this chapter, the reader will be able to:
1. identify important aspects of elbow and forearm structure and function for review.
2. establish a therapeutic exercise program to manage soft tissue and joint lesions in the elbow and forearm region related to stages of recovery following an inflammatory insult to the tissues.
3. establish a therapeutic exercise program to manage common musculoskeletal lesions, recognizing unique circumstances for their management.
4. establish a therapeutic exercise program to manage patients following common surgical procedures.

I. REVIEW OF THE STRUCTURE AND FUNCTION OF THE ELBOW AND FOREARM

   A. Bony Parts Are the Distal Humerus, Radius, and Ulna
      (see Figure 5-24)

B. Joints and Their Movements

1. The capsule of the elbow encloses three joints
a. the humeroulnar, which is the primary joint for flexion and extension
b. the humeroradial, which moves with flexion and extension but primarily affects pronation and supination
c. the proximal radioulnar, which participates in pronation and supination

2. The distal radioulnar joint
structurally separate from the elbow complex but moves with the proximal radioulnar joint as a functional unit for pronation and supination

3. Elbow joint characteristics
a compound, uniaxial hinge joint with a lax joint capsule, supported by two major ligaments: the medial (ulnar) and lateral (radial) collateral.
a. Humeroulnar articulation
   (1) The medially placed hourglass-shaped trochlea at the distal end of the humerus is convex. It faces anteriorly and downward 45 degrees from the shaft of the humerus. The concave trochlear fossa, on the proximal ulna, faces upward and anteriorly 45 degrees from the ulna[10] (see Figure 5-25).
   (2) The primary motion is flexion and extension; the concave fossa slides in the same direction in which the ulna moves.
   (3) There is also slight medial and lateral sliding of the ulna, allowing for full elbow ROM; it results in a valgus angulation of the joint with elbow extension and a varus angulation with elbow flexion. When the bone moves in a medial/lateral direction, the trochlear ridge provides a convex surface, and the trochlear groove a concave surface, so the sliding of the ulna is opposite the bone motion.

Physiologic Motion of Ulna	Direction of Slide of Ulna on Trochlea
Flexion	Distal/Anterior
Varus angulation	Lateral
Extension	Proximal/Posterior
Valgus angulation	Medial

b. The humeroradial joint
   (1) The laterally placed, spherical capitulum at the distal end of the humerus is convex. The concave bony partner, the head of the radius, is at the proximal end of the radius.
   (2) As the elbow flexes and extends, the concave radial head slides in the same direction as the bone motion. With pronation and supination of the forearm, the radial head spins on the capitulum.

Physiologic Motion of Radius	Direction of Slide of Radius on Capitulum
Flexion	Anterior
Extension	Posterior

4. Forearm joint characteristics

Both the proximal and distal radioulnar joints are uniaxial pivot joints that function as one joint to produce pronation and supination (rotation) of the forearm.

a. The proximal (superior) radioulnar joint

(1) It is within the capsule of the elbow joint but is a distinct articulation.

(2) The convex rim of the radial head articulates with the concave radial notch on the ulna so that, with rotation of the radius, the convex rim moves opposite to the bone motion.

Physiologic Motion of Radius	Direction of Slide of Proximal Radius on Ulna
Pronation	Posterior (dorsal)
Supination	Anterior (volar)

(3) With rotation of the radial head, it spins in the annular ligament and against the capitulum of the humerus.

b. The distal (inferior) radioulnar joint

(1) The concave ulnar notch on the distal radius articulates with the convex portion of the head of the ulna.

(2) With physiologic movements, the articulating surface of the radius slides in the same direction.

Physiologic Motion of Radius	Direction of Slide of Distal Radius on Ulna
Pronation	Anterior (volar)
Supination	Posterior (dorsal)

C. Muscle Function at the Elbow and Forearm

1. Elbow flexor muscles

a. Brachialis

The brachialis is a one-joint muscle that inserts close to the axis of motion on the ulna, so it is unaffected by the position of the forearm or the shoulder; it participates in all flexion activities of the elbow.

b. Biceps brachii

The biceps is a two-joint muscle that crosses both the shoulder and elbow and inserts close to the axis of motion on the radius, so it also acts as a supinator of the forearm. It functions most effectively as a flexor of the elbow between 80 and 100 degrees of flexion. For optimal length-tension relationship, the shoulder extends to lengthen the muscle when it contracts forcefully for elbow and forearm function.

c. Brachioradialis

With its insertion a great distance from the elbow on the distal radius, the brachioradialis mainly functions to provide stability to the joint, but it also participates as the speed of flexion motion increases and a load is applied with the forearm from midsupination to full pronation.[20]

2. Elbow extensor muscles

a. Triceps brachii

The long head crosses both the shoulder and elbow; the other two heads are uniaxial. The long head functions most effectively as an elbow extensor if the shoulder simultaneously flexes; this maintains an optimal length-tension relationship in the muscle.

   b. Anconeus
      This muscle stabilizes the elbow during supination and pronation and assists in elbow extension.

3. Forearm supinator muscles

   a. Biceps brachii
      See Section 1 a.
   b. Supinator
      This muscle pulls the distal end of the radius over the ulna.

4. Forearm pronator muscles

   a. Pronator teres
      This muscle pronates as well as stabilizes the proximal radioulnar joint and helps approximate the humeroradial articulation.[20]
   b. Pronator quadratus
      The pronator quadratus is a one-joint muscle and is active during all pronation activities.

D. Wrist and Hand Muscles

Many muscles that act on the wrist and hand are attached on the distal portion (epicondyles) of the humerus. This allows for movement of the fingers and wrist whether the forearm is in pronation or supination.

1. Originating on the medial epicondyle are the flexor carpi radialis, flexor carpi ulnaris, palmaris longus, and the flexor digitorum superficialis and profundus.
2. Originating on the lateral epicondyle are the extensor carpi radialis longus and brevis, extensor carpi ulnaris, and extensor digitorum.
3. The muscles provide stability to the elbow but contribute little to motion at the elbow. The position of the elbow will affect the length-tension relationship of the muscles during their actions on the wrist and hand.[20]

E. Major Nerves Subject to Pressure and Trauma Around the Elbow[12]

1. Ulnar nerve

The nerve is superficial to the olecranon fossa, posterior to the medial epicondyle, and is covered by a fibrous sheath, which forms the cubital tunnel; it then passes between the heads of the flexor carpi ulnaris. Pressure or injury to the nerve at these sites will cause sensory changes in the cutaneous distribution of the nerve (ulnar border of the hand, little finger, and ulnar half of the ring finger), with progressive weakness in the muscles innervated distal to the site of injury (flexor carpi ulnaris, ulnar half of the flexor digitorum profundus, hypothenar eminence, interossei, lumbricals III and IV, flexor pollicis brevis, and adductor pollicis).

2. Radial nerve

The nerve pierces the lateral muscular septum anterior to the lateral epicondyle and passes under the origin of the extensor carpi radialis brevis, then divides.

    a. The deep branch may become entrapped as it passes under the edge of the extensor carpi radialis brevis and the fibrous slit in the supinator, causing progressive weakness in the wrist and finger extensor and supinator muscles (except the extensor carpi radialis longus, which is innervated proximal to the bifurcation).

    b. The deep branch may also be injured with a radial head fracture.

    c. The superficial radial nerve may receive direct trauma that causes sensory changes in the lateral aspect of the forearm to the anatomic snuffbox, and the radial side of the dorsum of the wrist and hand and radial three and one-half digits.

3. Median nerve

The nerve courses deep in the cubital fossa, medial to the tendon of the biceps and brachial artery, then progresses between the ulnar and humeral heads of the pronator teres and dips under the flexor digitorum sublimis muscle. Entrapment may occur between the heads of the pronator muscle, causing sensory changes duplicating the carpal tunnel syndrome (palmar aspect of the thumb, index, middle, and half of the ring finger, and dorsal aspect of distal phalanges of index and ring fingers). Motor changes include the pronator teres, wrist flexors, extrinsic finger flexors, and the intrinsic thenar and lumbricals I and II. (Carpal tunnel syndrome involves just the intrinsic muscles of the thenar eminence and lumbricals I and II; see Chapter 9.)

II.   GUIDELINES AND THERAPEUTIC EXERCISE MANAGEMENT OF COMMON MUSCULOSKELETAL PROBLEMS IN THE ELBOW AND FOREARM

Note: To avoid redundancy, the reader is referred to Chapter 6 for general guidelines that should be followed when establishing therapeutic exercise programs during the acute, subacute, and chronic phases of inflammation and healing.

A. Joint Problems

1. Humeroulnar joint

    a. **Clinical picture**
With joint involvement, passive flexion is more limited than extension and there is a capsular end-feel. Pronation and supination are not restricted except in long-standing arthritis.[4] With an acute injury, there are signs of inflammation.

    b. **Management**

      (1) Traumatic injuries
Immobilize with follow-up therapy if there is limitation after healing.

      (2) Acute inflammatory arthritis
See section VII of Chapter 6.

      (3) Subacute or chronic capsular restrictions
Follow the outline as described for chronic conditions (sections V and IX C of Chapter 6) with emphasis on joint mobilization.

        (a) To increase flexion
Sustained distraction of the ulna (see Figure 5-26A)
Sustained distraction with distal glide of the ulna (see Figure 5-26B)

Sustained lateral glide or varus angulation of the ulna is used to gain the terminal degrees of flexion

(b) To increase extension

Sustained distraction of the ulna (see Figure 5-26A)

Medial glide or valgus angulation of the ulna is used to gain the terminal degrees of extension

Precaution: Following trauma, if the brachialis muscle is injured, ossification of the injured tissue is a potential complication; therefore, evaluate for signs of myositis ossificans (see Section C to follow). If myositis ossificans is not present, progress stretching carefully.

2. Humeroradial joint

a. Clinical picture

This joint limits flexion and extension only in long-standing arthritis or following prolonged periods of immobilization; then pronation and supination (rotation) will also be limited.

Precaution: If flexion and extension are limited, as well as rotation, and the condition is acute following trauma, there is usually a fracture,[4] so the part must be immobilized for healing; or there is a subluxation of the radial head, which requires special procedures depending of the type of subluxation (see numbers 3 and 4 below).

b. Management

Follow the outline as described for chronic conditions in sections V and IX C of Chapter 6

(1) To increase flexion

Sustained distraction of the radial head (see Figure 5-27)

Sustained volar glide head of radius (see Figure 5-28)

(2) To increase extension

Sustained distraction of the radial head

Sustained dorsal glide head of radius (see Figure 5-28)

(3) See also numbers 5 and 6 below to increase pronation and supination.

3. Proximal subluxation of radial head (pushed elbow)

a. Clinical picture

There may be limited flexion or extension of the elbow, limited wrist flexion, and limited pronation. It often occurs from falling on an outstretched hand.[24] The radial head is pushed proximally in the annular ligament and impinges against the capitulum. This sometimes accompanies a fracture of the distal radius (Colles' fracture) or scaphoid and is not considered a clinical problem until after healing of the fracture and removal of the cast. It is often overlooked because there is considerable soft-tissue and joint restriction caused by the period of immobilization. Bilateral palpation of the joint spaces will reveal the decreased space on the involved side.

b. Management

If acute (and no fracture), a distal traction of the radius will reposition the radial head. If chronic, it will require repetitive stretching with sustained Grade III distal traction to the radius (see Figure 5-27), in addition to the soft-tissue stretching and strengthening techniques needed for increasing motion.

4. **Distal subluxation of the radial head (pulled elbow)**
   a. **Clinical picture**
      There is limited supination with pain in the elbow region following a forceful traction to the forearm. This is usually seen as an acute injury in children and is sometimes labeled tennis elbow when it occurs in adults.[24]
   b. **Management**
      A quick compressive manipulation with supination to the radius (see Figure 5-29) will usually reposition the head. If it is an initial injury, there may be soft-tissue trauma from the injury, which is treated with cold and compression.

5. **Proximal radioulnar joint**
   a. **Clinical picture**
      With joint involvement there is limited pronation and supination with pain in the proximal forearm when overpressure is applied.
   b. **Management**
      For subacute or chronic capsular restrictions, follow the outline as described for chronic conditions (see Sections V and IX C of Chapter 6) emphasing mobilization.
      (1) To increase pronation
          Dorsal glide radial head (see Figure 5-30)
      (2) To increase supination
          Volar glide radial head (see Figure 5-30)

6. **Distal radioulnar joint**
   a. **Clinical picture**
      When this joint is involved there may be limited pronation or supination and pain in the distal forearm with overpressure following immobilization. With inflammatory arthritis there may be pain only at the extremes of rotation.
   b. **Management**
      For subacute or chronic capsular restrictions follow the outline as described for chronic conditions (sections V and IX C of Chapter 6) emphasizing mobilization.
      (1) To increase pronation
          Sustained volar glide distal radius (see Figure 5-31)
      (2) To increase supination
          Sustained dorsal glide distal radius (see Figure 5-31)
      (3) To treat for pain
          Grade I or II oscillations, dorsal-volar glides

Note: Following healing of fractures in the forearm, it is not unusual for there to be malunion, which prevents full range of pronation or supination. A bony block end-feel or an abnormal appearance of the forearm should alert the therapist. X-ray films are helpful in verifying the problem. No amount of stretching or mobilizing will change the patient's range. Indiscriminate stretching may lead to hypermobility of related joints, which could cause additional trauma and pain.

B. Limited Elbow Extension From Tight Elbow Flexor Muscles (Biceps or Brachialis)

1. Clinical picture

With tight muscles there is an elastic end-feel. Differentiate between the biceps and brachialis muscles by taking the elbow to maximum extension, then pronating the forearm and extending the shoulder. This will not change the length of the brachialis but will change the length of the biceps.

2. Management

If the brachialis is limited and tender over the distal muscle belly, stretching may precipitate myositis ossificans. Do not attempt to stretch (see section C below). To elongate the biceps, use active inhibition techniques (maximum range is pictured in Figure 2-8). Passive stretching, if done using a moderate- to high-intensity, short-duration stretch force, can traumatize soft tissues around the elbow. Very low-intensity, long-duration stretching with dynamic splinting holds promise as a safe and effective method for reducing elbow flexion contractures.[6]

C. Myositis Ossificans

1. Clinical picture

The brachialis muscle may be affected following trauma in the elbow region. Myositis ossificans is most commonly seen with a supracondylar fracture and posterior dislocation[11] or with a tear of the brachialis tendon.[4] It is distinguished from traumatic arthritis of the humeroulnar joint in that resisted elbow flexion causes pain, flexion is limited and painful when the inflamed muscle is pinched between the humerus and ulna, and resisted flexion in midrange causes pain in the brachialis muscle. Palpation of the distal brachialis muscle is tender. See comments in section B above.

2. Management

If the brachialis muscle is implicated following trauma, massage, passive stretching, and exercise should NOT be done. The elbow should be kept at rest.

D. Tendinitis

Pain is experienced in the elbow region with forceful movements of the wrist or fingers.

1. Typical lesions

a. When the common extensor tendons along the lateral epicondyle are involved, it is known as *lateral epicondylitis* or *tennis elbow*. The highest incidence is in the musculotendinous junction of the extensor carpi radialis brevis.[4,11]

Note: Pulled elbow, pushed elbow, rotated elbow, radial head fracture, pinched synovial fringe, meniscal lock, and periosteal bruise are also possible sources of pain at the elbow and are sometimes called tennis elbow.[24]

b. Common flexor tendon involvement at the tenoperiosteal junction near the medial epicondyle is known as *medial epicondylitis* or *golfer's elbow*.

2. Causes
a. Repetitive or excessive use of the muscle, causing microdamage to the tissue, which does not heal properly, is the most common cause.
b. Recurring problems are seen because the resulting immobile or immature scar is redamaged when returning to activities.

3. Clinical picture
a. There is gradually increasing pain in the elbow region following excessive activity of the wrist and hand.
b. Pain is experienced when the involved muscle is stretched or when it contracts against resistance while the elbow is extended.
c. Often, chronic recurrences of the inflammatory process are seen whenever the part is used excessively. The condition does not spontaneously resolve.

4. Management—Acute stage
Follow the outline for treatment considerations in Chapter 6, sections III, IV, and V.
a. To control pain, edema, or spasm
   (1) Rest the muscles in a splint. If the extensor muscles are involved, immobilize the wrist in a cock-up splint, while keeping the elbow free to move.
   (2) The patient should not perform strong gripping activities.
   (3) Cryotherapy also helps control edema and swelling.
b. To maintain soft tissue and joint mobility
   (1) Several times a day, remove the splint and gradually elongate the muscle within its pain-free range of motion. Have the patient do a gentle muscle-setting contraction with the muscle in its shortened position, then actively move the muscle through its range. Cyriax[4] suggests that it takes 10 days to gain full range of motion.
   POSITION OF THE PATIENT AND TECHNIQUE FOR EXTENSOR TENDONS The patient sits with his elbow flexed and forearm resting on a table. With the wrist in extension, provide a gentle resistance to the wrist extensor muscles; hold the contraction to the count of six, then slowly move the wrist towards flexion, just to the point where pain begins. No forcing is done when pain is acute. Progress by placing the elbow in greater degrees of extension until it is fully extended. For further progression see section c (1) below. The patient can be taught to apply gentle resistance with his other hand.
   (2) Electrical stimulation to the muscle may also keep it mobile.[13]
   (3) Gentle cross-fiber massage within tolerance to the site of the lesion.
   (4) Active ROM should be done in all other elbow, forearm, and wrist motions.

5. Management—Subacute or chronic stage
Note: If there is chronic inflammation, treat the inflammation first as described above.
a. To gradually increase the flexibility of the muscle and create a mobile scar as the pain and inflammation decrease
   (1) ACTIVE INHIBITION TECHNIQUE FOR THE EXTENSOR CARPI RADIALIS BREVIS

The patient begins with the elbow extended and forearm pronated. While holding this position, he ulnarly deviates the wrist and flexes the wrist and fingers. There should not be an increase in pain, just a stretching sensation.[11] Gentle contract-relax techniques can also be used.

(2) SELF-STRETCHING TECHNIQUE FOR THE EXTENSOR MUSCLE GROUP
The patient places the back of his hand against the wall, fingers pointed down. Keeping the elbow in extension and forearm in pronation, he moves the back of his hand up the wall[23] (Figure 8-1). When a pulling sensation in the extensors is felt, the position is maintained. Active inhibition can then be added by maintaining the position and having the patient flex his fingers.

(3) SELF-STRETCHING TECHNIQUE FOR THE FLEXOR MUSCLE GROUP
Elongate the muscles by placing the palm of the hand against the wall, fingers pointed down, then moving the hand up the wall in the same manner as described in number (2) above, keeping the elbow extended.[23]

(4) The intensity of the cross-fiber massage at the site of the scar formation is increased.

b. To gradually strengthen the muscle

(1) Progress the isometric exercises in various pain-free positions; when there is no pain through the range of motion progress to concentric resistance at an appropriate dosage.

(2) Progressive resistance exercises (PRE) using a hand-held weight are used for flexion, extension (Figure 8-2), pronation, and supination (Figure 8-3A and B). Elastic resistance is used for wrist flexion and extension by placing a loop of elastic material under the foot and holding the other end in the hand; the arm is held or supported in a horizontal position. When the forearm is pronated, resistance is against the wrist extensors; when supinated, the resistance is against the wrist flexors.

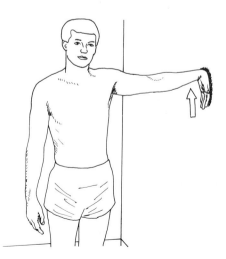

FIGURE 8-1. Self-stretching of the muscles of the lateral epicondyle.

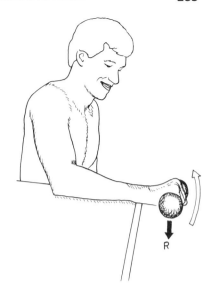

FIGURE 8-2. Mechanical resistance exercise using a hand-held weight for strengthening the muscles of the lateral epicondyle (wrist extensors).

        (3) Wall pulleys or elastic resistance can be used to simulate tennis swings (Figure 8-4A, B, and C).[13]

    c. To progress to functional training and conditioning

Include strength, endurance, power, and flexibility exercises in the arm and forearm. Of equal importance is reducing the overload forces that caused the problem and retraining for proper technique.[11,12,18]

        (1) Instruct the patient to apply friction massage and to stretch the involved muscle prior to using it.

        (2) Begin strength and power training sessions with warm-up exercises that include general flexibility exercises for the shoulder, elbow, wrist, and trunk.

        (3) Attain general strengthening and conditioning of any unused or underused part of the extremity or trunk before returning to the stressful activity.

        (4) Include exercises simulating the desired activity at high speeds with low resistance to improve timing.

        (5) Assess the patient's technique and advise him on how to modify it before returning to the stressful activity. (This may require taking tennis lessons to correct improper tennis techniques.) If equipment is used (as in tennis or with a hammer), it should also be analyzed and modified to reduce stress.[11,18]

E. Muscle Strength and Flexibility Imbalances

In addition to the conditions already described in this chapter, imbalances in length and strength of muscles crossing the elbow and forearm can result from a variety of causes such as nerve injury or following surgery, trauma, or immobilization. Selections of appropriate exercises following biomechanical evaluation can be made from the stretching and strengthening techniques described in the previous sections as well as in Chapters 3 and 4. For patients with elbow problems, exercises to the joints above (shoulder) and below (wrist

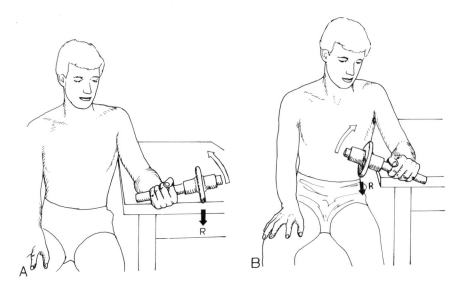

FIGURE 8-3. Mechanical resistance exercise using a small bar with asymmetrically placed weights for strengthening forearm pronators (*A*) and supinators (*B*).

and hand) should also be incorporated into the therapeutic program to prevent complications and aid in healing.

III. THERAPEUTIC EXERCISE MANAGEMENT FOLLOWING COMMON SURGICAL PROCEDURES OF THE ELBOW AND FOREARM

Surgical intervention at the elbow is often necessary following a variety of fractures that require open reduction and internal fixation.[9,15] Long-standing rheumatoid arthritis and osteoarthritis, which is usually the result of trauma, may also need to be treated surgically.

The goals of surgery and postoperative management in almost all procedures for the elbow are:[3,8,15]

1. relief of pain.
2. adequate joint stability.
3. sufficient range of motion and strength for all functions of daily living.

Procedures done to relieve pain and improve elbow stability tend to be more successful than procedures done solely to increase range of motion. Heterotopic bone formation, which leads to joint stiffness, is often a complication of elbow fractures and elbow joint surgery.[9] Therefore, the single goal of improving range of motion is rarely an indication for surgery.[8]

In the postoperative period, as with any other surgical procedure of the extremities, it is important to maintain range of motion and strength in all unoperated joints. Special attention should be given to the shoulder, wrist, and hand after elbow surgery. Elevation of the operated extremity and active range of motion of the shoulder and hand, as soon after surgery as possible, will prevent dysfunction in these unoperated joints.

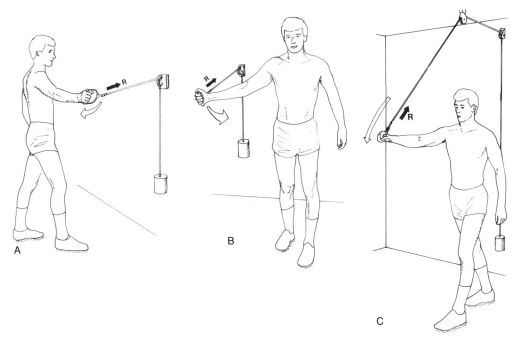

FIGURE 8-4. Mechanical resistance exercise using wall pullies to simulate tennis swings; backhand stroke (*A*), forehand stroke (*B*), and serve (*C*).

A. Elbow Synovectomy and Resection of the Radial Head (with or without Radial Head Implant)[16,19,21]

1. Indications for surgery
 a. Chronic synovitis of the elbow because of rheumatoid or traumatic arthritis.
 b. Pain on motion and marked limitation of flexion and extension of the elbow or supination and pronation of the forearm because of involvement of the humeroradial and proximal radioulnar joints.
 c. Tenderness on palpation and possible subluxation of the radial head.

2. Procedure
 a. Removal of the proliferated synovium of the elbow.
 b. Resection of the radial head usually through a lateral incision.
 c. Possible implantation of a silicone radial head.

3. Postoperative management[16,19,21]
 a. From the first to fourth postoperative day, the elbow is immobilized either in a cast or in a compression bandage and posterior plaster elbow splint. The elbow is held in a position of 90 degrees of flexion, and the forearm is held in midposition.
  (1) The arm is elevated for comfort and for prevention of edema distally.
  (2) Active finger motion is indicated to prevent stiffness.
 b. Between 3 and 5 days postoperatively, either the cast is bivalved or the compression dressing is removed.

(1) Active-assistive range of motion of the elbow and forearm is begun.
(2) The splint is replaced after exercise and worn at night for several weeks.
  c. Exercise is progressed from active-assistive to active exercise over the next 4 to 6 weeks. During that time, the patient must avoid lifting heavy objects with the operated arm and hand.
  d. By 6 weeks, full joint activity is allowed.
(1) Progressive resistance exercise may be implemented slowly and cautiously.
(2) Gentle stretching, using active inhibition and elongation techniques (see Chapter 4), may be necessary to increase range of motion.

B. Total Elbow Arthroplasty[3,5,8,22]
1. Indications for surgery
  a. Pain and articular destruction of the humeroulnar and humeroradial joints.
  b. Marked limitation of motion at the elbow, particularly in patients with bilateral ankylosis of the elbow.
  c. Gross instability of the elbow.
  d. Bone stock loss from trauma or tumors.

2. Procedure
  a. General Background
  Several humeroulnar joint replacements have been developed over the years. The early designs were hinged (constrained) metal prostheses, allowing only flexion and extension of the elbow joint. These implants eventually failed because no allowances for normal varus and valgus and rotational movements of the elbow were incorporated into these early designs, and hence, the prosthesis loosened. More recent implants now build in all appropriate elbow motions. The majority of total elbow replacements done today are either semiconstrained or unconstrained (resurfacing) replacements. The unconstrained designs do not provide additional elbow joint stability.
  b. Overview of the Procedure
(1) A longitudinal incision is made at the posterior aspect of the elbow.
(2) The triceps muscle is incised (split), and a small portion of the distal humerus and proximal ulna is resected.
(3) A stainless steel humeral replacement and a polyethylene ulnar component are cemented in place with methyl methacrylate. More recent implants, designed to minimize loosening, include an intramedullary cemented stem and extramedullary flange for osseus ingrowth.[17] In the future, cementless elbow components may minimize prosthetic loosening, which continues to be the most common cause of failure of elbow arthroplasty.
(4) If the head of the radius is removed, it may or may not be replaced with a prosthetic silicone implant.

3. Postoperative management[1,8,16,19,21]
  a. Immediately after surgery a soft compression dressing and posterior splint are applied to immobilize the elbow in approximately 90 degrees of flexion and a neutral position of the forearm.

    b. During this period (1 to 4 days) of immobilization of the elbow
       (1) The arm is elevated in bed or supported with a sling when the patient is upright.
       (2) Active finger, wrist, and shoulder exercises are done to minimize edema in the hand and maintain normal motion in the joints proximal and distal to the elbow.
    c. Between 5 to 7 days postoperatively the splint is removed, and active-assistive range of motion of the elbow is started with the patient in a supine position and the patient's arm at his side. The exercises include
       (1) active-assistive flexion and passive extension of the elbow with the forearm in supination, pronation, and midposition.
       Precaution: Avoid any *antigravity* elbow extension or stretch to the triceps to protect the re-attachment of the triceps mechanism.
       (2) active supination and pronation of the forearm with the elbow in 90 degrees of flexion.
       (3) The splint should be worn for 4 to 6 weeks when the patient is not exercising.
    d. Between 8 to 10 days, a new splint is fabricated with the elbow in maximum comfortable extension. The patient alternates wearing the extension and the flexion splints to maintain as much range of motion as possible.
    e. At 3 to 4 weeks, active antigravity elbow extension may be added to the patient's exercises.
    f. By 6 weeks postoperatively, when the triceps mechanism is secure, gentle isotonic resistance exercise may be started. This is continued until the patient is using his arm in all normal activities of daily living.

4. Long-term results[1,3,20]

    a. A good functional result gives the patient at least 90 degrees of pain-free elbow flexion and extension. The patient should strive for at least 110 degrees of flexion and as complete extension as possible.
    b. *Precaution:* the patient should avoid using the elbow joint for lifting and carrying heavy objects or using the operated arm for weight bearing during ambulation with crutches.

IV. SUMMARY

Following a brief review of anatomy and kinesiology of the elbow and forearm region, common musculoskeletal conditions that can be treated with therapeutic exercise were described. Suggestions and guidelines for treatment were outlined. The reader again is encouraged to use the information provided in Chapter 6 as the foundation for designing appropriate therapeutic exercise programs.

    Common surgical procedures of the elbow and the use of therapeutic exercises during the postoperative rehabilitation period were described. Guidelines for the progression of exercise and precautions during exercise were also included in this final section of the chapter.

REFERENCES

1. Bentley, JA: *Physiotherapy following joint replacements.* In Downie, PA: *Cash's Textbook of Orthopedics and Rheumatology for Physiotherapists.* JB Lippincott, Philadelphia, 1984.

2. Cailliet, R: *Soft Tissue Pain and Disability.* FA Davis, Philadelphia, 1977.
3. Cofield, RH, Morrey, BF, and Bryan, RS: *Total shoulder and total elbow arthroplasties: The current state of development*—Part II. J Contin Educ Orthop, Jan. 1979, p 17.
4. Cyriax, J: *Textbook of Orthopaedic Medicine, Volume One. Diagnosis of Soft Tissue Lesions,* ed 8. Bailliere Tindall, London, 1982.
5. Dee, R: *Total replacement arthroplasty of the elbow for rheumatoid arthritis.* J Bone Joint Surg (Br) 54:88, 1972.
6. Hepburn, G and Crivelli, K: *Use of elbow dynasplint for reduction of elbow flexion contractures: A case study.* J Orthop Sports Phys Ther 5:259, 1984.
7. Hoppenfeld, S: *Physical Examination of the Spine and Extremities.* Appleton-Century-Crofts, New York, 1976.
8. Inglis, AE (ed): *Symposium on Total Joint Replacement of the Upper Extremity* (1979). American Academy of Orthopedic Surgeons, CV Mosby, St Louis, 1982.
9. Iversen, LD and Clawson, DK: *Manual of Acute Orthopedic Therapeutics,* ed 2. Little, Brown & Company, Boston, 1982.
10. Kapadji, IA: *The Physiology of the Joints,* Volume I. Churchill-Livingstone, Edinburgh, 1970.
11. Kessler, R and Hertling, D: *Management of Common Musculoskeletal Disorders.* Harper & Row, Philadelphia, 1983.
12. Kopell, H and Thompson, W: *Peripheral Entrapment Neuropathies,* ed 2. Robert E. Krieger, Huntington, NY, 1976.
13. LaFreniere, J: *Tennis elbow: Evaluation, treatment and prevention.* Phys Ther 59:742, 1979.
14. Lehmkuhl, LD and Smith, LK: *Brunnstrom's Clinical Kinesiology,* ed 4. FA Davis, Philadelphia, 1983.
15. Marmor, L: *Surgery of the rheumatoid elbow.* J Bone Joint Surg 54A:573, 1972.
16. Melvin, J: *Rheumatic Disease: Occupational Therapy and Rehabilitation.* FA Davis, Philadelphia, 1977.
17. Morrey, BF and Kavanagh, BF: *Cementless joint replacement: Current status and future.* Bull Rheuma Dis 37:1, 1987.
18. Nerschl, R and Sobel, J: *Conservative treatment of tennis elbow.* Phys Sports Med 9.6:43, 1981.
19. Nickel, VL (ed): *Orthopedic Rehabilitation.* Churchill-Livingstone, New York, 1982.
20. Norkin, C and Levangie, P: *Joint Structure and Function: A Comprehensive Analysis.* FA Davis, Philadelphia, 1983.
21. Occupational Therapy Staff: *Upper Extremity Surgeries for Patients with Arthritis—A Pre and Post-operative Occupational Therapy Treatment Guide.* Rancho Los Amigos Hospital, California, 1979.
22. Pritchard, RW: *Semiconstrained elbow prosthesis: A clinical review of five years' experience.* Orthop Rev 8:33, 1979.
23. Sheon, R, Moskowitz R, and Goldberg, V: *Soft Tissue Rheumatic Pain: Recognition, Management, Prevention.* Lea & Febiger, Philadelphia, 1982.
24. Zohn, D and Mennell, J: *Musculoskeletal Pain: Principles of Physical Diagnosis and Physical Treatment.* Little, Brown & Company, Boston, 1976.

CHAPTER ——————————— 9

The Wrist and Hand

The wrist is the final link of joints that position the hand. It has the significant function of controlling the length-tension relationship of the multi-articular muscles of the hand as they adjust to various activities and grips.[19] The hand is a valuable tool through which we control our environment and express ideas and talents. It also has an important sensory function of providing feedback to the brain.

The anatomy and kinesiology of the wrist and hand is rather complex but is important to know in order to effectively treat hand problems. The first section of this chapter reviews highlights of the anatomy and function of those areas that the reader should know and understand. The reader is also referred to several texts for study of the material.[3,11,12,14,19] Chapter 6 presents information on principles of management; the reader should be familiar with that material before proceeding with establishing a therapeutic exercise program for the wrist or hand.

OBJECTIVES

After studying this chapter, the reader will be able to:
1. identify important aspects of wrist and hand structure and function for review.
2. establish a therapeutic exercise program to manage soft-tissue and joint lesions in the wrist and hand related to stages of recovery following an inflammatory insult to the tissues.
3. establish a therapeutic exercise program to manage common musculoskeletal lesions, recognizing unique circumstances in the wrist and hand for their management.
4. establish a therapeutic exercise program to manage patients following common surgical procedures.

I.   REVIEW OF THE STRUCTURE AND FUNCTION OF THE WRIST
     AND HAND

A. Bony Parts (see Figure 5-32)
   1. **Wrist**
      Distal radius, scaphoid (S), lunate (L), triquetrum (Tri), pisiform (P), trape-
      zium (Tm), trapezoid (Tz), capitate (C), and hamate (H).

   2. **Hand**
      Five metacarpals and 14 phalanges make up the hand and five digits.

B. Joints of the Wrist Complex and Their Movements
   1. **The wrist complex**
      The wrist complex is multi-articular and is made up of two compound
      joints. It is biaxial, allowing for flexion (volar flexion), extension (dorsiflex-
      ion), radial deviation (abduction), and ulnar deviation (adduction).

   2. **The radiocarpal joint**
      a. It is enclosed in a loose but strong capsule, reinforced by ligaments
         also shared with the midcarpal joint.
      b. The biconcave articulating surface is the distal end of the radius and
         radioulnar disk (discus articularis); it is angled slightly volarly and ul-
         narly.
      c. The biconvex articulating surface is the combined proximal surface of
         the scaphoid, lunate, and triquetrum. The triquetrum primarily articu-
         lates with the disk. These three carpals are bound together with numer-
         ous interosseous ligaments.
      d. With motions of the wrist, the convex proximal row of carpals slides in
         the direction opposite the physiologic motion of the hand.

Physiologic Motion of Wrist	Direction of Slide of Carpals on Radius or Disk
Flexion*	Dorsal
Extension	Volar
Radial deviation	Ulnar
Ulnar deviation*	Radial

   3. **The midcarpal joint**
      a. This is a compound joint between the two rows of carpals. It has a
         capsule that is also continuous with the intercarpal articulations.
      b. The combined distal surfaces of the scaphoid, lunate, and triquetrum
         articulate with the combined proximal surfaces of the trapezium, trape-
         zoid, capitate, and hamate.
         (1) The articulating surfaces of the capitate and hamate are in essence
             convex and slide on the concave articulating surfaces of a portion
             of the scaphoid, lunate, and triquetrum.
         (2) The articulating surfaces of the trapezium and trapezoid are con-
             cave and slide on the convex distal surface of the scaphoid.

---

*Greater movement in flexion and ulnar deviation than the other two motions occurs at this joint.[29]

    c. With physiologic motions of the wrist, a complex of motions occurs between the carpals. In summary:

Physiologic Motion of the Wrist	Direction of Slide of Distal Carpal Bones with Respect to to the Proximal Carpal Bones
Flexion	C and H—Dorsal Tm and Tz—Volar
Extension*	C and H—Volar Tm and Tz—Dorsal
Radial deviation*	C and H—Ulnar Tm and Tz—Dorsal
Ulnar deviation	C and H—Radial Tm and Tz—Volar

4. The pisiform

The pisiform is categorized as a carpal and is aligned volar to the triquetrum in the proximal row of carpals. It is not part of the wrist joint but functions as a sesamoid bone in the flexor carpi ulnaris tendon.

5. The ligaments

Stability and some passive movement of the wrist complex are provided by numerous ligaments: the ulnar and radial collateral, the dorsal and volar (palmar) radiocarpal, the ulnocarpal, and the intercarpal.

C. Joints of the Hand Complex and Their Movements

1. Carpometacarpal (CMC) joints of digits 2 through 5

    a. The joints are enclosed in a common joint cavity and include the articulations of each metacarpal with the distal row of carpals and the articulations between the bases of each metacarpal.

    b. The joints of 2, 3, and 4 are plane uniaxial joints; the joint of digit 5 is biaxial. They are supported by transverse and longitudinal ligaments. The fifth metacarpal is most mobile, with the fourth being the next mobile.

    c. The flexion of the metacarpals and additional adduction of the fifth contribute to the cupping (arching) of the hand.

Physiologic Motions of the Metacarpals	Direction of Slide of Metacarpals on Carpals
Flexion (cupping)	Volar
Extension (flattening)	Dorsal

2. Carpometacarpal joint of the thumb (digit 1)

    a. This joint is a saddle-shaped (sellar) biaxial joint between the trapezium and base of the first metacarpal. It has a lax capsule and wide ROM, which allows the thumb to move away from the palm of the hand for opposition in prehension activities.

---

*Greater movement in extension and radial deviation than the other two motions occurs at this joint.[29]

b. For flexion-extension of the thumb (components of opposition-reposition, respectively) occurring in the frontal plane, the trapezium surface is convex and the base of the metacarpal is concave; therefore, its surface slides in the same direction as the angulating bone.

c. For abduction-adduction, occurring in the sagittal plane, the trapezium surface is concave and the metacarpal is convex; therefore, its surface slides in the opposite direction of the angulating bone.

Physiologic Motion of the First Metacarpal	Direction of Slide of Base of Metacarpal
Flexion	Ulnar
Extension	Radial
Abduction	Dorsal
Adduction	Volar

3. **Metacarpophalangeal joints (MCP)**

a. They are biaxial condyloid joints with the distal end of each metacarpal convex and proximal phalanx concave, supported by a volar and two collateral ligaments. The collaterals become taut in full flexion and prevent abduction and adduction in this position.

b. The MCP of the thumb differs in that it is reinforced by two sesamoid bones and has minimal abduction and adduction even in extension.

Physiologic Motion of the First Phalanx	Direction of Slide of First Phalanx
Flexion	Volar
Extension	Dorsal
Abduction	Away from center of hand
Adduction	Toward center of hand

4. **Interphalangeal joints (IP)**

a. There is a proximal (PIP) and distal (DIP) interphalangeal joint for each digit, 2 through 5; the thumb has only one interphalangeal joint. Each is a uniaxial hinge joint. The articulating surface at the distal end of each phalanx is convex; the articulating surface at the proximal end of each phalanx is concave.

b. Each capsule is reinforced with collateral ligaments.

c. Going radial to ulnar, there is increasing flexion-extension range in the joints. This allows for greater opposition of the ulnar fingers to the thumb and also causes a potentially tighter grip on the ulnar side.

Physiologic Motion of Each Phalanx	Direction of Slide of Base of Phalanx
Flexion	Volar
Extension	Dorsal

D. Hand Function

1. **Length-tension relationships**

The wrist position controls the length of the extrinsic muscles to the digits.

a. As the fingers or thumb flex, the wrist must be stabilized by the wrist extensor muscles to prevent the flexor digitorum profundus and flexor digitorum superficialis or flexor pollicis longus from simultaneously flexing the wrist. As the grip becomes stronger, synchronous wrist extension lengthens the extrinsic flexor tendons across the wrist and maintains a more favorable overall length of the musculotendinous unit for a stronger contraction.

b. For strong finger or thumb extension, the wrist flexor muscles stabilize or flex the wrist so the extensor digitorum communis, extensor indices, extensor digiti minimi, or extensor pollicis longus muscles can function more efficiently. In addition, there is ulnar deviation; the flexor and extensor carpi ulnaris muscles are both active as the hand opens.[16]

2. Cupping and flattening

Cupping of the hand occurs with finger flexion, and flattening of the hand occurs with extension. Cupping improves the mobility of the hand for functional usage and flattening for release of objects.

3. Extensor mechanism

Structurally, the extensor hood is made up of the extensor digitorum communis tendon, its connective tissue expansion, and fibers from the tendons of the dorsal and volar interossei and lumbricals.[19] Each structure has an effect on the extensor mechanism.

a. An isolated contraction of the extensor digitorum produces clawing of the fingers (MCP hyperextension with IP flexion from passive pull of the extrinsic flexor tendons).

b. PIP and DIP extension occur concurrently and can be caused by the interossei or lumbrical muscles through their pull on the extensor hood.

c. There must be tension in the extensor digitorum communis tendon for there to be interphalangeal extension. This occurs by active contraction of the muscle, causing MCP extension concurrently as the intrinsic muscles contract, or by stretch of the tendon, which occurs with MCP flexion.

4. Grips and prehension patterns

The nature of the intended activity dictates the type of grip used.[15,16,18]

a. *Power grips* involve clamping an object with partially flexed fingers against the palm of the hand, with counterpressure from the adducted thumb. Power grips are primarily isometric functions. The fingers are flexed, laterally rotated, and ulnarly deviated. The amount of flexion varies with the object held. The thumb reinforces the fingers and helps make small adjustments to control the direction of the force. Varieties include cylindrical grip, spherical grip, hook grip, and lateral prehension.

b. *Precision patterns* involve manipulating an object that is not in contact with the palm of the hand between the opposing abducted thumb and fingers. The muscles primarily function isotonically. The sensory surface of the digits is used for maximum sensory input to influence delicate adjustments. With small objects, precise handling occurs primarily between the thumb and index finger. Varieties include pad-to-pad, tip-to-tip, and pad-to-side prehension.

c. *Combined grips* involve digits 1 and 2 performing precision activities, while digits 3 through 5 supplement with power.

E. Hand Control[16]

1. **Control of the unloaded (free) hand**

   Involves anatomic factors, muscular contraction, and viscoelastic properties of the muscles.
   a. Clawing motions occur with only extrinsic muscle contractions.
   b. Closing motions can occur only with extrinsic muscle contraction but
      also require the viscoelastic force of the bi-articular interossei.
   c. Opening motions require the synergistic contraction of the extrinsic ex-
      tensor and the lumbrical muscles.
   d. Reciprocal motion of MCP flexion and IP extension is caused by the
      interossei. The lumbrical removes the viscoelastic tension from the pro-
      fundus tendon and assists IP extension.

2. **Power grip**
   a. Extrinsic flexors provide the major gripping force.
   b. Extrinsic extensor provides a compressive force preventing sublux-
      ation of the finger joints.
   c. Interossei rotate the first phalanx for positioning to compress the exter-
      nal object, and also flex the MCP joint.
   d. Lumbricals do not participate in the power grip (except the fourth).
   e. The thenar muscles and adductor pollicis provide compressive forces
      against the object being gripped.

3. **Precision handling**
   a. Extrinsic muscles provide the compressive force to hold the objects be-
      tween the fingers and thumb.
   b. For manipulation of an object the interossei abduct and adduct the fingers,
      the thenar muscles control movement of the thumb, and the lumbricals
      help move the object away from the palm of the hand. The amount of
      participation of each muscle varies with the amount and direction of mo-
      tion.

4. **Pinch**

   Compression between the thumb and fingers is provided by the thenar
   eminence muscles, the adductor pollicis, the interossei, and extrinsic flexors. The lumbricals also participate.

F. Major Nerves Subject to Pressure and Trauma
   at the Wrist and Hand[4,13]

1. **Median nerve**

   Passes through the carpal tunnel at the wrist with the flexor tendons. The
   carpal tunnel is covered by the thick, relatively inelastic transverse carpal
   ligament. Entrapment in the tunnel causes sensory changes (over the radial two thirds of the palm, the palmar surfaces of the first three and one-
   half digits, and the dorsum of the distal phalanges) and progressive weakness in the muscles innervated distal to the wrist (opponens pollicis,
   abductor pollicis brevis, superficial head of the flexor pollicis brevis, and
   lumbricals I and II) resulting in ape-hand deformity (thenar atrophy and
   thumb in plane of hand). The branch innervating the opponens muscle
   hooks over the carpal ligament two thirds of the way up the thenar eminence and can be entrapped separately.

9 THE WRIST AND HAND ————————————————————————————— 295

2. Ulnar nerve

Enters the hand through a trough formed by the pisiform bone and hook of the hamate bone and is covered by the volar carpal ligament and palmaris brevis muscle. Trauma or entrapment causes sensory changes (ulnar third of the hand, entire fifth digit, and ulnar side of the fourth digit), and progressive weakness to muscles innervated distal to the site (palmaris brevis, muscles of the hypothenar eminence, lumbricals III and IV, interossei, adductor pollicis, and deep head of the flexor pollicis brevis) resulting in claw-hand deformity. Injury to the nerve after it bifurcates leads to partial involvement, depending on the site of injury.

3. Radial nerve

Enters the hand as the superficial radial nerve, which is sensory only. Injury to it in the wrist or hand causes sensory changes only (over the radial two thirds of the dorsum of the hand and thumb and the proximal phalanx of the second, third, and half of the fourth digit). Influence of the radial nerve on hand musculature is entirely proximal to the wrist. It innervates extrinsic wrist and hand muscles (see Chapter 8). Injury near the elbow results in wrist-drop.

II. GUIDELINES AND THERAPEUTIC EXERCISE MANAGEMENT OF COMMON MUSCULOSKELETAL PROBLEMS IN THE WRIST AND HAND

Note: Exercises applied to the wrist and hand during acute, subacute, and chronic phases of inflammation and healing follow the principles as described in Chapter 6, taking into account the unique anatomic and kinesiologic relationships of the region. This section will expand on the general guidelines.

A. Joint Problems—Distal Radioulnar (RU) Joint

This joint is often included in discussions of the wrist because of its proximity to the wrist, and because pain in the RU joint is experienced just proximal to the wrist. Restrictions affect the forearm functions of pronation and supination. See Chapter 8 for discussion of this joint and its treatment.

B. Joint Problems—Wrist Joint Complex

Passive flexion and extension are equally limited when the joint is involved.

1. Trauma

a. Following trauma, the therapist needs to be alert to signs of a fracture, which include swelling, muscle spasm when passive flexion and extension are attempted, increased pain when the wrist is deviated toward the side of the pain, and tenderness over the involved carpal when palpated.[5]

b. Management of traumatic arthritis with no fracture
Usually the joint reaction clears up after a couple of days of rest; therefore, therapeutic exercise is not indicated.

2. Rheumatoid arthritis (RA)

a. **Clinical picture**
RA commonly affects the wrists bilaterally. Joint swelling and increased

warmth are present. In advanced stages, there may be subluxation and deformities. Common deformities at the wrist include[28]

(1) Volar subluxation of the triquetrum with relation to the ulna; ultimately the extensor carpi ulnaris tendon displaces volarly and causes a flexor force at the joint.

(2) Ulnar subluxation of the carpals resulting in radial deviation.

b. **Management of RA in the wrist**

See section VII of Chapter 6 for general principles, goals, and plan of care for RA.

(1) To avoid progression of deformities in the wrist

In addition to the use of splints, the patient should avoid using strong grasps with resistance when the joints are reactive, since these cause radial deviation and wrist extension, which tend to reinforce the volar and ulnar subluxation of the carpals. (Strong grasps also accentuate the deforming forces at the MCP joints. See C 2 of the next section for the discussion on fingers.)

(2) To unlock the subluxed ulnomeniscal-triquetral (UMT) joint to allow for supination and wrist function

Volar glide the ulna on a stabilized triquetrum (similar to Figure 5-37).

(3) To teach the patient UMT self-mobilization

The patient grasps the distal ulna with the fingers of his opposite hand and places his thumb on the palmar surface of the triquetrum just medial to the pisiform. He then presses with his thumb, causing a dorsal glide of the triquetrum on the radioulnar disk and ulna (Figure 9-1).

(4) To manage additional mechanical restrictions, use appropriate mobilizations as summarized in the following section

3. **Management of general joint restrictions in the wrist**

a. Follow the outline as described for chronic conditions in Chapter 6, Sections V and IX C, with emphasis on joint mobilization.

b. To increase flexion

(1) traction on the carpals (see Figure 5-33)

(2) general dorsal glide of the carpals (see Figure 5-34)

(3) specific carpal glides as indicated

Stabilize the bone that has the convex articulating surface, and apply the mobilizing force against the bone with the concave articulating surface. The force is in a volar direction.

(a) stabilize lunate, volar glide radius (see Figure 5-37)

(b) stabilize capitate, volar glide lunate (see Figure 5-37)

(c) stabilize scaphoid, volar glide radius (see Figure 5-37)

(d) stabilize scaphoid, volar glide trapezium (see Figure 5-38)

c. To increase extension

(1) traction on the carpals (see Figure 5-33)

(2) general volar glide of the carpals (see Figure 5-35)

(3) specific carpal glides as indicated

Stabilize the bone that has the concave articulating surface, and apply the mobilizing force against the dorsal surface of the bone with the convex articulating surface. The force is in a volar direction.

(a) stabilize radius, volar glide lunate (see Figure 5-38)

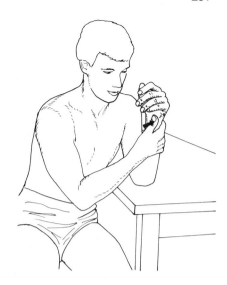

FIGURE 9-1. Self-mobilization of the ulnome-niscal-triquetral (UMT) joint.

        (b) stabilize radius, volar glide scaphoid (see Figure 5-38)
        (c) stabilize trapezium, volar glide scaphoid (see Figure 5-37)
        (d) stabilize lunate, volar glide capitate (see Figure 5-38)
        (e) stabilize scaphoid, volar glide capitate (see Figure 5-38)
    d. To increase radial deviation
        (1) traction on the carpals (see Figure 5-33)
        (2) general ulnar glide (see Figure 5-36)
        (3) specific carpal glides as indicated
           (a) stabilize trapezius, volar glide scaphoid (see Figure 5-37)
           (b) stabilize radius, volar glide scaphoid (see Figure 5-38)
    e. To increase ulnar deviation
        (1) traction on the carpals (see Figure 5-33)
        (2) general radial glide (opposite of Figure 5-36)

C. Joint Problems—Joints of the Hand and Fingers

Equal limitation of passive flexion and extension occurs with joint involvement. Passive rotation of the involved joint is painful.

1. Trauma

    a. Joint trauma is common in the hand; in addition to limited motion, joint swelling also occurs.
    b. Management of traumatic joint injuries with no fracture
        (1) Follow guidelines in Chapter 6 for acute injuries.
        (2) Move the joint as tolerated; immobility in the hand quickly leads to muscle imbalance and contracture formation.

2. Rheumatoid arthritis

    a. **Clinical picture**

    Signs of joint swelling often begin in the MCP joints or PIP joints; usually bilaterally. Often there is involvement of the tendons and their sheaths in the hand. As the disease progresses, deformities occur from muscle and ligamentous imbalances. Common deformities in the hand and fingers include[28]

(1) ulnar drift of the fingers at the MCP joints and volar subluxation of the proximal phalanx.

(2) swan-neck deformity (PIP hyperextension with DIP flexion).

(3) boutonnière deformity (PIP flexion with DIP extension)

b. **Management of RA in the hand and fingers**

(1) Follow guidelines in Chapter 6, Section VII for general principles, goals, and plan of care.

(2) To avoid progression of common deformities in the hand in addition to splinting[28]

(a) avoid strong grasping and pinching activities, which tend to accentuate ulnar drift of the fingers. Use the hand in nonprehensile functional ways or in motions opposite to those of the deforming forces. It may require opening jars with the left hand, cutting food with the blade of the knife protruding from the ulnar side of the hand, or stirring food with the spoon on the ulnar side of the hand.

(b) look for early signs of muscle tightness in the intrinsic muscles. If tight, elongate them, since one cause of swan-neck deformity is tight interossei muscles pulling on the extensor tendon, leading to hyperextension of the hypermobile PIP joints (see Section D b and c).

3. Osteoarthritis (DJD)

a. **Clinical picture**

This form of arthritis most often affects the large weight-bearing joints of the body. It may also affect the DIP joints of the fingers and the CMC joints of the thumb. Isolated joints of the hand may also become involved after prolonged occupational or recreational stress.

b. **Management**

See section VIII of Chapter 6 for general principles, goals, and plan of care for DJD. If joint restrictions are present, use appropriate mobilization techniques as summarized in the following section.

4. Management of joint or capsular restrictions in the hand and fingers

a. Follow the outline for goals and plan of care for chronic conditions in Chapter 6, sections V and IX C, with emphasis on joint mobilization.

b. To increase mobility of the CMC joint of the thumb

(1) joint traction

(2) To increase flexion
ulnar glide base of first metacarpal on stabilized trapezium (see Figure 5-40A)

(3) To increase extension
radial glide first metacarpal (see Figure 5-40B)

(4) To increase abduction
dorsal glide first metacarpal (see Figure 5-40C)

(5) To increase adduction
palmar glide first metacarpal (see Figure 5-40D)

c. To increase the arch of the hand

(1) joint traction of the carpometacarpal joints of the hand (see Figure 5-39)

(2) palmar glide base of each metacarpal on its fixated carpal
  d. To increase mobility of the MCP and IP joints of the digits
      (1) joint traction (see Figure 5-41)
      (2) rotation with traction (see Figure 5–43)
      (3) To increase flexion
          volar glide base of phalanx (see Figure 5-42)
      (4) To increase extension
          dorsal glide base of phalanx
      (5) To increase abduction or adduction
          glide radially or ulnarly, depending on digit and direction of limitation

D. Muscle Strength or Flexibility Imbalance

Note: No matter what the cause, muscle strength or flexibility imbalance can lead to poor hand mechanics. If there is nerve damage with motor loss or faulty mechanics from progressive joint degeneration, splinting is necessary to prevent contracture formation and to provide stabilization for the functioning of remaining muscles. (Techniques of functional splinting are beyond the scope of this textbook.)

  1. **Techniques to stretch tight muscles**
     Precautions: Before initiating stretching techniques to muscle or inert tissue, there should be normal gliding of the joint surfaces in order to avoid joint damage; if normal gliding is not present, joint-play techniques should be initiated first.
     Because there are many multi-joint muscles in the hand, stabilization and specific stretching techniques are critical to avoid joint damage or hypermobility.
       a. Active inhibition and passive stretching techniques for the muscles and soft tissues of the wrist and hand are described in Chapter 4.
       b. Self-stretching of tight lumbricale and interossei muscles
          The patient actively extends the MCP joints and flexes the IP joints. For reciprocal inhibition, manual resistance is applied against the fingertips with the fingers of the patient's other hand as the motion is performed.
       c. To stretch the extrinsic muscles
          Because they are multi-joint muscles, the final step is to elongate them over all the joints simultaneously, but DO NOT initiate stretching procedures in this manner because joint compression and damage can occur to the smaller or less stable joints. Begin by allowing the wrist and more proximal finger joints to relax; stretch the tendon unit over the most distal joint first. Stabilize the distal joint at the end of the range, then stretch the tendon unit over the next joint. Then stabilize the two joints as you stretch the tendon over the next joint and progress in this manner until the ultimate length is reached.
          Caution: Do not let the PIP and MCP hyperextend as you stretch the tendons over the wrist.
       d. Self-stretching of the flexor digitorum profundus and superficialis
          Have the patient begin by resting the palm of his involved hand on a table. He first extends the DIP joint, using his other hand to straighten the joint; keeping it extended, he then straightens the PIP and MCP joints in succession. If he can actively extend the finger joints to this point, he should do the motion unassisted. When extended, he places

his hand flat on the table, using his other hand to firmly fixate the hand on the table. He then begins to extend his wrist by actively bringing his arm up over his hand. He goes just to the point of feeling discomfort, holds the position, then progresses as the length improves (Figure 9-2).

e. Self-stretching of the extensor digitorum communis
The fingers are flexed to the maximum range, beginning with the distalmost joint first, and progressing until the wrist is simultaneously flexed. The patient should do this actively if possible.

f. Stretching techniques for wrist flexors and extensors
These were described in the section on medial and lateral epicondylitis (Chapter 8, Section II D).

g. Selective stretching
Patients with C-6 quadriplegia are able to use tendon action to flex their fingers for functional grasp if the extrinsic flexor muscles (profundus and superficialis) are allowed to tighten. This action is called tenodesis; it is the passive movement of the finger joints caused by the multi-joint muscles as they are stretched over the wrist. The fingers close as the wrist is actively extended and open as the wrist flexes.[14]

2. Techniques to strengthen weak muscles

If musculature is weak, progressive strengthening exercises are used to gain muscle balance (see Chapter 3 for descriptions of resistive exercise programs).

a. To strengthen wrist musculature
Allow the fingers to relax. The wrist muscles can be exercised as a group if their strength is similar. If one muscle is weaker, the wrist should be guided through the range desired to minimize the action of the stronger muscles. For example, with wrist flexion, if the flexor carpi radialis is stronger than the flexor carpi ulnaris, instruct the patient to attempt to flex his wrist toward the ulnar side as you guide the wrist into flexion and ulnar deviation. If the muscle is strong enough to tolerate resistance, place your manual resistance over the fourth and fifth metacarpals (similar to Figure 3-10).

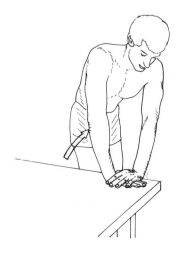

FIGURE 9-2. Self-stretching of the extrinsic finger flexor muscles, showing stabilization of the small distal joints.

b. To strengthen weak intrinsic musculature

Note: Imbalance from weak intrinsic muscles leads to a claw hand.

(1) MCP joint flexion with IP joint extension

Have the patient start with the MCP joints extended and PIP joints flexed, then actively push his finger tips outward, performing the desired combined motion (Figure 9-3A and B). If he tolerates resistance, have him push his fingers into the palm of his other hand (Figure 9-3C).

(2) Isolated or combined abduction/adduction of each finger

Have the patient rest the palm of his hand on a table. Give resistance at the distal end of the first phalanx, one finger at a time, for either abduction or adduction.

To resist adduction, the patient interlaces the fingers of both hands (or with your hand), and pinches his fingers together.

Place a rubber band around two digits and have the patient spread them apart.

(3) Abduction of the thumb

The patient rests the dorsum of his hand on a table, and resistance is applied at the base of the first phalanx of the thumb as the patient lifts his thumb away from the palm of this hand.

Place a rubber band around the thumb and index finger. The patient abducts his thumb against the resistance.

(4) Opposition of the thumb

For manual resistance, see Figure 3-12.

c. To strengthen weak extrinsic musculature of the fingers

Note: The wrist must be stabilized for the action of the extrinsic hand musculature to be effective. With inadequate wrist strength for stabilization, manually stabilize it during exercises and splint it for functional usage.

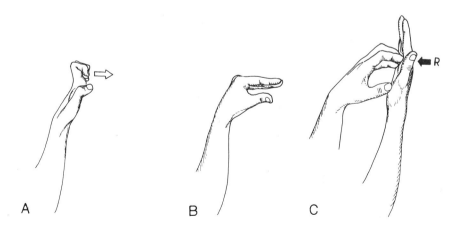

A B C

FIGURE 9-3. To strengthen intrinsic muscle function for combined MCP flexion and IP extension, the patient begins with MCP extension and IP flexion (*A*) and pushes his fingertips outward (*B*). The same motion is resisted by pushing the fingertips against the palm of the other hand (*C*).

(1) Metacarpophalangeal extension

Manual resistance is applied at the distal end of the proximal phalanx; the wrist is neutral or partially flexed.

For mechanical resistance, the hand rests on a table with the palm down and digits over the edge. Place a loop over the distal end of the proximal phalanx with the weight hanging down from it.

See also mechanical resistance techniques under d.

(2) Interphalangeal flexion

The profundus and superficialis actions can be isolated for manual resistance, as is done with manual muscle testing procedures,[6] or resisted together if their strength is similar. The wrist must be stabilized in midposition or partially extended.

With his hands pointing in opposite directions, the patient places the pads of each finger on one hand against the pads of each finger of the other hand (or against your hand). He then curls his fingers against the resistance provided by the other hand (Figure 9-4).

The same technique is used to resist thumb flexion.

See also mechanical resistance techniques under d.

d. Mechanical resistance techniques requiring intrinsic and extrinsic muscle function

Note: Proper stabilization is important; either the patient's stabilizing muscles must be strong enough, or the weakened areas must be supported manually. If a weight causes stress because the patient cannot control it, the exercise will be detrimental rather than beneficial.

(1) Spread a towel out on a table. The patient places the palm of his hand down at one end of the towel. While maintaining contact with the heel of his hand, he crumples the towel into his hand. The same exercise can be done by placing a stack of newspapers under the hand. The patient crumples the top sheet into a ball (and tosses it into a basket for coordination and skill practice), then repeats it with each sheet in succession.

(2) Using a disk weight as tolerated

Grasp the disk with the tips of all five digits spread around the outer edge. Lift with the forearm pronated and palm down. Hold the position for isometric resistance to grasp and wrist extension. Increase the effect of the resistance by extending one finger.

Pick up the side of the disk weight, either with fingertips or between the pads of the distal phalanx of thumb and individual fingers.

The hand is placed palm down on the table; place a weight on the dorsum of the fingers; the patient hyperextends the fingers by lifting the weight.

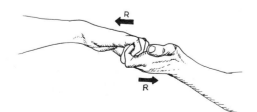

FIGURE 9-4. Self-resistance to strengthen extrinsic finger flexor muscles.

E. Ligamentous Injuries

1. Clinical picture

Following trauma (with or without fracture or subluxation), the patient experiences pain at the involved site whenever a stretch is placed on the ligament. A simple sprain heals in a few weeks. Severe trauma may result in ligamentous rupture, which leads to permanent instability.

2. Management

a. Follow the guidelines as outlined in Chapter 6, according to the stage of healing, emphasizing cross-fiber massage.
b. Avoid positions of stress and activities that provoke the symptoms while healing. Complete immobility is contraindicated.

F. Tendinitis

1. Clinical picture

Inflammation from overuse, from the effects of RA, and from roughening of the surface of the tendon or its sheath can cause pain on motion of the wrist or active contraction of the related muscle.

2. Management

a. Follow the guidelines as outlined in Chapter 6, according to the stage of healing. In some cases, cross-fiber massage helps smooth down roughened surfaces.
b. Use caution with RA, since there is accompanying tissue weakening.

G. Shoulder-Hand Syndrome

See discussion in Chapter 7.

H. Referred Pain and Nerve Injury Patterns

The hand is the terminal point for several major nerves. Injury or entrapment of these nerves may occur anywhere along their course, from the cervical spine to their termination. What the patient perceives as pain or sensory disturbance in the hand may be from injury of the nerve anywhere along its course, or the pain may be from irritation of tissue of common segmental origin. For treatment to be effective, it must be directed to the source of the problem, not to the site where the patient perceives the pain or sensory changes. Therefore, a thorough history is taken and a selective tension examination done when referred pain patterns or sensory changes are reported by the patient.[5]

1. Common sources of segmental sensory reference in the hand

a. Cervical spine
    (1) Vertebral joints between C-5 and C-6, between C-6 and C-7, or between C-7 and T-1 vertebrae.
    (2) C-6, C-7, or C-8 nerve roots.
b. Tissue derived from the same spinal segments as C-6, C-7, or C-8.

2. Common sources of extrasegmental sensory reference in the hand

a. Peripheral nerves
    Median, ulnar, or radial nerve entrapments
b. Brachial plexus
    Thoracic outlet syndrome

III. THERAPEUTIC EXERCISE MANAGEMENT OF COMMON SURGICAL PROCEDURES FOR THE WRIST AND HAND

Surgical repair of the wrist and hand may be indicated after a severe trauma causes laceration or rupture of tendons and subsequent loss of hand function. Chronic synovitis associated with rheumatoid arthritis of the hand and wrist can also cause rupture of tendons. Severe deterioration of articular surfaces of the wrist or fingers because of arthritis may necessitate joint reconstruction or replacement.

The goals of surgery and postoperative management, which are similar in most of these procedures, include

1. restoration of normal or adequate function of the hand.
2. relief of pain.
3. improved stability of the wrist and finger joints.
4. improved range of motion and strength for adequate grasp and pinch.
5. elimination of deformity.

Rehabilitation of the hand after surgery is complex. It is essential that postoperative management of the hand and wrist be based on an understanding of the principles of wound healing (Chapter 6) and thorough knowledge of the anatomic structures involved. In the early stages of rehabilitation, use of static and dynamic hand splints is common. It is important that the therapist become familiar with the fabrication, fit, and use of these splints. Melvin[17] and Trombly[28] provide specific information and references on this topic.

A. Tendon Repairs and Tendon Transfers in the Hand

Reconstructive surgery or transfer of tendons in the hand may be necessary to restore muscle balance and function of the hand after

—rupture of tendons due to chronic synovitis.
—tendon lacerations.
—peripheral nerve injuries.

1. General considerations for tendon repairs and transfers in the hand

Normal passive joint range of motion is necessary if a tendon repair or transfer is to be successful. Postoperative management must include a proper balance of immobilization of the operated areas to protect the repaired or transferred tendon and early range of motion to prevent joint and soft-tissue contractures.[1,10,21] As mentioned in Chapter 6, it is important to understand the physiology of tendon healing and the factors that affect healing. Immobilization of a repaired tendon is necessary, but it is also important to maintain the normal gliding action of the tendon through the tendon sheath as the tendon heals. Extensor and flexor tendons of the digits heal at different rates after surgical repair. Extensor tendons take longer to heal than flexor tendons. This may be due to differences in anatomic tissues surrounding the tendons. For example, synovial sheaths surround most of the lengths of the flexor tendons, but they surround the extensor tendons only at the wrist. Since synovial fluid provides nutrition to healing tendons, it is theorized that the flexors may receive better nutrition and therefore heal more rapidly than the extensor tendons. The extensor tendons are also protected with an immobilization device longer because of the potential stretch (lengthening) force that can be placed on them by contraction of the much stronger flexor muscles.[7,21] The duration and position of immobilization vary and depend upon the site of the laceration or avulsion of the tendon.

Excessive motion at a joint or a vigorous muscle contraction too soon after surgery can cause rupture of the transferred or repaired tendon. Passive stretching and progressive resistance exercises must be avoided for 6 to 8 weeks after surgery to allow complete healing of the repaired or transferred tendon. Initially, active exercises and, later, gentle resistance exercises must be carried out for 3 months to ensure maximum success from the procedure. A brief discussion of several procedures and recommendations and precautions for postoperative exercise follow.

2. **Repair of ruptured extensor tendons associated with RA**

   a. **Background of the problem**

      (1) Patients with long-term rheumatoid arthritis of the hand may experience rupture of one or more of the extensor digitorum communis or extensor pollicis longus tendons.

      (2) This may be caused by

         (a) chronic tenosynovitis that infiltrates and weakens the tendons.

         (b) pressure on the tendons from extensive proliferative synovitis at the MCP and PIP joints.

         (c) progressive deterioration of a tendon at the distal ulna because the tendon is rubbing against an irregular bony surface.[17,28]

   b. **Procedure**[17,20]

      (1) If the patient has good passive range of motion of the fingers, repair of the extensor tendons can restore active extension to the MCP joints of the hand. This procedure may also be done prior to or in conjunction with a flexible implant arthroplasty of an MCP joint (see discussion later in this section).

      (2) A tendon anastomosis to an adjoining, intact extensor tendon may be done. The ruptured extensor tendon is rewoven into the remaining extensor tendons.

      (3) Dorsal clearance (extensor tendon synovectomy) of the proliferated synovium along the extensor tendon sheaths of the wrist is also done.

      (4) A tendon graft or a tendon transfer, rather than a tendon anastomosis, can also be done to restore hand function.

   c. **Postoperative management**[17,20]

      (1) Immobilization

         (a) The wrist and hand are immobilized in a short arm cast for at least 4 weeks. All motion of the MCP joints must be avoided to protect the repaired tendon.

         (b) The wrist is held in slight extension and the MCP joints are held in 45 degrees of flexion.

         (c) The hand is elevated to minimize edema.

      (2) At 4 weeks postoperatively, the cast is bivalved and gentle active-assistive exercise of the fingers may be initiated.

         Precaution: It is essential not to place any stretch or resistance on the repaired extensor tendons for approximately 6 to 8 weeks.

         (a) Emphasis is placed on active-assistive extension of the MCP joints.

         Note: Wrist and PIP joints should be held in a neutral position.

         (b) No active or passive flexion of the MCP joints is done.

         (c) The patient remains in a volar splint made from the bivalved cast at all times except during exercise.

(3) The patient begins gentle active finger flexion at 5 weeks.

(4) The splint is removed during the day at 6 weeks, and the patient may use the hand for light functional activities.
Precaution: If the patient must use his hands for transfer activities, have him avoid putting pressure on the dorsum of the hand.

(5) Gentle stretching and resistance exercises may be added at 6 to 8 weeks to increase range of motion and strength.

(6) If a tendon transfer (such as transfer of the flexor digitorum superficialis) has been done to restore active MCP extension, the postoperative rehabilitation time is usually longer. Exercises may be combined with use of biofeedback and electrical stimulation for muscle re-education.

3. Repair of lacerated flexor tendons of the hand

a. Background of the problem[1,22,28]

Lacerations to the flexor tendons of the hand are common and can occur in various areas along the volar surface of the fingers, palm of the hand, and wrist. Each area presents specific problems of postoperative rehabilitation. An injury that occurs from the metacarpals to the middle phalanx often causes adhesions in the area. The space in which the tendons glide is very constricted, and there is very little room for scar tissue formation. It is very difficult to restore normal gliding of the tendon in the tendon sheath after injury in this area. Restoration of function after digital flexor tendon laceration is the most difficult of all tendon repairs.

b. Procedures[17,20,22,28]

(1) Simple flexor tendon lacerations are sutured and repaired in one surgical procedure.

(2) The wrist and hand are then immobilized in a bulky dressing with the wrist in 20 to 45 degrees of flexion and the MCP and PIP joints in 20 degrees of flexion. This position takes any mechanical stretch off the repaired flexor tendon.

(3) After surgery, elevation of the hand is essential to prevent edema.

c. Postoperative management

(1) At approximately 5 days postoperatively, the bulky dressing is removed. A traditional method of management is to place the patient's hand or wrist in a static splint that immobilizes the wrist and fingers in a flexed position. The splint is worn 24 hours per day for 3 weeks as repaired tendons heal. An alternative to this traditional approach is to have the patient wear a specially designed glove that allows early, *controlled* motion in the fingers. The glove passively holds the fingers in flexion with rubber bands but allows the patient to actively contract the extensors and *partially* extend the fingers against the resistance of the rubber bands. The bands then *passively* return the fingers to flexion when the extensors relax.
Precaution: Absolutely no active finger flexion or passive extension of the fingers is permissible at this time.

(2) At 3 weeks, the static splint or glove is removed for exercise, and *active* finger flexion may be begun. The splint or glove is replaced after exercise.

(3) At 6 to 8 weeks, the glove may be discontinued and mild resistance exercise to the flexors may be added. The patient may then use his

hand for stronger grasp activities. Full activity is allowed by 12 weeks.

(4) If flexion contractures occur, gentle stretching may be initiated at about 8 weeks postoperatively.

d. More complicated procedures with multiple stages of surgical reconstruction and tendon grafts are required for more severe lacerations of the flexors.[7,22,28]

4. Repair of lacerated extensor tendons of the hand

a. **Background of the problem**[1,22,28]

The extensor tendons of the digits glide in a synovial sheath only at the wrist joint. Therefore, these tendons are less likely to develop adhesions in the tendon sheath.[23] Depending on the location of the laceration, deformities of the fingers, such as a boutonnière deformity, can develop. Surgical repair and postoperative rehabilitation vary depending on where in the hand the laceration of the tendon(s) occurred. A laceration between the distal radius and the MCP joints will disrupt the common extensors and MCP extension. A laceration to the extensor surface at the PIP joint level disrupts the extensor hood mechanism. Laceration at the DIP joint involves disruption of terminal extension of a digit.

b. **Procedures**[1,22]

(1) Surgical suturing and repair of the tendon is followed by immobilization in some degree of wrist and finger extension for several weeks. Immobilization in extension minimizes the stretch to newly sutured tendons.

(2) In general, lacerations and repair of the common extensors require immobilization of the wrist and MCP joints in extension for at least 3 weeks.

(3) If the injury has occurred at the PIP joint and the extensor hood mechanism is disrupted, the PIP joint is immobilized for 4 to 6 weeks with a splint and/or K-wire. Active MCP and DIP flexion and extension may be permitted.

(4) If the laceration has occurred at the DIP joint, the DIP joint is immobilized for 6 to 8 weeks. Some surgeons splint the PIP joint in flexion and others splint the PIP joint in extension while the lacerated tendon heals and its tensile strength increases.

c. **Postoperative management**

(1) Injuries and repairs of extensor tendons at different levels require different periods of immobilization. The therapist must also determine if limited movement of joints is caused by capsular or tendinous restrictions.

(2) Active-assistive and active finger extension of the involved joints is begun when the immobilization device is removed. The joints above and below the lacerated area are held in a neutral position during exercise.

(3) Then approximately 1 week later, active flexion at the involved finger joints is begun.

Remember: the flexors are a much stronger muscle group than the extensors, so active flexion must be gentle and controlled to avoid a stretch to the repaired extensor tendon. A dynamic extension splint to assist extension and resist flexion sometimes is used for the first few weeks after the immobilization device is removed to protect the repaired extensor tendon.

Too much emphasis on flexion can also cause an extensor lag of the injured digit. This is caused by attenuation (secondary remodeling) of the tendon scar.

(4) Exercises and splinting are continued for approximately 8 to 10 weeks. Gentle resistive exercises can be added as healing progresses. The hand is used for progressively more vigorous daily functional activities.

B. Total Wrist Arthroplasty (Radiocarpal Implant Arthroplasty)

1. Indications for surgery[1,9,20,26,27]

a. Severe instability of the wrist joint and deterioration of the distal radius, carpals, and distal ulna as a result of chronic arthritis.

b. Marked limitation of motion of the wrist.

c. Subluxation or dislocation of the radiocarpal joint.

d. Severe pain at the wrist that compromises hand strength and function.

2. Procedures[1,9,26,27]

a. The total wrist replacement arthroplasty is an alternative to arthrodesis of the wrist. A successful total wrist replacement provides a balance of functional wrist motion combined with adequate joint stability.

b. There are two general types of radiocarpal implant arthroplasties. Both require a dorsal incision of the wrist.

(1) The flexible implant arthroplasty is a double-stemmed unit of silicone rubber. After removal of the proximal row of carpals and resection of the distal aspect of the radius and the base of the capitate, the proximal stem of the prosthesis is placed in the intramedullary canal of the distal radius. The distal stem is placed through the capitate and into the intramedullary canal of the third metacarpal. The prosthesis does not require cement but rather becomes encapsulated over time by a new fibrous capsule.

This procedure is often combined with synovectomy of the wrist, dorsal clearance of the extensor tendons, and possible repair of the extensor tendons.

(2) Various rigid (metal and high-density plastic), hinged total wrist prostheses have also been developed.[9] These prostheses are all cemented in place with methyl methacrylate. In most procedures, the distal radius, possibly the distal ulna, and adequate carpal bones are resected. The implant inserts proximally into the intramedullary canal of the distal radius and distally into the third and possibly second or fourth metacarpals.

c. In both types of procedures, the hand and wrist are placed in a bulky dressing for 3 to 6 days postoperatively and elevated to reduce edema.

3. Postoperative management

a. Immobilization

(1) Flexible implant arthroplasty requires approximately 4 weeks of immobilization in a short arm cast with the wrist in neutral or 20 degrees of extension. No wrist exercise is begun until there is adequate joint stability.[26,28]

(2) Hinged implants of rigid plastic and metal that are cemented in

place require a shorter period of immobilization, usually 1 to 2 weeks, before wrist exercise is begun.
b. Exercise[20,28]
   (1) During the period of immobilization, the patient is encouraged to carry out frequent active finger flexion exercises in the splint or cast to maintain finger mobility and reduce edema in the hand.
   (2) When wrist motion is allowed, the splint is removed and the patient begins
      (a) Active pronation and supination of the forearm.
      (b) Active radial and ulnar deviation of the wrist.
      (c) Active or active-assistive wrist extension with the fingers relaxed and flexed.
      (d) Active or active-assistive wrist flexion with the fingers relaxed and extended.
      (e) Active finger flexion and extension with the wrist in neutral.
      (f) Active opposition of the thumb to each of the digits.
   (3) The wrist splint is worn between exercise sessions during the day for at least 6 to 8 weeks. Light functional activities may be begun at 8 weeks without the splint. The splint is worn at night for up to 12 weeks.
   (4) Active exercises are continued until functional range of motion of the wrist is achieved.
   (5) Gentle resistance exercises may be begun at 6 to 8 weeks to improve grip strength.
c. **Precautions**
   (1) If a repair of extensor tendons has also been done, follow the precautions for tendon repair discussed earlier in this chapter.
   (2) The patient must be advised that heavy lifting or excessive weight bearing on the hand is contraindicated postoperatively.

4. Expected results[9,26]

Follow-up studies of total wrist arthroplasties indicate that a good result involves
a. Relief of pain.
b. Stability of the wrist for light functional activities.
c. Approximately 50 to 60 percent of full range of motion (45 degrees of flexion and 45 degrees of extension of the wrist and 45 degrees of supination of the forearm).
d. Adequate grip strength, although this is difficult to measure because finger joints are often also involved because of rheumatoid arthritis.

C. Metacarpophalangeal (MCP) Implant Arthroplasty

1. Indications for surgery[8,9,25,26]

a. Pain at the MCP joint(s) of the hand and deterioration of the joint, usually because of rheumatoid arthritis.
b. Instability and deformity (ulnar drift) of the fingers that cannot be corrected with soft-tissue releases alone.
c. Stiffness and decreased range of motion at the MCP joints.
d. Possible subluxation of the MCP joints.

2. Procedure

a. Prerequisites

In order for this implant arthroplasty to be successful, a patient must have an intact extensor digitorum communis, or repair of these tendons must be done prior to or at the time of surgery. (See section III A of this chapter.)

b. Dorsal clearance (removal of diseased synovium along the extensor tendon sheaths) may be done either as an earlier surgical procedure or at the same time as the implant arthroplasty.

c. Overview of the procedure

Note: The majority of implant arthroplasties done for the digits are one-piece, flexible, stemmed prostheses made of silicone. The implant acts as a dynamic spacer as the joint heals. Flexible implant arthroplasty was an improvement over the hinged metal prosthesis. Newer designs include a two-piece, plastic-to-metal articulated implant that is cemented in place and, most recently, a cementless, non-constrained implant made of pyrolite carbon.[24]

(1) A transverse incision is made over the dorsal aspect of the MCP joints.

(2) The thick, proliferated synovium is removed.

(3) Release of soft-tissue contractures (at the volar capsule or collateral ligaments) and repair of the extensor tendons are done if necessary.

(4) The heads of the involved metacarpals are excised and the intramedullary canals of the metacarpal and proximal phalanx are widened.

(5) The prosthesis is implanted.

(6) The wound is closed and a bulky compression dressing is placed around the hand; the MCP joints are held in extension and the distal joints in some flexion.

3. Postoperative management[1,8,17,20,24]

a. Immobilization

For the first 3 to 7 days the hand is elevated to prevent edema and remains in the compression dressing. Immobilization of the early metal-to-metal hinged prosthesis was necessary for 4 weeks. Gentle active motion was not begun until after the immobilization was removed. Very few metal, hinged prostheses are used today. Immobilization after flexible implant arthroplasty, cemented plastic and metal implants, or cementless pyrolite carbon implants is not as lengthy, and therefore exercises can be initiated within a few days to a week after surgery.

(1) If only an MCP implant has been done, the hand remains immobilized for about 3 days.

(2) If, in addition to the MCP implant, a repair of the extensor tendons has been done, the hand remains immobilized and elevated for at least 5 days or possibly 7 to 10 days.

b. Between 3 to 7 days postoperatively, the bulky dressing is removed and the patient is placed in a dynamic, extensor outrigger splint.

(1) The dynamic splint keeps the MCP joints in full extension. The patient wears the splint at all times except during exercise.

(2) The adjustable dynamic splint is worn to prevent any recurrent deformity, such as ulnar drift, and to control and guide joint motion during healing.

c. At this time, gentle active flexion and extension exercises of the MCP joints with the PIP joints flexed and extended may be performed several times a day.

   (1) Do not let the patient substitute with PIP flexion and extension.

   (2) Stabilize the PIP joints manually or with small splints to get isolated MCP movement.

   (3) Active exercise to the PIP joints should also be done with the MCP joints stabilized in extension.

   (4) Active wrist movement with the hand relaxed should be included.

   (5) Active opposition of the thumb to each finger should also be done.

   Precaution: During the first few postoperative weeks, do not apply any stretch or resistance to the extensors if an extensor tendon repair has been done.

d. Continue active flexion and extension exercises of the MCP joints for 2 to 3 weeks. The desired result will be at least 70 degrees of active flexion at the MCP joint, with a minimum of active extensor lag. It is important to attain this active range early.

   (1) If extensor lag is a persistent problem, place greater emphasis on active extension exercises.

   (2) By 3 weeks, if at least 60 to 70 degrees of MCP flexion has not been achieved, a flexor outrigger may be added to the splint or a flexor cuff may be worn 1 to 2 hours per day. MCP flexion is most important in the third, fourth, and fifth digits for a good functional grasp.

e. By 2 months, the patient may stop wearing the extensor splint during the day and may use the hand for light functional activities.

f. Exercise may include the use of small hand exercisers designed to improve grip strength. For optimal results, exercise should continue for at least 3 months.

D. Proximal Interphalangeal (PIP) Implant Arthroplasty

1. Indications for surgery[8,9,24,25]

a. Pain at the PIP joint(s) of the fingers and deterioration of the joint surfaces because of synovitis

b. Decreased range of motion at the PIP joints

c. Deformity of the fingers

   (1) swan-neck deformity

   (2) boutonnière deformity

2. Procedure[9,17,24,26]

a. The head of the involved proximal phalanx is excised and replaced with a flexible silicone implant.

b. The joint is realigned.

c. Repair may also be done to the extensor tendon mechanism if necessary.

d. If either swan-neck or boutonnière deformities exist, they are corrected at this time.

e. The wound is closed, and a bulky compression dressing is placed on the hand.

   (1) If a swan-neck deformity existed prior to surgery, the PIP joints are held in 10 to 20 degrees of flexion.

   (2) If a boutonnière deformity existed, the PIP joints are held in extension.

3. **Postoperative management**[8,20,24,27,28]
    a. Immobilization
       The period of time required for immobilization will vary, depending on whether or not extensor tendon reconstruction was part of the procedure.
       (1) If no tendon repair was done, only 3 to 5 days of immobilization will be necessary before exercises can be started.
       (2) If the extensor tendons have been repaired, a period of 14 to 21 days of immobilization will be required to protect the extensor mechanism.
    b. If no tendon reconstruction was done, the bulky dressing is removed at 3 to 5 days and active exercise to the hand may be started. This includes
       (1) active flexion and extension of the PIP joints with the MCP and DIP joints stabilized in neutral.
       (2) active flexion and extension of the MCP and DIP joints of the fingers.
       (3) active exercises of the thumb.
       (4) active range of motion of the wrist and forearm.
       (5) The PIP joints are immobilized in extension with a small aluminum splint between exercise sessions and at night.
    c. If a swan-neck deformity was corrected at the time the joint implant was done, it will be extremely important to avoid hyperextension of the PIP joint.
       (1) Active flexion and extension exercises to the PIP joints are begun at approximately 10 to 14 days postoperatively. Be sure to stabilize the DIP joints in neutral during exercise.
       (2) It may be appropriate to allow the patient to develop a slight (10 degrees) flexion contracture at the PIP joint. This will protect the volar aspect of the joint capsule and lessen the possibility that a recurrent hyperextension deformity will develop.
       (3) The PIP joint is immobilized in a splint in 10 to 20 degrees of flexion between exercises and at night.
    d. If a boutonnière deformity has been repaired at the time the joint arthroplasty was done, it will be important to maintain as much extension at the PIP joint as possible. Since the extensor tendons are repaired as a part of the procedure, stretching or heavy resistance to the extensor mechanism must be avoided for 6 to 8 weeks postoperatively.
       (1) At 14 to 21 days postoperatively, active flexion and extension exercises to the PIP joints may be started.
       (2) During active motion of the PIP joint, the MCP joints should be stabilized in neutral at the edge of a table or book.
       (3) After exercise, the PIP joints are held in full extension in an aluminum splint.
    e. In all variations of the PIP implant arthroplasty, active exercise is continued for 6 to 8 weeks postoperatively or until functional range of motion of the PIP joints (0 degrees of extension and 70 degrees of flexion) is attained.
       (1) A home program of exercises should be done everyday.
       (2) The patient may use a number of hand exercisers to add variety to the program.
    f. A splint is worn for protection for 8 to 12 weeks between exercise ses-

sions and at night. The splint may be discontinued in the daytime initially and later at night. (If no tendon repair was done, the splint may be discontinued as early as 6 to 8 weeks postoperatively.)
g. Mild stretching and gentle resistance exercises may be started at 6 to 8 weeks postoperatively. At that time the patient may use his hand for light functional activities.
h. Exercises should be continued for about 3 months to avoid recurrence of stiffness and contractures.

E. Carpometacarpal (CMC) Joint Replacement of the Thumb

1. Indications for surgery[8,9]
a. Pain at the carpometacarpal (CMC) joint of the thumb because of osteoarthritis or traumatic or rheumatoid arthritis. The majority of CMC arthroplasties are done for pain and instability associated with degenerative joint disease.
b. Dorsoradial subluxation or dislocation of the first metacarpal, leading to a hyperextension deformity of the thumb.
c. Limited range of motion, often an adduction contracture of the thumb.
d. Decreased pinch and grip strength because of pain in or subluxation of the CMC joint.
e. When arthrodesis of the CMC joint is inappropriate.

2. Procedures[9,26,27]
A number of procedures have been developed to replace the carpometacarpal joint. They may be classified into three broad categories:
a. Resection of the trapezium and replacement with a flexible silicone implant.
b. Carpometacarpal joint replacement with a flexible silicone intramedullary stemmed prosthesis.
c. Replacement of the CMC joint with a metal-to-plastic ball-and-socket prosthesis held in place with methyl methacrylate.

3. Postoperative management[9,26,27]
a. Immobilization
In all procedures, the thumb and hand are immobilized in a large bulky dressing for 3 to 6 days postoperatively and elevated to prevent edema.
b. Exercise
(1) Active range of motion exercises are begun 5 to 7 days postoperatively with procedures in which a metal-to-plastic ball-and-socket prosthesis has been held in place with cement.
(a) A protective splint is worn for 3 weeks.
(b) Full activity without the splint can be resumed by 4 weeks.
(2) If a flexible silicone implant has been used to replace the carpometacarpal joint, the bulky dressing is removed in 4 to 5 days. A short arm thumb spica cast is then applied and worn for 6 weeks.
(a) This prolonged immobilization ensures good healing of the capsule and lessens the likelihood of recurrent subluxation of the CMC joint.
(b) During this time, active motion of the fingers is encouraged.
(c) At 6 weeks when the cast is removed, the patient may begin active abduction, circumduction, and opposition of the thumb.

Precaution: Avoid hyperextension of the joint, particularly during the first 12 weeks.

(d) Gentle pinch and grasp activities may be added to increase strength.

(e) Unrestricted use of the hand is allowed at 12 weeks.

4. Expected results

(1) 50 percent of full motion of the thumb.

(2) Elimination or marked decrease in pain at the CMC joint.

(3) 50 percent of full, normal pinch by 1 year postoperatively, which is usually significantly greater than preoperative strength.

IV. SUMMARY

The anatomy and kinesiology of the wrist and hand were outlined in Chapter 9. Clinical application of this information included a discussion of hand control, grasp, and pinch. Guidelines for therapeutic exercise management of specific musculoskeletal problems of the wrist and hand were outlined. These guidelines included management of deformities of the wrist, fingers, and thumb secondary to arthritis, exercise for imbalance of strength and flexibility in the hand, and management of ligamentous injuries and tendinitis. An outline of common surgical procedures of the wrist and hand was also included. Tendon transfers and repairs, synovectomy, and joint replacement of the wrist and hand were discussed. Recommendations, precautions, and progression of exercise after surgery were also outlined.

REFERENCES

1. Beasley, RW: *Basic Considerations for Tendon Transfer Operations in the Upper Extremity.* In *AAOS Symposium on Tendon Surgery of the Hand.* CV Mosby, St Louis, 1975.
2. Bentley, JA: *Physiotherapy following joint replacements.* In Downie, PA: *Cash's Textbook of Orthopedics and Rheumatology for Physiotherapist.* JB Lippincott, Philadelphia, 1984.
3. Cailliet, R: *Hand Pain and Impairment,* ed 3. FA Davis, Philadelphia, 1982.
4. Chusid, J and McDonald, J: *Correlative Neuroanatomy and Functional Neurology,* ed 17. Lang Medical Publications, Los Altos, California, 1979.
5. Cyriax, J: *Textbook of Orthopaedic Medicine, Vol 1. Diagnosis of Soft Tissue Lesions,* ed 8. Bailliere Tindall, London, 1982.
6. Daniels, L and Worthingham, C: *Muscle Testing: Techniques of Manual Examination,* ed 4. WB Saunders, Philadelphia, 1980.
7. Hunter, JM: *Two stage flexor tendon reconstruction—A technique using a tendon prosthesis before tendon grafting.* In Hunter, JM (ed): *Rehabilitation of the Hand.* CV Mosby, St Louis, 1978.
8. Hyde, SA: *Physiotherapy in Rheumatology.* Blackwell Scientific Publications, Oxford, 1980.
9. Inglis, AE (ed): *Symposium on Total Joint Replacement of the Upper Extremity* (1979). American Academy of Orthopedic Surgeons, CV Mosby, St Louis, 1982.
10. Iversen, LD and Clawson, DK: *Manual of Acute Orthopedic Therapeutics,* ed 2. Little, Brown & Company, Boston, 1982.
11. Kapandji, IA: *The Physiology of the Joints,* Volume I. Churchill-Livingstone, Edinburgh, 1970.
12. Kessler, R and Hertling, D: *Management of Common Musculoskeletal Disorders.* Harper & Row, Philadelphia, 1983.
13. Kopell, H and Thompson, W: *Peripheral Entrapment Neuropathies,* ed 2. Robert E. Krieger, Huntington, NY, 1976.
14. Lehmkuhl, LD and Smith, LK: *Brunnstrom's Clinical Kinesiology,* ed 4. FA Davis, Philadelphia, 1983.

15. Long, R, et al: *Intrinsic-extrinsic muscle control of the hand in power grip and precision handling.* J Bone Joint Surg 52A:853, 1970.
16. Long, C: *Normal and Abnormal Motor Control in the Upper Extremities.* Final Report, Case Western Reserve University, Cleveland, 1970.
17. Melvin, J: *Rheumatic Disease: Occupational Therapy and Rehabilitation,* ed 2. FA Davis, Philadelphia, 1982.
18. Napier, JR: *The prehensile movements of the human hand.* J Bone Joint Surg 38B:902, 1956.
19. Norkin, C and Levangie, P: *Joint Structure and Function: A Comprehensive Analysis.* FA Davis, Philadelphia, 1983.
20. Occupational Therapy Staff: *Upper Extremity Surgeries for Patients with Arthritis—A Pre and Post-Operative Occupational Therapy Treatment Guide.* Rancho Los Amigos Hospital, Downey, California, 1979.
21. Omer, GE: *Tendon transfers for reconstruction of the forearm and hand following peripheral nerve injuries.* In Omer, GE and Spinner, M (eds): *Management of Peripheral Nerve Problems.* WB Saunders, Philadelphia, 1980.
22. Rosenblum, NI and Robinson, SJ: *Advances in flexor and extensor tendon management.* In Moran, CA (ed): *Hand Rehabilitation.* Churchill-Livingstone, New York, 1986.
23. Rosenthal, EA: *The extensor tendons.* In Hunter, JM (ed): *Rehabilitation of the Hand.* CV Mosby, St Louis, 1980.
24. Shurr, DG: *The therapist's role in finger joint arthrophasty.* In Moran, CA (ed): *Hand Rehabilitation.* Churchill-Livingstone, New York, 1986.
25. Swanson, AB: *Flexible implant athroplasty for arthritic finger joints: Rationale, technique and results of treatment.* J Bone Joint Surg 54A:535, 1972.
26. Swanson, AB: *Flexible implant resection arthroplasty in the hand and extremities.* CV Mosby, St Louis, 1973.
27. Swanson, AB, ET AL: *Upper limb joint replacement.* In Nickel, VL (ed): *Orthopedic Rehabilitation.* Churchill-Livingstone, New York, 1982.
28. Trombly, CA: *Occupational Therapy for Physical Dysfunction,* ed 2. Williams & Wilkins, Baltimore, 1983.
29. Zohn, D and Mennell, J: *Musculoskeletal Pain: Principles of Physical Diagnosis and Physical Treatment.* Little, Brown & Company, Boston, 1976.

CHAPTER ———————————— 10

THE HIP

The hip is often compared with the shoulder in that it is a triaxial joint, able to function in all three planes, and is also the proximal link to its extremity. In contrast to the shoulder, which is constructed for mobility, the hip is a stable joint, constructed for weight bearing. Forces from the lower extremities are transmitted upwards through the hips to the pelvis and trunk during gait and other lower extremity activities. The hips also support the weight of the head, trunk, and upper extremities.

     The initial section of this chapter reviews highlights of the anatomy and function of the hip and its relation to the pelvis and lumbar spine. The reader is referred to several texts for study of the material.[10,29,35] Chapter 6 presents information on principles of management; the reader should be familiar with that material before proceeding with establishing a therapeutic exercise program for the hip region.

OBJECTIVES

After studying this chapter, the reader will be able to:
1. identify important aspects of the hip structure and function for review.
2. establish a therapeutic exercise program to manage soft tissue and joint lesions in the hip that are related to stages of recovery following an inflammatory insult to the tissues.
3. establish a therapeutic exercise program to manage common musculoskeletal lesions, recognizing unique circumstances in the hip and pelvis for their management.
4. establish a therapeutic exercise program to manage patients following common surgical procedures for the hip.

I.   REVIEW OF THE STRUCTURE AND FUNCTION OF THE HIP

    A. Bony Parts are the Proximal Femur and the Pelvis (see Figure 5-44).

B. Hip Joint

1. Characteristics

A ball-and-socket (spheroidal) triaxial joint; supported by a strong articular capsule that is reinforced by the iliofemoral, pubofemoral, and ischiofemoral ligaments. The two hip joints are linked to each other through the bony pelvis and to the vertebral column through the sacrum and lumbosacral joint

2. The acetabulum

The concave bony partner, the acetabulum, is made up of the fusion of the ilium, ischium, and pubic bones and is deepened by a ring of fibrocartilage, the acetabulum labrum. It is located in the lateral aspect of the pelvis and faces laterally, anteriorly, and inferiorly. The articular cartilage is horseshoe-shaped, being thicker in the lateral region. The central portion of the acetabular surface is nonarticular.

3. The femoral head

The convex bony partner is the spherical head of the femur, which is attached to the femoral neck. It projects anteriorly, medially, and superiorly.

4. Motions of the femur

The convex head slides in the direction opposite the physiologic motion of the femur.

Physiologic Motions of the Femur	Direction of Slide of the Femoral Head
Flexion	Posterior
Extension	Anterior
Abduction	Inferior
Adduction	Superior
Internal rotation	Posterior
External rotation	Anterior

5. Motions of the pelvis

When the lower extremity is fixated, as in standing or during the stance phase of gait, the concave acetabulum moves on the convex femoral head, so the acetabulum slides in the same direction as the pelvis. (See section C below.)

Physiologic Motions of the Pelvis	Direction of Slide of of the Acetabulum
Anterior pelvic tilt	Anterior
Posterior pelvic tilt	Posterior
Lateral pelvic tilt:	
Pelvis elevated	Inferior
Pelvis dropped	Superior
Forward pelvic rotation	Anterior
Backward pelvic rotation	Posterior

Note: When the pelvis moves, it affects both hip joints, but the motion is not necessarily the same on the contralateral side.

6. Angle of inclination

The angle between the axis of the femoral neck and shaft of the femur. The normal is 125 degrees. A pathologically larger angle is called coxa valga, and a pathologically smaller angle is called coxa vara. Unilateral coxa valga results in a relatively longer leg on that side and associated genu varum. Unilateral coxa vara leads to a relatively shorter leg with associated genu valgum on that side. Compensations with unilateral differences usually occur in the pelvis, foot, and ankle.

7. Torsion

The angle formed by the transverse axis of the femoral condyles and the axis of the neck of the femur. The angle ranges from 8 to 25 degrees, with a normal angle of 12 degrees. An increase in the angle is called anteversion and causes the shaft of the femur to be rotated medially; a decrease in the angle is called retroversion and causes the shaft of the femur to rotated laterally. Anteversion often results in genu valgum and pes planus. Unilateral anteversion results in a relatively shorter leg on that side with compensations in the position of the pelvis. Retroversion causes the opposite effects.

C. Functional Relationships of the Hips, Pelvis, and Spine

1. With pelvic motion, the angle of the hip and lumbar spine changes

a. Anterior pelvic tilt (PT)

The anterior superior iliac spines of the pelvis move anteriorly and inferiorly and thus closer to the anterior aspect of the femur as the pelvis rotates forward around the transverse axis of the hip joints. This results in hip flexion and increased lumbar spine extension (hyperextension).

(1) Muscles causing this motion are the hip flexors and back extensors.

(2) When standing, with the line of gravity of the trunk falling anteriorly to the axis of the hip joints, the effect is an anterior PT.

b. Posterior PT

The posterior superior iliac spines of the pelvis move posteriorly and inferiorly, thus closer to the posterior aspect of the femur as the pelvis rotates backward around the axis of the hip joints. This results in hip extension and lumbar spine flexion. Muscles causing this motion are the hip extensors and trunk flexors.

c. Pelvic shifting

When standing, a forward translatory shifting of the pelvis results in extension of the hip and extension of the lower lumbar spinal segments. There is a compensatory posterior shifting of the thorax on the upper lumbar spine with increased flexion of these spinal segments. This is often seen with slouched or relaxed postures (see Chapter 14). Little muscle action is required; the posture is maintained by the iliofemoral ligaments at the hip, anterior longitudinal ligament of the lower lumbar spine, and posterior ligaments of the upper lumbar and thoracic spine.

d. Lumbar-pelvic rhythm[10,42]

A coordinated movement between the lumbar spine and pelvis occurs for maximal forward bending of the trunk as when reaching toward the floor or the toes. As the head and upper trunk initiate flexion, the pelvis shifts posteriorly to maintain the center of gravity balanced over the base of support. The trunk continues to forward bend, being controlled by the extensor muscles of the spine, until approximately 45 degrees. The ligaments are then taut and the facets oriented in the frontal plane approximated, both providing stability for the vertebrae, and the muscles relax. Once all of the vertebral segments are at the end of the range and stabilized by the posterior ligaments and facets, the pelvis begins to rotate forward (anterior pelvic tilt), being controlled by the gluteus maximus and hamstring muscles. The pelvis continues to rotate forward until the full length of the muscles is reached. Final range of motion (ROM) in forward bending is dictated by the flexibility in the various back extensor muscles and fascia as well as hip extensor muscles. The return to the upright position begins with the hip extensor muscles rotating the pelvis posterior through reverse muscle action (posterior pelvic tilt), then back extensor muscles extending the spine from the lumbar region upward. Variations in the normal synchronization of this activity occur due to faulty habits, restricted muscle or facsia length, or injury and faulty proprioception.

e. Lateral pelvic tilt
Frontal plane pelvic motion results in opposite motions at each hip joint. On the side that is elevated (hip hiking), there is hip adduction; on the side that is lowered (hip drop), there is hip abduction. When standing, the lumbar spine laterally flexes toward the side of the elevated pelvis (convexity of the lateral curve is toward the lowered side).

(1) Muscles causing lateral pelvic tilting include the quadratus lumborum on the side of the elevated pelvis and reverse muscle pull of the gluteus medius on the side of the lowered pelvis.

(2) With an asymmetric slouched posture, the person shifts his trunk weight onto one lower extremity and allows the pelvis to drop on the other side. Passive support comes from the iliofemoral ligament and iliotibial band on the elevated side (stance leg).

f. Pelvic rotation
Rotation occurs around one lower extremity that is fixed on the ground. The unsupported lower extremity swings forward or backward along with the pelvis. When the unsupported side of the pelvis moves forward, it is called forward rotation of the pelvis. The trunk concurrently rotates opposite, and the femur on the stabilized side concurrently rotates internally. When the unsupported side of the pelvis moves backward, it is called posterior rotation; the femur on the stabilized side concurrently rotates externally, and the trunk rotates opposite.

2. **Motions and postures of the lower extremity affect the pelvis and spine**

a. Active hip flexion will result in anterior pelvic tilt and increased lumbar extension unless the pelvis is stabilized by the abdominal musculature. The opposite occurs with active hip extension.

b. Tight hip muscles or joints will cause weight-bearing forces and movement to be transmitted to the spine rather than being absorbed in the pelvis. Tight hip extensors will cause increased lumbar flexion when the thigh is flexed. Tight hip flexors will cause increased lumbar extension as the thigh extends. Hip flexion contractures with incomplete hip extension on weight bearing will also place added stresses on the knee since the knee cannot lock while the hip is in flexion unless the trunk is bent forward. Tight adductors cause lateral pelvic tilt opposite and side bending of the trunk toward the side of tightness when weight bearing. The opposite occurs with tight abductors.

    c. A unilateral short leg will cause lateral pelvic tilting (drop on the short side) and side bending of the trunk away from the short side (convexity of lateral lumbar curve towards side of short leg). This may lead to a functional or eventually a structural scoliosis (Chapter 17). Causes of a short leg could be unilateral lower extremity asymmetries such as flat foot, genu valgum, coxa vara, tight hip muscles, anterior rotated innominate bone, poor standing posture, or asymmetry in bone growth.

3. The hip and gait[35,36]

    a. During the normal gait cycle, the hip goes through a range of motion of 40 degrees (10 degrees extension at terminal stance to 30 degrees flexion at midswing and initial contact). There is also some lateral pelvic tilt and rotation (about 8 degrees) which requires hip abduction/adduction and hip internal/external rotation. Loss of any of these motions will affect the smoothness of the gait pattern.

    b. Muscle control during gait

        (1) Hip flexors

        Control hip extension at the end of stance, then contract concentrically to initiate swing. With loss of flexor function, a posterior lurch of the trunk to initiate swing is seen. Contractures in the hip flexors will prevent complete extension during the second half of stance; the stride is shortened. The person increases the lumbar lordosis or walks with the trunk bent forward.

        (2) Hip extensors

        Control the flexor moment at initial foot contact, then the gluteus maximus initiates hip extension. With loss of extensor function, a posteror lurch of the trunk occurs at foot contact to shift the center of gravity of the trunk posterior to the hip. With contractures in the gluteus maximus, there will be some decrease in the terminal swing as the femur comes forward, or the person may compensate by rotating the pelvis more forward. The lower extremity may rotate outward due to the external rotation component of the muscle, or place greater tension on the iliotibial band through its attachment, leading to irritation along the lateral knee with excessive activity.

        (3) Hip abductors

        The gluteus medius controls the lateral pelvic tilt during swinging of the opposite leg. With loss of function, lateral shifting of the trunk occurs over the weak side during stance when the opposite leg swings. This lateral shifting also occurs with a painful hip, since it minimizes the torque at the hip joint during weight bearing. The tensor fascia lata also functions as an abductor and may become tight and affect gait with faulty use.

    c. Bony and joint deformities will change alignment of the lower extremity and therefore the mechanics of gait. Painful conditions cause antalgic gait patterns, which are characterized by minimum stance on the painful side to avoid the stress of weight bearing.

4. Hip muscle imbalances commonly affecting gait[40]

Muscles function through habit. Faulty mechanics from inadequate or excessive length and imbalanced strength cause hip, knee, or back pain. Overuse syndromes, soft-tissue stress, and joint pain develop in response to continued abnormal stresses.

a. Tight iliotibial (IT) band with tight tensor fascia lata (TFL) or tight gluteus maximus
Often there are associated postural dysfunctions of an anterior pelvic tilt posture, slouched posture, or flat back posture (see Chapter 14).

(1) Anterior pelvic tilt posture; hip musculature imbalances
—tight TFL and IT band
—general limitation of hip external rotation
—weak, stretched posterior portion of the gluteus medius and piriformis
—excessive medial rotation of femur during first half of stance with increased stresses on the medial structures of the knee
—associated lower extremity compensations including medial rotation of the femur, genu valgum, lateral tibial torsion, pes planis, and hallix valgus

(2) Slouched posture; hip musculature imbalances
—tight rectus femoris and hamstrings
—general limitation of hip rotators
—weak, stretched iliopsoas
—weak and tight posterior portion of the gluteus medius
—weak, poorly developed gluteus maximus
—associated lower extremity compensations including hip extension, sometimes medial rotation of femur, genu recurvatum, genu varum, pes valgus

(3) Flat back posture; hip musculature imbalances
—tightness in the rectus femoris, IT band, and gluteus maximus
—variations of the above two postures

b. Overuse of the two-joint hip flexor muscles (TFL, rectus femoris, and sartorius) rather than iliopsoas.
This may cause faulty hip mechanics or knee pain from overuse of these muscles as they cross the knee.

c. Overuse of the TFL rather than gluteus medius.
This leads to lateral knee pain from IT band tension, or medial rotation of the femur with medial knee stresses from increased bowstring effect.

d. Overuse of hamstring muscles rather than gluteus maximus.
The gluteus maximus becomes tight and range of hip flexion decreases; compensation occurs with excessive lumbar spine flexion whenever flexing the thigh. Tightness in the gluteus maximus also causes increased tension on the IT band with associated lateral knee pain. Overuse of the hamstring muscles causes muscle tightness as well as muscle imbalances with the quadriceps femoris muscle at the knee. The hamstrings dominate the stabilizing function by pulling posterior on the tibia to extend the knee in closed-chain activities. This alters the mechanics at the knee and may lead to overuse syndromes in the hamstring tendons or anterior knee pain from imbalances in quadriceps pull.

e. Lateral trunk muscles for hip abductors. This results in excessive trunk motion and increased stress in the lumbar spine.

D. Equilibrium and Posture Control

The joint capsule is richly supplied with mechanoreceptors that respond to variations in position, stress, and movement for control of posture, balance, and movement. Joint pathologies could lead to problems with balance and posture control.[21]

E. Nerves in the Hip and Buttock Region[28]

1. Major nerves subject to entrapment

a. Sciatic nerve

Forms in the posterior region of the pelvis from the sacral plexus (L-4, L-5, S-1, S-2, and S-3 nerve roots), and leaves the pelvis across the lower edge of the greater sciatic notch. It then passes deep to the piriformis muscle. (Occasionally, it passes over or through the piriformis.) Entrapment results in sensory changes along the lateral and posterior portion of the leg and dorsal and plantar surface of the foot. Progressive weakness in the hamstring muscles, a portion of the adductor magnus muscle, and all the muscles of the leg and foot also develops.

b. Obturator nerve

Forms within the psoas muscle from nerve roots of L-2, L-3, and L-4 and enters the pelvis anterior to the sacroiliac joint. It then courses through the obturator canal along with the obturator vessels; there, it divides into the anterior and posterior branch. Injury or entrapment results in sensory changes along the medial aspect of the thigh and weakness primarily in the adductor muscles.

2. The hip is innervated primarily from the L-3 spinal level; hip joint irritation is usually felt along the L-3 dermatome reference from the groin, down the front of the thigh to the knee.[13]

II. GUIDELINES AND THERAPEUTIC EXERCISE MANAGEMENT OF COMMON MUSCULOSKELETAL PROBLEMS IN THE HIP

Note: Exercises applied to the hip during acute, subacute, and chronic phases of inflammation and healing follow the same principles as those described in Chapter 6, taking into account the unique anatomic and kinesiologic relationships of the hip region (including the low back and pelvis). This section will expand on these guidelines for common hip problems.

A. Joint and Capsule Restrictions of the Hip

1. Clinical picture

With early joint involvement, only internal rotation is painful or restricted. In advanced joint dysfunctions, the hip may be fixed in adduction, have no internal rotation or extension past neutral, be limited to 90 degrees of flexion, and full external rotation.[13]

a. Osteoarthritis (degenerative joint disease, DJD)

DJD commonly affects the hip as part of the aging process, or as a result of trauma from injury, deformity, or disease. There may be osteophyte formation at the joint margins, capsular fibrosis, and articular cartilage degeneration, usually occurring in regions undergoing greatest stress, such as along the superior weight-bearing surface.

(1) In early stages, the patient may experience pain on weight bearing during gait or at the end of the day after a lot of activity. The pain

may be in the groin but is often experienced in the L-3 dermatome along the anterior thigh and knee.

(2) With further degeneration, functional activities become difficult (such as climbing stairs, dressing, squatting) and a compensated gluteus medius gait (abductor limp) develops, which requires the use of an assistive device.

(3) Limitation of hip extension often leads to backache because attempted extension will rotate the pelvis anteriorly and cause excessive hyperextension of the lumbar spine. In addition, limited hip extension may prevent the knee from extending completely during gait.

(4) The mechanoreceptor system may be affected with capsular tissue changes so that equilibrium and balance are impaired.[21]

b. Other forms of joint dysfunction such as RA and aseptic necrosis may occur and are treated according to the signs and symptoms they present.

2. Management of joint lesions

See section VIII of Chapter 6 for general principles and plan of care in the treatment of osteoarthritis as well as the other information in Chapter 6 on general management of joints during acute, subacute, and chronic stages of tissue repair. Restoration of faulty mechanics is an integral part of decreasing pain in the hip, since faulty use of the joint in standing and walking provokes symptoms. In the hip, faulty mechanics may be caused by conditions such as obesity, differences in leg length, muscle imbalance, tight joint capsule, and poor posture.

a. **Procedures to decrease effects of stiffness (maintain available motion)**

(1) Instruct the patient in the importance of moving his hips through their ROM every day. This should be done actively if the patient can control the motion, or with assistance if necessary.

(2) Apply Grade I or II joint-play techniques (sustained or oscillation) in a pain-free position.

b. **Procedures to decrease the pain by decreasing mechanical stress**

(1) Use of assistive devices for ambulation helps reduce stress on the hip joint. If the pain is asymmetric, the patient is taught to walk with a cane or crutch on the side opposite the painful joint.

(2) If a short leg creates asymmetry, gradually elevate the extremity with lifts in the shoe.

(3) Evaluate for muscle-length imbalances and develop an appropriate flexibility program if indicated. (See section B.)

(4) Increase strength in supporting muscles. Begin with isometric resistance; progress to isotonic resistance as the patient tolerates movement.

c. **Procedures to increase the range of motion**

(1) Joint mobilization procedures; use sustained Grade III techniques.

(a) To distract the weight-bearing surface, use long-axis traction (see Figure 5-45)

(b) To increase flexion and internal rotation, apply a posterior glide to the femoral head (see Figure 5-46)

(c) To increase extension and external rotation, apply an anterior glide to the femoral head (see Figure 5-47)

(2) Active inhibition techniques to tight muscles (see Chapter 4).
(3) Self-stretching procedures (see section B below)
(4) Self-mobilization
    (a) Distraction of the weight-bearing surface
        Fixate a strap around the patient's ankle or over his foot. Place the other end of the strap under a box or movable step; the remaining strap length should be (approximately) the same height as the step. The patient then places his opposite foot on the step. When in position, he extends the hip and knee on the step until the strap tightens. The fixated strap will pull the lower extremity, and thus, glide the femur caudally (Figure 10-1).
    (b) Posterior glide of the femoral head
        The patient sits in a chair and arches (extends) his low back to stabilize the spine. He then grasps the front of the chair seat and pulls himself forward, keeping his back arched so the motion occurs only at his hips.
d. **Procedures to decrease pain at rest**
    (1) Grade I or II oscillation techniques with the joint in the resting position
    (2) Rock in a rocking chair (provides gentle oscillations to the lower extremity joints as well as stimulates the mechanoreceptors in the joints).[44]

B. Muscle Strength or Flexibility Imbalance

Note: No matter what the cause, muscle strength or flexibility imbalance in the hip can lead to poor lumbopelvic mechanics as well as poor hip mechanics, which predisposes the patient to or perpetuates low back, sacroiliac, or hip pain. See Chapters 14 and 15 for discussion and treatment of poor posture and low back pain. Poor hip mechanics can also affect the knee and ankle in weight-bearing activities, thus causing stress to these joints.

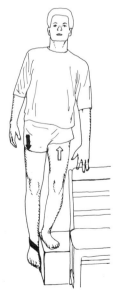

FIGURE 10-1. Self-mobilizing technique for long-axis traction. The weight-bearing surface of the hip joint is distracted as the patient stands up on a step and the strap pulls on the lower extremity.

1. **Techniques for self-stretching of tight muscles**

   Flexibility or self-stretching exercises, chosen according to the degree of limitation and ability of the patient to participate, can be valuable to reinforce therapeutic measures done by the therapist. Active inhibition and passive stretching techniques are described in Chapter 4. Not all of the following exercises are appropriate for every patient; the therapist should choose the exercise and intensity appropriate for the level of patient function, and progress them when indicated. Whenever the patient is able to contract the muscle opposite the tight muscle, there are the added benefits of reciprocal inhibition of the tight muscles as well as training the agonist to function for effective control in the gained range of motion.

   a. **To stretch tight hip flexor muscles and soft tissue anterior to the hip**

      (1) Position of patient: prone. The patient presses his thorax upward, allowing the pelvis to sag (see Figure 14-16A).

      Precaution: This exercise also stretches the lumbar spine into extension; if it causes pain to radiate down the patient's leg, rather than just a stretch sensation in the anterior trunk, hip and thigh, it must not be done.

      (2) Position of patient: supine. He flexes the hip and knee opposite the tight muscle, clasps his hands around the thigh, and holds it against his chest thus stabilizing the pelvis. The extremity with the tight hip flexor muscles is placed in hip and knee flexion and is slowly lowered toward the table in a controlled manner. The thigh should not be allowed to rotate outward or abduct. The patient attempts to relax the tight muscles at the end of the available range and allow the weight of the leg to cause a pulling sensation in the anterior hip region.

      (3) To progress the range as well as include stretching of the two-joint hip flexor muscles (rectus femoris and tensor fascia lata), the patient is positioned with the hips at the end of the treatment table. The tight hip can then extend beyond neutral and the knee can flex. The contract-relax technique is added by applying resistance to the distal femur as the patient attempts to flex the hip. Following relaxation, the hip is moved into greater extension as allowed (see Figure 4-8).

      The patient can attempt to further extend his hip by contracting the extensor muscles against the resistance of his own tissues, against manual resistance from the therapist, or against mechanical resistance from a pulley system.

      (4) Position of patient: standing. The patient assumes a fencer's squatlike posture, with the back leg in the same plane as the front leg and the foot pointing forward. As the patient shifts his body weight on the anterior leg, he should feel a stretch sensation in the anterior hip region of the back leg (Figure 10-2). If the heel of the back foot is kept on the floor, this exercise may also stretch the gastrocnemius muscle.

   b. **To isolate stretch to the rectus femoris muscle**

      (1) Position of patient: prone, with the knee flexed on the side to be stretched. The patient grabs the ankle on that side and pulls the hip into extension as he flexes the knee until the stretch is felt in the anterior thigh. The patient may also place a strap around the ankle

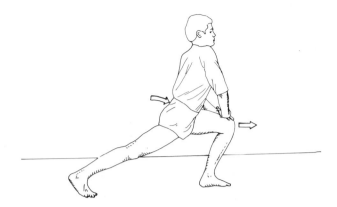

FIGURE 10-2. Self-stretching of hip flexor muscles and soft tissue anterior to the hip, using a modified fencer's squat posture.

and pull on the strap to flex the knee. Do not let the hip abduct or laterally rotate or let the spine hyperextend.

(2) Position of patient: sitting on the floor, with one lower extremity forward and the one to be stretched abducted as far as possible with the knee flexed. The patient extends the hip on that side by leaning down onto the opposite elbow and rolling the trunk back until a pull is felt proximally in the anterior thigh (Figure 10-3).

Precaution: If done incorrectly, this exercise places significant stress on the medial supporting structures of the knee and therefore should be monitored carefully if a patient has instability or pain.

c. **To stretch tight gluteus maximus muscles and soft tissue posterior to the hip**

(1) Position of patient: supine. He brings both his knees toward his chest and grasps the thighs firmly. He flexes his hips until he feels the stretch sensation in his posterior hip, then holds the position. (If he flexes further, he would begin flexing the lumbar spine.) The therapist should monitor this exercise to influence where the stretch is applied.

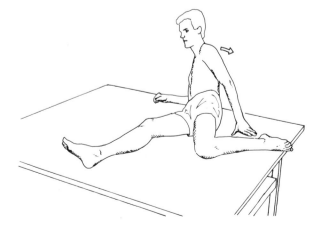

FIGURE 10-3. Rectus femoris self-stretch. The leg to be stretched is abducted as far as possible with the knee flexed. The hip is then extended by leaning down onto the opposite elbow and rolling the trunk back. A pull should be felt in the anterior thigh, not medial to the knee.

(2) Position of patient: supine. He brings one knee to his chest and grasps the thigh firmly. This isolates the stretch force to the hip being flexed. To progress this stretch, pull the knee toward the opposite shoulder.

(3) Position of patient: on hands and knees (all 4's position). He rocks his pelvis into an anterior tilt, causing lumbar extension, then maintains lumbar extension, while shifting his buttocks back in an attempt to sit on his heels. The hands remain forward. It is important not to let the lumbar spine flex while holding the stretch position (Figure 10-4 A and B).

d. **To stretch the hamstring muscle group**

(1) Position of patient: supine, with one leg brought into hip flexion with knee extension (straight leg-raising: SLR). If the patient can do this actively, the therapist then adds a stretch force, using the contract-relax technique, or resists the SLR through the entire range of motion.

(2) Position of patient: supine, on the floor with one leg through a doorway and the other leg (the one to be stretched) propped up against

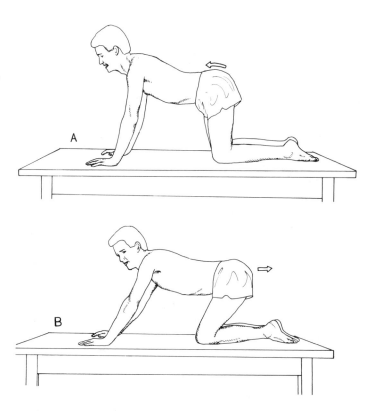

FIGURE 10-4. Gluteus maximus self-stretch with lumbar spine stabilization. (A) The patient on all 4's rocks into an anterior pelvic tilt causing lumbar extension. (B) While maintaining the lumbar extension, he shifts his buttock back attempting to sit on his heels. When lordosis can no longer be maintained, the end range of hip flexion is reached and held for the stretch.

the door frame. The knee should be kept extended. To increase the stretch, move the buttock closer to the door frame, keeping the knee extended (Figure 10-5A). The patient can be taught to do the contract-relax technique by forcing the heel of the leg being stretched against the door frame, causing an isometric contraction, relaxing it, then lifting the leg away from the frame (Figure 10-5B).

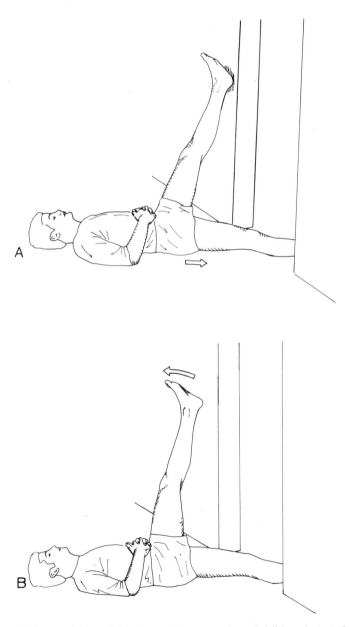

FIGURE 10-5. Self-stretching of the hamstring muscles. Additional stretch can occur if the person either moves the buttock closer to the door frame (A) or lifts the leg away from the door frame (B).

For an effective stretch, the pelvis and opposite leg must remain on the floor with the knee extended.

(3) Position of patient: sitting, with the leg to be stretched extended across to another chair, or sitting at the edge of a treatment table, with the leg to be stretched extended along the treatment table and the opposite foot on the floor. The patient leans his trunk forward toward his thigh, keeping his back extended, so that there is motion only at the hip joint (Figure 10-6).

(4) Position of patient: supine, with both hips flexed 90 degrees, knees extended, and legs and buttocks against the wall. He alternately flexes each leg away from the wall.

(5) Bilateral toe-touching exercises are often used to stretch the hamstring muscles. The therapist must recognize that having the patient reach for his toes does not selectively stretch the hamstrings but stretches the low- and midback as well. Toe-touching is considered a general flexibility exercise and tends to mask tightness in one region and overstretch areas already flexible. Whether a person can touch his toes depends on many factors such as body type, arm, trunk, and leg length, flexibility in thoracic and lumbar regions, as well as hamstring and gastrocnemius length.[27]

e. **To stretch tight hip adductor and internal rotator muscles**

(1) Position of patient: sitting, with soles of feet together and hands on the inner surface of his knees. He pushes his knees down toward the floor with a sustained stretch. The amount of stretch can be increased by pulling the feet closer to the trunk.
Alternate position: supine with soles of feet together. He lets his knees fall outward toward the floor, with the force of gravity applying the stretch force at the end of the available range.

(2) Position of patient: supine, with both hips flexed 90 degrees, knees extended, and legs and buttocks against the wall. The hips are abducted bilaterally as far as possible (Figure 10-7).

(3) Patient in fencer's squatlike position, with the hind leg externally rotated. As the patient shifts his weight on the front leg, he should feel a stretch along the medial thigh in the hind leg.

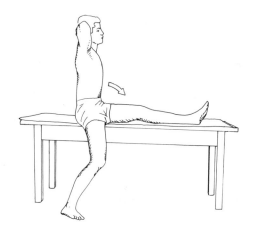

FIGURE 10-6. Self-stretching of the hamstring muscles by leaning the trunk towards the extended knee, flexing at the hips.

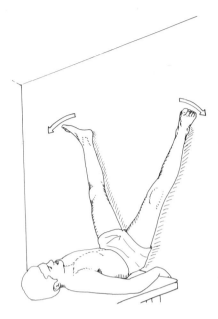

FIGURE 10-7. Self-stretching of the adductor muscles with the hips at 90 degrees of flexion.

   f. **To stretch tight iliotibial band and tensor fasciae latae**
     (1) Position of patient: standing on the normal extremity, with the tight extremity crossed behind. Keeping both feet on the floor, he side bends away from the tight side, shifting the pelvis toward the tight side, allowing his normal knee to bend slightly. To place additional stretch on the tensor fasciae latae, position the extremity in external rotation as it is placed behind the normal extremity (Figure 10-8).
     (2) Position of patient: side lying, with the leg to be stretched uppermost; the bottom leg is flexed for support. The top leg is abducted and aligned in the plane of the body in extension. While maintaining this position, the patient externally rotates the hip and then gradually lowers (adducts) his thigh to the point of stretch. If the extended and externally rotated position is not maintained, the iliotibial tract will slip in front of the greater trochanter and there will not be an effective stretch. Additional stretch can be obtained by having the knee flexed during this activity (Figure 10-9).

2. Techniques to strengthen weak muscles

Begin at the functional level for each muscle group. A muscle that has not been properly used or has been stretched due to antagonistic muscle tightness will require training by making the patient aware of it contracting in its new range as the antagonist is lengthened. On a manual muscle test, the patient may have good isometric strength, yet coordination and timing of muscle contractions may not be satisfactory as a result of faulty posture, poor gait habits, pain, improper lower extremity usage, or other problems. As a muscle is strengthened, it should be exercised as closely as possible in a manner similar to its intended functional use. For gait, the hip functions in both an open and closed kinematic chain and so should be exer-

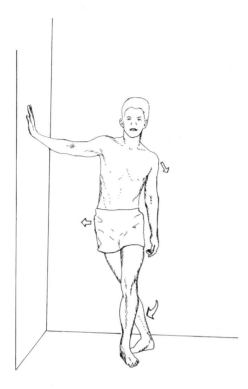

FIGURE 10-8. Self-stretching of the tensor fascia lata and iliotibial band occurs as the trunk bends away from and the pelvis shifts towards the tight side. Increased stretch occurs when the extremity is positioned in external rotation prior to the stretch.

cised, if possible, with the extremity free as well as with the extremity fixed. Manual and mechanical resistance exercise techniques are described in Chapter 3.

a. **To train and strengthen the hip abductor (gluteus medius) and hip hiker (quadratus lumborum) muscles**
   (1) Position of patient: standing, with one leg on a 2- to 4-inch block. Have him alternately lower and elevate the pelvis on the side of the unsupported leg (Figure 10-10).
   (2) Position of patient: standing. He abducts one leg, then the other. The motion should be only in the hips; there should be no side bending of the trunk. Adding ankle weights provides additional resistance.
   (3) Position of patient: sidelying, with the bottom leg flexed for balance. Have him abduct the top leg, keeping the hip neutral to rotation and in slight extension. Do not allow the hip to flex or the trunk to roll backward. If this is too difficult, begin with the patient supine and have him concentrate on isolated hip abduction movements while keeping the trunk still. Adding ankle weights in the side-lying position provides resistance as the patient progresses in strength.

b. **To train and strengthen the hip extensor (gluteus maximus) muscle**
   (1) Position of patient: prone or supine. He is first taught gluteal setting exercises to increase awareness of the contracting muscle.
   (2) Position of patient: prone. He extends the hip by lifting one leg several inches off the mat. Resistance can be added with ankle weights.

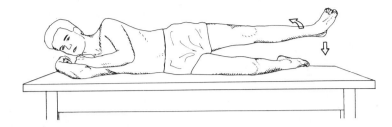

FIGURE 10-9. Tensor fascia lata and iliotibial band self-stretching; side lying. The leg is abducted in the plane of the body, and the hip is externally rotated then slowly lowered. Additional stretch can occur by flexing the knee.

(3) Patient stands at the edge of the treatment table then flexes his trunk over on to the table with his hips at the edge. He alternately extends one hip then the other. This is done with the knee flexed to train the gluteus maximus while relaxing the hamstrings. If the hamstrings cramp from active insufficiency, the patient is attempting to use them and should practice relaxing them before progressing with this exercise. Progress by adding weights or elastic resistance to the distal thigh.

(4) Position of patient: on hands and knees in an all-4's position. He then alternately extends his hips keeping the knee flexed. Care is taken not to attempt extension beyond the available range in the hip causing stress in the sacroiliac joint or lumbar spine (Figure 10-11).

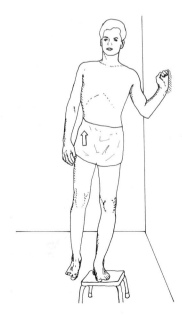

FIGURE 10-10. Training the hip abductor and hiker muscles.

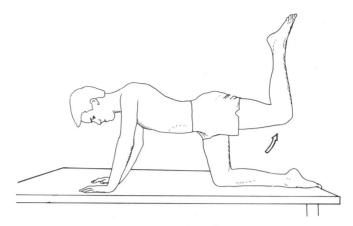

FIGURE 10-11. Isolated training and strengthening of the gluteus maximus. Starting in the all 4's position, the knee is flexed to rule out substitution by the hamstring muscles. Care is taken not to hyperextend the back causing stress to the sacroiliac or lumbar spinal joints.

(5) Position of patient: hook lying. Bridging exercises are done by having the patient press his upper back and feet into the mat and elevate his hips (Figure 10-12). Manual resistance can be applied against the pelvis, or mechanical resistance can be applied by strapping a weighted belt around the pelvis.

c. **To train and strengthen the external rotators of the hip**

(1) Position of patient: prone with knees bent and about 10 inches apart. He presses his heels together causing an isometric contraction of the external rotators.

(2) Position of patient: standing, with feet parallel, about 4 inches apart. Have him flex his knees slightly, then externally rotate his thighs (so that the knees are pointing laterally), keeping his feet stationary on the floor. He maintains the external rotation as he extends his knees, then relaxes the rotation slightly until the patellae point forward. This activity is useful when the patient has functional medial rotation of the femur.[14]

(3) Position of patient: sitting, with knees flexed over the edge of the treatment table, with an elasticized material around his ankle and the table leg on the same side. He moves his foot toward the opposite side, pulling against the resistance, causing external rotation at the hip.

d. **To train and strengthen the hip adductor muscles**

(1) Position of patient: side lying, with the bottom leg aligned in the plane of the trunk, the top leg is flexed forward with the foot on the floor, or with the thigh resting on a pillow. The patient lifts his bottom leg upward in adduction. Weights can be added to the ankle to progress strengthening (Figure 10-13A).

(2) Position of patient: side lying, with both legs aligned in the plane of the trunk. The patient holds his top leg in abduction and adducts the bottom leg up to meet it (Figure 10-13B).

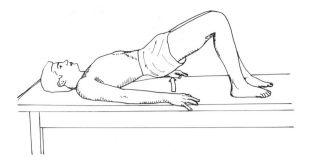

FIGURE 10-12. Training and strengthening the hip extensor muscles using bridging exercises. Resistance can be added against the pelvis.

C. Bursitis

1. Clinical picture of common lesions in the hip region

a. Trochanteric bursitis

Pain is experienced over the lateral hip and possibly down the lateral thigh to the knee when the iliotibial band rubs over the trochanter. Discomfort may be experienced after standing asymmetrically for long periods of time with the affected hip elevated and adducted and pelvis dropped on the opposite side. Ambulation and climbing stairs aggravates the condition.

b. Psoas bursitis

Pain is experienced in the groin or anterior thigh and possibly into the

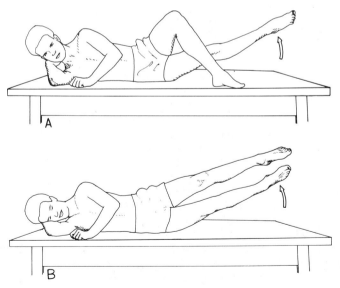

FIGURE 10-13. Training and strengthening the hip adductors. (*A*) The top leg is stabilized by flexing the hip and resting the foor on the mat while the bottom leg is adducted against gravity. (*B*) The top leg is isometrically held in abduction while the bottom leg is adducted against gravity.

patellar area. It is aggravated during activities requiring excessive hip flexion.

c. Ischiogluteal bursitis (tailor's or weaver's bottom)
Pain is experienced around the ischial tuberosities, especially when sitting. If the adjacent sciatic nerve is irritated from the swelling, symptoms of sciatica may occur.

2. Management

a. Rest the region during an acute flair by not stressing or putting pressure on the bursa.

b. When the pain diminishes, determine if there is a biomechanical cause that can be altered, such as stretching the gluteus maximus, iliotibial tract, or the hip flexor muscles, or changing faulty postural habits.

c. Educate the patient as to the cause of the irritation and correct the faulty activity patterns to avoid recurrences.

D. Referred Pain

1. Common sources referring pain into the hip region include

a. nerve roots and tissues derived from spinal segments L1-, L-2, L-3, and S-1 and S-2.

b. lumbar vertebral joints

c. sacroiliac joints

2. Treatment of the source of irritation is necessary to relieve the pain.

Therapeutic exercise to the hip region is beneficial only in preventing disuse of the part that feels painful to the patient; primary treatment must be directed to the source of the irritation.

III. THERAPEUTIC EXERCISE MANAGEMENT OF COMMON SURGICAL PROCEDURES FOR THE HIP

Fractures, dislocations, and chronic arthritis of the hip often require surgical treatment. Therapists are involved in the postoperative management of many patients after open reduction and internal fixation of a hip fracture or after total or partial replacement of the hip joint. Therefore, it is important to have a basic understanding of common surgical procedures for the hip and the postoperative management of these patients.

In order to achieve normal hip function postoperatively, the following goals must be met:

1. A pain-free hip.
2. A stable extremity for weight bearing.
3. Adequate range of motion and strength of the hip for functional activities.

An appropriate postoperative exercise plan can help achieve these goals.

A. Open Reduction and Internal Fixation of Hip Fractures

One of the more common orthopedic problems that occurs in the elderly is fracture of the hip or, more correctly, fracture of the very proximal portion of the femur. Osteoporosis, a condition associated with aging, weakens bone. A sudden twisting motion can cause a fracture in bone that is osteoporotic. The neck of the femur is very susceptible to osteoporosis. An elderly person may fall and break the hip, but in many patients the fall may occur as the result of a hip fracture.

The signs of hip fracture are pain in the groin or hip region with passive or active motion or weight bearing, and shortening and external rotation of the involved extremity.

In most cases reduction of the fracture and internal fixation to stabilize the fracture site is indicated. Only patients who are very poor surgical risks will be treated with external immobilization (traction or cast) and confined to bed or a wheelchair for an extended period of time.

1. Indications for surgery[24,26,43]

a. Intertrochanteric fracture (extracapsular)
b. Subcapital femoral neck fracture (intracapsular)
c. Subtrochanteric fracture
d. Fracture of the proximal femur

2. Procedures[3,26]

a. A variety of internal fixation devices can be used to reduce and stabilize many different types of hip fractures. The type and severity of the fracture and the age and physical abilities of the patient are all considered by the surgeon.
b. Internal fixation devices are chosen for their maximum stabilization of the fracture site.
   (1) multiple pins.
   (2) screws.
   (3) nail-plate fixation.
c. Prosthetic replacement is indicated for subcapital fractures where the vascular supply to the head of the femur is disturbed.

3. Postoperative management[5,23,24,26,38,43]

a. The primary goal of postoperative care is to get the patient up and moving as quickly as possible. Internal fixation of the fracture site allows early movement and weight bearing on the involved extremity, which minimizes the complications of bed rest, edema, muscle atrophy, soft-tissue contractures, and osteoporosis.
b. With most forms of internal fixation, there is no need for external immobilization (i.e., a cast). If stabilization of the fracture site can only be achieved with external immobilization, a hip spica cast will have to be worn for 8 to 12 weeks, and the patient will have to avoid weight bearing on the involved leg. It is important for these patients that limited ambulation with a walker, independence in transfers, and wheelchair mobility all are a part of their plan of care.
c. After internal fixation of a hip fracture, the following activities should be initiated:
   (1) active assisted and active ROM of the involved hip to maintain mobility and prevent contractures. Continuous passive motion (CPM) may also be used in the early postoperative period.
   (2) muscle-setting exercises (gluteal and quadriceps setting) and neuromuscular electrical stimulation to minimize muscle atrophy.
   (3) active ankle exercises to maintain circulation and to decrease the possibility of thromboembolitic disease.
   (4) resisted knee flexion and extension and possibly light manual resistance exercises to the involved hip to maintain strength postoperatively.

Note: There is lack of agreement whether or not light resistance exercise (2 to 3 lb of resistance) for the involved hip should be done before the fracture site has healed. (Bony healing may take 4 to 6 months.) Some therapists and surgeons believe that resistance to hip musculature may put undesirable stress on the internal fixation and jeopardize the stability of the fracture site. Others believe that light manual resistance will minimize postoperative weakness without undue stress at the fracture site. Close communication between the therapist and surgeon is necessary before resistance to the involved hip is added to a postoperative exercise program.

    (5) early protected weight bearing and ambulation with a walker or crutches whenever the internal fixation device adequately stabilizes the fracture site to prevent complications associated with long-term bed rest.

    (6) active resistive exercises, emphasizing strengthening of the uninvolved lower extremity and the scapular depressors and triceps, to enhance gait training and ADL.

B. Total Hip Replacement

1. Indications for surgery[7,11,15,19,31,37]

  a. Severe hip pain with motion and weight bearing because of rheumatoid or traumatic arthritis, osteoarthritis, ankylosing spondylitis, or aseptic necrosis

  b. Marked limitation of hip motion

  c. Instability or deformity of the hip

  d. Failure of previous hip surgery (femoral stem hemiarthroplasty or resurfacing arthroplasty)

  e. A hemireplacement of the hip may be done for fractures of the neck of the femur

2. Procedures

  a. General background

    (1) Total hip replacements have been performed since the early 1960s. Charnley[11] and McKee,[31] surgeons from England, are credited with the early research. Earlier procedures, such as the Smith-Petersen cup arthroplasty,[16,20] required long postoperative periods of rehabilitation. Successful methods of prosthetic fixation such as the use of methyl methacrylate cement or cementless procedures using bioingrowth fixation have dramatically improved arthroplasty of the hip.

    (2) There are a variety of designs of total hip replacement components that have been developed since the early 1960s. Early designs included the Charnley,[11] the McKee-Ferrar,[31] and the Charnley-Mueller[34] replacements. Today all designs are made up of an inert metal (cobalt-chrome alloy, stainless steel) femoral stem and a high-density polyethylene acetabular replacement. In the 1960s and 1970s, the prosthetic components were cemented in place with an acrylic cement, methyl methacrylate. This revolutionized joint replacement surgery, because the use of cement allowed very early weight bearing and shortened the patient's period of rehabilitation.

        The main postoperative complication after total hip arthroplasty has been loosening of the prosthetic components, which leads to recurrent hip pain and the need for surgical revision. The patients in which loosening is a significant problem are those who are young and physically active. Loosening has not been a particular problem in elderly patients or in young patients with multiple joint involvement who tend to limit their physical activities.[17,18,30,33]

The long-term problem of loosening of the cemented prostheses at the bone-cement interface has given rise to the development of porous-coated total hip replacements. The porous-coated surfaces (beaded or wire mesh) of the femoral and acetabular components allow ingrowth of bone into the prostheses for fixation. This is sometimes called biologic fixation. Weight bearing is more restricted over a longer period of time postoperatively with bioingrowth fixation than with cemented total hip arthroplasty, but it is anticipated that there will be a lower incidence of future loosening and less need for revision of the arthroplasty.[17,18,22,33]

b. Overview of procedures[7,11,32,34,37]
   (1) A lateral, posterolateral, or anterolateral incision is made along the affected hip.
   (2) The head of the femur is removed and replaced with an intramedullary femoral stem prosthesis.
   (3) The acetabulum is remodeled and replaced with a high-density polyethylene cup.
   (4) The greater trochanter may or may not be removed. If a trochanteric osteotomy is performed, the greater trochanter is often repositioned and then reattached (wired in place) in a more distal position. This is done to improve the function of the gluteus medius, which stabilizes the pelvis during weight bearing.

3. Preoperative instruction[4,6,8,9,15,19]

If possible, preoperative contact should be made with the patient to
a. Evaluate the patient.
b. Begin gait training with assistive devices to be used after surgery in order to prevent pulmonary complications.
c. Teach basic precautions for early bed mobility so the patient will avoid excessive flexion and adduction of the operated hip postoperatively.
d. Teach deep breathing and coughing exercises to be started directly after surgery in order to prevent pulmonary complications.
e. Teach ankle pumping exercises to decrease the risk of thrombophlebitis.

4. Postoperative management[6,8,9,12,19,25,39]

a. During the first 2 to 4 days after surgery, the patient remains in bed. The operated extremity is held in slight flexion, abduction, and neutral rotation. This may be done with an abduction pillow or splint, or the patient may be placed in a balanced sling suspension, with the thigh and calf supported.
b. If the patient is in a sling-pulley system, exercise during the first 2 to 4 postoperative days consists of
   (1) Active-assistive flexion and extension of the hip with the thigh supported in a sling. An overhead pulley system, attached to the sling, is used by the patient during exercise. The patient can then flex the hip through a limited range, usually only to 45 degrees.
   (2) Active knee flexion and extension while in the suspension sling.

      (3) Bilateral ankle pumping exercise to decrease the possibility of thrombophlebitis and pulmonary embolism.

      (4) Active, active-assistive, or mild resistive exercise to other joints in the body, particularly if the patient has multiple joints affected by arthritis.

  c. If the patient is using an abduction splint or pillow, rather than a sling-pulley system, exercises in the first 2 to 4 days are done in bed and include

      (1) Muscle-setting exercises to the hip and knee extensors: gluteal setting and quadriceps setting.

      (2) Active-assistive hip flexion to 45 degrees and hip extension to neutral with assistance by the therapist.

      (3) Ankle pumping exercises.

      (4) Exercise to unoperated joints and extremities.

  d. When the patient is allowed out of bed, usually by the third to fifth postoperative day, the following activities are begun.

      (1) Short periods of sitting at the edge of the bed with the hips in no more than 45 degrees of flexion and the legs abducted.

      (2) Gait training with crutches or a walker or in the parallel bars with the patient partially weight bearing on the operated hip.

      Note: If the prosthetic components have been cemented in place and no trochanteric osteotomy has been done, full weight bearing on the operated side can be achieved very early. If a trochanteric osteotomy has been done, weight bearing will be partially limited for at least 6 weeks postoperatively. If a cementless arthroplasty has been performed, the patient will be restricted to a touch-down (minimal weight-bearing) gait with crutches or a walker for approximately 1 month. Full weight bearing may not be possible for 3 months. Bioingrowth fixation requires the use of assistive devices during ambulation for a longer period of time than cemented arthroplasty.[22,23]

      (3) Transfer activities to chairs, toilet, and so forth. Be sure the patient avoids hip adduction beyond neutral or hip flexion beyond 45 degrees.

  e. Exercises include

      (1) Active and active-assistive hip flexion and extension exercises.

      (2) Active hip abduction exercises, done in a gravity eliminated position (supine) with therapist assistance, on a powder board or on a skateboard.

      Note: Patients with a trochanteric osteotomy must avoid antigravity abduction for at least 6 weeks, to allow time for bony healing.

  f. Ambulation with assistive devices and exercises are continued to the time of discharge, usually 2 to 3 weeks postoperatively. The patient may continue to walk with crutches for as long as 6 to 12 weeks and then may progress to a cane.

5. Precautions

In the early postoperative days, the patient must avoid full ROM of the operated hip. The hip joint will be unstable, and the patient will be at risk for dislocation or subluxation of the prosthetic hip until soft tissues around the joint have healed.[22,41]

  a. If a posterior or posterolateral incision has been done, excessive hip flexion and adduction can cause subluxation or dislocation of the prosthesis. During the first few weeks, avoid hip flexion beyond 45 degrees and hip adduction across the midline.

    (1) Have the patient avoid sitting in low soft chairs and suggest that he use a raised toilet seat.[32]

    (2) Do not allow the patient to excessively bend the trunk over the operated hip when rising from a chair. This will cause excessive flexion of the hip.

    (3) Do not allow the patient to cross his legs.

    (4) Suggest to the patient that he sleep with an abduction pillow for at least 8 to 12 weeks postoperatively.

    (5) A stationary bicycle can be used for general conditioning and endurance exercises, if the seat of the bicycle is raised.

  b. Excessive hip rotation must also be limited after surgery.

    (1) If an anterolateral incision has been made, avoid excessive external rotation.

    (2) If a posterolateral incision has been made, avoid excessive internal rotation.

  c. Patients with an anterior or anterolateral incision should avoid hyperextension of the operated hip.

C. Hemireplacement of the Hip

1. Indications for surgery[3,37]

  a. Subcapital fractures of the femur in the elderly.

  b. Pain, deformity, and instability of the hip associated with the fracture or disease.

2. Procedure[3,37,43]

  a. Replacement of the head of the femur after femoral neck fracture.

    (1) The head of the femur is removed and replaced with a metal intramedullary stemmed prosthesis.

    (2) The prosthesis is held in place with acrylic cement as with many total hip replacements.

  b. This procedure has replaced the Austin-Moore procedure commonly used in the 1950s and early 1960s to treat subcapital fractures of the femur in elderly patients.

  c. Since some young, active patients are candidates for hemireplacement arthroplasty, a new bipolar prosthesis with a polyethylene covering over the metal femoral head has been developed. The polyethylene covering is designed to minimize wear and tear of the patient's acetabulum from the metal femoral head.[37]

3. Postoperative management

  a. Early ambulation with partial weight bearing on the operated extremity.

  b. Active and active-assistive exercises to the operated lower extremity as early as possible (see Section III B in this chapter).

D. Resurfacing Arthroplasty of the Hip

1. Indications for surgery[16,20,37]

  a. This procedure is rarely done today because of the advent of the total hip replacement.

  b. It may be a conservative surgical alternative to total hip replacement for the very young patient with severe pain and immobility of the hip because of chronic juvenile rheumatoid arthritis or degenerative joint disease secondary to aseptic necrosis of the head of the femur.

2. Procedure[19,20,37]

a. A resurfacing (interpositional) arthroplasty involves resurfacing one or both joint surfaces with minimal loss of bone stock.

b. The cup arthroplasty (Smith-Peterson) was developed in the 1930s and involved smoothing the head of the femur and covering it with a metallic cup. The acetabulum was also shaped to fit the cup. The main problems with this procedure were the necessity for a long rehabilitation period, and after a period of time, the bone beneath the cup deteriorated, causing recurrence of hip pain.

c. Recently, a double-cup resurfacing system has also been developed.[1,2] This is sometimes referred to as the THARIES procedure (total hip articular replacement by internal eccentric shells). The components are cemented in place, allowing more rapid rehabilitation.

3. Postoperative management[16,19,37]

a. Active exercises, similar to those done after a total hip arthroplasty without trochanteric osteotomy, must be carried out daily to maintain flexibility and strength of the operated lower extremity (see Section III B in this chapter).

b. Cement fixation of the resurfacing arthroplasty permits early weight bearing.

IV. SUMMARY

The anatomy and kinesiology of hip structure and function, as well as the functional relationships between hip motion and pelvic motion, were reviewed. The action of the hip during gait, including hip motion and muscular control, and the role of the hip in relation to balance and coordination were also discussed.

Guidelines for therapeutic exercise management of common musculoskeletal problems, such as joint and muscle lesions, and common surgical procedures, such as hip pinnings and hip replacements, were outlined. Specific descriptions of self-stretching techniques and strengthening procedures for the hip were described and illustrated in this chapter.

REFERENCES

1. Amstutz, HC, et al: *Total hip articular replacement with internal eccentric shells.* Clin Orthop 128:261, 1977.
2. Amstutz, HC: *Surface replacement of the hip.* In Riley, LH (ed): *The Hip.* Proceedings of the Hip Society, 1980, CV Mosby, St Louis, 1980.
3. Apley, AG: *System of Orthopedics and Fractures,* ed 5. Butterworth, London, 1977.
4. Ball, PB, Wroe, MC, and MacLeod, L: *Survey of physical therapy preoperative care in total hip replacement.* Phys Ther Health Care 1:83, 1986.
5. Barnes, B: *Ambulation outcomes after hip fracture.* Phys Ther 64:317, 1984.
6. Beber, C and Convery, R: *Management of patients with total hip replacement.* Phys Ther 52:823, 1972.
7. Benke, GJ: *Joint replacement.* In Downie, PA (ed): *Cash's Textbook of Orthopedics and Rheumatology for Physiotherapists.* JB Lippincott, Philadelphia, 1984.
8. Bentley, JA: *Physiotherapy following joint replacement, etc.* In Downie, PA: *Cash's Textbook of Orthopedics and Rheumatology for Physiotherapists.* JB Lippincott, Philadelphia, 1984.

9. Burton, D and Imrie, S: *Total hip arthroplasty and postoperative rehabilitation.* Phys Ther 53:132, 1973.
10. Cailliet, R: *Low Back Pain Syndrome,* ed 3. FA Davis, Philadelphia, 1981.
11. Charnley, J: *Total hip replacement by low friction arthroplasty.* Clin Orthop 72:721, 1974.
12. Cullen, S: *Physical therapy program for patients with total hip replacement.* Phys Ther 53:1293, 1973.
13. Cyriax, J: *Textbook of Orthopaedic Medicine, Volume One. Diagnosis of Soft Tissue Lesions,* ed 8. Bailliere Tindall, London, 1982.
14. Daniels, L and Worthingham, C: *Therapeutic Exercise for Body Alignment and Function,* ed 2. WB Saunders, Philadelphia, 1977.
15. Eftekhar, N: *Preoperative management of total hip replacement.* Orthop Rev 3:17, 1974.
16. Egil, H: *Exercise routine for patients with cup arthroplasty.* Phys Ther 37:447, 1957.
17. Engh, CA: *Bone ingrowth into porous coated canine acetabular replacements: The affect of pore size, apposition and dislocation.* Hip 13:214, 1985.
18. Engh, CA, Bobyn, JD, and Matthews, JCH: *Biological fixation of a modified Moore prosthesis.* In *Hip Society: The Hip. Proceedings of the Twelfth Open Scientific Meeting of the Hip Society.* CV Mosby, St Louis, 1984.
19. Fortune, W: *Lower limb joint replacement.* In Nickel, VL (ed): *Orthopedic Rehabilitation.* Churchill-Livingstone, New York, 1982.
20. Friedebold, G: *The Smith-Petersen cup arthroplasty: An analysis of fractures.* In Chapchal, G: *Arthroplasty of the Hip.* Georg Thieme, Stuttgart, 1973.
21. Grieve, G: *Manual Mobilizing Techniques in Degenerative Arthrosis of the Hip.* Bulletin of the Orthopaedic Section, American Physical Therapy Association, 2:7, 1977.
22. Harris, WH: *The porous total hip replacement system.* In Harris, WH (ed): *Advanced Concepts in Total Hip Replacement.* Slack Publishing, Thorofare, NJ, 1985.
23. Hielema, F and Summerfore, R: *Physical therapy for patients with hip fracture or joint replacement.* Phys Ther Health Care 1:89, 1986.
24. Hielema, FJ: *Epidemiology of hip fracture.* Phys Ther 59:1221, 1979.
25. Hyde, SA: *Physiotherapy in Rheumatology.* Blackwell Scientific Publication, Oxford, 1980.
26. Iversen, LD and Clawson, DK: *Manual of Acute Orthopedic Therapeutics,* ed 2. Little, Brown & Company, Boston, 1982.
27. Kendall, F: *Criticism of current tests and exercises for physical fitness.* Phys Ther 45:187, 1965.
28. Kopell, H and Thompson, W: *Peripheral Entrapment Neuropathies,* ed 2. Robert E. Krieger, Huntington, NY, 1976.
29. Lehmkuhl, LD and Smith LM: *Brunnstrom's Clinical Kinesiology,* ed 4. FA Davis, Philadelphia, 1983.
30. Ling, RSM (ed): *Current Problems in Orthopedics: Complications of Total Hip Replacement.* Churchill-Livingstone, New York, 1984.
31. McKee, G: *Development of total prosthetic replacement of the hip.* Clin Orthop 72:85, 1970.
32. Melvin, J: *Rheumatic Disease: Occupational Therapy and Rehabilitation.* ed 2. FA Davis, Philadelphia, 1982.
33. Morrey, RF and Kavanagh, BF: *Cementless joint replacement: Current status and future.* Bull Rheum Dis 37:1, 1987.
34. Muller, WE: *Total hip prosthesis.* Clin Orthop 72:460, 1970.
35. Norkin, C and Levangie, P: *Joint Structure and Function: A Comprehensive Analysis.* FA Davis, Philadelphia, 1983.
36. *Normal and Pathological Gait Syllabus.* Physical Therapy Department, Rancho Los Amigos Hospital, Downey, California, 1977.
37. Nunley, JA and Oser, ER: *Surgical treatment of arthritis of the hip.* Phys Ther Health Care 1:59, 1986.
38. Patton, F: *Treament of hip fractures in the geriatric patient.* J Am Phys Ther Assoc 42:314, 1962.
39. Richardson, R: *Physical therapy management of patients undergoing total hip replacement.* Phys Ther 55:984, 1975.
40. Sahrmann, SA: *Diagnosis and treatment of muscle imbalances associated with musculoskeletal pain.* Lecture outline. Ohio State Chapter, APTA Conference, Columbus, 1988.

41. Schamerloh, C and Ritter, M: *Prevention of dislocation or subluxation of total hip replacements.* Phys Ther 57:1028, 1977.
42. Taylor, JR and Twomey, LT: *Age changes in lumbar zygapophyseal joint.* Spine 11(7):739, 1986.
43. Trombly, CA: *Occupational Therapy for Physical Dysfunction,* ed 2. Williams & Wilkins, Baltimore, 1983.
44. Wyke, B: *Neurological aspects of pain for the physical therapy clinician.* Physical Therapy Forum, 1982, Columbus, 1982.

CHAPTER ——————————— 11

The Knee

The knee joint is designed for mobility and stability; it functionally lengthens and shortens the lower extremity to raise and lower the body or to move the foot in space. Along with the hip and ankle, it supports the body when standing, and it is a primary functional unit in walking, climbing, and sitting activities.

Highlights of the anatomy and function of the knee complex are reviewed in the first section of this chapter. For further study the reader is referred to several texts and references.[4,8,35,40,47,52] In order to design a therapeutic exercise program for a patient's knee, the reader should be familiar with the principles of management presented in Chapter 6.

OBJECTIVES

After studying this chapter, the reader will be able to:
1. identify important aspects of the knee structure and function for review.
2. establish a therapeutic exercise program to manage soft-tissue and joint lesions in the knee region related to stages of recovery following an inflammatory insult to the tissues.
3. establish a therapeutic exercise program to manage common musculoskeletal lesions, recognizing unique circumstances in the knee and patella for their management.
4. establish a therapeutic exercise program to manage patients following common surgical procedures for the knee.

I. REVIEW OF THE STRUCTURE AND FUNCTION OF THE KNEE

A. Bony Parts Include the Distal Femur, Proximal Tibia, and Patella (see Figure 5-48).

B. Knee Joint Complex
The lax joint capsule encloses two articulations: the tibiofemoral and the pa-

tellofemoral joints. Recesses from the capsule form the suprapatellar, sub-popliteal, and gastrocnemius bursae. Folds or thickenings in the synovium persist from embryologic tissue in up to 60 percent of individuals, and may become symptomatic with micro or macro traumas.[5,37]

1. The tibiofemoral joint

a. Characteristics

The knee joint is a biaxial modified hinge joint with two interposed menisci, supported by ligaments and muscles. Anterior-posterior stability is provided by the posterior and anterior cruciate ligaments, respectively; medial-lateral stability is provided by the medial (tibial) and lateral (femoral) collateral ligaments, respectively.

b. The convex bony partner is composed of two asymmetric condyles on the distal end of the femur. The medial condyle is longer than the lateral, which contributes to the locking mechanism at the knee.

c. The concave bony partner is composed of two tibial plateaus on the proximal tibia with their respective fibrocartilaginous menisci. The medial plateau is larger than the lateral.

d. The menisci improve the congruency of the articulating surfaces. They are attached to the joint capsule by the coronary ligaments. The medial meniscus is firmly attached to the joint capsule as well as to the medial collateral ligament, anterior cruciate ligament, and the semimembranosus muscle; therefore, it is subject to injury when there is a lateral blow to the knee.

e. With motions of the tibia (open kinematic chain), the concave plateaus slide in the same direction as the bone motion.

Physiologic Motions of the Tibia	Direction of Slide of the Tibia
Flexion	Posterior
Extension	Anterior

f. With motions of the femur on a fixated tibia (closed kinematic chain), the convex condyles slide in the direction opposite to the bone motion.

g. Rotation occurs between the femoral condyles and the tibia during the final degrees of extension. This is called the locking, or screw-home, mechanism.

(1) When the tibia is free (open kinematic chain), terminal extension results in the tibia rotating externally on the femur. To unlock the knee, the tibia rotates internally.

(2) When the tibia is fixed with the foot on the ground (closed kinematic chain), terminal extension results in the femur rotating internally (the medial condyle slides further posteriorly than the lateral). Concurrently, the hip goes into extension. If a person lacks hip extension, knee locking cannot occur when the foot is fixed. As the knee is unlocked, the femur rotates laterally. Unlocking of the knee occurs indirectly with hip flexion and directly from action of the popliteus muscle.

2. The patellofemoral joint

a. Characteristics

The patella is a sesamoid bone in the quadriceps tendon. It articulates with the intercondylar (trochlear) groove on the anterior aspect of the distal portion of the femur. Its articulating surface is covered with smooth hyaline cartilage. The patella is embedded in the anterior portion of the joint capsule and is connected to the tibia by the ligamentum patellae. Many bursae surround the patella.

b. With flexion of the knee, the patella slides caudally along the intercondylar groove; with extension, it slides cranially. If patellar movement is restricted, it interferes with the range of knee flexion and may contribute to an extensor lag in active knee extension.[71]

C. Knee and Patellar Function

1. Patellar alignment

Normal alignment of the patella is defined as a 15-degree Q-angle. The Q-angle is the angle formed by two intersecting lines; one from the anterior superior iliac spine to the mid-patella; the other from the tibial tubercle through the mid-patella. The Q-angle describes the lateral tracking or bowstring effect that the quadriceps muscles and patellar tendon have on the patella.

a. Forces maintaining alignment
Lateral fixation of the patella is provided by the iliotibial band and lateral retinaculum; these are opposed by the active medial pull of the vastus medialis muscle. The patellar ligament fixates the patella inferiorly against the active pull of the quadriceps muscle superiorly.[56]

b. Factors leading to malalignment (increased Q-angle) of the patella as it tracks in the trochlear groove are those that increase the quadriceps bowstring effect such as wide pelvis, genu valgum, laterally placed tibial tubercle, patella alta, lax medial capsular retinaculum, inefficient vastus medialis muscle (high insertion on the patella or weakness or atrophy from disuse), and tight lateral capsular retinaculum.[56]

2. Patellar compression

Compression of the posterior aspect of the patella against the femur rises sharply after 30 degrees knee flexion. Near 30 degrees, it approximates body weight; it rises to greater than 3 times body weight during stair climbing and 8 times body weight during squatting and deep knee-bending activities.[52,56]

3. Extensor muscles

a. The quadriceps femoris muscle group is the only muscle crossing anterior to the axis of the knee and is the prime mover for knee extension. Other muscles that can act to extend the knee require the foot to be fixated, creating a closed kinematic chain. In this situation, the hamstrings and also soleus muscles can cause or control knee extension by pulling the tibia posteriorly.

b. During standing and the stance phase of gait, the knee is an intermediate joint in a closed kinematic chain. The quadriceps muscle controls the amount of flexion at the knee as well as causes knee extension through reverse muscle pull on the femur. In the erect posture, when the knee is locked, the quadriceps need not function when the gravity line falls anterior to the axis of motion (see Chapter 14). In this case, tension in the hamstring and gastrocnemius tendons supports the posterior capsule.

c. The patella improves the leverage of the extensor force by increasing the distance of the quadriceps tendon from the knee joint axis. Its greatest effect on the leverage of the quadriceps is during extension of the knee from 60 to 30 degrees.[52] A recent cadaver study reported the peak effective moment arm of the quadriceps is at 20 degrees, with the moment arm rapidly diminishing from 15 to 0 degrees of full extension.[25]

d. The peak torque of the quadriceps muscle occurs between 70 and 50 degrees.[7] The physiologic advantage of the quadriceps rapidly decreases during the last 15 degrees of knee extension due to its shortened length. This, combined with its decreased mechanical advantage in the last 15 degrees, requires the muscle to significantly increase its contractile force when large demands are placed on the joint during terminal extension.[25] During standing, assistance probably comes from the hamstrings and soleus muscles, as well as from the mechanical locking mechanism of the knee. During knee extension exercises in the sitting or supine position, when the resistive force is maximum in terminal extension due to the moment arm of the resistance, very strong contraction of the quadriceps muscle is required to overcome both the physiologic and mechanical disadvantages of the muscle to complete the final 15 degrees of motion.[25]

4. Flexor muscles

a. The hamstring muscles are the primary knee flexors and also influence rotation of the tibia on the femur. Because they are 2-joint muscles, they contract more efficiently when they are simultaneously lengthened over the hip (during hip flexion) as they flex the knee. In closed chain activities, the hamstring muscles can act to extend the knee by pulling on the tibia.

b. The gastrocnemius muscle can also function as a knee flexor, but its prime function at the knee on weight bearing is to support the posterior capsule against hyperextension forces.

c. The popliteus muscle supports the posterior capsule and acts to unlock the knee.

5. The knee and gait[52,53]

a. Range of motion of the knee during gait
   During the normal gait cycle, the knee goes through a range of 60 degrees (0 degrees extension at initial contact or heel strike, to 60 degrees at the end of initial swing). There is some medial rotation of the femur as the knee extends at initial contact and just prior to heel off.

b. Muscle control of the knee during gait
   (1) The quadriceps muscle controls the amount of knee flexion during initial contact (loading response), then extends the knee toward mid-stance. It again controls the amount of flexion during pre-swing (heel off to toe off), and prevents excessive heel rise during initial swing. With loss of quadriceps function, the patient lurches his trunk anteriorly during initial contact to move his center of gravity anterior to the knee so it is stable, or he rotates the extremity outward to lock the knee.[69] With fast walking, there may be excessive heel rise during initial swing.
   (2) The hamstring muscles primarily control the forward swinging leg

during terminal swing. Loss of function may result in the knee snapping into extension during this period. The hamstrings also provide posterior support to the knee capsule when the knee is extended during stance. Loss of function results in progressive genu recurvatum.[69]

(3) The uni-joint ankle plantarflexor muscles (primarily the soleus) help control the amount of knee flexion during pre-swing by controlling the forward movement of the tibia. Loss of function results in hyperextension of the knee during pre-swing (also loss of heel rise at the ankle and thus a lag or slight dropping of the pelvis on that side during the pre-swing phase).

(4) The gastrocnemius muscle provides tension posterior to the knee when it is in extension (end of loading response or foot flat, and just prior to pre-swing or heel off). Loss of function results in hyperextension of the knee during these periods (as well as loss of plantarflexion during pre-swing or push off).

c. Because the knee is the intermediate joint between the hip and foot, problems in these two areas will interfere with knee function during gait. Examples:

(1) Inability to extend the hip will prevent the knee from extending just before terminal stance (heel off).

(2) Most of the muscles functioning to control the hip are two-joint muscles and also cross the knee. With asymmetries in length and strength, imbalanced forces may stress various structures in the knee, giving rise to pain when walking or running (see Chapter 10).

(3) The position and function of the foot and ankle affect the stresses transmitted to the knee. For example, with pes planus or pes valgus there is medial rotation of the tibia and an increased bowstring effect on the patella, increasing the lateral tracking forces.

II. GUIDELINES AND THERAPEUTIC EXERCISE MANAGEMENT OF COMMON MUSCULOSKELETAL PROBLEMS IN THE KNEE

Note: Exercises applied to the knee during acute, subacute, and chronic phases of inflammation and healing follow the same principles as described in Chapter 6, taking into account the unique anatomic and kinesiologic relationships of the knee and patella. This section will expand on these guidelines for common knee problems.

A. Joint Problems and Capsule Restrictions of the Knee

1. Clinical picture

With joint involvement, the pattern of restriction at the knee is more loss of flexion than extension. When there is effusion (swelling within the joint), the joint assumes a position near 25 degrees of flexion, where there is greatest capsular distensibility. Little motion is possible because of the swelling. Symptoms of joint involvement, such as distension, stiffness, pain, and reflex muscle weakness, may cause *extensor lag* (the active range of knee extension is less than the passive range).[68]

a. Rheumatoid arthritis (RA)

Early in the disease, the hands and feet are usually involved first; with progression, the knees may become involved. The joints become warm and swollen, with limitation as described above. In addition, a genu valgum deformity commonly develops in the advanced stages of this disease. See Section VIII of Chapter 6 for clinical and treatment considerations for RA. Because the knees are weight-bearing structures, they should be protected during ambulation by using assistive devices and minimizing weight-bearing activities during the acute stage. With joint pain, there is reflex muscle inhibition and progressive muscle weakness resulting in less muscle support for the joint. With progression, functional activities such as stair climbing, rising up from a chair (or commode), and stooping to lift become difficult.

b. Osteoarthritis (degenerative joint disease, DJD)
See Section VII of Chapter 6 for a description of the disease and clinical and treatment considerations. Pain, muscle weakness, and joint limitations progressively worsen. Genu varum commonly develops. Joint replacement surgery is an alternative treatment in the advanced stages.

c. Joint trauma
Swelling in the joint following trauma frequently accompanies other problems such as ligament and meniscal tears. Swelling results in limited motion and should be treated as an acute joint lesion. When the swelling recedes, check for ligamentous and meniscal tears and, if present, treat them accordingly (see Sections D and E).

d. Joint restrictions after a period of immobilization
When the knee has been immobilized for several weeks or longer, such as following healing of a fracture or soft tissue, the capsule, muscles, and soft tissue become restricted. The condition is no longer acute. Treatment begins at the patient's functional level.

2. **Management of acute joint lesions**
See Chapter 6 for general guidelines as well as specific guidelines for RA and DJD as noted above.

a. **To control the pain**
In addition to using modalities and providing rest with an elastic wrap or splint, gentle joint-play oscillation techniques (Grade I) may inhibit the pain. If these techniques increase the pain or swelling, they should not be done for several days.

b. **To minimize stiffness**
(1) Passive or active assistive ROM within the limits of pain and available motion are performed.
(2) If tolerated, Grade I or II tractions or glides, with the joint in resting position (25 degrees flexion), are done; stretching is contraindicated at this stage.

c. **To minimize muscle atrophy and prevent patellar adhesions** (see description of exercise techniques in Section F)
(1) Gentle quadriceps femoris muscle-setting (quad sets) is repeated many times a day, but not to the point of increasing joint irritability. Quad sets also assist circulation.
(2) If the patient has adequate extensor muscle strength to hold the knee in extension, have him set the muscle, then do straight leg raising.
(3) Active extension of the knee through a pain-free range is done if tolerated. It is important to recognize that the quadriceps muscle must generate a large force during the last 15 degrees of terminal extension when the knee is extending against gravity; so if pain

increases, active knee extension exercises in an antigravity position should not be done at this stage.

   d. **To prevent deformity and to protect the joint**

      (1) If necessary use crutches, canes, or a walker to distribute forces through the upper extremities while walking.

      (2) Instruct the patient and family members in good bed positioning to avoid flexion contractures.

      (3) Make functional adaptations to reduce the amount of knee flexion and patellar compression when the person moves from flexion to extension in activities such as standing up from sitting or stair climbing. Instruct the patient to minimize stair climbing, to use elevated seats on commodes, and to avoid deep-seated or low chairs.

3. Management during the subacute and chronic period of joint problems

   a. **To decrease the effects of stiffness from inactivity**

   Instruct the patient to do active ROM.

   b. **To decrease pain from mechanical stress**

      (1) Continue use of assistive devices for ambulation, if necessary. The patient may progress to using less assistance or continue for periods without assistance. Continue use of elevated seats on commodes and chairs if needed to reduce the mechanical stresses imposed when attempting to stand up.

      (2) Strengthen the quadriceps femoris muscle with minimum stress to the patellofemoral joint.[60] (See description of exercises in Section F.)

         (a) Progress setting exercises to resisted isometric exercises with the knee fully extended, since there is less patellar compression in extension. Direct the patient's attention to the sensation of the vastus medialis muscle contracting, since this portion of the quadriceps helps align the patella. Continue to progress by providing isometric resistance at multiple angles in the range (multiple-angle isometrics), avoiding any ranges where there is increased joint pain.

         (b) When tolerated, resistance is applied at the ankle and straight leg-raising exercises are done.

         (c) As the patient gains control of the vastus medialis and can maintain isometric knee extension with straight leg raising, short-arc terminal extension exercises are initiated (See Figure 11-2). Light resistance is added at the ankle, as tolerated, if the motion is not painful. Strengthening in the terminal extension ranges forces the patient to train the muscle to function where it is least efficient.

         Precaution: Applying resistance to knee extension at an angle greater than 45 degrees of knee flexion creates excessive compression of the patellofemoral joint.[60]

         (d) Initiate training of closed-chain, weight-bearing functional activities by using closed-chain elastic resistance exercises. Have the patient stand on the elastic resistance and hold the free ends in his hands, then do small-range flexion and extension (See Figure 11-3). He should concentrate on contracting the quadriceps muscle to control the motion. Deep knee bends should not be done.

(e) Resistance through full ROM can be initiated when no symptoms of pain or crepitis are experienced. If symptoms are present, strengthen on either side of the symptomatic range, but avoid provoking the symptoms. This could be done using manual resistance in the pain-free ranges, limiting the range with mechanical resistance exercises, as well as using a range-limiting device on an isokinetic unit.

c. **To improve knee function**

(1) Begin functional training. With improved strength, the patient increases his level of functional activities, beginning with swimming and bicycling and progressing to unassisted walking when the muscle is functioning at a "good" strength grade (4/5 or 80 percent) on a manual muscle test.

(a) When bicycling, adjust the seat so that the knee goes into complete extension when the pedal is down.[44] Resistance from pedaling should be minimal.

(b) For some patients, progression to running or jumping rope and other faster paced or more intense activities can be done as long as the joint remains asymptomatic. If joint deformity is present and proper biomechanics cannot be restored, the patient probably cannot progress to these activities.

(2) Balance strength in the quadriceps muscle with strength in the hamstring muscles (see Section F for exercise suggestions.)

(3) With degenerative and rheumatoid arthritis, the patient should be cautioned to alternate activity with rest.

d. **To increase range of motion (ROM)**

(1) When there is loss of joint play and decreased mobility, joint mobilization techniques should be used.

Precaution: Do not increase ROM unless the patient has strength to control the motion already available. A mobile joint with poor muscle control causes knee instability and makes lower extremity function difficult.

(a) To increase flexion of the joint
Long-axis traction to the tibia (see Figure 5-49A, B, and C)
Posterior glide to the tibia (see Figures 5-50 and 5-51A and B)
Caudal glide of the patella if restricted (see Figure 5-53)

(b) As the available range of flexion plateaus, progress by flexing the knee to the limit of its motion, then apply a posterior glide to the tibia, or position the tibia in medial rotation then apply a posterior glide.

(c) To increase extension of the joint
Long-axis traction (see Figure 5-49A, B, and C)
Anterior glide of the tibia (see Figure 5-52)
Progress by positioning the tibia in lateral rotation then apply an anterior glide.

(2) When there is decreased flexibility in the muscles affecting knee motion, muscle elongation (inhibition) techniques should be used.

Precaution: Strong muscle contractions may exacerbate joint symptoms; adapt the dosage according to the patient's tolerance level.

(3) When there is decreased flexibility in the noncontractile soft tissue

preventing knee motion, passive stretching techniques should be used.

(a) Apply low-intensity, long-duration stretch within the patient's tolerance.

Precaution: Passive stretching using the tibia as a lever tends to exacerbate joint symptoms; use these techniques only when there is joint play available.

(b) Apply soft-tissue massage or friction massage to loosen adhesions or contractures.

B. Patellar Restrictions

1. Clinical picture

Following periods of immobilization (in a splint or cast or following surgery), adhesions may restrict patellar mobility. Usually, this will limit knee flexion and may cause pain as the patella is compressed against the femur. With lack of superior gliding of the patella, there may be an extensor lag with active knee extension even though there is full passive knee extension.[71] This usually occurs after operative repairs of some knee ligaments, when the knee has been immobilized in flexion for a prolonged period of time.

2. Management

a. The best therapy is prevention. To keep the patella mobile whenever the knee is to be immobilized, the patient should be taught quadriceps setting exercises to be done frequently every day (see Section F).

b. To increase mobility of the patella
Caudal glide of the patella (see Figure 5-53)
Medial-lateral glide of the patella (see Figure 5-54)
Deep massage around the border of the patella
Superior glide the patella if restricted in a caudal position

c. Active ROM and frequent quadriceps setting exercises are used to maintain mobility after stretching.

C. Patellofemoral Pain Syndrome

1. Chondromalacia patellae

a. Description

Proposed explanations of the origins of chondromalacia are degeneration of the cartilage of the patella from surface degeneration (particularly on the odd facet), which may eventually predispose the joint to degenerative arthritis, or basal degeneration of the middle and deep zones of the cartilage.[23] Causes of the degeneration may include trauma, surgery, prolonged or repeated stress, or lack of normal stress, such as during periods of immobilization.[56]

b. Clinical picture

The patient may initially complain of anterior knee pain, usually when descending stairs, and pain or crepitation when the patella is compressed against the femur, as when sitting or squatting for prolonged periods of time. The patella femoral grinding test is positive,[29] and palpation elicits tenderness along the medial part of the articular surface of the patella.[23] It is common in young people, and girls have a greater tendency to develop symptoms than boys.[23] In older people, it is associated with osteoarthritis. An increased Q-angle is often seen.

c. **Management**

(1) When symptoms are acute, treat as any acute joint with rest, gentle motion, and muscle-setting exercises.

(2) Assess mechanical factors to see if they could be the cause of abnormal stress on the patella. Causes that can be managed conservatively include weak vastus medialis, foot pronation (leading to lateral displacement of the tibial tubercle), tight iliotibial band, and excessive stressful trauma to the knee (such as deep knee bends and inappropriate exercising).

(3) Treat the faulty mechanics

(a) Strengthen the quadriceps femoris muscle in terminal extension so there is minimal stress to the patellofemoral joint. The patient should concentrate on the sensation of the vastus medialis muscle contracting to emphasize its medial pull on the patella. High repetitions with low resistance to the point of muscle fatigue is less traumatic to the joint than low repetitions with high resistance. Begin and progress exercises as described under Section A 3 b and c of this section.

(b) Stretch the iliotibial band (see Figures 4-16 and 10-6)

(c) If necessary, construct a foot orthosis to control foot pronation.

(d) Educate the patient to avoid positions and activities that provoke the symptoms. Avoid stair climbing and descending until the muscles are strengthened and the joint is symptom free. The patient should not sit with the knees flexed excessively for prolonged periods. If on a training program, he should not do heavy resistance exercises through the full range of knee flexion to extension.

2. **Plica syndrome (plica synovialis, medial shelf syndrome suprapatellar plica synovitis, medial plica synovitis)[5]**

a. **Description**

Remnants of embryologic synovial tissue around the patella may become irritated with micro or macro trauma, leading to anterior knee pain. With chronic irritation, the tissue becomes an inelastic fibrotic band and may cause secondary knee stresses. It is sometimes associated with chondromalacia patellae and quadriceps atrophy.

b. **Clinical picture**

The symptoms of pain are similar to those in chondromalacia. When acute, the tissue is painful on palpation; when chronic, the plical band is tender and palpable. Tests that pinch the plica are painful.[5] The band is usually palpable medial to the patella, although there are variations in location of the band.[5,37]

c. **Management**

The conservative treatment approach is the same as with chondromalacia patellae. With the quad sets and terminal extension exercises, the patient concentrates on the sensation of drawing the patella upward through action of the vastus intermedius and thus affecting the articularis genus muscle. (This deep portion of the vastus intermedius attaches to the synovial membrane of the knee and acts to keep it from being pinched as the knee extends). Stretching tight muscles such as the hamstrings is also indicated. Surgical intervention, with excision of the plica is indicated if the conservative approach does not relieve symptoms.

D. Sprains and Minor Ligamentous Tears

1. Onset

Ligamentous injuries occur most often in individuals between 20 and 40 years of age as the result of sport injuries (e.g., skiing and football). The anterior cruciate ligament (ACL) is the most commonly injured ligament. The injury occurs when the knee is forcefully hyperextended. The medial collateral ligament, as well as the ACL, can be injured with a valgus strain and external rotation of the tibia when the foot is planted. The posterior cruciate ligament can be injured with a forceful blow to the anterior portion of the tibia while the knee is flexed. Often more than one ligament is damaged as the result of a single injury.[34]

2. Clinical picture

Following trauma, the joint usually does not swell for several hours. Once swollen, motion is restricted. The joint assumes a position of minimum stress, usually around 25 degrees of flexion. If tested when the joint is not swollen, the patient feels pain when the injured ligament is stressed. If there is a complete tear, instability is detected when the torn ligament is tested.

3. Management

Acute sprains and partial ligamentous tears of the knee can be treated conservatively with rest, joint protection, and exercise. After the acute stage of healing, exercises should be geared toward regaining normal ROM and strength to the muscles supporting and stabilizing the joint during functional activities. The degree of instability with ligamentous tears will affect the demands the patient can place on the knee when returning to full activity. See Chapter 6 for principles of treatment during stages of inflammation and repair.

a. If possible, evaluate and treat the problem with cold, wrapping, and quadriceps setting exercises before effusion sets in.

b. When the joint is swollen, treat it like an acute joint lesion as described in Section II A. The knee may not fully extend for muscle-setting exercises, so begin the exercises in the range most comfortable for the patient.

c. As the swelling decreases, initiate active range of motion and strengthening exercises to the flexors and extensors of the knee.

d. If the collateral or coronary ligaments are involved, cross-fiber massage to the structure helps align the healing fibers and maintain mobility in them.

e. Protective bracing may be necessary in weight-bearing activities to decrease stress to the healing ligament or to provide stability where ligament integrity has been compromised. The patient must be instructed to decrease vigorous activities until appropriate stability is obtained.

4. Complete tears

When complete tears lead to chronic instability of the knee and the patient complains of the knee "giving way," or when the patient cannot return to a level of activity that he is satisfied with without re-injury, surgical repair may be indicated. (see Section III.)

E. Meniscal Tears

1. Onset

Most frequently injured is the medial meniscus. Insult may occur when the foot is fixed on the ground and the femur is rotated internally, as when pivoting, getting out of a car, or receiving a clipping injury. An anterior cruciate ligament injury often accompanies a medial meniscus tear. Lateral rotation of the femur on a fixed tibia may tear the lateral meniscus. Simple squatting or trauma may also cause a tear.

2. Clinical picture

Meniscal tears can cause an acute locking of the knee as well as chronic sympoms with intermittent locking, pain along the joint line from stress to the coronary ligament, joint swelling, and some degree of quadriceps atrophy. When there is joint locking, the knee does not fully extend and there is a springy end-feel when passive extension is attempted. If the joint is swollen, there is usually slight limitation of flexion or extension. The McMurrey or Appley grinding tests may be positive.[29]

3. Management

a. Often the patient can actively move the leg to "unlock" the knee, or the unlocking happens spontaneously. If a passive manipulation is necessary, the following techniques may be used:

(1) Manipulative reduction of the medial meniscus.
Position of patient: supine. Passively flex the involved knee and hip as you simultaneously internally and externally rotate the tibia. When the knee is fully flexed, laterally rotate the tibia and apply a valgus stress at the knee. Hold the tibia in this position as you extend the knee. The meniscus may click into place[29] (Figure 11-1). Once reduced, the knee will respond as an acute lesion; treat as described in section II A in this chapter.

(2) Surgical intervention may be necessary; see section III.

F. Muscle Strength and Flexibility Imbalances

Note: Strength and flexibility imbalances in muscle can occur from a variety of causes, some of which are disuse, faulty joint mechanics, surgery, immobilization (from fracture, surgery, trauma), and nerve injury. Besides the hamstrings and rectus femoris, most of the 2-joint muscles crossing the knee primarily function either at the hip or at the ankle, yet they have an effect on knee function. If there is an imbalance in length or strength in the hip or ankle muscles, there are usually altered mechanics throughout the lower extremity. See also the chapters on the hip and the foot for a complete picture. When attempting to increase ROM and strength, the mechanics of the tibiofemoral and patellofemoral joints and their importance in lower extremity function must be respected (see section I of this chapter). When the patient has chondromalacia or when predisposing factors that could lead to articular cartilage degeneration exist, such as immediately following immobilization of the joint or following surgery or trauma, heavy resistance against the quadriceps with the knee in greater than 30 degrees of flexion should be avoided.[56,60] In addition, special mechanical adaptations must be made with spe-

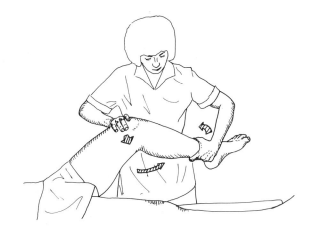

FIGURE 11-1. Manipulative reduction of a medial meniscus. Internally and externally rotate the tibia as you flex the hip and knee (not shown), then laterally rotate the tibia and apply a valgus stress at the knee as you extend it. The meniscus may click into place.

cific surgical procedures. These are highlighted in the surgical section. Because the knee is a weight-bearing joint, the need for stability takes precedence over the need for mobility, although with adequate strength, mobility is necessary for normal function.

1. **Techniques to train and strengthen weak muscles**

   Strengthening exercises at the knee begin at the level of the patient's ability, with stability and safe patellofemoral and extensor mechanics as primary concerns. High repetitions with low resistance is safer and results in less painful joint reactions than low repetition with heavy resistance.[44] In addition, during immobilization of the knee there is deterioration of type I and IIA (oxidative) fiber types. High-repetition exercises with low weights is a good way to selectively recruit and increase the metabolic capacity of Type I fibers when movement can be initiated. Once stability and patellar mechanics are good, coordination and timing of the muscle contraction along with endurance are emphasized in functional activities. The knee functions both in an open and closed kinematic chain, with the quadriceps contracting either concentrically or eccentrically, so exercises in all these situations should be incorporated into the final program.

   a. **To train and strengthen the knee extensor (quadriceps femoris) muscles**

      (1) Quad sets (muscle-setting exercises to the quadriceps)
         Position of patient: supine or long-sitting, with the knee in extension, if possible. The patient contracts the muscle, causing the patella to glide proximally, then holds it to the count of six. If he cannot contract the muscle on command, some cues that can be used are: "Try to push your knee down and tighten your thigh muscle"; "Attempt to lift your leg just enough to tense the thigh muscle"; or "Try to tighten your muscle and move your knee cap up." When the patient sets the muscle properly, immediately offer verbal reinforcement and have him repeat it.

      (2) Straight leg raising (SLR), hip flexion with knee extension.
         This is a progression of isometric exercise to the quadriceps mus-

cle when the patient can maintain the knee extended while lifting the extremity. To stabilize the pelvis and back, the opposite leg is flexed and the foot is placed flat on the exercise table. Instruct the patient to set the quadriceps muscle, then lift the leg with the knee extended to about 45 degrees of hip flexion, hold it to the count of 6, then lower it. As the patient progreses, have him lift it to only 30 degrees, hold to the count of 6, then lower it. The most effective resistance to the quadriceps is during the first few degrees of SLR.

If the patient cannot do SLR because of quadriceps weakness, begin by passively placing the involved extremity at 90 degrees of SLR (or as far as the flexibility of the hamstrings allows) and have the patient gradually lower it. Be prepared to control the descent of the leg with your hand under the heel as the torque created by gravity increases. If the knee begins to flex as the extremity is lowered, have the patient stop at that point, then raise the extremity upward toward 90 degrees. Repeat the motion, attempting to lower the extremity a little further each time. Once the patient can lower the extremity full range, he can begin SLR activities.

(3) Isometric exercises against resistance
   (a) When tolerated, resistance is applied at the ankle, either manually, or mechanically with Velcro weights, or by using an elasticized material. The patient then attempts SLR against the resistance.
   (b) Isometric exercises may also be applied with the knee at various angles, being careful not to use a resistance too heavy for the condition (multiple angle isometrics).
(4) Short-arc terminal extension (Figure 11-2)
   (a) The patient is supine or long-sitting. Place a bolster or rolled towel under his knee to support it in flexion. Begin with the knee in a few degrees of flexion. Progress the degrees of flexion as tolerated by the patient or dictated by the condition. The patient extends his knee initially against only the resistance of gravity. Resistance is added at the ankle, as tolerated, if the motion is not painful. This can be combined with an isometric hold and/or SLR when the knee is in full extension.
   (b) If the patient sits with the knee at the edge of the treatment table, a chair should be placed under the heel to stop knee flexion at the desired angle.

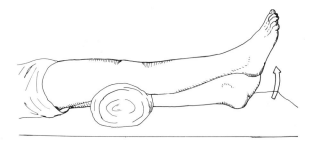

FIGURE 11-2. Short-arc terminal extension exercise to strengthen the quadriceps femoris muscle. When tolerated, resistance is added proximal to the ankle.

(c) **Precaution:** When adding resistance to the distal leg, the amount of force generated by the quadriceps muscle increases significantly in the terminal ranges of extension because of its poor mechanical advantage and poor physiologic length while having to contract against an external resistance force that has a long lever arm. The amount of muscle force causes an anterior gliding force on the tibia, which is restrained by the anterior cruciate ligament. These exercises are not appropriate for strained or unstable anterior cruciate ligaments or following surgical repair of the ligament until the ligament is fully healed.[25]

(5) Closed-chain knee extension (Figure 11-3)

To train the quadriceps to contract in the weight-bearing position, using short arc terminal extension motions, begin by having the patient stand and bend both knees up to 30 degrees, then extend them. Progress by using elastic resistance placed under both feet, the ends being held in the patient's hands. As he flexes and extends his knees through the short-arc motion, have him maintain his trunk upright and concentrate on the sensation of the quadriceps muscle contracting. This is important since the knee extension can be done by the hamstrings or soleus muscles pulling on the tibia, causing a faulty substitute muscle function to develop.

(6) Full-arc extension

Resistance is applied through the arc of 90 degrees of flexion to 0 degrees of extension. This should be done only if the knee is pain free and asymptomatic. If there is pain within the range, resistance may be applied through those parts of the range where there are no symptoms.

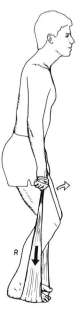

FIGURE 11-3. Closed-chain knee extension. Elastic resistance to knee extension is provided for short-arc motion. It is important to use the quadriceps femoris muscles rather than substitute with the hamstring muscles for proper strengthening.

(7) Step-ups

To progress weight-bearing knee extension exercises through greater ROM, the patient begins using steps. The patient stands sideways to a step and places the extremity to be exercised on a step. He then steps up until the knee is extended, then lowers himself until the opposite heel is again on the floor. The patient should maintain his trunk upright and concentrate on the sensation of the quadriceps muscle contracting rather than substituting with the hamstrings pulling the tibia backwards. The exercise is begun with a low step (4 inches) and is progressed by increasing the height of the step and therefore range of knee flexion.

(8) Mechanical resistance

(a) Various kinds of mechanical equipment are available to build strength in the quadriceps muscle: Weighted boots, pulleys, NK table, and isokinetic or variable resistance are just a few examples of commonly available pieces. The ease of application, stress to the supporting structures, and effective resistance to the muscle at various ranges of motion should be taken into account when making a choice for equipment.

(b) A weighted boot placed on the foot will cause distraction of the joint and stress to the ligaments when the person sits with the knee flexed 90 degrees over the edge of the treatment table.[8] To avoid this stress to ligaments, place a stool under the foot so it can be supported when the leg is in the dependent position.

(c) Use of a wedge under the knee while doing knee extension exercises is a matter of individual preference. It has been found that it does not increase the effectiveness of the resistance significantly, but it does concentrate pressure (and therefore discomfort) on the distal posterior thigh.[15]

(d) High repetition with low resistance causes less joint pain and swelling in knee disorders than the high-resistance, low-repetition techniques.[44,60]

(e) Resistance through a full arc of motion (as in isotonic and isokinetic exercises) often exacerbates a symptomatic knee and therefore should not be done until the patient is pain free.

(9) Functional training for coordination, timing, and endurance

(a) Walking (unassisted if the patient is at that level), stair climbing and descending, bicycling, and swimming are begun at the patient's functional level; distance and intensity are progressed as tolerated.

(b) Training on a balance board may be appropriate to stimulate proprioception and coordination.

(c) Depending on the patient and the level of function desired and if adequate strength and endurance permits, running, sprinting, jumping rope, jumping jacks, and similar fast-paced activities are initiated and monitored for correct mechanics.

b. **To train and strengthen the knee flexor muscles (primarily the hamstrings)**

Balance of the ratio between flexor and extensor strength should be obtained for functional usage of the knee in a variety of activities.[8,9] Normally, knee flexor force is about 67 percent of knee extensor force.[51]

(1) Hamstring sets (muscle-setting exercises to the hamstrings)

Position of patient: supine or long-sitting with the knee in extension, if possible. The patient contracts the muscle by gently pushing his heel into the treatment table, holds to the count of 6, then relaxes.

(2) Isometric exercises against resistance
   (a) When tolerated, resistance is applied at the ankle, either manually or mechanically, and the patient attempts to flex his knee.
   (b) Isometric exercises may also be applied with the knee at various angles, using a resistance appropriate for the condition.

(3) Active knee flexion against gravity
   (a) Position of patient: standing, holding on to a solid object for balance. The patient picks up his foot and flexes the knee (Figure 11-4). Maximum resistance from gravity occurs when the knee is at 90 degrees flexion. Add resistance with ankle weights or a weighted boot. If the patient flexes his hip, stabilize it by having him place his anterior thigh against a wall or solid object.
   (b) Position of patient: prone. Place a small towel roll or foam rubber under the femur just proximal to the patella in order to avoid compression of the patella between the treatment table and femur. The patient then flexes the knee only to 90 degrees; maximum resistance from gravity occurs when the knee first starts to flex at 0 degrees. Resistance can be applied manually or mechanically with ankle weights or a boot.

(4) Mechanical resistance can also be applied using a weight-and-pulley system, an NK table, or isokinetic resistance equipment.

2. Techniques to stretch tight muscles

a. To stretch tight hamstring muscles

Flexibility in the hamstring muscle group is necessary for knee extension as well as many functional activities in which the muscle group is elongated over the hip and knee simultaneously.

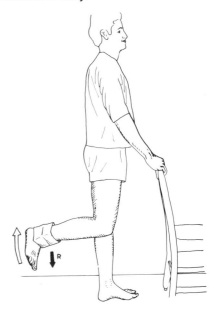

FIGURE 11-4. Resistance exercises to the knee flexors with the patient standing. Maximum resistance occurs when the knee is at 90 degrees.

(1) If the knee extends to 0 degrees but the hamstrings limit straight leg raising (the knee begins to flex as the hip is flexed), active stretching techniques for the hamstrings, as described in Chapters 4 and 10 (Hip), should be used.

(2) If the knee cannot extend because of extreme tightness in the hamstrings, active inhibition techniques are used, but emphasis is placed on knee extension rather than hip flexion.

    (a) Position of patient: supine, with the hip extended as much as possible. Resist knee extension for reciprocal inhibition, or resist knee flexion with your hand proximal to the ankle, have the patient relax, and then extend the knee for contract-relax maneuvers.

    (b) Position of patient: prone. This places the hip in extension. Padding must be placed under the femur, proximal to the patella, in order to avoid patellar compression. Contract-relax or reciprocal inhibition techniques can then be used with the resistance being applied against the distal tibia.

b. **To stretch tight quadriceps femoris muscles**

Before stretching the muscle, be sure the patella is mobile (see Section II B), so it can glide in the trochlear groove as the knee flexes.

(1) Active inhibition techniques

Position of patient: sitting, with the knee at the edge of the treatment table and flexed as far as possible. Resist knee flexion for reciprocal inhibition, or resist knee extension isometrically; have the patient relax, then flex the knee for contract-relax maneuvers.

(2) Self-stretching wall slide (Figure 11-5)

Position of patient: supine with buttocks against wall and lower extremities vertical resting against the wall (hips flexed, knees extended). Slowly flex the involved knee by sliding the foot down the wall, hold in a comfortable stretch position, then slide the foot back up the wall.

(3) Self-stretching rock on step (Figure 11-6)

Position of patient: standing with foot of involved knee on a step. The patient rocks forward over the stabilized foot, flexing the knee to the limit of its range. He can rock back and forth in a slow rhythmic manner or apply a sustained stretch. Begin with a low step or stool; progress the height as more range is obtained.

(4) Self-stretching prone-lying

Position of patient: Prone with the knee flexed to the end of its range. The patient grasps his foot and pulls the heel towards his buttocks.

(5) Self-stretching while sitting (Figure 11-7)

Position of patient: Sitting in a chair with the involved knee flexed to the end of its available range and the foot firmly planted on the floor. Have the patient move forward in the chair, not allowing the foot to slide. Have him hold the stretch position for a comfortable, sustained stretch to the knee extensors.

G. Referred Pain

1. Common sources for referred pain to the knee include[16]

    a. nerve roots and tissues derived from spinal segments L-3, referring to the anterior aspect, and from S-1 and S-2, referring to the posterior

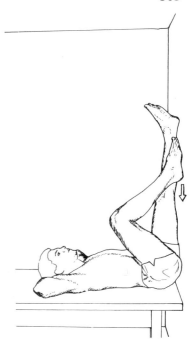

FIGURE 11-5. Self-stretching wall slide. The patient flexes the knee to the limit of its range and holds it there for a sustained stretch to the quadriceps femoris muscle.

aspect of the knee.
   b. the hip joint (which is primarily L-3)
2. Treatment of the source of irritation is necessary to relieve the pain. Therapeutic exercise to the knee is beneficial only in preventing disuse of the part; primary treatment must be directed to the source of the irritation.

III. THERAPEUTIC EXERCISE MANAGEMENT OF COMMON SURGICAL PROCEDURES FOR THE KNEE

Acute traumatic injuries or chronic lesions and deterioration of the knee joint can cause severe pain, gross joint instability, deformity, and limitation of motion of the knee. The

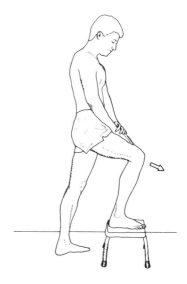

FIGURE 11-6. Self-stretching rock on step. The patient places the foot on the involved side on a step, then rocks forward over the stabilized foot to the limit of knee flexion to stretch the quadriceps femoris muscle. Use a higher step for greater flexion.

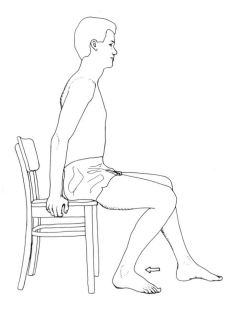

FIGURE 11-7. Self-stretching in a chair. The patient fixates the foot of the involved leg on the floor, then moves forward in the chair over the stabilized foot to place a sustained stretch on the quadriceps femoris muscle and increase knee flexion.

knee must be pain free and stable for normal weight bearing and walking. Adequate motion of the knee is necessary in many functional and recreational activities.

Surgical intervention is often indicated for repair of soft-tissue injuries to the knee. Torn ligaments or menisci and malalignment of the extensor mechanism or plica syndrome may have to be managed surgically. Procedures such as synovectomy, osteotomy and total joint replacement may be necessary in the management of arthritis of the knee. Rehabilitation of the knee after any of these procedures should meet the following goals:

1. Restore normal function to the knee.
2. Eliminate pain during motion and weight bearing.
3. Improve stability and increase strength of the knee structures.
4. Improve range of motion.
5. Prevent further injury or deterioration of the knee.

Most of the exercises outlined in this section that are used to meet these postoperative goals have been described in detail in section II of this chapter. Guidelines for the progression of exercise after surgery are emphasized in this section.

A. Surgical Management of Soft-Tissue Injuries of the Knee—General Considerations

The soft-tissue structures that surround the anatomically unstable knee joint are highly vulnerable to acute or chronic injury.[10] These structures are[28,29] (1) the extensor mechanism, that is, the quadriceps muscle, patellar tendon, and the patella; (2) the menisci; and (3) the ligaments. Acute injury or chronic insufficiency of any of these structures can cause severe pain, limited motion, and gross instability of the knee.

Surgical intervention is often considered if an injury significantly impairs an individual's level of functional activity. The type of surgical procedure that is chosen to repair the damaged soft tissue will depend on the diagnosis, the severity of the problem, and the philosophy of the surgeon. Some acute injuries may result in so much swelling, pain, and muscle spasm that a diagnosis of the problem may not be possible until several days after the injury has occurred. Surgery is indicated in severe injuries as soon as a diagnosis has been made.[30,34,44] The surgery will involve either an arthroscopic removal or repair of the tissue or an open procedure in which an arthrotomy of the knee is necessary.

The goals of soft-tissue surgery and postoperative rehabilitation are to restore normal stability and strength to the knee and provide relief of pain on movement and weight bearing. Therapeutic exercise is a key component of the postoperative plan of care of patients who have undergone repair of soft tissue of the knee. The exercises that are indicated in the early postoperative period after arthroscopic surgery or arthrotomy of the knee are very similar. The intensity and progression of exercises carried out during the later rehabilitative period differ considerably from procedure to procedure. A thorough understanding of each surgical procedure and the precautions and contraindications associated with each procedure is necessary to plan a safe and effective exercise program for each patient.

1. **Preoperative management of soft-tissue lesions**

Patients with acute or chronic injuries of the extensor mechanism, menisci, plica, or ligaments of the knee can benefit from preoperative supervision and instruction. In a knee with acute symptoms, several days of splinting, cold packs, and muscle-setting exercises will help decrease joint effusion, hemarthrosis, and muscle spasm so a diagnosis of the problem can be made.[34,39,44] Many patients who have recurrent dysfunction of the knee from chronic lesions have a more successful result from surgery and are able to return to normal and vigorous physical activities sooner after surgery if they participate in a preoperative exercise program.[34,39,44]

The preoperative exercises in both these situations are similar to the exercises that are used for conservative (nonoperative) treatment of soft-tissue injuries of the knee. (See section II of this chapter.)

a. The necessary components of a preoperative program for patients with an acute injury are
   (1) Compression and ice to the injured knee and elevation of the lower extremity to minimize pain and inflammation.
   (2) External support with a splint or support wrap to immobilize the knee.
   (3) Decreased weight bearing, using crutches or a cane.
   (4) Exercise.
      (a) Quadriceps or hamstrings setting performed regularly during the day.
      (b) Straight leg raising several times a day. This should be done without the splint or wrap, if possible.
      (c) Active short-arc terminal extension of the knee, that is, extension of the knee from 45 degrees of flexion to full extension, if comfortable.
      (d) *Note:* Some of these exercises may have to be modified to avoid additional stress to the injured soft tissues. For example, after an acute injury of the anterior cruciate ligament, hamstrings-setting exercises may be emphasized more than quad sets. If performed, quad sets may have to be done with a small wedge under the knee so that the patient does not hyperextend

the knee.[1] Further modifications of exercises will be explained under postoperative management of specific soft-tissue injuries later in this section.

b. Preoperative management of chronic lesions of the knee when surgery is several weeks away, can include
   (1) External support of the knee and assistive devices during ambulation, if necessary.
   (2) Exercises for the knee as described above under acute management, and the addition of:
      (a) Gentle stretching of the hamstrings, if tight.
      (b) Short-arc terminal knee extension and straight leg-raising against light resistance.
      (c) Full-arc extension of the knee (from 90 degrees of flexion to full extension). This may be done actively or against very low resistance if there is no pain or irritation to the knee.
      (d) Hamstrings strengthening against low resistance.
      (e) In general, low-intensity (low-resistance) exercise, carried out for a high number of repetitions, is preferable to exercise done at high intensity for a low number of repetitions. Low-intensity exercise appears to be less irritating to the knee joint and more tolerable for the patient.[10,12,44]
   (3) Exercises to strengthen hip musculature, such as the hip extensors, abductors, adductors, and possibly the flexors. Resisted straight leg raising can be done with the patient prone, side lying, and supine to strengthen hip musculature while protecting the knee.
   (4) Daily bicycling, preferably on a stationary bicycle for safety, with the seat raised to promote maximum hip and knee extension.

c. **Preoperative precautions during exercise**
   (1) Precautions and contraindication to exercise during the preoperative period will vary depending on the type and severity of the injury.
   (2) Exercises should not further irritate the injured tissues or cause additional swelling or pain.

2. **Early postoperative rehabilitation after arthrotomy of the knee**

After most open repairs of soft-tissue structures of the knee (when an arthrotomy has been performed), there is a period of time when the knee is immobilized in a splint, cast, or bulky compression dressing. The period of immobilization will vary from a few days to 6 to 8 weeks, depending on the type of surgery that was done. One exception is when continuous passive motion (CPM) is used immediately after surgery. Early motion has been used safely after repair of the anterior cruciate ligament[54] and will be discussed later in this section.

During the early postoperative period after an arthrotomy, patients must restrict weight bearing on the involved extremity to protect incised or repaired tissues. After some procedures, such as ligamentous repair or reconstruction, non–weight bearing is necessary. After other procedures, such as repair of the extensor mechanism, early weight bearing to patient tolerance is permissible.[12,30,34,44,58,59]

The exercises that are performed during the early postoperative period after soft-tissue repairs do not vary greatly from surgery to surgery.

Differences in the progression and intensity of exercise after the immobilization device is removed, amount of weight bearing during ambulation, and special precautions will be discussed later in this section with the descriptions of specific surgical procedures.

The early postoperative exercises performed while the knee is immobilized are

a. **Quadriceps-, hamstrings-, and gluteal-setting exercises and ankle-pumping exercises.** These are begun on the first day after surgery and repeated periodically during the day.
   (1) Electrical stimulation to the quadriceps or hamstring muscles, or both, is also used to decrease early muscle atrophy.
   (2) Quad sets are often very uncomfortable during the first few postoperative days. A modification of the quad set may make the early contractions more comfortable. Have the patient actively dorsiflex the foot, if possible, before doing a quad set. This will decrease the force of the quadriceps contraction, which will make the contraction less painful.[1]

b. **Upper extremity push-ups, while sitting in bed or in a wheelchair, in preparation for crutch walking.** This may be started whenever the patient can move about in bed with relative comfort, usually by the end of the first or on the second postoperative day.

c. **Straight leg raising (SLR) exercises in the cast or splint.**
   (1) After a meniscectomy, SLR may be started within the first few days after surgery, depending on the patient's tolerance.
   (2) After extensor mechanism repairs, SLR is not started until 7 to 10 days postoperatively.

d. **Hip strengthening exercises.** These are begun as soon as the patient can perform
   (1) hip extension, while standing or lying prone.
   (2) hip abduction, while side lying.

e. *Precaution:* After any knee surgery, a patient will experience considerable discomfort during exercise. Soft tissues disturbed during surgery will be irritated and painful. Exercises begun during this early postoperative period must be done cautiously and within the patient's pain tolerance.

3. **Early postoperative rehabilitation after arthroscopic surgery of the knee**

   a. Rehabilitation after most arthroscopic surgeries of the knee moves very quickly. The knee is placed in a soft compression dressing postoperatively. Immobilization may only be necessary for 1 day after some arthroscopic procedures, such as partial meniscectomy or excision of the plica. After arthroscopic meniscus or ligament *repairs,* immobilization may be required for several weeks to protect the sutured and repaired structures.

   b. After arthroscopic surgery, the exercises that are performed in the early postoperative period while immobilization is necessary are the same as the exercises performed after an arthrotomy of the knee. The intensity of the exercises is usually greater and the progression more rapid after arthroscopic surgery because the soft tissues around the knee have been subjected to less trauma.

B. **Realignment of the Extensor Mechanism for Recurrent Dislocation of the Patella**
   1. **Indications for surgery**[28,34,59]
      a. Chronic or recurrent dislocation of the patella occurring with sudden contraction of the quadriceps mechanism.
      b. Associated problems include
         (1) chronic patellar subluxation.
         (2) malalignment and abnormal tracking of the patella.
         (3) chondromalacia.
         (4) patella alta.
         (5) genu valgum.
         (6) laxity of the medial aspect of the joint capsule.

   2. **Procedure**[34,44]
      a. An arthrotomy of the knee is performed.
      b. The patellofemoral joint is inspected for chondromalacia, and the underside of the patella is shaved, if necessary.
      c. A proximal or distal reconstruction involving the patellar tendon and realignment of the extensor mechanism is done. There are numerous variations of this procedure. The primary purpose is to alter the line of pull of the quadriceps mechanism or decrease the Q-angle of the patella. To accomplish this, the patellar tendon and extensor mechanism are realigned to a more medial and distal position.
      d. The soft tissues on the anterolateral aspect of the joint are released, and the tissues on the anteromedial aspect of the joint are tightened.

   3. **Postoperative management**[34,44,59]
      a. The patient is immobilized in a long leg cast or tight compression dressing, with the knee extended for approximately 2 to 4 weeks. During that time, setting exercises of the knee and hip SLRs and isotonic ankle pumping exercises are begun.
         (1) As noted previously, to make quadriceps-setting exercises more comfortable in the early postoperative days have the patient dorsiflex the foot prior to the quad set to lessen the force of the contraction and the discomfort associated with the contraction.
         (2) Use electrical stimulation to the vastus medialis muscle to decrease atrophy.
      b. While the knee is immobilized, the patient may begin ambulation with crutches, bearing only minimal weight on the operated leg.
      c. When the cast or splint is removed, very gentle active flexion and extension exercises are begun to restore knee motion and strength.
         (1) To increase knee flexion and prevent a knee extension contracture, reciprocal inhibition of the quadriceps and a caudal glide of the patella can be used. Passive stretching is contraindicated. The patient should have 90 degrees of knee flexion by 4 to 6 weeks postoperatively.
         (2) To increase active knee extension and prevent a quadriceps lag[41,44,59]
            (a) Continue setting and SLR exercise begun while the patient's knee was immobilized and begin multiple-angle, isometric knee extension exercises against light resistance.

(b) Add 5 to 10 lb of weight to straight leg raising if the patient can actively extend the knee to at least 10 or 15 degrees from the zero position.

(c) Before initiating short-arc knee extension exercises, have the patient perform isometric contractions of the hip adductors (squeeze a pillow). This will facilitate contraction of the vastus medialis muscle because fibers of this muscle originate, in part, from the fascia overlying the adductor magnus muscle.[1]

(d) Begin short-arc active extension of the knee in about 45 degrees of knee flexion. When the knee is flexed to this angle, the patella is seated better in the femoral groove, and there will be less lateral shear and discomfort as the patient actively extends the knee. Beginning in 45 degrees of flexion also allows more time for the vastus medialis to fire and provide better stability to the patella.

(e) Later add very low weight during short-arc extension if the patient does not experience pain, swelling, or increased crepitation. Light weights will keep the compressive forces on the patella low as the patient approaches knee extension in the terminal range.

(f) Progress to full-arc knee extension exercises if the movement is comfortable. After patellar realignment surgery, it may also be more comfortable for the patient to do short-arc or full-arc knee extension with the foot dorsiflexed and inverted. Inversion of the foot decreases excessive external tibial rotation with full knee extension and reduces the lateral shear forces to the patella which, in turn, reduces parapatellar pain.[1]

(g) Closed-chain short-arc knee extension (see Figure 11-3) against elastic resistance can also be initiated when the patient is allowed to bear full weight on the operated extremity.

(3) As range of motion improves, resistance is also added during active knee flexion to increase the strength of the hamstrings.

(4) Isokinetic exercises at intermediate and fast velocities are appropriate in the later stages of rehabilitation to develop a balance of knee extensor and flexor muscle strength and endurance.

d. A quadriceps lag of 10 to 15 degrees because of knee effusion, quadriceps atrophy, or poor mechanical advantage of the quadriceps mechanism may persist for 6 months or more after surgery.[31,52]

e. Bicycling may be started with the seat raised to allow for full knee extension as soon as full passive range of motion has been achieved.

f. *Precautions*

(1) Avoid exercise against resistance in the portions of the ROM where there is crepitus or pain.

(2) Avoid the use of heavy weights in an isotonic program or maximal effort at slow speeds during isokinetic exercise. Both will cause excessive compressive forces on the patellofemoral joint.

C. Arthroscopic Meniscectomy

1. Indications[34,39,44,76]

a. Partial or complete tear or rupture of the medial or lateral meniscus

b. Displacement of the meniscus associated with locking of the knee

c. *Note:* The majority of uncomplicated injuries to the medial or lateral meniscus are managed by arthroscopic meniscectomy. Some meniscal repairs are also done arthroscopically.

2. Procedure[34,39,44,76]

a. Endoscopic removal of the torn portion of the meniscus
b. Multiple portals (usually three) are required in this procedure. The lesion is identified, grasped, and divided endoscopically by knife or scissors, and removed by vacuum.
c. A soft compression dressing is applied.

3. Postoperative management after removal of meniscus

Note: The following guidelines are for postoperative management of complete or partial *removal* of a torn meniscus. If a *repair* of the meniscus is done, rehabilitation will progress much more slowly. Postoperative management after arthroscopic repair of a meniscus will be discussed later in this section.

a. Immobilization
  (1) It may only be necessary to immobilize the knee for 1 day after surgery.
  (2) During this time, the involved leg is elevated, and ice is applied several times per day.
  (3) Have the patient ambulate with crutches bearing weight to tolerance while wearing the immobilization device.
b. Exercise
  (1) On the first postoperative day, begin with quadriceps-setting and ankle-pumping exercises while the knee is immobilized.
  (2) Straight leg raising (SLR) is done in supine, prone, and side-lying positions to strengthen hip and knee muscles as soon as the patient can tolerate this.
  (3) Exercises to increase ROM of the knee. Active knee flexion and is initiated on the second or third postoperative day after uncomplicated arthroscopic meniscectomy.
    (a) *Heel slides:* the patient assumes a supine position and slides the heel up the bed to flex the knee.
    (b) Active ROM: the patient can begin short-arc active knee extension and flexion in a sitting position by the second or third postoperative day. The patient may increase the ROM as quickly as tolerable. Most patients achieve full knee motion by 7 days postoperatively.
  (4) Exercises to increase strength
    (a) Resistance can be added to SLRs and multiple-angle isometrics as long as this does not cause pain or increase effusion.
    (b) Light isotonic resistance exercise or *submaximal* isokinetic exercise are begun when the patient has 90 degrees of knee flexion.
    (c) As healing continues, isokinetic exercises are done with maximal effort at medium and, later, at fast velocities to improve strength but minimize compressive forces to the joint.[72]
  (5) Exercises to increase muscle endurance. Stationary bicycling can often be started at the end of 1 week and progressed during the rehabilitation process.
  (6) Exercises to increase joint proprioception and balance. As soon as

the patient can tolerate full weight bearing, he may stand on a balance board and shift his weight forward, backward, and from side to side to improve balance and agility (see Figure 12-5).

(7) *Precautions:* Patients who have undergone arthroscopic meniscectomy must be cautioned not to push themselves too rapidly. Too rapid progression of exercises will cause recurrent joint effusion and possible re-injury to the knee. Young, active patients should avoid activities such as jogging for about 3 months. Jogging places abnormally high compressive loads on the articular surfaces of the knee at heel strike and will cause joint irritation and effusion.[44] An alternative to jogging could include swimming or bicycling. When the patient does initially return to jogging, some therapists advocate jogging on the toes for a period of time to avoid excessive joint loading.

4. Postoperative management after arthroscopic repair of the meniscus

If a repair of the torn meniscus is performed where the fragments of the meniscus are sutured together, a much longer period of immobilization and protected weight bearing is necessary than after removal of the meniscus to allow the sutured cartilage to heal. The repaired meniscus takes about 6 weeks to heal. The knee is immobilized in 30 to 40 degrees of knee flexion for 6 weeks, and the patient must remain non–weight bearing during that time. Therefore, arthroscopic meniscal repair is managed very conservatively.[39]

D. Open Meniscectomy (Arthrotomy)

1. Indications[30,34,39,55]

a. Repair of a torn meniscus

b. Complete tear of a meniscus that requires full meniscectomy

c. Tears of menisci associated with ligament injury

2. Procedure[34,55]

a. An arthrotomy of the knee is done through a longitudinal or transverse incision along the anterior aspect of the knee.

b. Complete removal of the meniscus or repair of torn fibers is done.

3. Postoperative management

a. Immobilization

The knee is initially immobilized in a bulky compression dressing for several days after open meniscectomy. If the meniscus is repaired, the knee is immobilized in 30 to 40 degrees of knee flexion for 6 weeks as noted previously.

b. Exercise

(1) Exercises as described for early postoperative rehabilitation after arthrotomy earlier in this section are begun immediately after surgery while the knee is immobilized. Ambulation with crutches and weight bearing to tolerance are permissible the day after surgery.

(2) Exercises to increase ROM

(a) Active-assisted and active ROM are initiated as soon as the immobilization device is removed.

(b) *Precaution:* Knee flexion is limited to 90 degrees for 7 days

postoperatively to protect the incision.
(3) Exercises to increase strength
    (a) A progression of resisted SLR, multiple-angle isometrics, and resisted isotonic exercises are begun between 7 to 14 days postoperatively.
    (b) Isokinetic exercises are progressed from submaximal to maximal with the patient's response closely monitored.[72]
    (c) Overall, strengthening exercises for the knee are progressed more slowly after open meniscectomy than after arthroscopic meniscectomy.
    (d) **Note:** Most patients tend to regain normal strength of the knee flexors before the knee extensors after meniscectomy.[9]
    (e) Be sure to continue hip-strengthening exercises as the patient progresses through his rehabilitation.
(4) Balance exercises
These may be started when the patient is bearing full weight. The patient can practice quick movements and weight shifts on a tilt board to improve proprioception and balance in a closed kinematic chain (see Figure 12-5).
(5) Functional activities
    (a) Bicycling may be done routinely after 1 month.
    (b) The same precautions apply to jogging as discussed under arthroscopic meniscectomy.

E. Ligament Repair or Reconstruction

1. Indications for surgery[28,30,34,38,64]

a. Acute or chronic lesions of one or several ligamentous structures of the knee, that is, the collaterals, cruciates, oblique, or capsular ligaments.
    (1) Acute injuries that are severe are usually repaired as soon as an accurate diagnosis is made. Acute injuries that are less severe are treated conservatively in the hope that surgery can be avoided.
    (2) Chronic injuries are repaired only after a conservative treatment program of protective weight bearing and exercise has failed.
b. Instability (buckling) of the knee: medial/lateral, anterior/posterior, or rotary (anteromedial, anterolateral, or posterolateral).
c. Pain with weight bearing or joint motion or with specific stress tests.
    (1) Incomplete tears are often associated with a great deal of pain.
    (2) Complete tears may not be painful.[30]
d. Injury to the anterior cruciate ligament (ACL) is the most common ligamentous injury to the knee. The injury may also be coupled with an injury to the medial collateral ligament or medial meniscus.

2. Procedures[6,19,30,34,38,58]

a. The procedures vary with the type of ligamentous lesion, the severity of knee instability, and the philosophy of the surgeon.
b. Most procedures involve an arthrotomy of the knee through a medial parapatellar approach and removal, repair, or reconstruction of pathologic structures.
c. Recently some ligamentous injuries such as partial ACL tears have been managed by arthroscopic repair.[38,54]
d. Repair or reconstruction of the ACL is the most common ligamentous

surgery performed.

(1) Intra-articular surgery for ACL repair may involve a primary repair of the torn ACL fibers or substitution of the ACL with other inert structures from the patient such as part of the patellar tendon, iliotibial band, or semitendinosus tendon. This is known as an *autograft.* Intra-articular repair may also be achieved by use of *prosthetic implants,* such as Gore-Tex, or use of an *allograft,* which is freeze-dried patellar tendon from a cadaver.

(2) Extra-articular repair of the knee after ACL injury may involve transferring an inert structure around the knee, such as the iliotibial (IT) band, to a new position to improve joint stability.

(3) Some surgeries involve intra-articular reconstruction augmented by an extra-articular procedure.

(e) In almost all cases after repair or reconstruction of a ligament, the knee is immobilized for 4 to 8 weeks in a position that places the least amount of stress on the repaired ligaments as it heals.

3. Postoperative management[6,10,18,38,39,44,58,64,72]

Note: Postoperative management of ligamentous repairs usually includes a series of stages or phases beginning with a stage of maximal protection to the repaired tissues. The stages and progression outlined here are simply suggestions to consider in a treatment plan. Many variations and modifications are possible, depending on the type of surgery performed and the philosophy of the surgeon. This outline represents the main concepts of rehabilitation after ligament surgery and an overview of the progression of postoperative activities.

a. **Immobilization after ligament surgery**

(1) Position of immobilization

(a) After ACL reconstruction, some surgeons may immobilize the knee in 30 to 45 degrees of flexion. This position places very little tension on the reconstructed ligament but allows some anterior displacement of the tibia on the femur during quad sets or weight bearing. Other surgeons immobilize the knee in 5 to 10 degrees of knee flexion because this position virtually eliminates anterior displacement of the tibia during quad sets and allows earlier weight bearing

(b) After posterior cruciate ligament (PCL) repair, the knee is immobilized in full extension.

(c) After medial collateral ligament repair, the knee is placed in 20 to 30 degrees of flexion.

(2) Types of immobilization

(a) Long leg cast with the foot enclosed

(b) Hinged cast or hinged long leg brace placed on the patient immediately after surgery or after a period of complete immobilization in a cast. This allows early motion in a safe range but may not fit tightly enough to prevent anterior displacement of the tibia.

(3) Duration of immobilization

(a) After most ligament repairs and reconstructions, the knee is completely immobilized for as little as 1 week or as long as 8 weeks postoperatively to allow time for repaired tissues to heal. The average period of immobilization is 4 to 6 weeks.[6,38]

(b) In a recent study[54] continuous passive motion (CPM) was applied 8 hours per day beginning on the second postoperative day after intra-articular ACL repair. The allowable passive motion was 90 degrees of knee flexion to full extension, or from 90 to 20 degrees of flexion, depending on the type of reconstruction necessary. An equal number of patients with open (arthrotomy) and with closed (arthroscopy) procedures were placed in CPM. The use of early CPM after intra-articular ACL repair was found to be safe and caused no increase in joint effusion or hemarthrosis. CPM was not recommended for 4 weeks after extra-articular repair of the collateral ligament or repair of the meniscus.

(c) A delicate balance exists in the early postoperative period between adequate immobilization to avoid a stretch to the repaired tissues and early knee motion to minimize postoperative contractures, atrophy, and articular degeneration.

(4) Some therapists use electrical stimulation to the thigh muscles through a window in the cast to minimize muscle atrophy during the period of immobilization.

b. **Weight bearing**

(1) After some ligament repairs, the patient must be non–weight bearing on the involved lower extremity for 6 to 8 weeks.

(2) After other surgeries such as arthroscopic repair of the ACL, partial weight bearing may be permitted shortly after surgery while the knee is immobilized in a full leg or hinged cast with locks.

c. **Exercise**

(1) *Stage of maximal protection*

During immobilization, the patient performs quadriceps and hamstrings sets, and straight leg raising in several positions as described earlier in this section on early postoperative rehabilitation (see Section III A 2). If the knee is immobilized in flexion and the patella is accessible, patellar mobilization in a superior direction should be done to prevent *patella baja*. Inferior positioning of the patella can occur when the knee is immobilized in a flexed position for a prolonged period of time and has been identified as a cause of extensor lag.[71]

(2) *Stage of controlled motion*

When the immobilization device is removed or when motion is allowed in a hinged cast or brace, the key to a successful rehabilitation program after ligament repair is a *very slow and cautious* progression of exercise and weight bearing. The primary concern the therapist should have at this time is protection of the reconstructed ligament. Even though early movement will create a stronger, better-oriented scar in the healing ligament, too vigorous exercise or too rapid progression of weight bearing can stretch and damage the repaired structures. This period of protected movement is necessary so that proper vascularization and organization of collagen fibers can occur during healing and so that the tensile strength of the collagen fibers of the ligament can increase.[6,38]

Specific exercises during the stage of controlled motion

(a) Continuation of exercises initiated in the stage of maximal protection such as quadriceps or hamstrings setting and SLR in multiple positions for hip strengthening. Emphasis is placed on hamstrings sets after ACL repair or reconstruction and on quad sets after PCL repair.

(b) In some cases, the patient may begin to bear minimal weight on the operated extremity while the knee is immobilized.

(c) Exercises to increase knee flexion such as *gravity-assisted wall slides* (see Figure 11-5) with the knee in a hinged brace and gravity-assisted knee flexion with the patient sitting in a chair. The lower leg is passively extended to the starting position by the uninvolved leg or by the therapist to avoid excessive quadriceps activity in this early stage of rehabilitation.[6,38]

(d) Exercises to increase knee extension such as active-assisted knee extension within a protected range. A dial lock on the hinged brace or cast can be adjusted weekly so that more active knee extension is possible each week. In most cases after ACL repair, the range of knee extension must be increased more slowly than the range of knee flexion.[44]

(e) Exercises to increase muscle strength such as resisted isometrics and isotonic knee flexion *(hamstring curls)* against light resistance. Emphasis is placed on strengthening the hamstrings more than the quadriceps after ACL repair so that the hamstrings can serve as a dynamic stabilizer to minimize anterior tibial displacement. After PCL repair, the patient should refrain from early hamstrings exercises because the hamstrings pull the tibia posteriorly and could overstretch and damage the repaired ligament.

(3) *Stage of moderate protection*

(a) As the repaired ligament becomes stronger, the patient may begin to bear more weight on the involved lower extremity while the knee is protected in an immobilizer (around 12 to 16 weeks postoperatively).[6,38]

(b) Exercises to increase the strength of the quadriceps after ACL repair can now be initiated and progressed very slowly. Antigravity knee extension and then knee extension against light resistance can now be done safely.

(c) Short-arc *submaximal* velocity spectrum isokinetic exercises can also be initiated late in this stage (16 to 24 weeks postoperatively).

(4) *Stage of minimal protection*

(a) By the end of the fourth to the sixth month postoperatively, stretching can be initiated to decrease any contractures that exist. Even at this point, stretching in the last 5 to 10 degrees of knee extension after ACL repair is usually contraindicated. A reasonable goal for motion during this stage is 120 degrees of knee flexion and 5 to 10 degrees short of full knee extension.

(b) Isokinetic and isotonic exercise against resistance can be progressed. It is still advisable at this time to avoid full knee extension against resistance.

(c) During the period of minimal protection, full weight bearing in a brace (usually a Lenox Hill brace) with the knee in slight flexion is sometimes permissible.

(d) Stationary bicycling or swimming using a flutter kick with emphasis on hip motion can be started for general conditioning.

   (5) *Return to activity*

     (a) By 6 months, the patient may gradually increase his level of functional activities. If full weight bearing was not initiated previously, it is begun at this time.

     (b) Full-arc, active-resisted knee extension is now allowed after ACL repairs. A progression of isotonic and isokinetic exercises is used for the knee and hip muscles.

     (c) A light jogging program may be started at 6 months or when there is no joint effusion and when the patient has regained 75 to 80 percent of strength in the knee musculature. A brace should be worn to provide additional protection to the knee.

     (d) The patient often requires a full year of rehabilitation before returning to a pre-injury level of activity.

     (e) The total rehabilitation time for multiple reconstructions and repairs such as ACL, MCL, and medial meniscus repairs will be at least 1 year.

  d. **Precautions**

    (1) Avoid full weight bearing on the operated extremity until the patient has almost full active knee extension. This will take many weeks because the patient is often immobilized in as much as 45 to 60 degrees of flexion for a 6- to 8-week period of time.

    (2) Achieve active flexion and active extension *very* slowly. It is not unusual for a patient to take 6 to 8 weeks, or even 12 to 16 weeks, after the cast has been removed to achieve full active extension.[6,44]

    (3) Heavy resistance exercise for the knee is not recommended for 3 to 4 months postoperatively. When it is begun, weights should be kept at a very low level (no more than 10 to 15 percent of body weight), emphasizing a high number of repetitions rather than heavy resistance.[44]

    (4) If a weight boot is used for resistance exercise, do not allow the patient's foot and lower leg to dangle, because it will cause stress to the capsular ligaments. Instead, have the patient rest his foot on a footstool when he is in 90 degrees of knee flexion.[44] Isokinetic equipment can also be used to avoid this problem.

    (5) An orthosis is usually worn during progressive ambulation and functional activities to protect the repaired ligament and to compensate for decreased internal stability of the knee.

    (6) Specific precautions during exercise will vary with the type of ligamentous lesion, amount of knee instability, and the exact type of surgical repair or reconstruction. It is the responsibility of the therapist to understand the biomechanics of the reconstruction and discuss any specific precautions for postoperative exercise and weight bearing with the surgeon.

F. Synovectomy of the Knee

  1. **Indications for surgery**[2,21,34,48]

    a. Chronic synovitis secondary to rheumatoid or degenerative arthritis of the knee, that cannot be controlled by medical management

    b. Minimal or no deterioration of the articular surfaces

    c. Joint pain

    d. Decreased range of motion

2. Procedure[21,34,48]

a. A longitudinal incision is made along the anteromedial aspect of the knee to allow access to the anterior and posteromedial compartments of the joint.
b. The capsule and deep fascia are incised.
c. As much of the synovium as possible is removed.
d. A synovectomy can also be performed arthroscopically, using multiple portals.

3. Postoperative management[33,48]

a. The knee is immobilized for several days postoperatively, usually 3 to 5 days, in a bulky, compression dressing and posterior splint.
 (1) During this time, quadriceps-setting exercises and straight leg raising and ankle-pumping exercises may be done.
 (2) Hip abduction and extension exercises can also be done in the knee splint.
b. Ambulation with crutches is begun the first few days after surgery. The patient may bear partial weight on the involved extremity and must wear the splint during ambulation.
c. The splint is removed for exercise, and the patient may begin range of motion exercises of the knee at 3 to 10 days postoperatively.
d. Progressive repetitions of active flexion and extension exercises of the knee, in addition to quadriceps setting and straight leg raising, are carried out several times a day.
e. Exercise and weight bearing are progressed over a 6-week period of time to increase the range of motion and strength of the knee.
f. The patient may return to a full level of functional activities by 6 weeks postoperatively.
g. After arthroscopic synovectomy, the patient is allowed to actively move the knee 1 day postoperatively. The patient may regain full knee extension and at least 90 degrees of flexion within a few days after surgery. He often will require protected weight bearing for only a few days after surgery.[34]

G. Total Knee Replacement

1. Indications for surgery[11,20,21,34,62,67]

a. Severe pain
b. Destruction of articular surfaces of the knee secondary to arthritis
c. Gross instability or limitation of motion
d. Marked deformity of the knee, such as genu varum or genu valgum
e. Failure of a previous surgical procedure

2. Procedures

a. **Background of the development of total knee replacements**
 Prosthetic replacement of one or both surfaces of the knee joint has been seen clinically since the late 1950s and early 1960s.
 (1) MacIntosh[42,43] and then McKeevor[46] suggested replacement of the tibial plateau with an acrylic and, later, a metal implant as a treatment for severe degenerative arthritis and varus or valgus deformities of the knee.
 (2) In 1951, Walldius[36,49,73] developed the first constrained total knee prosthesis, which consisted of a stemmed and hinged (articulated)

metal replacement for the distal femur and proximal tibia. The original design was press-fit into the intramedullary canals. The prosthetic design could be aligned easily and provided its own stability to the knee. Therefore, all the ligaments and soft-tissue stabilizers of the knee were removed. This prosthesis allowed 90 degrees of flexion and full extension of the knee but did not take into account the rotatory motion between the femur and tibia. Consequently, this procedure had a high failure rate because of eventual loosening of the prosthesis. This procedure also required a very long period of complete immobilization after surgery. Today, the hinged prosthesis, which is cemented in place with acrylic cement, is used only in cases of articular destruction with severe joint instability or failure of a previous prosthetic implant.

(3) A nonarticulated, unconstrained, multi-condylar replacement was developed by Gunston[27] in the late 1960s, with all the normal motions of the knee built into the design. This is sometimes referred to as a polycentric or compartmental knee replacement. It consisted of two high-density polyethylene, troughlike tibial components and two inert metal disklike femoral components held in place with acrylic cement.[20,21,34,57,62,67] This condylar resurfacing system allows approximately 130 degrees of knee flexion and full extension. The patient must have intact collateral ligaments, because this type of total knee replacement does not provide its own internal stability. The patient must also have an intact extensor mechanism and a flexion contracture of less than 15 degrees for the procedure to be successful.

(4) Other early designs of nonarticulated knee replacements such as the geometric and the duocondylar knees were made up of two components. These systems consisted of a polyethylene tibial prosthesis and metal femoral prosthesis, also cemented in place with acrylic cement. The nonarticulated design allowed for a small amount of rotation between the tibia and femur and retained the cruciate ligaments. The patellafemoral joint was not resurfaced.

(5) A unicondylar design was developed to resurface only one femoral and one tibial condyle with a metal femoral runner and plastic tibial trough.

(6) Current classifications
Many variations of total knee replacements have been developed from these early designs. Today there are two basic classifications of prostheses: *resurfacing* (unconstrained) and *constrained.*

   (a) *Resurfacing prostheses* can be unicondylar, unicompartmental, bicondylar, or total condylar. Bicondylar and total condylar replacements can be cruciate-retaining or cruciate-existing. The convex femoral component is made of a cobalt-chrome alloy and the concave or flat tibial component is a high-density polyethylene material. In a total condylar replacement, the patella is also resurfaced with a polyethylene dome-shaped component.

   (b) *Constrained protheses* can have a fixed-axis metal hinge or can be somewhat loose (semiconstrained) with some degree of rotation and varus or valgus motions. Constrained replacements are used only in patients with severe joint instability and deterioration.

(7) Fixation

The very early total knee replacements, such as the Walldius hinged prosthesis were press-fit into the intramedullary canals. Gunston was the first to hold his total knee replacements with methylmethacrylate, an acrylic cement. In the 1960s and 1970s, almost all total knee arthroplasties used cement fixation. Some designs, such as the rigid articulated prostheses or replacements with separate tibial components, were prone to loosening at the bone-cement interface.

Biologic cementless fixation utilizes the rapid, postoperative growth of bone into a porous-coated prosthesis.[51,61,62] This type of fixation has been used in some total knee replacements since 1980. One type of prosthesis using biologic fixation is the PCA (porous-coated anatomic) knee replacement developed by Hungerford. To date, there are no long-term studies that have evaluated the effectiveness of biologic fixation. Short-term (up to 5 years) follow-up of patients has shown that biologic fixation is as effective as cemented fixation.[31,32,50,51,61,62]

b. **Overview of the procedures**

(1) A longitudinal incision is made along the anteromedial aspect or midline of the knee.

(2) A synovectomy, if necessary, is performed.

(3) The posterior aspect of the patella may also be resurfaced with a patellar button if the patellofemoral joint has significantly deteriorated.

(4) Implants are held in place with acrylic cement or are coated with a porous metal that allows rapid bony fixation postoperatively.

(5) The knee may be immobilized in a bulky dressing and a posterior splint or in a cylinder cast, which is later bivalved for easy removal prior to ROM exercises, or the patient may be placed on a continuous passive motion (CPM) device immediately after surgery.

3. **Postoperative management**[3,13,20,24,45,48,66,74,75]

a. **Early management during period of immobilization**

(1) The knee is immobilized for several days to several weeks. Most procedures require only a few days of immobilization. In general, cementless arthroplasties must be immobilized for a slightly longer period of time than cemented arthroplasties to allow ingrowth of bone into the prosthesis.

(2) While the patient's knee is immobilized, the following exercises are carried out numerous times each day:

(a) Quadriceps-setting exercise on the first postoperative day

(b) Straight leg raising on the first or second postoperative day

(c) Ankle-pumping exercises immediately after surgery to promote circulation

(3) Ambulation (partial weight bearing with crutches) is begun by the third to fifth day after surgery. The patient must wear the splint or cast during ambulation. The amount of weight bearing is increased over time, based on the patient's tolerance and the type of prosthetic fixation used. Patients who have undergone cementless fixation must limit the intensity and progression of weight bearing more than patients with cemented replacements.

b. **Early management with continuous passive motion (CPM)**[3,22,24]

In the 1980s, CPM has been used extensively after total knee replacement surgery to decrease postoperative pain, promote wound healing, and prevent contractures. In some instances, the patient is placed on the CPM unit in the recovery room. No postoperative immobilization is used. Other surgeons recommend immobilization of the knee for several days, followed by the use of CPM until the patient is discharged. The number of hours per day that the patient is on the CPM device varies. The rate and degrees of movement can be adjusted. In one study,[3] a maximum of 15 hours per day was as effective as 20 hours or more per day. In most situations, CPM is used as an adjunct to, not a replacement for, postoperative physical therapy.

c. **Neuromuscular electrical stimulation**[13]

In an attempt to get the best possible postoperative result after total knee replacement, neuromuscular electrical stimulation is begun as soon as the bulky dressing is removed. Stimulation is applied to the quadriceps and hamstring muscles to minimize muscle atrophy and loss of strength.

d. **Exercises to increase ROM**

When the splint has been removed or when adequate healing has occurred, active ROM exercises can be initiated. Most exercises are done with the patient in a supine position or sitting on the edge of a mat table.

(1) Exercise to increase the range of knee flexion

After a patient has been immobilized with the knee in an extended position, it will be difficult to flex the knee because of soft-tissue pain and muscle spasm. Reciprocal inhibition of the quadriceps is used to decrease muscle spasm in the quadriceps and to increase flexion of the knee.

(2) Exercise to increase the range of knee extension

Active extension of the knee is equally important. Start with the patient in as much knee flexion as is available and have him fully extend the knee actively or with assistance.

Precaution: Passive stretching to increase knee flexion or extension is contraindicated during this very early stage of rehabilitation while the knee is still healing.

e. **Exercises to increase strength**

Sufficient strength for ambulation and for moderate physical activities is also important. A proper balance of strength is needed between the quadriceps and hamstrings.

(1) Quadriceps and hamstrings setting and straight leg raising with weights are continued for several more weeks but are now done outside the splint. Isotonic resistance exercises are contraindicated for several weeks to allow adequate time for soft tissues to heal.

(2) When light weights are used during straight leg-raising, short-arc (terminal) extension, and knee flexion exercises, the emphasis should be placed on low-intensity exercises performed for a high number of repetitions.

Precaution: Heavy resistance exercises are not recommended after a total knee replacement because it places excessive stress on the prosthetic components.

(3) Include resistance exercises to strengthen hip musculature.

(4) Exercise on a stationary bicycle against mild resistance can also

increase muscular and total body endurance. Begin with the bicycle seat raised as high as possible. Progressively lower the seat as the patient develops better knee flexion.

f. Active stretching, using the contract-relax technique or passive stretching using a low-intensity, long duration stretch, may be used to increase motion of the knee after soft tissues have healed, usually by 6 weeks postoperatively.

g. Assistive devices, such as crutches or a cane, are used during ambulation for at least 6 to 12 weeks after surgery.

h. The posterior splint is worn during ambulation, until the patient has full active extension of the knee, and at night for at least 8 to 12 weeks postoperatively.

4. **Expected results**

a. Almost all patients who have total knee replacements report a significant relief of pain with knee motion and weight bearing.

b. A patient is encouraged to achieve functional range of motion of the knee (full active extension and at least 90 degrees of flexion) before or by the time he is discharged from the hospital.

(1) Long-term postoperative follow-up of patients after total knee replacement suggests that improvement of range of motion may be the poorest result of surgery. Patients with very restricted knee motion preoperatively will usually have the poorest ROM postoperatively. Some patients may achieve as little as 45 degrees of motion postoperatively if they have had severe, chronic contractures preoperatively.[26,34,45,66,75]

(2) Therapists have suggested that a more vigorous exercise program after surgery could improve these results.[45,66,75]

c. It may take at least 3 months postoperatively for a patient to regain strength in the quadriceps and hamstrings to a preoperative level. Quadriceps weakness tends to persist longer after total knee arthroplasty than knee flexor weakness. As the patient's level of activity continues to increase, he may see further gains in strength for over a year postoperatively.[66,75]

IV. SUMMARY

The anatomy and kinesiology of knee structure and function were briefly reviewed, including the tibiofemoral and patellofemoral relationships, muscle function, and muscle control of the knee during gait.

Guidelines for therapeutic exercise management of common musculoskeletal problems such as joint, muscle, meniscus, and ligamentous lesions, as well as common surgical procedures for the knee and techniques for pre- and postoperative management, were outlined. Similarities and differences in the management of various surgical procedures and precautions during exercise were delineated.

Descriptions of self-stretching techniques and strengthening procedures for the knee region were described and illustrated in this chapter.

REFERENCES

1. Antich, TJ and Brewster, CE: *Modification of quadriceps femoris muscle exercises during knee rehabilitation.* Phys Ther 66:1246, 1986.

2. Arthritis & Rheumatism Council, British Orthopaedic Association: *Controlled trial of synovectomy of the knee and MCP joints in rheumatoid arthritis.* Ann Rheum Dis 35:437, 1976.
3. Basso, DM and Knapp, L: *Comparison of two continuous passive motion protocols for patients with total knee implants.* Phys Ther 67:360, 1987.
4. Blackburn, T and Craig, E: *Knee anatomy.* Phys Ther 60:1556, 1980.
5. Blackburn, TA, Eiland, WG, and Bandy, WG: *An introduction to the plica.* JOSPT 3:171, 1982.
6. Brewster, CE, Moynes, DR, and Jobe, FW: *Rehabilitation for anterior cruciate reconstruction.* JOSPT 5:121, 1983.
7. Brownstein, BA, Lamb, RL, and Mangine, RE: *Quadriceps, torque, and integrated electromyography.* JOSPT 6:309, 1985.
8. Cailliet, R: *Knee Pain and Disability.* FA Davis, Philadelphia, 1973.
9. Campbell, D and Glenn, W: *Foot-pounds of torque of the normal knee and the rehabilitated postmeniscectomy knee.* Phys Ther 59:418, 1979.
10. Campbell, D and Glenn, W: *Rehabilitation of knee flexor and knee extensor muscle strength in patients with meniscectomies, ligamentous repairs and chondromalacia.* Phys Ther 62:10, 1982.
11. Convery, RF: *Total knee arthroplasty: Indications, evaluation and post-operative management.* Clin Orthop 94:42, 1973.
12. Costill, DL, Fink, WJ, and Habansky, AJ: *Muscle rehabilitation after knee surgery.* The Physician and Sports Med 5:71, 1977.
13. Coutts, RD, Stewart, WT, et al: *The effect of muscle stimulation in the rehabilitation of patients following total knee replacement.* In Rand, JA and Dorr, LD (eds): *Total Arthroplasty of the Knee: Proceedings of the Knee Society, 1985–1986.* Aspen Publishers, Rockville, MD, 1987.
14. Coventry, MB, et al: *A new geometric knee for total knee arthroplasty.* Clin Orthop 83:157, 1972.
15. Currier, D: *Evaluation of the use of a wedge in quadriceps strengthening.* Phys Ther 55:870, 1975.
16. Cyriax, J: *Textbook of Orthopaedic Medicine, Volume One. Diagnosis of Soft Tissue Lesions,* ed 8. Bailliere Tindall, London, 1982.
17. Davies, G, Malone, T, and Bassett, F: *Knee examination.* Phys Ther 60:1565, 1980.
18. DePalma, BF and Zelko, RR: *Rehabilitation following anterior cruciate ligament surgery.* Athletic Train 21:200, 1986.
19. Erikson, E: *Reconstruction of the anterior cruciate ligament.* Orthop Clin North Am 7:167, 1976.
20. Fortune, WP: *Lower limb joint replacement.* In Nickel, VL (ed): *Orthopedic Rehabilitation.* Churchill-Livingstone, New York, 1982.
21. Freeman, MAR: *Arthritis of the knee: Clinical features and surgical management.* Springer-Verlag, New York, 1980.
22. Goll, SR, Lotke, PA, and Ecker, ML: *Failure of CPM as prophylaxis against deep venous thrombosis after total knee arthroplasty.* In Rand, JA and Dorr, LD (eds): *Total Arthroplasty of the Knee.* Aspen Publishers, Rockville, MD, 1987.
23. Goodfellow, J, Hungerford, D, and Woods, C: *Patellofemoral joint mechanics and pathology of chondromalacia patellae.* J Bone Joint Surg 58(Br): 291, 1976.
24. Gose, JC: *CPM in the postoperative treatment of patients with total knee replacements.* Phys Ther 67:39, 1987.
25. Grood, ES, et al: *Biomechanics of the knee: Extension exercise.* J Bone Joint Surg 66A:725, 1984.
26. Gunston, FH: *Complications of polycentric knee arthroplasty.* Clin Orthop 120:11, 1976.
27. Gunston, FH: *Polycentric knee arthroplasty: Prosthetic stimulation of normal knee movement.* J Bone Joint Surg 53(Br):272, 1971.
28. Helfet, AJ: *Disorders of the Knee.* JB Lippincott, Philadelphia, 1982.
29. Hoppenfeld, S: *Physical Examination of the Spine and Extremities.* Appleton-Century-Crofts, New York, 1976.
30. Hughston, JC: *Knee surgery: A philosophy.* Phys Ther 60:1611, 1980.
31. Hungerford, DS, Krackhow, KA, and Kenna, RV: *Two to five years experience with cementless, porous-coated total knee prosthesis.* In Rand, JA and Dorr, LD (eds): *Total Arthroplasty of the Knee.* Aspen Publishers, Rockville, MD, 1987.

32. Hungerford, DS, Kenna, RV, and Krackhow, KA; *The porous-coated anatomic total knee.* Orthop Clin North Am 13:103, 1982.
33. Hyde, SA: *Physiotherapy in Rheumatology.* Blackwell Scientific Publications, Oxford, 1980.
34. Insall, JN: *Surgery of the Knee.* Churchill-Livingstone, New York, 1984.
35. Kapandji, IA: *The Physiology of the Joints,* Vol. II. Churchill-Livingstone, Edinburgh, 1970.
36. Kluge, L: *The Walldius prosthesis: A total treatment program.* Phys Ther 52:26, 1972.
37. Kegerreis, S, Malone, T, and Ohnson, F: *The diagonal medical plica: An underestimated clinical entity.* JOSPT 9:305, 1988.
38. King, S and Butterwick, D: *The anterior cruciate ligament: A review of recent concepts.* JOSPT 8:110, 1986.
39. Kuland, DN: *The Injured Athlete,* ed 2. JB Lippincott, Philadelphia, 1988.
40. Lemkuhl, LD and Smith, LK: *Brunnstrom's Clinical Kinesiology,* ed 4. FA Davis, Philadelphia, 1983.
41. Lennington, KR and Yanchuleff, TT: *The use of isokinetics in the treatment of chondromalacia patellae—A case report.* JOSPT 4:176, 1983.
42. MacIntosh, DL and Hunter, GA: *The use of the hemiarthroplasty prosthesis for advanced osteoarthritis and rheumatoid arthritis of the knee.* J Bone Joint Surg 54(Br):244, 1972.
43. MacIntosh, DL: *Hemiarthroplasty of the knee using a space-occupying prosthesis for painful varus and valgus deformities.* J Bone Joint Surg (Am) 40:1431, 1958.
44. Malone, T, Blackburn, R, and Wallace, L: *Knee rehabilitation.* Phys Ther 60:1602, 1980.
45. Manske, PR and Gleason, P: *Rehabilitation program following polycentric total knee arthroplasty.* Phys Ther 57:915, 1977.
46. McKeaver, DC: *Tibial plateau prosthesis.* Clin Orthop 18:86, 1960.
47. McLeod, W and Hunter, S: *Biomechanical analysis of the knee.* Phys Ther 60:1561, 1980.
48. Melvin, J: *Rheumatic Disease: Occupational Therapy And Rehabilitation,* ed 2. FA Davis, Philadelphia, 1982.
49. Merriweather, R: *Total knee replacement: The Walldius arthroplasty.* Orthop Clin North Am 4:585, 1973.
50. Miller, J: *Fixation in total knee arthroplasty.* In Insall, JN: *Surgery of the Knee.* Churchill-Livingstone, New York, 1984.
51. Morrey, RD and Kavanagh, BF: *Cementless joint replacement: Current status and future.* Bull Rheum Dis 37:1, 1987.
52. Norkin, C and Levangie, P: *Joint Structure and Function: A Comprehensive Analysis.* FA Davis, Philadelphia, 1983.
53. *Normal and Pathological Gait Syllabus.* Physical Therapy Department, Rancho Los Amigos Hospital, Downey, California, 1977.
54. Noynes, FR and Mangine, RE: *Early knee motion after open and arthroscopic anterior cruciate ligament reconstruction.* Am J Sports Med 15:149, 1987.
55. O'Donoghue, DH: *Meniscectomy: Indications and management.* Phys Ther 60:1617, 1980.
56. Outerbridge, RE, and Dunlop, J: *The problem of chondromalacia patellae.* Clin Orthop Rel Res 110:177, 1975.
57. Paradis, D and Hamlin, C: *Geometric and polycentric knee prosthesis.* Phys Ther 53:762, 1973.
58. Paulos, L, et al: *Knee rehabilitation after anterior cruciate ligament reconstruction and repair.* Am J Sports Med 9:140, 1981.
59. Paulos L, Rusche, K, Johnson, C, et al: *Patellar malalignment: A treatment rationale.* Phys Ther 60:1624, 1980.
60. Pevsner, D, Johnson, J, and Blazina, M: *The patellofemoral joint and its implications in the rehabilitation of the knee.* Phys Ther 59:869, 1979.
61. Rand, JA, Bryan, RS, and Chao, EYS: *A comparison of cemented versus cementless porous-coated anatomic total knee arthroplasty.* In Rand, JA and Dorr, LD (eds): *Total Arthroplasty of the Knee.* Aspen Publishers, Rockville, MD, 1987.
62. Rand, JA and Dorr, LD (eds): *Total Arthroplasty of the Knee: Proceedings of the Knee Society, 1985–1986.* Aspen Publishers, Rockville, MD, 1987.
63. Riley, LH: *Geometric total knee replacement.* Orthop Clin North Am 4:561, 1973.
64. Sandor, SM, Hart, JAL, and Oakes, BW: *Case study: Rehabilitation of a surgically repaired medial collateral knee ligament using a limited motion cast and isokinetic exercise.* JOSPT

7:154, 1986.

65. Skolnick, MD, Coventry, MB, and Ilstrop, OM: *Geometric total knee arthroplasty.* J Bone Joint Surg 58(Am):749, 1976.

66. Smidt, GL, Albright, JP and Deusinger, RH: *Pre- and postoperative functional changes in total knee patients.* JOSPT 6:25, 1984.

67. Sonstegard, D, et al: *The surgical replacement of the human knee joint.* Scientific American 238:1, 1978.

68. Sprague, R: *Factors related to extension lag at the knee joint.* JOSPT 3:178, 1982.

69. Steindler, A: *Kinesiology of the Human Body Under Normal and Pathological Conditions.* Charles C Thomas, Springfield, Ill, 1955.

70. Stratford, P: *Electromyography of the quadriceps femoris muscles in subjects with normal and acutely effused knees.* Phys Ther 62:279, 1982.

71. Tamburello, et al: *Patella hypomobility as a cause of extensor lag.* Research presentation, Overland Park, KS, May 1985.

72. Timm, KE and Patch, DG: *Case study: Use of Cybex II velocity spectrum in the rehabilitation of postsurgical knees.* JOSPT 6:347, 1985.

73. Walldius, B: *Arthroplasty of the knee using an endoprosthesis.* Acta Orthop Scand 30:137, 1960.

74. Waters, EA: *Physical therapy management of patients with total knee replacement.* Phys Ther 54:936, 1974.

75. Wigren, A, et al: *Isokinetic muscle strength and endurance after knee arthroplasty with the modular knee in patients with osteoarthritis and rheumatoid arthritis.* Scand J Rheum 12:145, 1983.

76. Zarins, B: *Arthroscopy and arthroscopic surgery.* Bull Rheum Dis 34:1, 1984.

CHAPTER ——————————— 12

THE ANKLE AND FOOT

The joints and muscles of the ankle and foot are designed to provide stability as well as mobility in the terminal structures of the lower extremity. The foot must bear the body weight when standing, with a minimum of muscle energy expenditure. The foot also must be able to adapt in order to absorb forces and to accommodate uneven surfaces, and then it must be able to become a rigid structural lever to propel the body forward when walking or running.

The anatomy and kinesiology of the ankle and foot are complex, but it is important to understand them in order to effectively treat problems in that area. The first section of this chapter reviews highlights of these areas that the reader should know and understand. For greater depth and explanation, the reader is referred to several texts and articles for study of the material.[2,15,17,19,30,32] Chapter 6 presents information on principles of management; the reader should be familiar with that material before proceeding with establishing a therapeutic exercise program for the ankle and foot.

OBJECTIVES

After studying this chapter, the reader will be able to:
1. identify important aspects of the structure and function of the ankle and foot for review.
2. establish a therapeutic exercise program to manage soft-tissue and joint lesions in the ankle and foot related to stages of recovery following an inflammatory insult to the tissues.
3. establish a therapeutic exercise program to manage common musculoskeletal lesions, recognizing unique circumstances in the ankle and foot for their management.
4. establish a therapeutic exercise program to manage common surgical procedures in the ankle and foot.

I. **REVIEW OF THE STRUCTURE AND FUNCTION OF THE ANKLE AND FOOT**

A. **Bony Parts (see Figures 5-48 and 5-57)**

   1. **Leg**
      Tibia and fibula

   2. **Hindfoot (posterior segment)**
      Talus and calcaneus

   3. **Midfoot (middle segment)**
      Navicular, cuboid, and three cuneiforms

   4. **Forefoot (anterior segment)**
      Five metatarsals and 14 phalanges, which make up the 5 toes (3 phalanges for each toe except the large toe, which has 2 phalanges).

B. **Motions of the Foot and Ankle**

   1. **Primary plane motions defined**
      a. Sagittal plane motion is *dorsiflexion* (in a dorsal direction) and *plantarflexion* (in a plantar direction)
      b. Frontal plane motion is *inversion* (turning inward) and *eversion* (turning outward)
      c. Transverse plane motion is *abduction* (away from midline) and *adduction* (toward the midline)

   2. **Triplanar motions occurring about oblique axes defined**
      a. *Pronation* is a combination of dorsiflexion, eversion, and abduction.
      b. *Supination* is a combination of plantarflexion, inversion, and adduction.
      Note: The terms inversion and supination, as well as eversion and pronation, are often interchanged.[32] This text will use the terms as defined above.

C. **Joints and Their Characteristics**

   1. **The tibiofibular joints**
      Anatomically, the superior and inferior tibiofibular joints are separate from the ankle but provide accessory motions, which allow greater movement at the ankle; fusion or immobility in these joints may impair ankle function.
      a. *Superior tibiofibular joint*
         A plane synovial joint made up of the fibular head and a facet on the posterolateral aspect of the rim of the tibial condyle; the facet faces posteriorly, inferiorly, and laterally.
      b. *Inferior tibiofibular joint*
         A syndesmosis with fibroadipose tissue between the two bony surfaces; it is supported by the crural tibiofibular interosseous ligament and the anterior and posterior tibiofibular ligaments.
      c. With dorsiflexion and plantarflexion of the ankle, there are slight accessory movements of the fibula.[15]
         (1) As the ankle plantarflexes, the lateral malleolus (fibula) rotates medially and is pulled inferiorly, and the two malleoli approximate. At the superior joint, the fibula slides inferiorly. The opposite occurs with dorsiflexion.

(2) As the foot supinates, the head of the fibula slides distally and posteriorly (external rotation); with pronation, the head of the fibula slides proximally and anteriorly (internal rotation).

2. The ankle (talotibial) joint

This is a synovial hinge joint supported by a structurally strong mortice and medial (deltoid) and lateral collateral ligaments (anterior and posterior talofibular and calcaneofibular ligaments).

a. The concave articulating surface is the mortice, which is made up of the distal tibia and the tibial and fibular malleoli. The fibular malleolus extends further distally than the tibial malleolus. The combined surfaces are congruent with the body of the talus. Integrity of the mortice is provided by the tibiofibular joints and their associated ligaments.

b. The convex articulating surface is the body of the talus. The surface is wedge-shaped, being wider anteriorly, and is also cone-shaped, with the apex pointing medially. As a result, when the foot dorsiflexes, the talus also abducts and slightly everts; and when the foot plantar flexes, the talus also adducts and slightly inverts around an oblique axis.

c. With physiologic motions of the foot, the body of the talus slides in the opposite direction.

Physiologic Motion	*Direction of Slide of the Talus*
Dorsiflexion	Posterior
Plantarflexion	Anterior

See also accessory motions of the fibula listed in section 1 c above.

3. Subtalar (talocalcaneal) joint

This is a uniaxial joint with an oblique axis of motion lying approximately 42 degrees from the transverse plane and 16 degrees from the sagittal plane, which allows the calcaneus to pronate and supinate in a triplanar motion on the talus. Frontal plane inversion (turning heel inward) and eversion (turning heel outward) can be isolated only with passive motion. The subtalar joint is supported by the medial and lateral collateral ligaments, which support the talocrural joint; by the interosseous talocalcaneal ligament in the tarsal canal; and by the posterior and lateral talocalcaneal ligaments. In closed-chain activities, the joint attenuates the rotatory forces between the leg and foot so that normally there is not excessive inward or outward turning of the foot.

a. There are three articulations between the talus and calcaneus; the posterior is separated from the anterior and middle by the tarsal canal. The canal divides the subtalar joint into two joint cavities.

b. The posterior articulation has its own capsule; the facet on the bottom of the talus is concave, whereas the opposing facet on the calcaneus is convex.

c. The anterior articulations are enclosed in the same capsule as the talonavicular articulation, forming the talocalcaneonavicular joint.[30] Functionally, these articulations work together. The facets of the anterior and middle articulations on the talus are convex, whereas the opposing facets on the calcaneus are concave.

d. With physiologic motions of the subtalar joint, the convex posterior portion of the calcaneus slides opposite to the motion; the concave anterior and middle facets on the calcaneus slide in the same direction.

Physiologic Motion	Direction of Slide of Posterior Articulation
Supination with inversion	Lateral
Pronation with eversion	Medial

4. Talonavicular joint

Anatomically and functionally part of the talocalcaneonavicular joint, this joint is supported by the spring, the deltoid, the bifurcate, and the dorsal talonavicular ligaments. The triplanar motions of the navicular on the talus function with the subtalar joint resulting in pronation and supination. With pronation, the accessory motions of the navicular are dorsal sliding with abduction and eversion. The opposite accessory motions occur with supination. Supination results in an increased medial longitudinal arch; pronation results in a decreased medial longitudinal arch.

a. The head of the talus is convex; the proximal articulating surface of the navicular is concave.
b. With physiologic motions of the foot, the navicular slides in the same direction as the motion of the forefoot.
c. In the weight-bearing foot (closed chain), the motions of the talus and navicular are in the opposite directions, so that if the head of the talus drops plantarward and rotates medially, the navicular slides dorsally and rotates laterally.

Physiologic Motion of the Foot	Direction of Slide of the Navicular on the Head of the Talus
Supination	Plantar (and medial)
Pronation	Dorsal (and lateral)

5. Transverse tarsal joint

A functionally compound joint including the anatomically separate talonavicular and calcaneocuboid joints.

a. *Talonavicular joint* (see Section 4 above).
b. The *calcaneocuboid joint* is saddle-shaped. The articulating surface of the calcaneus is convex in a dorsal to plantar direction and concave in a medial to lateral direction; the articulating surface of the cuboid is reciprocally concave and convex.
c. The transverse tarsal joint participates in the triplanar pronation-supination activities of the foot and makes compensatory movements to accommodate variations in the ground. Passive accessory motions include abduction-adduction, inversion-eversion, and dorsal-plantar gliding.

6. The remaining intertarsal and tarsometatarsal joints

These are plane joints whose functions reinforce those of the hind foot (see Section D).

7. **The metatarsophalangeal (MTP) and interphalangeal (IP) joints of the toes**

These joints are the same as the metacarpophalangeal and interphalangeal joints of the hand except that, in the toes, extension range of motion is more important than flexion (the opposite is true in the hand). Extension of the MTP joints is necessary for normal walking. Also, the large toe does not function separately as does the thumb.

D. Functional Relationships of the Ankle and Foot

1. Normally, an external torsion exists in the tibia, so that the ankle mortice faces approximately 15 degrees outward.[12] With dorsiflexion, the foot moves up and slightly laterally; with plantarflexion, the foot moves down and medially.[30] Dorsiflexion is the closed-pack, stable position of the talocrural joint. Plantarflexion is the loose-pack position. This joint is more vulnerable to injury when walking in high heels due to the less stable plantarflexed position.

2. In a closed-chain, weight-bearing foot, supination of the subtalar and transverse tarsal joints with a pronation twist of the forefoot (plantarflexion of the first and dorsiflexion of the fifth metatarsals) increases the arch of the foot and is the closed-pack or stable position of the joints of the foot. This is the position the foot assumes when a rigid lever is needed for propelling the body forward during the push off phase of ambulation.[30]

3. During weight bearing, pronation of the subtalar and transverse tarsal joints causes the arch of the foot to lower, and there is a relative supination of the forefoot with dorsiflexion of the first and plantarflexion of the fifth metatarsals. This is the loose-pack or mobile position of the foot and is assumed when the foot absorbs the impact of weight bearing and rotational forces of the rest of the lower extremity, and when the foot conforms to the ground.[30]

4. In the weight-bearing foot, subtalar motion and tibial rotation are interdependent. Supination of the subtalar joint results in or is caused by lateral rotation of the tibia, and conversely, pronation of the subtalar joint results in or is caused by medial rotation of the tibia.

5. The arches of the foot are visualized as a twisted osteoligamentous plate,[30] with the metatarsal heads being the horizontally placed anterior edge of the plate, and the calcaneus being the vertically placed posterior edge. The twist causes the longitudinal and transverse arches. When bearing weight, the plate tends to untwist and flatten the arches slightly.

   a. Primary support of the arches comes from the spring ligament, with additional support from the long plantar ligament, the plantar aponeurosis, and short plantar ligament. During push off in gait, as the foot plantarflexes and supinates and the metatarsal phalangeal joints go into extension, increased tension is placed on the plantar aponeurosis, which helps increase the arch (windlass effect).

   b. In the normal static foot, muscles do little to support the arches. They contribute to support during ambulation.

6. A person with a varus deformity of the calcaneus (observed non–weight bearing) may compensate by standing with a pronated (or everted) calcaneus posture. *Pes planus, pronated foot,* and *flat foot* are terms often interchanged to mean a pronated posture of the hindfoot and decreased medial longitudinal arch. *Pes cavus* and *supinated foot* describe a high-arched foot.[32]

E. Muscle Function in the Ankle and Foot

1. Plantarflexion is primarily caused by the two-joint gastrocnemius muscle and the one-joint soleus muscle; they attach to the calcaneus via the Achilles tendon.
2. Other muscles passing posterior to the axis of motion for plantarflexion contribute little to that motion, but they do have other functions:
   a. Tibialis posterior is a strong supinator and invertor that helps to control and reverse pronation during gait.
   b. Flexor hallucis longus and flexor digitorum longus flex the toes and help support the medial longitudinal arch. To prevent clawing of the toes (MTP extension with IP flexion), intrinsic muscles must also function at the MTP joints.
   c. Peroneus longus and brevis primarily evert the foot, and the longus gives support to the transverse and lateral longitudinal arches.
3. Dorsiflexion of the ankle is caused by the tibialis anterior muscle (which also inverts the ankle), the extensor hallucis longus and extensor digitorum longus muscles (which also extend the toes), and the peroneus tertius.
4. Intrinsic muscles of the foot are similar to the hand in the functioning of the toes (except there is no thumblike function in the foot), and they also provide support of the arches during gait.
5. In normal standing, the gravitational line falls anterior to the axis of the ankle joint, creating a dorsiflexion moment. The soleus muscle contracts to counter the gravitational moment through its pull on the tibia. Other extrinsic foot muscles help stabilize the foot during postural sway.
6. The ankle and foot during gait[30,31]
   a. During the normal gait cycle, the ankle goes through a range of motion of 35 degrees; 15 degrees of dorsiflexion occurs at the end of mid-stance and 20 degrees of plantarflexion occurs at the end of stance.
   b. Shock-absorbing, terrain-conforming, and propulsion functions of the ankle and foot.
      (1) From heel strike to foot flat (loading response), the anterior tibialis muscle contracts to control the foot as it lowers to the ground and also to untwist the forefoot to its loose-pack position.[19] The entire lower extremity rotates inward, which reinforces the loose-pack position of the foot. With the joints in a lax position, they can conform to variations in the ground contour as the foot is lowered and absorb some of the impact forces.
      (2) Once the foot is fixed on the ground, dorsiflexion begins as the tibia comes up over the foot; the tibia continues to rotate internally, which reinforces pronation of the subtalar joint and loose-pack position of the foot.
      (3) During mid-stance, the tibia begins to rotate externally, which initiates supination of the hindfoot and locking of the transverse tarsal joint. This brings the foot into its closed-pack position, which is reinforced as the plantar aponeurosis tightens. This stable position converts the foot into a rigid lever, ready to propel the body forward as the ankle plantarflexes from the pull of the gastrocsoleus muscle group.
   c. Muscle control of the ankle during gait
      (1) The ankle dorsiflexors function during the initial foot contact and loading response (heel strike to foot flat) to counter the plantarflex-

ion torque and to control the lowering of the foot to the ground. They also function during the swing phase to keep the foot from plantarflexing and dragging on the ground. With loss of the dorsiflexors, foot slap occurs at initial foot contact, and the hip and knee flex excessively during swing (or else the toe drags on the ground).

(2) The ankle plantarflexors begin functioning near the end of midstance and during terminal stance and pre-swing (heel off to toe off) to control the rate of forward movement of the tibia and also to plantarflex the ankle for push off. Loss of function results in slight lag of the lower extremity during terminal stance with no push off.

F. Major Nerves Subject to Pressure and Trauma[21]

1. Common peroneal nerve

After it bifurcates from the sciatic nerve, it passes between the biceps femoris tendon and lateral head of the gastrocnemius muscle then comes laterally around the fibular neck and passes through an opening in the peroneus longus muscle. Pressure or force against the nerve in this region can cause a neuropathy. Sensory changes occur in the distal lateral surface of the leg and dorsum of the foot (except the little toe); muscles affected may include the dorsiflexors of the ankle and evertors of the foot (peroneus longus and brevis, tibialis anterior, extensor digitorum longus and brevis, extensor hallucis longus, and peroneus tertius).

2. Posterior tibial nerve

Occupies a groove behind the medial malleolus along with the tendons of the tibialis posterior, flexor and flexor d. longus muscles; the groove is covered by a ligament, forming a tunnel. Entrapment usually from a space-occupying lesion is known as a tarsal tunnel syndrome. Sensory innervation includes the plantar surface of the foot and toes and the dorsum of the distal phalanges. Muscles affected include intrinsic muscles of the foot (abductor hallucis, flexor hallucis brevis, lumbricals, interossei, and quadratus plantae); weakness and postural changes in the foot (pes cavus and clawing of the toes) may occur.

3. Plantar and calcaneal nerves

These branches of the posterior tibial nerve may become entrapped as they turn under the medial aspect of the foot and pass through openings in the abductor hallucis muscle. Overpronation presses the nerves against these openings. Irritation of the nerves may elicit symptoms similar to acute foot strain (tenderness at the posteromedial plantar aspect of the foot), painful heel (inflamed calcaneal nerve), and pain in a pes cavus foot. The degree of muscle weakness will depend on which of the branches is involved.

II. GUIDELINES AND THERAPEUTIC EXERCISE MANAGEMENT OF COMMON MUSCULOSKELETAL PROBLEMS IN THE ANKLE AND FOOT

Note: Exercises applied to the ankle and foot during acute, subacute, and chronic phases of inflammation and healing follow the principles described in Chapter 6, taking into account the unique anatomic and kinesiologic relationships of the region. This section will expand on the general guidelines.

A. Joint Problems and Restrictions

1. Clinical picture (general)

a. With arthritic joint involvement in the ankle, passive plantarflexion is more limited than dorsiflexion (unless the gastrocsoleus muscle group is also tight, then dorsiflexion will be limited accordingly). In the subtalar joint, there is progressive limitation of supination until eventually the joint fixes in pronation. The transverse tarsal joint reinforces the pronation and flattening of the medial longitudinal arch, so that the closed-pack position of the tarsals (supination) becomes more and more difficult to assume during the push-off phase of gait. Involvement of the first metatarsophalangeal joint results in gross limitation of extension and some limitation of flexion; the other joints are variable.[3]

b. Following periods of immobility, depending on the reason for immobilization and length of time, the joints and soft-tissue structures around the joints loose their mobility. Loss of mobility in the proximal and distal tibofibular joints will also limit ankle and subtalar joint motion.[22]

2. Rheumatoid arthritis (RA)

RA commonly affects the subtalar and other joints of the foot, leading to painful deformities that increase with the stress of weight bearing. Joint swelling and increased warmth are present over the involved joints (see Chapter 6, Section VII for general discussion of RA). Common deformities of the foot include[6]

a. **Pronated foot**

Instability leading to malalignment of the subtalar and talonavicular joints shifts weight bearing medially. This increases the depression of the medial longitudinal arch and outward rotation of the calcaneus. The foot becomes unable to supinate and thus cannot develop the rigid lever necessary for push off during gait.

b. **Hallux valgus**

The phalanges of the great toe shift laterally toward the second toe. Eventually the flexor and extensor muscles of the great toe shift laterally and further accentuate the deformity. The bursa over the medial aspect of the metatarsal head may become inflamed, causing a painful bunion.

c. **Dorsal dislocation of the proximal phalanges on the metatarsal heads**

This causes the fat pad, which is normally under the metatarsal heads, to migrate dorsally with the phalanges and thus the protective cushion on weight bearing is lost, leading to pain, callus formation, and potential ulceration.

d. **Claw toe** (MTP hyperextension and IP flexion) **and hammer toe** (MTP hyperextension, PIP flexion, and DIP hyperextension)

These result from muscle imbalances in the flexors and extensors of the toes. Friction from shoes may cause calluses to form where the toes rub.

3. Other forms of arthritis that affect the feet

Symptoms of arthritis may occur from a variety of causes such as

a. traumatic arthritis; seen with ankle sprains or overuse syndromes in the foot

    b. osteoarthritis, degenerative joint disease (DJD); seen in joints that are continually traumatized

    c. gout; commonly affecting the great toe

4. Management of joint problems and restrictions

Management will depend on the signs and symptoms present. Follow the general outline as presented in Chapter 6 for acute, subacute, and chronic joint problems. Protection from deforming weight-bearing forces and additional trauma imposed by improperly fitting footwear is an integral part of managing arthritis in the ankles and feet. Use of orthotics and well-constructed shoes may be necessary to help protect the joints by realigning forces or providing support from faulty foot postures.[26,27]

    a. **Procedures to manage acute symptoms**

        (1) Treat the pain and maintain mobility with Grade I or II distraction and oscillation techniques.

        (2) Gentle cross-fiber massage to associated ligaments will keep them mobile while the joint is restricted in movement.

        (3) Decrease mechanical stress with use of assistive devices for ambulation.

        (4) Active-assistive (or active, if tolerated) ROM through the available range; no stretch force or resistance is used when acute.

        (5) Muscle-setting to associated muscles

    b. **Procedures to manage subacute and chronic joint or capsular restrictions in the ankle and foot**

        (1) Evaluate for signs of muscle tightness, joint restrictions, or muscle weakness, and initiate exercises and mobilization procedures at a level appropriate for the condition of the patient.

        (2) To increase mobility of the talocrural joint

            (a) general mobility: joint traction (see Figure 5-58)

            (b) to increase plantarflexion: anteriorly glide the talus (see Figure 5-60)

            (c) to increase dorsiflexion: posteriorly glide the talus (see Figure 5-59)

            (d) to increase accessory motions of the fibula: anteriorly glide the fibular head (see Figure 5-55) and glide the fibular malleolus (see Figure 5-56)

        (3) To increase mobility of the subtalar joint

            (a) general mobility: joint traction (see Figure 5-61)

            (b) to increase inversion: laterally glide the calcaneus (see Figure 5-62B)

            (c) to increase eversion: medially glide the calcaneus (see Figure 5-62A)

        (4) To increase mobility of intertarsal and tarsometatarsal joints

            (a) for the accessory motion of plantarflexion, necessary for supination and increasing the longitudinal arches: plantar glide the distal articulating bone on the stablized proximal bone at the restricted joint (see Figure 5-62).

            (b) for the accessory motion of dorsiflexion, necessary for pronation and decreasing the longitudinal arches: dorsal glide the distal articulating bone on the stabilized proximal bone at the restricted joint (see Figure 5-63).

(5) To increase mobility of the MTP and IP joints of the toes, glide the distal articulating bone on the stabilized proximal bone in the direction of restriction, as is done with the joints of the fingers (see Figures 5-41, 5-42, and 5-43).

(6) To increase mobility in the soft tissue and muscles once joint play is available, passive stretching and active inhibition techniques are done as described in Chapter 4. Self-stretching techniques are described later in this chapter.

(7) To regain a balance in muscle strength, begin resistive exercises at a level appropriate for the weakened muscles. Begin with isometric resistance in pain-free positions and progress to isotonics through pain-free ranges. Additional resistive exercises are described later in this chapter.

(8) To protect the joint from deforming forces in degenerative or systemic arthritic conditions, proper orthotic devices should be fabricated to support the patient's foot, and proper shoe fit should be emphasized. Continued use of assistive devices for ambulation may be necessary.

(9) To stimulate balance and proprioception, use of a balance or rocker board may be beneficial.

B. Sprains and Minor Tears of Ligaments

1. Clinical picture

Following trauma, the ligaments of the ankle may be stressed or torn. The most common type of ankle sprain is caused by an inversion stress and can result in a partial or complete tear of the anterior talofibular ligament;[13,18] the posterior talofibular ligament is torn only with massive inversion stresses. If the inferior tibiofibular ligaments are torn following stress to the ankle, the mortice becomes unstable. Rarely do the components of the deltoid ligament become stressed; there is greater likelihood of an avulsion from or fracture of the medial malleolus with an eversion stress. Depending on the severity, the joint capsule may also be involved resulting in symptoms of acute (traumatic) arthritis. The patient feels pain when the injured ligament is stressed; with a complete tear, excessive motion is detected. Many people also experience a kinesthetic deficit manifested as decreased ability to perceive passive motion and increased balance problems following sprains.[9]

2. Management

See Chapter 6 for principles of treatment during stages of inflammation and repair.

a. Acute injury

(1) If possible, evaluate and treat the problem before swelling or joint effusion begins. To minimize the swelling use compression, elevation, and cold.

(2) Grades I and II (mild and moderate) sprains do not cause gross instability of the ankle and are treated conservatively. The ankle is usually immobilized in neutral or in slight dorsiflexion and eversion.

(3) While symptoms are acute, decrease the stress of weight bearing with crutches for ambulation.[34,42]

b. **Subacute and chronic**

(1) As the acute symptoms decrease, continue to provide protection for the involved ligament with a splint. Fabricating a stirrup out of thermoplastic material and holding it in place with an elastic wrap or Velcro straps provide stability to the joint structures while allowing for the stimulus of weight bearing for proprioceptive feedback and proper healing.[34] Commercial splints such as an air splint are also available to provide medial-lateral stability while allowing dorsiflexion and plantarflexion.[20]

(2) Begin cross-fiber massage to the ligaments as tolerated.

(3) Use joint mobilization techniques to maintain or regain mobility of the joint.

(4) As the swelling decreases, increase flexibility. Begin mild passive stretching to the healing ligament by having the patient actively move the ankle opposite the line of pull of the ligament within the pain-free range. For the anterior talofibular ligament, the motion would be plantarflexion and inversion. Stretch to the gastrocsoleus muscle group is important so that adequate dorsiflexion can be obtained. Progress the stretching to weight-bearing stretches (see Section C) as indicated by the patient's recovery.

(5) Increase strength in the supporting muscles. Resistance exercises to the peroneal muscles are important for lateral ankle support.[17] Any other muscles that test weak on evaluation should also be strengthened. (See Section C for exercise suggestions.)

(6) Training to improve proprioceptive feedback for ankle stability, coordination, and reflex response begins with use of a rocker or balance board and progresses to other balance activities. (See Section E for additional suggestions.) Depending on the final goals for rehabilitation, train the ankle when weight-bearing activities such as walking, jogging, and running, and agility activities such as controlled twisting, turning, and lateral weight shifting.

(7) When the patient is involved in sports activities, the ankle should be splinted, taped, or wrapped and proper shoes should be worn to protect the ligament from reinjury.[17]

C. Muscle Strength and Flexibility Imbalance

Note: Causes of strength and flexibility imbalances in the ankle and foot include disuse, nerve injury, and progressive joint degeneration. In addition, imbalances occur from the weight-bearing stresses that are imposed on the feet. Imbalances can be the cause or the effect of faulty lower extremity mechanics. Because the lower extremities bear weight, realignment by strengthening exercises alone is of limited value. Exercising done in conjunction with conscious correction, appropriate stretching, and other necessary measures (such as using orthopedic inserts or adaptations for shoes, bracing, splinting, or surgery) improves alignment so that structurally safe weight bearing is possible. In addition, observation of the types of shoes and surfaces that the person uses for walking or sports activities may lead to the source of faulty mechanics, which can then be adjusted. (Techniques of orthopedic adaptations for shoes, bracing, and splinting are beyond the scope of this text.) When attempting to gain balance in strength and flexibility of the muscles, appropriate precautions should be followed as outlined in Chapter 3 and Chapter 4. These chapters also describe manual stretching and resistive techniques that may be appropriately used early in a rehabilitation program.

1. Techniques for self-stretching of tight muscles

a. **Self-stretching tight ankle plantarflexor muscles.**

  Precaution: When the patient uses weight-bearing exercises to stretch the plantarflexor muscles (as in 4 and 5 below), he should wear shoes with arch supports or place a folded washcloth under the medial border of the foot[28] to minimize the stress to the arches of the foot.

  (1) Position of patient: long-sitting (knees extended). The patient strongly dorsiflexes his feet, attempting to keep his toes relaxed.

  (2) Position of patient: long-sitting. The patient places a towel or belt under his forefoot and pulls it dorsally.

  (3) Position of patient: sitting with involved foot on a rocker or balance board; rocking the heel downward will stretch the soleus. The soleus can also be stretched while sitting by placing the foot flat on the floor and sliding the foot backward, keeping the heel on the floor (see Figure 11-7).

  (4) Position of patient: standing. The patient strides forward with one foot, keeping the heel of the back foot flat on the floor. To provide stability to the foot, the patient partially rotates the hind leg inward so the foot assumes a supinated position and locks the joints. He then shifts his body weight forward on to the front foot (similar to Figure 10-2). To stretch the gastrocnemius muscle, the patient keeps the knee of the back leg extended; to stretch the soleus, he flexes the knee of the back leg.

  (5) Position of patient: standing, facing a wall, with his hands placed against the wall at shoulder level. The patient leans into the wall, keeping his heels on the floor. To increase the stretch force, increase the distance the feet are placed from the wall. Stretch either the gastrocnemius or the soleus muscle by keeping the knees extended or flexed, respectively.

  (6) Position of patient: standing on an inclined board with feet pointing upward and heels downward (Figure 12-1) Greater stretch will occur if the patient leans forward.

  (7) Position of patient: standing, with forefoot on the edge of a step or stool and heel over the edge. The patient slowly lowers his heel over the edge.

b. **Self-stretching the evertor muscles of the ankle and foot**

  (1) Position of patient: sitting, with the foot to be stretched placed across the opposite knee. The patient uses his opposite hand and lifts his foot into inversion. Emphasize to the patient that the heel must be turned inward and not to twist only the forefoot (similar to the position in Figure 2-34).

  (2) Same as above except the patient does the motion actively.

  (3) Position of patient: standing, with feet pointing forward. The patient rolls his weight to the lateral border of the feet, and if possible, walks a short distance on the lateral borders.

  (4) Position of patient: standing or walking, with his foot on a slanted board, placing the lateral aspect of the foot to be stretched on the lower side and the medial side of his foot on the top side of the board. Bilateral stretching can be done if hinged planks are placed in an inverted-V position and the patient stands or walks on them.

c. **Self-stretching the extrinsic muscles of the toes**

  (1) Position of patient: sitting, with his foot crossed on to the opposite

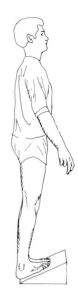

FIGURE 12-1. Self-stretching the ankle plantarflexor muscles.

knee. The patient stabilizes the foot under the metatarsophalan-geal (MTP) joints with his thumbs and passively flexes the MTP joints by applying pressure against the proximal phalages. Or he attempts active flexion of the MTP joints, assisting the motion if necessary.

(2) Position of patient: standing, with the toes over the edge of a stool or book. The MTP joints are at the edge. The patient attempts to flex the MTP joints, keeping the IP joints of the toes extended.

2. Procedures to train and strengthen muscles necessary for postural control of the ankle and foot

Most functional demands on the ankle and foot occur in weight-bearing postures. Kinesthetic input from skin, joint, and muscle receptors and the resulting joint and muscle responses are different in open and closed kine-matic chain activities; therefore, whenever possible, lower extremity exer-cises should be progressed to closed-chain positions.

Note: The cause of *toeing in*, or *pigeon-toed feet*, may not be from poor ankle posture; it may be due to internal rotation at the hips (anteversion), internal torsion of the tibia, or excessive adduction of the forefoot (metatar-sus varus). *Toeing out* may be associated with external rotation of the hips (retroversion), external torsion of the tibia, or flat feet. The problems may be congenital or acquired and may or may not be correctable with stretch-ing and training (see comments at the beginning of Section C). If related, the entire lower extremity needs to be included in the exercise and training program, not just the feet. See additional suggestions in the chapters on the hip and knee.

a. **Training activities**

(1) Position of patient: long-sitting. First the patient dorsiflexes and in-verts his feet to emphasize the anterior tibialis muscles, then plan-tarflexes and inverts to emphasize the posterior tibialis muscles.

    (2) Position of patient: sitting, with feet on the floor. The patient curls his toes against the resistance of the floor. A towel is placed under his feet, and he attempts to wrinkle it up by keeping his heel on the floor and flexing his toes. This may also be done with the patient standing.

    (3) Position of patient: sitting, with feet on the floor. The patient attempts to raise the medial longitudinal arches while keeping both the forefeet and hindfeet on the floor (lateral rotation of the tibia should occur but not abduction of the hips). He repeats the activity until he has good control, then progresses to doing the motion while standing.

    (4) Patient practices walking, concentrating on the placement of his feet and the shifting of his body weight with each step. The patient begins by accepting the body weight on the heel, then shifts his weight along the lateral border of the foot to the fifth metatarsal head and across to the first metatarsal head and great toe for the push off.

  b. **Strengthening activities**

    (1) The activities listed in section a above can also be used as strengthening exercises if the principles of strengthening are used. Since most of the activities provide low resistance, high repetition to fatigue is necessary to strengthen the muscles.

    (2) Position of patient: sitting, with a tennis ball placed between the soles of his feet. The patient rolls the tennis ball back and forth from heel to forefoot.

    (3) Position of patient: sitting. A number of small objects, such as marbles or dice, are placed to one side of the patient's foot. He picks up one object at a time by curling his toes around it, then places it in a container on the other side of his foot. This emphasizes the plantar muscles as well as inversion and eversion.

    (4) Position of patient: sitting, progressing to standing. Sand, foam, or other distensible material in a box can be used to offer resistance to the various foot motions as the patient rocks forward, backward, and side to side, or curls his toes.

    (5) Position of patient: long-sitting, holding on to an elasticized material which is also placed under his forefoot. The patient plantarflexes his foot against the resistance (Figure 12-2).

    (6) Position of patient: long-sitting or supine, with a loop of elasticized material placed around both feet. The patient everts one or both feet against the resistance (Figure 12-3).

    (7) Position of patient: long-sitting or supine. An elasticized material is tied to the foot end of the bed (or other object) and is placed over the dorsum of the patient's foot. He then dorsiflexes against the resistance (Figure 12-4).

    (8) Position of patient: standing. The patient begins with bilateral toe raises, heel raises, and rocking outward to the lateral borders of the feet; and then progresses to unilateral toe raises, heel raises, and lateral border standing to train and strengthen the muscles in a weight-bearing position. Training advances to walking on heels, toes, then lateral borders of his feet, progressively increasing the distance.

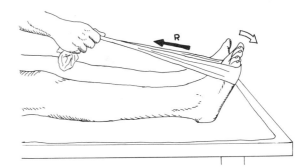

FIGURE 12-2. Resisting the ankle plantarflexor muscles with an elasticized material.

D. Overuse Syndromes[10]

1. Clinical picture

An overuse syndrome is a local inflammatory response to stresses from repetitive microtrauma, which may be from faulty alignment problems in the lower extremity, muscle imbalances or fatigue, changes in exercise or functional routines, training errors, improper footwear for the ground or functional demands placed on the feet, or a combination of several of these factors. The syndrome occurs because continued demand is placed on the tissue before it is adequately healed, so the pain and inflammation continue. A common cause predisposing the foot to overuse syndromes is abnormal pronation of the subtalar joint. The abnormal pronation could be related to a variety of causes including leg-length discrepancy, femoral anteversion, external tibial torsion, genu valgum, or muscle flexibility and strength imbalances. *Tendinitis, tenosynovitis, plantar fascitis,* and *shin splints* are examples of overuse syndromes.

a. **Tendinitis or tenosynovitis**

Any of the tendons of the extrinsic muscles to the foot may become irritated as they approach and cross over the ankle or where they attach in the foot. Pain occurs during or following repetitive activity. When the foot and ankle are tested, pain is experienced at the site of the lesion as resistance is applied to the muscle action and also when the

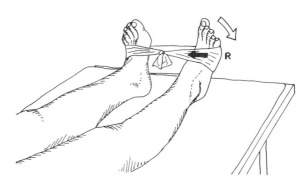

FIGURE 12-3. Resisting the evertor muscles of the foot with an elasticized material.

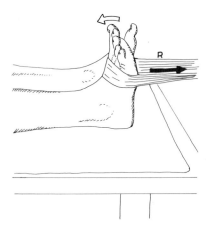

FIGURE 12-4. Resisting the ankle dorsiflexor muscles with an elasticized material.

involved tendon is placed on a stretch or palpated.[3] A common site for symptoms is proximal to the calcaneus in the Achilles tendon. For example, symptoms may develop when the person switches from high-heeled shoes to low-heeled shoes and then does a lot of walking.[23] Symptoms are also associated with high-impact sports. Usually there is a tight gastrocsoleus complex and abnormal foot pronation.

b. **Plantar fascitis**

Pain is usually experienced along the plantar aspect of the heel where the plantar fascia inserts on the medial tubercle of the calcaneus. The site of the injury is very tender to palpation. Excessive pronation of the subtalar joint, which may be reinforced by tight gastrocsoleus muscles, predisposes the foot to abnormal forces and irritation of the plantar fascia. Conversely, stress forces on the fascia can also occur with an excessively high arch (cavus foot). Pressure to the irritated site with weight bearing or stretch forces to the fascia as when extending the toes during push-off causes pain.

c. **Shin splints**

This term is used to describe pain along the posterior medial or anterior lateral aspects of the proximal two thirds of the tibia, and may include different pathologic conditions. Most common is overuse of the anterior tibialis muscle. A tight gastrocsoleus complex and a weak anterior tibialis muscle, as well as foot pronation, are associated with anterior shin splints. Pain increases with active dorsiflexion and when the muscle is stretched into plantarflexion. A tight gastrocsoleus complex and a weak posterior tibialis muscle, along with foot pronation, are associated with posterior medial shin splints. Pain is experienced when the foot is passively plantarflexed with eversion and with active supination. Muscle fatigue with vigorous exercise, such as running or aerobic dancing, may precipitate the problem.

2. **Management**

a. **Acute phase**

While inflamed, the foot problem should be treated as an acute condition with rest and appropriate modalities (see Chapter 6). Immobilization in a cast or splint with the foot slightly plantarflexed or the use of a heel lift inside the shoe may be used to relieve stress.[28]

(1) Apply cross-friction massage to the site of the lesion.

(2) Initiate gentle muscle-setting contractions or electrical stimulation to the involved muscle in pain-free positions.

(3) Teach active ROM within the pain-free ranges.

(4) Instruct the patient to avoid the activity that provokes the pain.

b. **Subacute phase**

When symptoms become subacute, the entire lower extremity as well as the foot should be evaluated for abnormal alignment or muscle flexibility and strength imbalances. Eliminating or modifying the cause is important to prevent recurrences.

(1) Correct abnormal foot alignment with appropriate foot orthoses if necessary.[7,26]

(2) Stretch tight structures such as the gastrocsoleus complex (See section C for suggestions.)

(3) Strengthen the muscles in dysfunction, beginning with resistive isometric and progressing to resistive isotonic and isokinetic exercises. This usually involves strengthening the dorsiflexors but should also include the invertors (especially the posterior tibialis) and evertors for proper medial and lateral support.

(4) As the patient gains a balance between flexibility and strength, emphasis needs to be placed on endurance in the involved muscle.

(5) When returning to the previously stressful activity, the patient should be taught prevention, which includes stretching, gentle repetitive warm-ups, and use of proper foot support. The importance of allowing time for recovery from fatigue and microtrauma after high-intensity workouts also must be emphasized.

E. Poor Balance

Following trauma to the ankle joint, there may be some loss of proprioceptive feedback from the mechanoreceptors and therefore some interference in balance. The joint and muscles should be rehabilitated in the weight-bearing position to stimulate proper functioning.[9,24] These activities may also be beneficial in hip and knee rehabilitation programs.

1. Many of the weight-bearing exercises listed in Section II C can also be used to train the patient's balance and timing of muscle contraction.

2. Use a rocker board or balance board and have the patient shift his weight from side to side and front to back while attempting to control the ankle. A variety of commercial exercise boards are available with gradations in size of the rocker or half-sphere, as well as adaptations for resistance. Gradations in difficulty can be adapted according to the patient's ability. Beginning with sitting, the patient learns to control the direction of motion of the board. Standing, the patient can support himself with both hands on a solid object and use both feet on the board, then progress to one-legged support (Figure 12-5). Additional progression would be to change the amount of motion allowed by the board (use a larger sphere or rocker), then to balancing without hand support with both feet, then with one foot at a time. Reactions the patients must make on the balance board are similar to quick muscular adjustments needed when walking on uneven ground.

3. Progress the patient with weight-bearing activities such as walking on uneven surfaces, side-to-side weight shifting, walking on a balance beam,

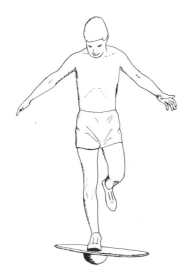

FIGURE 12-5. Advanced training for balance and co-ordination on a balance board requires that the patient does not hold on and balances with one leg.

and agility drills and obstacle maneuvering.
4. Finally, progress to training the patient in functional patterns and activities using repetitive motions for endurance.

F. Referred Pain and Nerve Injury Patterns

The foot is where several major nerves terminate. Injury or entrapment of the nerves may be anywhere along their course, from the lumbosacral spine to near their termination. For treatment to be effective, it must be directed to the source of the problem. Therefore, a thorough history and selective tension examination is done when referred pain patterns or sensory changes are reported by the patient.[3,12,19]

1. Common sources of segmental sensory reference in the foot
   a. Lumbosacral spine
      (1) Vertebral joints between L-4 and L-5 or between L-5 and S-1 vertebrae
      (2) Nerve roots L-4, L-5, and S-1
   b. Dermatomal reference from tissue derived from the same spinal segments as L-4, L-5, and S-1

2. Peripheral nerve cutaneous sensation in the foot
   a. Branches of the common peroneal nerve: superficial and deep peroneal nerves
   b. Terminal branches of the tibial nerve: medial and lateral plantar nerves
   c. Sural nerve
   d. Terminal branch of the femoral nerve: saphenous nerve

III. THERAPEUTIC EXERCISE MANAGEMENT OF COMMON SURGICAL PROCEDURES FOR THE ANKLE AND FOOT

Surgical management of severe pain, limitation of motion, and gross instability of the ankle as the result of rheumatoid or degenerative arthritis is primarily limited to arthrodesis or arthroplasty of the ankle. Pain with weight bearing and deformities of the foot or toes must often be managed surgically. Severe injuries to soft tissue such as complete rupture of the Achilles tendon or severe tears of ligaments may also require surgical management if conservative management fails.

In general the goals of surgery and postoperative exercise for the foot or ankle include

1. Relief of pain with weight bearing and joint motion
2. Stability of the ankle for ambulation and functional activities
3. Improvement in joint motion and strength
4. Correction of deformity at the foot and ankle

The postoperative exercise program required for most patients is minimal. Gait training with some type of assistive device is important. After surgery, it is also helpful for the therapist to educate the patient about shoe fit and selection.

A. Total Ankle Joint Replacement

1. Indications for surgery[8,38,39,40]

a. Severe pain in the tibiotalar joint, secondary to rheumatoid or traumatic arthritis
b. Marked limitation of ankle motion
c. Avascular necrosis of the ankle joint, secondary to repeated ankle injuries
d. An alternative to arthrodesis for the patient with good ligamentous stability at the ankle. (The components of a total ankle replacement do not improve stability of the ankle.)

Note: Patients with a very unstable ankle, vascular deficiency, or muscle imbalance are not good candidates for this type of surgery.

2. Procedures[36,43]

a. An anterior midline incision or sometimes a posterior incision is made.
b. Minimal bone is excised from the tibiotalar joint.
c. An all plastic tibial replacement (the Mayo prosthesis) or a metal-stemmed tibial prosthesis with a polyethylene articulating surface (the Waugh UCI prosthesis) is implanted and cemented in place.
d. A talar component made of metal is affixed to the talus with cement.

3. Postoperative management[38]

a. The ankle and foot are immobilized in a bulky compression dressing and sometimes a splint to hold the foot in a neutral position for 3 to 5 days. The foot is elevated at all times while the patient is in bed.
   (1) Elevation prevents or minimizes edema, which can cause poor wound healing.
   (2) Isometric dorsiflexion and plantarflexion should be started while the patient is still in the bulky dressing and splint.
   (3) Quadriceps and gluteal setting exercises should also be done in preparation for walking.
b. The patient must be non–weight bearing during transfers in the first 5 postoperative days.
c. The bulky dressing is removed on about the fifth postoperative day.
   (1) Active plantarflexion and dorsiflexion should be started if wound healing is sufficient. The patient will need about 25 degrees of total dorsiflexion and plantarflexion for normal walking and about 50 to 60 degrees for ascending and descending stairs.[39]

      (2) If the arthroplasty allows for some varus and valgus, as the UCI components do, gentle active circumduction should also be started.

   d. The patient should try partial weight bearing to tolerance with crutches when the bulky dressing is removed.

   e. By 12 to 14 days, the patient should be ambulating with a cane.

   f. By 6 to 12 weeks the patient should return to full activities without a cane.

B. Arthrodesis at the Ankle and Foot

1. Indications for surgery[14,33,41]

   a. Severe pain with weight bearing at any number of joints of the ankle or foot secondary to rheumatoid, degenerative, or traumatic arthritis

   b. Instability of a weight-bearing joint

   c. Deformity of the toes, foot, or ankle

2. Procedures[14,33,41]

   a. The procedures, all of which provide bony ankylosis, will vary depending on the joints involved.

   b. Some common procedures include

      (1) Triple arthrodesis of the ankle.

         (a) Fusion of the talocalcaneal, calcaneocuboid, and talonavicular joints.

         (b) Provides permanent medial-lateral stability and relief of pain in the subtalar joint.

         (c) Eversion and inversion of the ankle are lost.

      (2) Arthrodesis of the tibiotalar joint

         (a) Fusion of the tibia and talus in approximately 5 degrees of plantarflexion provides relief of pain and stability at the tibiotalar joint.

         (b) Dorsiflexion and plantarflexion are lost, significantly affecting the biomechanics of gait.

         (c) The forefoot must be stable and pain free in order to compensate for the loss of motion at the ankle.

      (3) Arthrodesis of the first toe

         (a) Fusion of the first metatarsophalangeal (MTP) joint for hallux rigidus and hallux valgus

         (b) Provides relief of pain during ambulation in the MTP joint of the first toe

      (4) Arthrodesis of the interphalangeal joints of the toes

         (a) Fusion of the proximal and middle or distal joints of the toes for hammer toes, usually occurring in the second and third toes

         (b) Provides relief of pain during ambulation.

3. Postoperative management[14]

   a. The fused joints are immobilized in plaster or with skeletal pins for approximately 6 to 12 weeks.

   b. During this time the patient must be non- or partially weight bearing. Gait training with assistive devices is necessary.

   c. Active range of motion exercises must be done to maintain mobility in any other joints affected by arthritis.

    d. The patient should be advised of proper shoe selection and fit when the immobilization device is removed.

C. Excision Arthroplasty for Metatarsalgia

1. Indications for surgery[14,33,35,41]

    a. Metatarsalgia involves severe pain in the metatarsophalangeal (MTP) region of the foot with weight bearing and ambulation.

        (1) Chronic synovitis of the MTP joints secondary to rheumatoid arthritis causes erosion and deterioration of the joint surfaces.

        (2) Metatarsalgia is associated with volar subluxation of the heads of the metatarsals because of destruction of the joint capsule and stretching of the plantar intertarsal ligaments.

    b. Hammer toes develop because of shortening of the long extensor muscles of the toes and pull on the long toe flexor muscles.[29]

    c. Hallux valgus of the first toe is also an associated deformity of the foot seen with metatarsalgia.

    d. Surgery is indicated when conservative management such as shoe modifications and foot orthoses[29] no longer relieve MTP pain during ambulation.

2. Procedures[14,33,35,41]

    a. The involved metatarsal heads and the proximal portion of the proximal phalanges are resected (Fowler procedure).

    b. If the first toe is primarily involved, the exostosis is removed from the medial aspect of the first metatarsal, and the proximal third to half of the first proximal phalanx is resected (Keller procedure).

3. Postoperative management

    a. Weight bearing is limited for several weeks. Gait training with assistive devices is necessary.

    b. Active exercise to the intrinsic muscles of the foot is begun at approximately 1 month.[14]

    c. The patient may be fitted with a metatarsal pad of polyethylene foam to be worn on the inside of the shoe. Use of the pad will equalize the pressure forces on the plantar aspect of the foot and will transfer the weight proximal to the metatarsal heads during weight bearing.[11,37]

D. Repair of Complete Tendon Ruptures and Severe Ligament Tears

Rupture of the Achilles tendon occurs most frequently in older adults with compromised blood supply to the tendon. In young, active individuals, a rupture can also occur after a forceful contraction of the gastrocnemius and soleus muscles against resistance. Although a rupture of the Achilles tendon is often managed conservatively, surgery is indicated when the torn fragments cannot be reopposed by positioning and conservative management.[23,28]

    A third-degree sprain of the ankle, which generally occurs as the result of a severe inversion injury, often tears both the anterior talofibular ligament and the calcaneofibular ligament. A severe tear of these ligaments causes marked instability of the ankle and will significantly impair an individual's functional activities.[16,20,23] Surgical intervention is often indicated in patients with third-degree ligament injuries, in patients who wish to return to very vigorous activities and sports, and in patients in whom gross instability of the ankle persists and continues to disrupt function after a trial of conservative management.[18,23,27]

1. Indications for surgery

a. Complete rupture of a tendon in which end-to-end opposition cannot be achieved by nonsurgical means[23,27]

b. Gross instability of the ankle as the result of a complete tear of the supporting ligaments[16,23,27]

2. Procedures[16,23]

a. After tendon rupture, the retracted ends of the tendon are gently pulled and opposed. An end-to-end anastomosis of the tendon is performed. A plantaris tendon graft may be used to reconstruct the tendon. The ankle is immobilized for 3 to 4 weeks with as much tension as the newly sutured tendon can withstand. Then a new cast or splint is applied with slightly more tension on the tendon for 3 to 4 more weeks.

b. When a torn ligament is grossly separated, the torn tissues are opposed and sutured. The patient is immobilized in a neutral position in a cast or bulky dressing and splint for 6 weeks.

3. Postoperative management[13,23,28]

a. Immobilization
   (1) Initial elevation of the foot for 48 hours will minimize postoperative edema.
   (2) Gentle muscle-setting exercises in the cast or splint can be initiated as soon as it is comfortable for the patient. As healing progresses, the intensity of the isometric setting exercise should be increased.
   (3) Electrical stimulation can also be done when the foot and ankle are immobilized to minimize muscle atrophy if the muscles are accessible.

b. Exercise
   (1) When the immobilization device is removed, begin exercise to increase ROM. Start with gentle joint mobilization. After a ligament repair, avoid stretch mobilizations (grade III) in the direction of the corrected instability.
   (2) Begin stretching the musculotendinous unit with gentle contract-relax procedures or manual stretching.
       (a) Initially, open-chain stretching is advisable in the early stages of rehabilitation. Closed-chain stretching (with the patient standing and the involved foot on the floor) produces significant ground reaction forces on the repaired soft tissues.
       (b) Gentle closed-chain stretching can be started with the patient sitting and the involved foot on a balance board or rocker board.
       (c) Closed-chain stretching can be done later with the patient standing for a more forceful stretch.
   (3) Progressively strengthen the muscles of the foot and ankle.
       (a) Continue isometric exercises and add resistance. This can be done by having the patient resist all ankle motions with his hands or with the opposite foot. After repair of lateral ligaments, strength of the evertors is particularly important for increased

support of the ankle. Isometric eversion can be achieved by having the patient cross his ankles and press the lateral borders of his feet together.

(b) Add isotonic and isokinetic resistance exercises.

(c) Progress to functional activities for closed-chain strengthening. Walking, bilateral toe raises, unilateral toe raises, jogging, straight running, and running in circles all progressively strengthen the ankle, foot, and lower extremity musculature and ligaments.

(4) Retrain balance with kinesthetic exercises using a rocker board or balance board. (See Section II E for additional suggestions.)

IV. SUMMARY

The anatomy, joint characteristics, and functional relationships of joints and muscles of the ankle and foot were briefly reviewed for background information in the first section of this chapter. Therapeutic exercise management of common musculoskeletal problems was presented, including joint problems, sprains, minor tears, imbalances of muscle strength and flexibility, and muscle overuse syndromes. Exercise techniques for the ankle and foot not previously described in other chapters were included. A discussion of total ankle joint replacement surgery, arthrodesis of several joints of the ankle and foot, excision arthroplasty for metatarsalgia, and repair of soft tissues concluded this chapter.

REFERENCES

1. Bistevins, R: *Footwear and footwear modifications.* In Kottke, FJ, Stillwell, GK, and Lehmann, JF (eds): *Krusen's Handbook of Physical Medicine and Rehabilitation,* ed 3. WB Saunders, Philadelphia, 1982.
2. Cailliet, R: *Foot and Ankle Pain.* FA Davis, Philadelphia, 1968.
3. Cyriax, J: *Textbook of Orthopaedic Medicine, Volume One. Diagnosis of Soft Tissue Lesions,* ed 8. Bailliere Tindall, London, 1982.
4. DeLacerda, F: *A study of anatomical factors involved in shinsplints.* JOSPT 2:55, 1980.
5. DeLacerda, F: *Iontophoresis for treatment of shinsplints.* JOSPT 3:183, 1982.
6. Dimonte, P and Light, H: *Pathomechanics, gait deviations and treatment of the rheumatoid foot.* Phys Ther 62:1148, 1982.
7. Donatelli, R, et al: *Biomechanical foot orthotics: A retrospective study.* JOSPT 10:205, 1988.
8. Fortune, WP: *Lower limb joint replacement.* In Nickel, VL (ed): *Orthopedic Rehabilitation.* Churchill-Livingstone, New York, 1982.
9. Garn, SN and Newton, RA: *Kinesthetic awareness in subjects with multiple ankle sprains.* Phys Ther 68:1669, 1988.
10. Greenfield, B: *Evaluation of overuse syndromes in the lower extremities.* In Donatelli, R (ed): *Mechanics of the Foot and Ankle.* FA Davis, Philadelphia, 1990.
11. Haslock, DI and Wright, V: *Footwear for arthritic patients.* Arch Phys Med 10:236, 1970.
12. Hoppenfeld, S: *Physical Examination of the Spine and Extremities.* Appleton-Century-Crofts, New York, 1976.
13. Howell, DW: *Therapeutic exercise and mobilization.* In Hunt GC (ed): *Physical Therapy of the Foot and Ankle.* Churchill-Livingstone, New York, 1988.
14. Hyde, SA: *Physiotherapy in Rheumatology.* Blackwell Scientific Publications, Oxford, 1980.
15. Kapandji, IA: *The Physiology of the Joints,* Vol II, ed 5. Churchill-Livingstone, Edinburgh, 1987.
16. Kaplan, EG, et al: *A triligamentous reconstruction for lateral ankle instability.* J Foot Surg 23:24, 1984.
17. Kaumeyer, G and Malone, T: *Ankle injuries: Anatomical and biomechanical considerations necessary for the development of an injury prevention program.* JOSPT 1:171, 1980.
18. Kay, DB: *The sprained ankle: Current therapy.* Foot and Ankle 6:22, 1985.

19. Kessler, R and Hertling, D: *Management of Common Musculoskeletal Disorders.* Harper & Row, Philadelphia, 1983.
20. Kimura, IF, et al: *Effect of the air stirrup in controlling ankle inversion stress.* JOSPT 9:190, 1987.
21. Kopell, H and Thompson, W: *Peripheral Entrapment Neuropathies,* ed 2. Robert E. Krieger, Huntington, NY, 1976.
22. Kramer, P: *Restoration of dorsiflexion after injuries to the distal leg and ankle.* JOSPT 1:159, 1980.
23. Kuland, DN: *The Injured Athlete.* JB Lippincott, Philadelphia, 1988.
24. Lattanza, L, Gray, GW, and Kantner, R: *Closed vs open kinematic chain measurements of subtalar joint eversion: Implications for clinical practice.* JOSPT 9:310, 1988.
25. Lehmkuhl, LD and Smith, LK: *Brunnstrom's Clinical Kinesiology,* ed 4. FA Davis, Philadelphia, 1983.
26. Lockard, MA: *Foot orthoses.* Phys Ther 68:1866, 1988.
27. McPoil TG: *Footwear.* Phys Ther 68:1857, 1988.
28. McPoil, TG and McGarvey, TC: *The foot in athletics.* In Hunt, GC (ed): *Physical Therapy of the Foot and Ankle.* Churchill-Livingstone, New York, 1988.
29. Moncur, C and Shields, M: *Clinical management of metatarsalgia in patients with arthritis.* Clinical Management 3:7, 1983.
30. Norkin, C and Levangie, P: *Joint Structure and Function: A Comprehensive Analysis.* FA Davis, Philadelphia, 1983.
31. *Normal and Pathological Gait Syllabus.* Physical Therapy Department, Rancho Los Amigos Hospital, Downey, California, 1977.
32. Oatis, CA: *Biomechanics of the foot and ankle under static conditions.* Phys Ther 68:1815, 1988.
33. Opitz, JL: *Reconstructive surgery of the extremities.* In Kottke, FJ, Stillwell, GK, and Lehmann, JF (eds): *Krusen's Handbook of Physical Medicine and Rehabilitation,* ed 3. WB Saunders, Philadelphia, 1982.
34. Quillen, W: *An alternative management protocol for lateral ankle sprains.* JOSPT 2:187, 1981.
35. Salter, RB: *Textbook of Disorders and Injuries of the Musculoskeletal System,* ed 2. Williams & Wilkins, Baltimore, 1983.
36. Samuelson, K, Tuke, M, and Freeman, MAR: *A replacement arthroplasty for the three articular surfaces of the ankle, utilizing a posterior approach.* J Bone Joint Surg 59(Br):376, 1977.
37. Schnell, MD, Bowker, JH, and Bunch, WH: *The orthotist.* In Nickel, VL (ed): *Orthopedic Rehabilitation.* Churchill-Livingstone, New York, 1982.
38. Smith, CL: *Physical therapy management of patients with total ankle replacement.* Phys Ther 60:303, 1980.
39. Stauffer, RN, Choco, E, and Brewster, R: *Force and motion analysis of the normal, diseased & prosthetic ankle.* Clin Orthop 127:189, 1977.
40. Stauffer, RN: *Total ankle joint replacement.* Arch Surg 112:105, 1977.
41. Thomas, WH: *Surgery of the foot in rheumatoid arthritis.* Orthop Clin North Am 6:831, 1975.
42. Wallace, L, Knortz, K, and Esterson, P: *Immediate care of ankle injuries.* JOSPT 1:46, 1979.
43. Waugh, TR and Evanski, PM: *Irvine ankle arthroplasty: Prosthetic design and surgical technique.* Clin Orthop 114:180, 1976.
44. Woodman, R and Pare, L: *Evaluation and treatment of soft tissue lesions of the ankle and forefoot using the Cyriax approach.* Phys Ther 62:1144, 1982.

CHAPTER ———————————— 13

Vascular Disorders of the Extremities

Vascular disorders, which cause disturbances of circulation to the extremities, can result in significant loss of function of either the upper or lower extremities. Disturbances of circulation may be caused by a number of acute or chronic medical conditions known as peripheral vascular diseases (PVD). Peripheral vascular diseases can affect the arterial, venous, or lymphatic circulatory systems. Surgical procedures that interfere with the lymphatic system may also lead to vascular disorders. For example, surgical removal or radiation of lymphatic vessels is a part of some mastectomy procedures. One or both may be necessary in the effective treatment of many types of breast cancer but can also lead to chronic lymphedema of the upper extremity.

A therapist must have a general understanding of these clinical problems to effectively evaluate and develop a plan of care for patients with a variety of vascular disorders. Although therapeutic exercise is just one procedure used in the management of vascular disorders of the extremities, emphasis will be placed on this aspect of treatment when appropriate in this chapter.

OBJECTIVES

After studying this chapter, the reader will be able to:
1. define common acute and chronic vascular disorders of the extremities that occur as a result of a variety of medical or surgical conditions and that affect the arterial, venous, and lymphatic circulatory systems.
2. describe the clinical problems associated with peripheral vascular disease.
3. explain evaluation and screening procedures used for patients with known or suspected vascular disorders affecting the extremities.
4. describe the rationale and principles involved in the specific treatment procedures for patients with vascular disorders.
5. outline appropriate treatment goals and plan of care for patients with acute or chronic peripheral vascular disease resulting in arterial, venous, or lymphatic circulatory dysfunction.

6. describe the vascular, musculoskeletal, respiratory, and functional problems of patients after a mastectomy.
7. outline the treatment goals and postoperative plan of care for a patient with a mastectomy.
8. explain any precautions or contraindications to treatment of patients with vascular disorders.

I. ARTERIAL DISORDERS

A. Types of Arterial Disorders

1. **Acute arterial occlusion**[11,13,21,28]
   a. May be caused by a thrombus (blood clot), embolism, or trauma to an artery
   b. Will result in absent or diminished pulses and complete or partial interruption of circulation to an extremity
   c. The severity of the problem is dependent upon the location of the occlusion and the availability of collateral circulation.
   d. If little or no collateral circulation is available, an acute arterial occlusion will cause tissue ischemia and possibly gangrene of the distal limb.

2. **Chronic arteriosclerotic vascular disease (ASVD)**[11,13,21]
   a. This disorder is also called *arteriosclerosis obliterans* (ASO).
   b. Circulation progressively deteriorates because of narrowing, fibrosis, and occlusion of the large and medium arteries, usually in the lower extremities.
   c. This disease is most often seen in elderly patients and is commonly associated with diabetes mellitus.

3. **Thromboangiitis obliterans (Buerger's disease)**[11]
   a. An inflammatory reaction of the arteries to nicotine in patients who smoke
   b. Usually occurs in the small arteries of the feet and hands and progresses proximally
   c. Results in decreased arterial circulation to the extremities
   d. The inflammatory reaction can be controlled if the patient stops smoking.

4. **Raynaud's disease (Raynaud's phenomenon)**[16,23]
   a. Functional arterial disease caused by vasospasm, most often affecting the arteries of the fingers
   b. Caused by an abnormality of the sympathetic nervous system
   c. Usually seen in young adults
   d. Characterized by
      (1) sensitivity to cold
      (2) blanching and cyanosis of the finger tips and nail beds
      (3) severe pain, sensory loss (tingling or numbness), and decreased function in the hands
   e. Symptoms are slowly relieved by warmth.

B. Clinical Signs and Symptoms of Arterial Disease

1. Changes in skin color and temperature[13,19,21,28]
a. Pallor—a chalky, white color, blanching of the skin
b. Shiny and waxy appearance of the skin and decreased hair growth distal to the insufficiency
c. Decreased skin temperature
d. Dryness of the skin
e. Ulcerations, particularly at weight-bearing areas and bony prominences
f. Gangrene

2. Sensory disturbances[28]
a. Decreased tolerance to hot or cold temperatures
b. Paresthesia
   (1) tingling and eventual numbness in the distal portion of the extremities
   (2) makes the patient more susceptible to wound infections after minor skin abrasions

3. Pain[13,21,28]
a. Intermittent claudication (exercise pain)
   (1) Exercise pain is due to cramping of muscles with exercise when there is ischemia.
   (2) Cramping usually occurs in the calf muscles during walking and is caused by insufficient blood supply to the involved limb.
   (3) Pain slowly diminishes with rest.
   (4) Exercise tolerance progressively decreases, and ischemic pain occurs more readily as the disease progresses.
b. Pain at rest[28]
   (1) A burning, tingling pain in the extremities occurs as a result of severe ischemia.
   (2) It frequently occurs at night because the heart rate and volume of blood flow to the extremities decreases with rest.
   (3) Partial or complete relief of pain may be achieved if the leg is placed in a dependent position, for example, over the edge of the bed.
   (4) Elevation of the limb will cause an increase in pain.

4. Paralysis
a. Atrophy of muscles
b. Eventual loss of motor function, particularly in the hands and feet
c. Loss of motor function is further compounded by pain

C. Evaluation of Arterial Disorders[6,15,18,19,21,27]

In order to establish the type and current status of an arterial disease and to determine the effectiveness of any subsequent treatment, a complete evaluation of arterial blood flow is necessary. Some evaluative procedures and screening tests may be done by the therapist; others are done exclusively by the physician. An understanding of test procedures and their interpretation is important so the therapist can plan an effective treatment program.

1. **Palpation of pulses**
   a. The basis of any evaluation of the integrity of the arterial system is the detection of pulses in the distal portion of the extremities.
   b. Pulses are described as normal, diminished, or absent. Pulselessness is a sign of severe arterial insufficiency.
   c. The femoral, popliteal, dorsalis pedis, and posterior tibial pulses are commonly palpated in the lower extremity.
   d. The radial, ulnar, and brachial pulses are often palpated in the upper extremity.

2. **Skin temperature**
   a. Temperature of the skin can be grossly assessed by palpation. A limb with diminished arterial blood flow will be cool to the touch.
   b. If a discrepancy exists between an involved and an uninvolved extremity, a quantitative measurement of skin temperature should be made with an electronic thermometer.[21]

3. **Test for rubor**
   a. Changes in skin color that occur with elevation and dependency of the limb are evaluated.
   b. Procedure
      (1) The legs are elevated for several minutes above the level of the heart while the patient is lying supine.
      (2) Pallor of the skin will occur in the feet if arterial circulation is poor.
      (3) The time necessary for blanching to develop is noted.
      (4) The legs are then placed in a dependent position, and the color of the feet is noted.
      (5) Normally, a pinkish flush appears in the feet after several seconds.
      (6) In occlusive arterial disease, a bright reddening or rubor of the distal legs and feet occurs.
      (7) The rubor may take as long as 30 seconds to appear.

4. **Reactive hyperemia**
   a. Blood flow to the distal extremity is temporarily restricted by a blood pressure cuff.
      (1) This restriction causes an accumulation of CO_2 and lactic acid in the extremity.
      (2) These metabolites are vasodilators and affect the vascular bed.
   b. When the cuff is released, blood flow resumes to the extremity.
   c. A normal hyperemia (flushing) of the extremity should occur within 10 seconds.
   d. In arterial vascular disorders, it may take as long as 1 to 2 minutes for a flush to appear.

5. **Doppler ultrasound**
   a. This assessment uses the Doppler principle to determine the relative velocity of blood flow in the major arteries and veins.[13,18]
   b. A sound head, covered with coupling gel, is placed on the skin directly over the artery to be evaluated. An ultrasonic beam is directed transcutaneously to the artery.
   c. Blood cells moving in the path of the beam cause a shift in the frequency of the reflected sound.

    d. The frequency of the reflected sound emitted varies with the velocity of blood flow.

    e. This information is transmitted visually, onto an oscilloscope or printed tape, or audibly, via a loudspeaker or stethoscope.

    f. Systolic pressure can also be measured at various points in arterial vessels.

Note: Although Doppler ultrasonic evaluations are not commonly performed by therapists, a recent study indicates that therapists who have been trained in the use of the technique have demonstrated competence and accuracy.[12]

6. Oscillometry

    a. This test measures the expansion of an artery caused by the thrust of blood during cardiac systole.

    b. Blood volume and flow to an extremity can then be determined.

    c. This test is not very reliable and has been replaced by the highly reliable Doppler ultrasound evaluation.

7. Arteriography

    a. This is an invasive procedure and is usually the last test to be done. It is performed by a vascular surgeon prior to reconstructive vascular surgery.

    b. A radiopaque dye is injected in an artery.[21]

    c. A series of x-ray examinations are taken to detect any restriction of movement of the dye, indicating a complete or partial occlusion of blood flow.

    d. Although this is an invasive procedure, it gives the most accurate picture of the location and extent of arterial obstruction.[6]

    e. It is a necessary procedure prior to any vascular surgery.

D. Treatment of Acute Arterial Occlusion

The treatment of acute arterial occlusion is often a medical or surgical emergency. The viability of the limb will depend on the location and extent of the occlusion and the availability of collateral circulation. Medical or surgical measures must be taken to reduce ischemia and restore circulation. If circulation cannot be significantly improved or restored, gangrene will develop in a very short time, and amputation of the extremity will be necessary.[11,13] Thus, therapeutic exercise is contraindicated and the use of physical therapy procedures, such as reflex heating, is limited in the treatment of acute arterial occlusion.[13,21]

General Treatment Goals

1. Decrease ischemia by restoration or improvement of blood flow

Plan of Care

1. Medical: bed rest; complete systemic anticoagulation therapy.

Physical: reflex heating of the torso or opposite extremity.[16]

Precautions: Local, direct heating of the extremity is contraindicated, because it can easily cause a burn to ischemic tissue.

General Treatment Goals	*Plan of Care*
	Positioning the patient in bed, with the head slightly raised, will increase the blood flow to the distal portion of the extremity.[11,13]
	Surgical: embolectomy; reconstructive arterial or bypass graft surgery[11,13]
2. Protection of the limb	2. The limb must be protected from any trauma. Pressure on skin must be minimized by special mattresses and periodic repositioning of the patient.[21]

E. Treatment of Chronic Arterial Disease[2,6,11,13,21,22,29]

Chronic arteriosclerotic vascular disease can often be conservatively treated by medical and physical means. Arteriosclerotic vascular disease does not usually require emergency medical or surgical care, except in the very advanced stages. Conservative measures are also useful in the management of thromboangiitis and Raynaud's disease.

In all cases, a patient must be advised to stop smoking and alter his diet to lower his cholesterol level and the use of salt, sucrose, and alcohol. These measures may not cure chronic arterial disorders but will minimize the risk factors.

Related medical disorders are also treated. Diabetes is commonly associated with chronic arteriosclerotic vascular disease and must be recognized and appropriately controlled. Hypertension is also managed with medication.

Reconstructive vascular surgery, such as bypass grafts, may be indicated for patients with pain at rest. Patients with vasospastic disease may benefit from sympathetic blocks or sympathectomies to increase blood flow. If patients develop ulcerations and gangrene that cannot be treated medically or with conservative surgical procedures, amputation of the limb will be necessary.[6]

General Treatment Goals	*Plan of Care*
1. Improve collateral circulation and increase vasodilation	1. Daily graded ambulation Buerger-Allen exercises **Note:** Although these exercises are often included in the plan of care of patients with chronic arterial disease, they have been shown to be ineffective in altering circulation.[32] Vasodilation by iontophoresis[1] Vasodilation by reflex heating[16] Vasodilation with medication is controversial and in many cases has not been shown to be helpful.[8]

General Treatment Goals	*Plan of Care*
2. Improve exercise endurance and decrease intermittent claudication	2. Have the patient pace himself during a graded walking program so as not to cause claudication. Gradually increase the duration of exercise, such as the distance walked.
3. Relieve pain at rest	3. Sleep with the legs in a dependent position over the edge of the bed or with the head of the bed slightly elevated.
4. Prevent joint contractures and muscle atrophy, particularly if the patient is confined to bed	4. Active or mild resistive range of motion exercises to the extremities
5. Prevent skin ulcerations	5. Patient education in the proper care and protection of the skin, particulary the feet Proper shoe selection and fit
6. Promote healing of any skin ulcerations that develop	6. A wide variety of procedures for treating ischemic ulcers are used clinically.[28]

F. Principles and Procedures of Treatment of Arterial DIsorders

1. Reflex heating[1]

  a. Heat is applied to the torso or opposite extremity, not directly to the involved extremity.
  b. This causes vasodilation and a general increase in blood flow.
  c. Blood flow then increases to the ischemic extremity.[1]
    (1) There is no documentation that blood flow increases in muscles.
    (2) It has been suggested that the increased blood flow primarily affects skin, not muscles.
  d. Reflex heating is safer than local heating, because it does not increase local tissue temperature or metabolism.
    (1) The risk of burns with the application of local heat is greater in a limb with arterial vascular disease. Metabolic demands increase when heat is applied to a limb. If adequate circulation is not available to meet these increased demands, necrosis of tissue may occur.[16]
    (2) The patient with diabetes is at even greater risk of burns due to hypesthesia (decreased sensation) in the distal portion of the extremities.

2. Daily graded ambulation or bicycling program

  a. Rationale for graded exercise[2,10,21,22]
    (1) During an active contraction of a muscle, blood flow temporarily decreases, but a rapid increase in blood flow occurs immediately after the muscle contraction.
    (2) After exercise is ended, there is a rapid decrease in blood flow during the first 3 to 4 minutes. This is followed by a slow decline to resting levels within 15 minutes.

        (3) With repeated, moderate-level exercise, blood flow in muscles can be increased 10 to 12 times the resting values for blood flow.

        (4) It has been suggested that regular daily exercise will increase walking endurance before the onset of exercise pain. Increased collateral circulation develops to meet increased oxygen demands of muscle tissue.

  b. Procedure[11,21]

        (1) The patient should be encouraged to walk or bicycle as far as possible, without causing intermittent claudication.

        (2) The graded endurance exercise should be carried out 3 to 5 days per week.

        (3) The patient should perform mild warm-up activities prior to initiating walking or bicycling. Warm-up activities could include static stretching of calf muscles and active isotonic pumping exercises of the ankle and toes.

  c. **Precautions**

        (1) A maximum target heart rate should be established. A discussion of maximum target heart rate can be found in Chapter 21.

        (2) The patient should avoid exercising outside during very cold weather.

        (3) The patient must wear shoes that fit properly and will not cause skin irritations, blisters, or sores.

        (4) Patients with a history of cardiac disease must be monitored closely. An outline of these evaluation procedures can also be found in Chapter 21.

  d. **Contraindications**

        (1) Graded ambulation or bicycling is discontinued if leg pain increases over time.

        (2) Patients with resting pain should not participate in an ambulation or bicycling program.

        (3) Patients with ulcerations of the feet and wound or fungal infections should not participate in a walking program.

3. Buerger-Allen exercises[2,9,13,21]

  a. Rationale

  A series of positional changes of the affected limb are coupled with active foot exercises to progressively increase collateral circulation.

  b. The effectiveness of this procedure is, at best, questionable and not necessarily advocated by the authors of this text.

        (1) It has been shown that Buerger-Allen exercises temporarily increase blood flow to an extremity rather than improve collateral circulation on a permanent basis.

        (2) This exercise regimen is included in this chapter so the therapist will understand the procedure and can judge its effectiveness in a clinical situation.

  c. Procedure[2,21]

  A three-stage exercise procedure is carried out three times per day.

        (1) First position

        The patient lies supine with legs elevated and supported at a 45- to 60-degree angle. This position is maintained for 1 to 3 minutes, or until blanching of the extremity occurs. The patient actively dorsiflexes and plantarflexes his feet against resistance from the wall.

(2) Second position
The patient sits up and dangles his feet over the edge of the bed. He actively dorsiflexes, plantarflexes, and circumducts his ankles and flexes and extends his toes for 3 minutes or until rubor in the feet develops.
(3) Third position
The patient lies supine with his feet and legs covered with a blanket for warmth and rests for 5 minutes.
(4) The entire three-stage procedure is repeated 3 to 6 times during each treatment session.
   d. **Precaution**
   Exercise and elevation of the limbs are discontinued if pain or cramping of the calf muscles occurs.
   e. **Contraindications**[2]
   (1) Recent acute thrombosis or embolus
   (2) Increased swelling in the lower extremities

II. VENOUS DISORDERS

A. Types of Venous Disorders[2,9,11,14,21]

1. Acute thrombophlebitis

   a. An acute inflammatory condition with occlusion of a superficial or deep vein by a thrombus
   (1) Superficial venous thrombosis
   If a blood clot is lodged in one of the superficial veins, the condition usually resolves without long-term complications.[11,14]
   (2) Deep venous thrombosis
   Thrombophlebitis of one of the deep veins can result in a pulmonary embolism and is life threatening.[11,14]
   b. *Phlebothrombosis* is another term used to describe the occlusion of a vein by a blood clot.[15,26]
   c. Acute venous disorders usually affect the lower extremities.
   d. Risk factors associated with thrombophlebitis[11,26]
   (1) immobility and bed rest over a prolonged period of time
   (2) obesity
   (3) age of the patient (risk increases with age)
   (4) orthopedic injuries
   (5) postoperative patients
   (6) congestive heart failure
   (7) malignancy
   (8) use of oral contraceptives
   (9) pregnancy

2. Chronic venous disorders[11,14,21]

   a. Varicose veins
   b. Chronic venous insufficiency
   c. These chronic disorders are associated with venous stasis in the lower extremities and inadequate return of blood to the heart.
   (1) The venous valves are not competent, and exercise no longer increases venous return.
   (2) Chronic venous insufficiency may follow an acute episode of thrombophlebitis.

B. **Clinical Signs and Symptoms of Venous Disorders**

1. **Acute thrombophlebitis**[11,14,27]

   Note: Symptoms are most notable if a deep vein is involved.

   a. Swelling of the extremity

   b. Pain

   c. Tenderness of the calf muscles that increases when the ankle is dorsiflexed[19]

   d. Inflammation and discoloration of the extremity

2. **Chronic venous insufficiency**[11,14,27]

   a. Dependent edema

      (1) Associated with standing and sitting for prolonged periods of time

      (2) Usually worse at the end of the day

      (3) Edema decreases if the leg is elevated while the patient lies supine.

   b. Aching or tiredness in the legs

   c. Increased pigmentation and stasis of the limb

   d. Skin ulcerations and secondary infection, which can lead to cellulitis

C. **Evaluation of Venous Disorders**

1. **Phlebography**[11,14,21,25]

   a. A test used by the physician in addition to observation and the physical examination to diagnose venous disorders

   b. An invasive procedure similar to arteriography, using x-ray study and radiopaque dye injected into the venous system. The procedure is used to detect a venous thrombosis.

2. **Girth measurements of the extremity**

   a. Circumferential measurements of the involved extremity are made to detect edema (or atrophy).

      (1) The girth of the involved extremity may be compared with the girth of the uninvolved extremity.

      (2) If consistent methods are used in taking measurements, the therapist can determine the effectiveness of treatment over a period of time.

   b. One accepted method is to take circumferential measurements every 2 inches along the entire length of the extremity.[21]

3. **Competence of the greater saphenous vein**[19]

   a. A test used for patients with varicose veins

   b. Procedure

      (1) Ask the patient to stand until the varicosities in the leg fill with blood.

      (2) Palpate a portion of the saphenous vein below the knee and then sharply percuss the vein above the knee.

      (3) If a thrust of blood is felt with the palpating finger below the knee, the valves are incompetent.

4. **Tests for possible deep venous thrombophlebitis**

   a. Homans' sign[19,21]

      (1) With the patient supine, forcefully dorsiflex the foot and squeeze the posterior calf muscles.

(2) Many patients, but not all, with thrombophlebitis will experience significant pain in the calf muscles.
    b. Application of a blood pressure cuff around the calf[19]
       (1) Inflate the cuff until the patient experiences pain in the calf.
       (2) Patients with acute thrombophlebitis usually cannot tolerate pressures above 40 mm Hg.

D. Prevention of Thrombophlebitis[2]

1. Every effort should be made to *prevent* the occurrence of thrombophlebitis in patients at risk.
2. It is well established that venous return decreases with prolonged periods of bed rest.
3. Bed rest is the primary cause of acute postoperative thrombosis in the deep veins of the legs.
4. The risk of postoperative thrombophlebitis can be minimized by early ambulation and exercise, such as
    a. Active pumping exercises (dorsiflexion, plantarflexion, and circumduction of the ankle) done regularly throughout the day while the patient is in bed.
    b. Active or mild resistive range of motion to both lower extremities if the postoperative condition permits.
    c. Daily passive ROM if active exercise is not possible because of a neuromuscular or medical condition.

E. Treatment of Acute Thrombophlebitis[11,14,21]

Immediate medical management is essential in this life-threatening disorder. During the initial stages of treatment, the patient will be on complete bed rest and systemic anticoagulant therapy, and the involved extremity will be elevated. Movement of the extremity will cause pain and increase congestion in the venous channels in the early inflammatory period.
Note: Passive or active range of motion exercises are contraindicated during this initial inflammatory period.

General Treatment Goals	*Plan of Care*
1. Relieve pain during the acute inflammatory period.	1. Application of moist heat, such as hot packs, to the entire length of the involved extremity
2. In later stages, as the symptoms subside, regain functional mobility.	2. Graded ambulation with legs wrapped in elastic bandages or when pressure gradient support stockings are worn
3. Prevent recurrence of the acute disorder.	3. The patient should avoid sitting or standing still for any length of time. Either resting with the legs elevated or walking is encouraged.

F. Treatment of Chronic Venous Insufficiency and Varicose Veins[11,14,21]

Patient education is primary in the treatment of these chronic disorders. The patient must be advised on how to prevent dependent edema, skin ulceration, and infections. The therapist may be involved in (1) measuring and fitting a patient for a pressure gradient support stocking; (2) teaching the patient how to put on the stocking before getting out of bed; (3) setting up a program of regular active exercise; and (4) teaching the patient proper skin care.

General Treatment Goals	*Plan of Care*
1. Increase venous return and reduce edema.	1. Individually tailored pressure-gradient support stockings should be worn during ambulation. Manual massage of the extremity in a distal to proximal direction Use of intermittent compression pump Regular ambulation or an active exercise program. ***Note:*** Instruct the patient to elevate the lower extremities after graded ambulation until the heart rate returns to normal. Avoid prolonged periods of standing still and sitting with legs dependent. Elevation of the foot of the bed during rest
2. Prevent skin ulcerations and wound infections.	2. Proper skin care

III. LYMPHATIC DISORDERS

A. Disorders of the Lymphatic System Possible Causes[11,14,21] that Lead to Lymphedema

1. a primary or congenital obstruction of the lymphatic system
2. an obstruction of the lymphatic system secondary to infection
3. surgical removal of lymphatic vessels
   a. The most common surgery in which lymph vessels are removed is the modified radical or radical mastectomy.
   b. The postoperative problems associated with mastectomy include more than just lymphedema of the upper extremity. For this reason, mastectomy will be covered separately and in detail in section IV of this chapter.

B. Lymphedema—Background of the Problem[15]

1. Lymphedema is an excessive accumulation of extravascular and extracellular fluid in tissue spaces. It is caused by a disturbance of the water and protein balance across the capillary membrane.
   a. The lymphatic system is specifically designed to remove plasma proteins that filter into tissue spaces.
   b. Obstruction or removal of lymphatic vessels causes retention of proteins in tissue spaces.

      c. The increased protein concentration draws greater amounts of water into the interstitial space leading to lymphedema.

  2. Signs and symptoms of lymphatic disorders[11,15]

      a. Lymphedema of the distal extremity, most often seen over the dorsum of the hand or foot

      b. Increased weight or heaviness of the extremity

      c. Sensory disturbances of the hand or foot

      d. Stiffness of the fingers or toes

      e. Tautness of skin

      f. Susceptibility to skin breakdown

      g. Decreased resistance to infection, causing frequent episodes of cellulitis

C. Evaluation of Lymphatic Disorders

1. Girth measurements of the extremity[21]
2. Volumetric measurements of the extremity

    a. The involved extremity is immersed in a tank of water.[3,21]

    b. The amount of water displaced as the extremity is lowered into the water is measured.

D. Treatment of Lymphedema[11,14,21,30]

The majority of patients seen by therapists in clinical settings have lymphedema secondary to obstruction of the lymphatic system from trauma, infection, radiation, or surgery. If a patient is at risk for developing lymphedema, prevention is the best goal.

    In order to increase lymphatic drainage, the hydrostatic pressure of tissues must be increased. This is accomplished by external compression of the skin. Lymphatic and venous return can also be increased by elevation of the limb. Lymphedema caused by lymphatic disorders does not diminish as readily with elevation as does edema secondary to venous disorders.

General Treatment Goals	*Plan of Care*
1. Reduce lymphedema.	1. Intermittent mechanical compression with a pneumatic pump and sleeve or bag for several hours daily
	Elevation of the extremity above the level of the heart (about 30 to 45 degrees) while sleeping and as often as possible during the day
	Manual massage from distal to proximal along the length of the extremity
	Isometric and isotonic pumping exercises of the distal muscles.
2. Prevent further edema.	2. Elastic support stocking or sleeve, individually measured and fitted to the patient.
	Regular elevation of the extremity

General Treatment Goals	*Plan of Care*
	Avoidance of sources of increased load on the lymphatics such as:
	—static, dependent positioning of the limb
	—application of local heat
	—prolonged use of muscles for even light tasks
	—hot environments
3. Prevention of infections and cellulitis	3. Care of skin abrasions, small burns, and insect bites
	Avoidance of harsh chemicals and detergents
	Frequent application of moisturizers to skin
	Use of antibiotics

IV. MASTECTOMY

According to the American Cancer Society carcinoma of the breast is the most common form of cancer in white females over the age of 40. About 1 out of 10 women will develop breast cancer sometime during her life.[9] Tumors that are detected early and are localized can be successfully treated by mastectomy (removal of the breast). Although the use of less deforming surgical procedures, such as the lumpectomy and quadrectomy, is increasing, mastectomy is still the most common procedure in preventing the spread of breast cancer and in ensuring a high rate of survival.

After a mastectomy and the accompanying excision or radiation of adjacent axillary lymph nodes, a patient is at risk of developing upper extremity lymphedema and loss of shoulder motion. Therapists often become involved in the postoperative management of patients who have undergone a mastectomy. Therapeutic exercise is an important part of the patient's postoperative plan of care to prevent or minimize lymphedema or loss of shoulder motion.

All therapists should be aware of Reach to Recovery, a one-to-one patient education program, sponsored by the American Cancer Society. Representatives of this program provide emotional support to the patient and family as well as current information on breast prostheses and reconstructive surgery.

A. Surgical Procedures[4,5,20]

1. Radical mastectomy

    a. A radical mastectomy involves removal of the breast, the pectoralis muscles, and the ipsilateral axillary lymph nodes, as well as radiation therapy to the involved area.

    b. Radical mastectomy was the treatment of choice until the 1970s.

    c. Lymphedema, upper extremity weakness, and significant disfigurement results.

2. Modified radical mastectomy

    a. The entire breast and axillary lymph nodes are removed.

    b. The pectoralis muscles remain intact.

    c. This reduces cosmetic deformity and muscular weakness.

    d. The modified radical mastectomy is used far more frequently today for most breast cancers than the more severe radical mastectomy.

3. Simple mastectomy

    a. A simple mastectomy involves surgical removal of the entire breast.

    b. The lymphatic system and pectoralis muscles are preserved.

    c. Postoperative radiation therapy is usually used to decrease the regional recurrence of the disease.

B. Clinical Problems of the Postmastectomy Patient[12,20,31]

1. Postoperative pain

    a. Incisional pain

        (1) A transverse incision across the chest wall is made to remove the breast tissue.

        (2) Secondary chest wall adhesions can result in

            (a) increased risk of postoperative pulmonary complications.

            (b) loss of range of motion of the shoulder on the involved side.

            (c) postural deformity of the trunk.

    b. Posterior cervical and shoulder girdle pain[5]

        (1) Pain and muscle spasm may occur in the neck and shoulder region as a result of muscle guarding.

        (2) The levator scapulae, teres major and minor, and the infraspinatus are often tender with palpation and can restrict active shoulder motion.

        (3) Decreased use of the involved upper extremity after surgery sets the stage for the patient to develop a chronic frozen shoulder and increases the likelihood of lymphedema in the hand and arm.

2. Lymphedema[4,5,31,35]

    a. Removal of the axillary chain of lymph nodes disrupts the normal circulation of lymph and causes swelling of the upper extremity.

    b. Radiation therapy may lead to the formation of scar tissue in the axilla and obstruct lymphatic vessels.

    c. Accumulation of extravascular and extracellular fluids in the upper extremity on the side of the surgery leads to

        (1) increased size of the extremity.

        (2) stiffness and decreased range of motion in the fingers.

        (3) sensory disturbances in the hand.

        (4) decreased function of the involved upper extremity.

3. Weakness of the involved upper extremity[4,5,20]

    a. Weakness of the horizontal adductors of the shoulder

        (1) If a radical mastectomy is performed, the pectoralis major muscle is removed.

        (2) This results in decreased strength and function of the upper extremity on the involved side.

    b. Weakness of the serratus anterior[5]

        (1) In a modified radical and radical mastectomy, the axillary lymph nodes are removed.

    (2) The long thoracic nerve can be temporarily traumatized during axillary dissection and removal of the axillary lymph nodes.

    (3) This results in weakness of the serratus anterior and compromised shoulder stabilization and function.

    (4) Without the stabilization and upward rotation of the scapula that the serratus anterior normally supplies, active flexion and abduction of the arm will be limited.

4. Chest wall adhesions

    a. Are due to restrictive scarring of overlying tissue on the chest wall.

    b. May form postoperatively due to wound infection or radiation.

    c. Contribute to decreased function and range of motion in the involved upper extremity.

C. Physical Therapy Treatment Goals and Plan of Care[4,5,20,31]

General Treatment Goals	*Plan of Care*
1. Prevent postoperative pulmonary complications.	1. Preoperative instruction in deep-breathing exercises and effective coughing (see Chapter 19)
2. Prevent or minimize postoperative lymphedema.	2. Elevation of the involved upper extremity on pillows (about 30 degrees) while the patient is in bed or sitting in a chair. Wrapping the involved upper extremity with elastic bandages or wearing an elastic pressure-gradient sleeve. Pumping exercises of the arm on the side of the surgery. Early range of motion exercises
3. Decrease lymphedema if or when it develops.	3. Daily use of a mechanical pneumatic pressure pump for at least 1½ to 2 hours, twice a day. Continual elevation of the involved upper extremity at night and use of elastic sleeve during the day
4. Prevent postural deformities.	4. Instruction in proper bed positioning preoperatively or on the first postoperative day, emphasizing midline and symmetric positioning of the shoulders and trunk. Carryover of symmetric posture to sitting and standing
5. Prevent muscle tension in cervical musculature.	5. Active range of motion to the cervical spine to promote relaxation

General Treatment Goals	*Plan of Care*
	Shoulder shrugging and shoulder circle exercises
	Gentle massage to cervical musculature
6. Maintain normal range of motion of the involved upper extremity.	6. Begin active exercise to the elbow and hand on the involved side as soon as possible. When the drainage tubes have been removed, begin daily active-assistive and active range of motion exercises to the involved shoulder.
	Pendulum (Codman's) exercises
	Wand exercises to maintain active shoulder motion bilaterally
7. Maintain or increase strength in the involved shoulder.	7. Isometric exercises to the shoulder musculature, initiated on the first postoperative day with the patient in bed
	Manual isotonic resistance exercise may be initiated about 1 week postoperatively.
	Resistance may be applied during shoulder exercise with a light hand-held weight (approximately 2 to 3 pounds).

Note: Although control of lymphedema and exercise are often suggested for patients who have undergone mastectomies, few studies have analyzed the effectiveness of specific rehabilitation procedures. In addition, some patients who have undergone mastectomies are not referred to physical therapy for participation in postoperative rehabilitation because of physicians' doubts of the benefits of therapy or concerns that early motion may increase the incidence of postoperative complications such as poor wound healing.[12,17]

In one study,[31] the efficacy of a postoperative physical therapy program (consisting of active-assisted, active, and resisted ROM exercises; proprioceptive neuromuscular facilitation; functional activities; and hand and arm care) and its impact on postoperative ROM, circumferential measurements, and functional use of the involved upper extremity were analyzed. Patients who received postoperative physical therapy had better ROM and function of the involved upper extremity than the group that did not receive postoperative rehabilitation. There was no significant difference in circumferential measurements of the involved arm in the treatment and control groups. The article did not describe what, if any, activities the patients performed to prevent or decrease lymphedema. Postoperative physical therapy did not prolong hospital stay or increase the incidence of postoperative complications.

D. Postoperative Precautions

1. To ensure proper healing of the incision
   a. Begin active-assistive and active shoulder exercises only after drain-

age tubes have been removed.
  b. Do not place undue stress on the scar or cause blanching of the scar during shoulder range of motion. Observe the incision during exercise.
  c. Initially, shoulder abduction may have to be limited until the sutures are removed. Joint mobilization techniques can be used to maintain joint play in the glenohumeral and scapulothoracic joints when arm movement must be restricted.
  2. If the patient has received radiation therapy postoperatively, wound healing may be delayed.
  3. Avoid positioning the arm in any gravity-dependent positions for prolonged periods of time.

V. SUMMARY

An overview of peripheral vascular disease was presented with specific discussion of arterial, venous, and lymphatic disorders. The signs and symptoms of acute and chronic vascular disorders were outlined. Basic evaluation and diagnostic procedures used to assess peripheral vascular disease were briefly explained. Outlines of treatment goals and plan of care were included for patients with acute or chronic arterial or venous disorders and lymphatic dysfunction. Because the postmastectomy patient is at risk for developing lymphedema and associated loss of function of the involved upper extremity, an expanded discussion of mastectomy and associated postoperative problems was included in this chapter.

REFERENCES

1. Abramson, DI: *Physiologic basis for the use of physical agents in peripheral vascular disorders.* Arch Phys Med Rehab 46:216, 1965.
2. Basmajian, JV (ed): *Therapeutic Exercise,* ed 3. Williams & Wilkins, Baltimore, 1978.
3. Beach, RB: *Measurement of extremity volume by water displacement.* Phys Ther 57:286, 1977.
4. Beeby, J and Broeg, PE: *Treatment of patients with radical mastectomies.* Phys Ther 50:40, 1970.
5. Bork, BE: *Physical therapy for the post mastectomy patient.* University of Iowa, Educational Program in Physical Therapy, 1980.
6. Burgess, EM: *Amputations of the lower extremities.* In Nickel, VL (ed): *Orthopedic Rehabilitation.* Churchill-Livingstone, New York, 1982.
7. *Cancer Facts And Figures: 1988.* American Cancer Society, New York, 1988.
8. Coffman, JD: *Vasodilator drugs in peripheral vascular disease.* N Engl J Med 300:713, 1979.
9. Correlli, F: *Buerger's disease: Cigarette smoker's disease may always be cured by medical therapy.* J Cardiovasc Surg 14:28, 1973.
10. Ekroth, R et al: *Physical training of patients with intermittent claudication: Indications, methods, and results.* Surgery 84:640, 1978.
11. Fell, G and Strandness, DE: *Management of vascular disease.* In Kottke, FJ, Stillwell, GK, and Lehmann, JF (eds): *Krusen's Handbook of Physical Medicine and Rehabilitation,* ed 3. WB Saunders, Philadelphia, 1982.
12. Fell, TJ: *Wound drainage following radical mastectomy. The effect of restriction of shoulder movement.* Br J Surg 66:302, 1979.
13. Hurst, PAE: *Peripheral vascular disease—Assessment and treatment.* In Downie, PA (ed): *Cash's Textbook, of Chest, Heart and Vascular Disorders for Physiotherapists,* ed 4. JB Lippincott, Philadelphia, 1987.
14. Hurst, PAE: *Venous and lymphatic disease—Assessment and treatment.* In Downie, PA (ed): *Cash's Textbook of Chest, Heart and Vascular Disorders for Physiotherapists,* ed 4. JB Lippincott, Philadelphia, 1987.

15. Kottke, FJ: *Common cardiovascular problems in rehabilitation.* In Kottke, FJ, Stillwell, GK, and Lehmann, JF (eds): *Krusen's Handbook of Physical Medicine and Rehabilitation,* ed 3. WB Saunders, Philadelphia, 1982.

16. Lehmann, JF and Delateur, BJ: *Diathermy: Superficial heat and cold therapy.* In Kottke, FJ, Stillwell, GK, and Lehmann, JF (eds): *Krusen's Handbook of Physical Medicine and Rehabilitation,* ed 3. WB Saunders, Philadelphia, 1982.

17. Lotze, MT, et al: *Early versus delayed shoulder motion following axillary dissection. A randomized prospective study.* Am Surg 193:288, 1981.

18. MacKinnon, JL: *Study of Doppler ultrasonic peripheral vascular assessment performed by physical therapists.* Phys Ther 63:30, 1983.

19. McCulloch, JM: *Examination procedure for patients with vascular system problems.* Clinical Management, 1:17, 1981.

20. Neel, DI: *Physical therapy following radical mastectomy.* Phys Ther Rev 40:371, 1960.

21. O'Sullivan, SB, Cullen, KE, and Schmitz, TJ: *Physical Rehabilitation: Evaluation and Treatment Procedures,* ed. 2. FA Davis, Philadelphia, 1988.

22. Ruell, PA et al: *Intermittent claudication. The effect of physical training on walking tolerance and venous lactate concentration.* Eur J Appl Physiol 52:420, 1984.

23. Spencer-Green, G: *Raynaud's phenomenon.* Bull Rheum Dis 33:1, 1983.

24. Stillwell, GK and Redford, JWB: *Physical treatment of postmastectomy lymphedema.* Proc Mayo Clin 33:1, 1958.

25. Strandness, DE, JR: *Invasive and noninvasive techniques in the detection and evaluation of acute venous thrombosis.* Vasc Surg 11:205, 1977.

26. Vallbona, C: *Bodily responses to immobilization.* In Kottke, FJ, Stillwell, GK, and Lehmann, FJ, (eds): *Krusen's Handbook of Physical Medicine and Rehabilitation,* ed 3. WB Saunders, Philadelphia, 1982.

27. Vogel, M, et al: *The role of the physical therapist in the diagnosis of peripheral vascular disease.* Phys Ther Rev 36:384, 1956.

28. Wagner, FW: *The dysvascular lower limb.* In Nickel, VL (ed): *Orthopedic Rehabilitation.* Churchill-Livingstone, New York, 1982.

29. Whitaker, R: *Peripheral vascular disease—The place of physiotherapy.* In Downie, PA: *Cash's Textbook of Chest, Heart and Vascular Disorders for Physiotherapists,* ed 4. JB Lippincott, Philadelphia, 1987.

30. Wing, MT: *Conservative management of peripheral edema.* Phys Ther Forum 6:1, October 21, 1987.

31. Wingate, L: *Efficacy of physical therapy for patients who have undergone mastectomies.* Phys Ther 65:896, 1985.

32. Wisham, LH, Abramson, AS, and Ebel, A: *Value of exercise in peripheral arterial disease.* JAMA 153:10, 1953.

33. Zeissler, RH, Rose, GB and Nelson, PA: *Postmastectomy lymphedema: Late results of treatment in 385 patients.* Arch Phys Med Rehabil 53:159, 1972.

CHAPTER ——————————————————— 14

The Spine: Posture

In theory, treating musculoskeletal conditions of the spinal column and trunk is the same as treating musculoskeletal conditions of the extremities. The complex functional relationships of the facet joints, the intervertebral joints, the muscles, and the nervous system in the axial skeleton provide a challenge for the therapist in evaluation, assessment of the problems, and development of a therapeutic exercise program that deals with the problems. Treating back problems has all too often been simplified into standard exercise routines that are used to prevent or correct all conditions. To the anxiety of the patient and frustration of the therapist, success has not been consistent. The etiology of many of the pain syndromes is unclear, but the importance of an evaluation and identification of problems cannot be overstressed. Most painful conditions of the spine and related areas can be categorized as being the result of stresses to pain-sensitive structures from poor posture, dysfunctions in soft tissue or joints, or an acute injury or pathologic process. Often there is a combination of problems.

Highlights of the anatomy and function of the spinal complex are reviewed in the first section of this chapter. The remainder of this chapter addresses principles and techniques of treating patients with postural faults and dysfunctions. Principles and techniques for treating spinal conditions with acute symptoms are in Chapter 15; principles and techniques of applying spinal traction are in Chapter 16; and Chapter 17 deals with scoliosis.

Therapists involved in posture screening programs or as consultants to physical fitness or education programs can contribute immeasurably to the prevention of painful postural syndromes through early posture awareness and development of exercise programs that are balanced for strength and flexibility and that do not accentuate faulty postures (see Chapter 22).

OBJECTIVES

After studying this chapter, the reader will be able to:
1. identify major components of spinal structure and function for review.
2. describe the dynamics of posture.

---

3. identify characteristics of common postural faults and dysfunctions in each region of the spine.
4. identify principles and techniques to use for treating posture problems in the cervical, thoracic, and lumbar regions.
5. establish a therapeutic exercise program to manage pain and soft-tissue dysfunctions caused by or related to posture problems.

I.   REVIEW OF THE STRUCTURE AND FUNCTION OF THE SPINE

A. Functional Units of the Spinal Column[3,15]

1. The anterior pillar, made up of the vertebral bodies and intervertebral disks, is the hydraulic, weight-bearing, shock-absorbing portion.
2. The posterior pillars, made up of the articular processes and facet joints, are the gliding mechanism for movement. Also part of the posterior unit are the two vertebral arches, two transverse processes, and a central posterior spinous process. Muscles attach to the processes from which they cause and control motion.

B. Physiologic Curves: Description and Function

1. Anterior curves are in the cervical and lumbar regions. *Lordosis* is a term also used to denote anterior curve, although some sources reserve the term lordosis to denote abnormal conditions such as those that occur with sway back.[4]
2. Posterior curves are in the thoracic and sacral regions. *Kyphosis* is a term used to denote a posterior curve. Kyphotic posture refers to an excessive posterior curving of the thoracic spine.[4]
3. The line of gravity transects the spinal curves, which are balanced anteriorly and posteriorly. Deviation of one portion of the spinal column results in shifting of another portion to compensate and maintain balance.
4. The flexibility of the curves gives the vertebral column 10 times the resistance to axial compression forces as that of a straight column.[15,28] Flexibility and balance in the spinal column are necessary to withstand the effects of gravity and other external forces.

C. Inert Structures Influencing Movement and Stability in the Spinal Column[3,15]

When a structure limits movement in a specific direction, it provides stability in that direction.

1. The slant and direction of the articulating facets

a. In the cervical region, the facets are generally in the frontal plane, with some oblique angulation toward the transverse plane, allowing relatively free forward bending (flexion) and backward bending (extension). From the second cervical vertebra to the third thoracic vertebra, side bending and rotation of the vertebrae always occur together and are toward the same side whether the upright position or in the forward-bent position.
b. In the upper thoracic region, the facets are in the frontal plane with slight angulation toward the sagittal plane. In the lower thoracic region, they lie more in the sagittal plane. Rotation, side bending, and forward

bending are allowed to various degrees by the facets, but restricted by the ribs. The facets markedly restrict backward bending along with the spinous processes. When upright, side bending of the vertebrae results in vertebral rotation in the opposite direction for the vertebrae below the third thoracic level.

   c. In the lumbar region, the facets are typically in the sagittal plane with some curvature in the frontal plane, although variations in shape and orientation occur,[2,25] allowing some forward, backward, and side bending, but limiting rotation except in the lower lumbar segments. At the end of the range of forward bending, the facet surfaces in the frontal plane approximate and provide stability against further movement.[27] When upright, side bending occurs with rotation in opposite directions. When forward bent, side bending and rotation of the vertebrae occur together in the same direction.

2. The ligaments

   a. The ligaments posterior to the axis of motion limit forward bending (flexion) of the spinal segments. Ligaments subjected to highest strains on forward bending are the interspinous and supraspinous ligaments. The capsular ligaments, ligamentum flavum, and posterior longitudinal ligament also become taut and stabilize the spine at the end of the flexion range.[21]

   b. The anterior longitudinal ligament limits backward bending.

   c. The contralateral intertransverse ligaments, as well as ligamentum flavum and capsular ligaments, limit side bending.[21]

   d. The capsular ligaments limit rotation.[21]

3. The thoracolumbar (lumbodorsal) fascia

   a. The thoracolumbar fascia reinforces the posterior ligamentous system through the orientation of its fibers and attachments in the lumbar spine and pelvic region.

   b. Passive tension in the posterior layer of the fascia occurs with forward bending of the lumbar spine on the pelvis or posterior tilt of the pelvis. The increased tension supports the lower lumbar vertebra by stabilizing against flexion moments.[2]

   c. The thoracolumbar fascia also provides dynamic trunk stability in conjunction with its muscular attachments as described in Section D to follow.

4. The shape and slant of the spinous processes limit extension.

5. The relative size of the intervertebral disks and bodies

The greater the ratio of disk thickness to vertebral body height, the greater the mobility. The cervical spine ratio is 2:5 and is most mobile; the thoracic ratio is 1:5 and is least mobile; the lumbar ratio is 1:3.[15]

6. The annulus fibrosis of the intervertebral disk

The organized concentric rings of the annulus provide tensile strength to the disk. Movement is allowed, yet some fibers will be taut, whichever direction the spinal column bends, twists, or shears, and therefore behave like ligaments. (See Chapter 15 for additional information on the intervertebral disk.)

7. The ribs in the thoracic region
  a. The ribs limit all motions of the thorax.
  b. During side bending, the thorax is elevated and enlarged on the contra-lateral side (side of the convexity) and is compressed on the ipsilateral side.
  c. During rotation, the ribs protrude posteriorly on the side on which the vertebral body rotates and are flattened on the contralateral side. See Chapter 17 for information on scoliosis.

8. Muscles

Muscles with normal elasticity do not cause limitations to spinal movement. When tight, they restrict movement opposite to their direction of contraction. Muscles provide dynamic stability and control of the spine as described in the following section.

D. Muscle Function: Dynamic Stabilization in the Spinal Column

1. Eccentric control

Muscles of the neck and trunk primarily act as stabilizers (guy wires) of the spinal column in upright posture. They are the dynamic control against the force of gravity as the weight of various segments shifts away from the base of support.[18]
  a. When the line of gravity shifts forward, control is provided by the extensor muscles. They are the erector spinae group and the posterior cervical muscles, including the upper trapezius.
  b. When the line of gravity shifts backward, control is provided by the flexor muscles, which are the abdominal and intercostal muscles, as well as psoas major, longus colli, longus capitis, rectus capitis, anterior scalenes, and sternocleidomastoid.
  c. When the line of gravity shifts laterally, the contralateral muscles provide control. They include the psoas major, quadratus lumborum, scalenes, sternocleidomastoid, erector spinae, internal and external obliques, and intercostal muscles.

2. Postural tone

Little muscle activity is required to maintain upright posture, but with total relaxation of muscles, the spinal curves become exaggerated and passive structural support is called on to maintain the posture.
  a. Continual exaggeration of the curves leads to faulty posture and muscle strength and flexibility imbalances, as well as other soft-tissue tightness or hypermobility.
  b. Muscles that are habitually kept in a stretched position beyond the physiologic resting position tend to weaken; this is known as *stretch weakness*.[16]
  c. Muscles kept in a habitually shortened position tend to loose their elasticity. These muscles test strong only in the shortened position but become weak as they are lengthened.[6] This is known as *tight weakness*.[13]

3. Effect of limb muscles on spinal stability
  a. Without adequate stabilization of the spine, contraction of the limb-girdle musculature will transmit forces proximally and cause motions of the spine that will place excessive stresses on spinal structures and the supporting soft tissue. For example, stabilization of the pelvis and lum-

bar spine by the abdominal muscles against the pull of the iliopsoas muscle is necessary when flexing the hip in order to avoid increased lumbar lordosis and anterior shearing of the vertebrae. Stabilization of the ribs by the intercostal and abdominal muscles is necessary for an effective pushing force from the pectoralis major and serratus anterior muscles.

b. Localized fatigue in the stabilizing spinal musculature may occur in unconditioned individuals when a lot of repetitive activity or heavy exertion is done with the extremities. There is greater chance of injury in the supporting structures of the spine when the stabilizing muscles fatigue.

c. Imbalances in the flexibility of hip, shoulder, and neck musculature will cause asymmetric forces on the spine.

4. **Dynamic support for the lumbar spine and intervertebral disks**[1,2,7,8,9,22,24,25,27]

a. The thoracolumbar (lumbodorsal) fascia consists of three layers of fascia and the aponeuroses of several muscles—the latissimus dorsi, serratus posterior inferior, internal obliques, and transverse abdominis[1,2] (Figure 14-1).

(1) The posterior layer of the fascia attaches to the spinous processes in a triangular pattern and covers the back muscles (Figure 14-2A and B). It blends with the other layers of fascia at the **lateral raphe,** along the lateral border of the iliocostalis lumborum.

(2) The middle layer is posterior to the quadratus lumborum and attaches to the tips of the transverse processes and intertransverse ligaments. Laterally, it blends with the lateral raphe and is continuous with the transversus abdominis. It, with the posterior layer, envelops the erector spinae muscles.

(3) The anterior layer is a thin sheet anterior to the quadratus lumborum and attaches to the anterior aspect of the transverse processes and intertransverse ligaments.

b. The muscle attachments are designed to converge forces via the fascia into the ligamentous system to provide stability and support as they function in the dynamics of the lumbar spine. Increased tension in, or participation of any of the muscles attached to or surrounded by, the fascia increases the support and equalizes forces at the lumbar spine.

FIGURE 14-1. Transverse section in the lumbar region showing the relationships of the three layers of the thoracolumbar fascia to the muscles in the region and their attachments to the spine. (ES = erector spinae, TA = transversus abdominis, IO = internal obliques, EO = external obliques, LD = latissimus dorsi, PM = psoas major, and QL = quadratus lumborum muscles.)

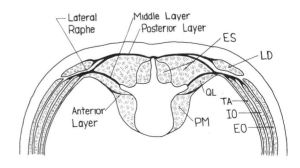

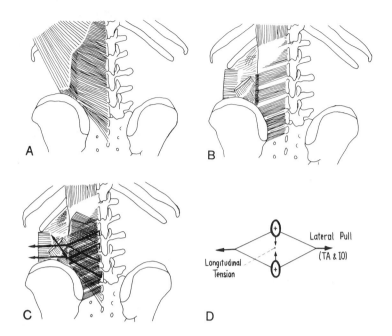

FIGURE 14-2. Orientation and attachments of the posterior layer of the thoracolumbar fascia. From the lateral raphe, (*A*) the fibers of the superficial lamina are angled inferiorly and medially, (*B*) and the fibers of the deep lamina are angled superiorly and medially. (Adapted from Bogduk and MacIntosh,[1] pp. 166-167, 1984), (*C*) Tension in the angled fibers of the posterior layer of the fascia is transmitted to the spinous processes in opposing directions, resisting separation of the spinous processes. (Adapted from Bogduk and MacIntosh,[1] p. 169, 1984), (*D*) Diagramatic representation of a lateral pull at the lateral raphe, resulting in a tension between the lumbar spinous processes that oppose separation thus creating an anti-flexion moment. (Adapted from Gracovetsky, Farfan, and Helleur,[7] p. 319, 1985)

(1) Tension in the posterior layer of the fascia is transmitted upward and downward through the angled fibers, resulting in opposing vectors that resist separation of the lumbar spinous processes, thus opposing any flexion moment (Figures 14-2C and D).

(2) Because the posterior and middle layers of the thoracolumbar fascia envelope the erector spinae muscles of the lumbar spine, when these muscles contract they expand against the fascial envelope, thereby increasing tension in the fascia. This creates a hydraulic amplifier mechanism (which is like filling a flexibile tube with fluid, resulting in greater stability of the tube).[7] This increased fascial tension reinforces the back extensor muscles in countering the flexion moment on the spine during forward bending and extending against gravity.

(3) Contraction of the transversus abdominis and internal oblique muscles increases the intra-abdominal pressure. The increased intra-abdominal pressure pushes out against these muscles, increasing their tension and pull on the lateral raphe, which is transmitted to the angled fibers of the lumbodorsal fascia (Figure 14-3).[9,23] This pressure mechanism, coupled with the pull of the muscles and increased tension in the lumbodorsal fascia, helps counter the flexion moment in the lumbar spine with lifting activities (see also Figure 14-2C and D).

(4) Contraction of the latissimus dorsi with lifting activities results in the force being transmitted through the thoracolumbar fascia to reinforce the anti-flexion moment of the fascia, thus providing additional support for the lumbar spine when bending and lifting.

(5) With flexion of the spine, the deep lamina of the posterior layer of the fascia becomes taut and thus supports the L4 and L5 vertebral segments via the attachments of the fascia from the spinous processes to the ilium. This is in addition to the ligamentous system supporting the entire lumbar spine.

II. THE DYNAMICS OF POSTURE

A. Posture defined

Posture is "a position or attitude of the body, the relative arrangement of body parts for a specific activity, or a characteristic manner of bearing one's body."[18]

1. Ligaments, fascia, bones, and joints are inert structures that support the body, whereas muscles and their tendinous attachments are the dynamic structures which maintain the body in a posture or move it from one posture to another.

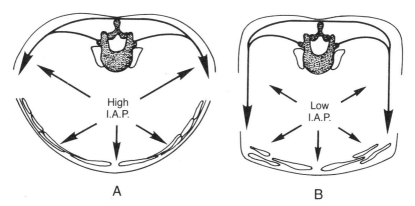

A　　　　　　　　　　　　　　　B

FIGURE 14-3. (*A*) Increased intra-abdominal pressure (IAP) pushes outward against the transversus abdominis and internal obliques, creating increased tension on the thoracolumbar fascia, resulting in an anti-flexion moment. (*B*) Reduced pressure allows flexion of the spine. (Adapted from Gracovetsky,[9] p. 114, 1986)

2. Gravity places stress on the structures responsible for maintaining the body upright in a posture. Normally, the gravitational line goes through the physiologic curves of the spinal column and they are balanced. If the weight in one region shifts away from the line of gravity, the remainder of the column compensates to regain equilibrium.

B. The Equilibrium of Posture[18,20]

For a weight-bearing joint to be stable, or in equilibrium, the gravity line of the mass must fall exactly through the axis of rotation, or there must be a force to counteract the force of gravity. In the body, the counter force is either muscle or inert structures. Upright posture usually involves a slight anterior-posterior swaying of the body of about 4 centimeters.[11]

In the standing posture, the following occur:

1. Ankle

The gravity line is anterior to the joint so it tends to rotate the tibia forward about the ankle. Stability is provided by the plantarflexor muscles, primarily the soleus muscle.

2. Knee

The normal gravity line is anterior to the joint, which tends to keep the knee in extension. Stability is provided by the anterior cruciate ligament, posterior capsule (locking mechanism of the knee), and tension in the muscles posterior to the knee (the gastrocnemius and hamstring muscles). The soleus provides active stability by pulling posteriorly on the tibia. With the knees fully extended, no muscle support is required at that joint to maintain upright posture, but if the knees flex slightly, the gravity line shifts posterior to the joint and the quadriceps femoris muscle must contract to prevent the knee from buckling.

3. Hip

The gravity line varies with the swaying of the body. When it passes through the hip joint, there is equilibrium and no external support is necessary. When the gravitational line shifts posterior to the joint, some posterior rotation of the pelvis occurs but is controlled by tension in the hip flexor muscles (primarily the iliopsoas); then passive tension in the iliofemoral ligament prevents further motion. In relaxed standing, the iliofemoral ligament provides passive stability to the joint and no muscle tension is necessary. When the gravitational line shifts anteriorly, stability is provided by active support of the hip extensor muscles.

4. Trunk

Normally, the gravity line goes through the bodies of the lumbar and cervical vertebrae; then the curves are balanced. Some muscle activity in the erector spinae helps maintain the balance. As the trunk shifts, contralateral muscles contract and function as guy wires. Extreme or sustained deviations are supported by inert structures.

5. Head

The center of gravity of the head falls anterior to the atlanto-occipital joints. The posterior cervical muscles contract to keep the head balanced. In postures in which the head is forward, greater demand is placed on these muscles. At the extreme of flexion, tension in the ligamentum nuchae prevents further motion.

C. Etiology of Pain in Postural Problems

1. The ligaments, facet capsules, periosteum of the vertebrae, muscles, anterior dura mater, dural sleeves, epidural areolar adipose tissue, and walls of blood vessels are innervated and responsive to nociceptive stimuli.[17]
2. Mechanical stress to pain-sensitive structures, such as sustained stretch to ligaments or joint capsules, or compression of blood vessels, causes distension or compression of the nerve endings that leads to the experience of pain. This type of stimulus occurs in the absence of an inflammatory reaction. It is not a pathologic problem but a mechanical one. Relieving the stress to the pain-sensitive structure relieves the pain stimulus, and the person no longer experiences pain. (For acute problems with inflammation, see Chapter 15.) If the mechanical stresses exceed the supporting capabilities of the tissues, breakdown will occur. If this continues without adequate healing, overuse syndromes with inflammation and pain will affect function without an apparent injury. Relieving the mechanical stress along with decreasing the inflammation is important.

D. Pain Syndromes Related to Poor Posture

1. **Postural fault and the postural pain syndrome**

   A postural fault is a posture that deviates from normal alignment but has no structural limitations. The postural pain syndrome refers to the pain that occurs from mechanical stress when a person maintains a faulty posture for a prolonged period; the pain is usually relieved with activity. There are no abnormalities in muscle strength or flexibility, but if the faulty posture continues, strength and flexibility imbalances will eventually develop.

2. **Postural dysfunction**

   This differs from the postural pain syndrome in that adaptive shortening of soft tissues and muscle weakness are involved. The cause may be prolonged poor posture habits, or it may be a result of contractures and adhesions formed during the healing of tissues after trauma or surgery. Stress to the shortened structures causes pain. In addition, strength and flexibility imbalances may predispose the area to injury or overuse syndromes that a normal musculoskeletal system could sustain (see Chapter 15).

3. **Postural habits**

   Good postural habits in the adult are necessary to avoid postural pain syndromes and postural dysfunctions. Also, careful follow-up in terms of flexibility and posture training exercises is important following trauma or surgery to prevent dysfunctions from contractures and adhesions. In the child, good postural habits are important in order to avoid abnormal stresses on growing bones and adaptive changes in muscle and soft tissue.

III. CHARACTERISTICS AND PROBLEMS OF COMMON FAULTY POSTURES

A. Pelvic and Lumbar Region

1. **Lordotic posture (Figure 14-4A)**

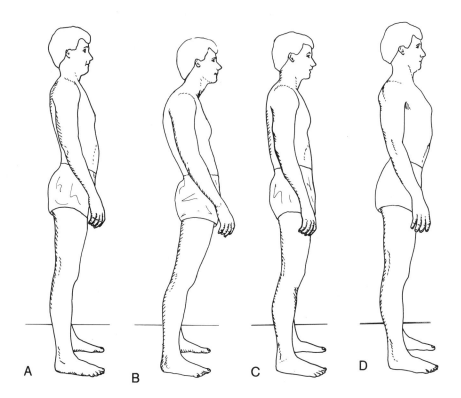

FIGURE 14-4. (*A*) Lordotic posture characterized by an increase in the lumbosacral angle, an increased lumbar lordosis, an increased anterior tilting of the pelvis, and hip flexion; (*B*) Relaxed or slouched posture characterized by an excessive shifting of the pelvic segment anteriorly, resulting in hip extension, and shifting of the thoracic segment posteriorly, resulting in flexion of the thorax on the upper lumbar spine. A compensatory increased thoracic kyphosis and forward head placement are also seen; (*C*) Flat low-back posture characterized by a decreased lumbosacral angle, a decreased lumbar lordosis, and a posterior tilting of the pelvis; (*D*) Flat upper back and cervical spine characterized by a decrease in the thoracic curve, depressed scapulae, depressed clavicle, and an exaggeration of axial extension (flexion of the occiput on atlas and flattening of the cervical lordosis).

Characterized by an increase in the lumbosacral angle (the angle that the superior border of the first sacral vertebral body makes with the horizontal, which optimally is 30 degrees), an increase in the lumbar lordosis, an increase in the anterior pelvic tilt and hip flexion.[3] This is often seen with an increased thoracic kyphosis and forward head and is called a *kypholordotic posture*.[16]

    a. Potential sources of pain
       (1) stress to the anterior longitudinal ligament
       (2) narrowing of the posterior disk space and narrowing of the intervertebral foramen. This may compress the dura and blood vessels of the related nerve root or the nerve root itself, especially if there are degenerative changes in the vertebra or disk.[3]
       (3) approximation of the articular facets. The facets may become weight bearing, which may cause synovial irritation and joint inflammation.
    b. Muscle imbalances observed[16]
       (1) tight hip flexor muscles (iliopsoas, tensor fasciae latae, rectus femoris), and lumbar extensor muscles (erector spinae).
       (2) stretched and weak abdominal muscles (rectus abdominis, internal and external obliques).
    c. Common causes
    Sustained faulty posture, pregnancy, obesity, weak abdominal muscles.

2. Relaxed or slouched posture (Figure 14-4B)

This posture is also called *swayback,*[16] which is a shifting of the entire pelvic segment anteriorly resulting in hip extension, and shifting of the thoracic segment posteriorly resulting in flexion of the thorax on the upper lumbar spine. This results in an increased lordosis in the lower lumbar region, an increased kyphosis in the lower thoracic region, and usually a forward head. The position of the mid- and upper lumbar spine depends on the amount of displacement of the thorax. When standing for prolonged periods, the person usually assumes an asymmetric stance in which most of the weight is borne on one lower extremity, with periodic shifting of weight to the opposite extremity.

    a. Potential sources of pain
       (1) stress to the iliofemoral ligaments, the anterior longitudinal ligament of the lower lumbar spine, and the posterior longitudinal ligament of the upper lumbar and thoracic spine. With asymmetric postures there is also stress to the iliotibial band on the side of the elevated hip.
       (2) narrowing of the intervertebral foramen in the lower lumbar spine that may compress the blood vessels, dura, and nerve roots, especially with arthritic conditions.
       (3) approximation of articular facets in the lower lumbar spine.
    b. Muscle imbalances observed[16]
       (1) tight upper abdominal muscles (upper segments of the rectus abdominis and obliques), internal intercostal, hip extensor, and lower lumbar extensor muscles and related fascia.
       (2) stretched and weak lower abdominal muscles (lower segments of the rectus abdominis and obliques), extensor muscles of the lower thoracic region, and hip flexor muscles.
    c. Common causes
    As the name implies, this is a relaxed posture in which the muscles are not used to provide support. The person yields fully to the effects of gravity, and only the passive structures at the end of each joint range (such as ligaments, joint capsules, and bony approximation) provide stability. Causes may be attitudinal (the person feels comfortable when

slouching), from fatigue (seen when required to stand for extended periods), from muscle weakness (the weakness may be the cause or the effect of the posture), or from a poorly designed exercise program (one which emphasizes thoracic flexion; see Chapter 22).

3. **Flat low-back posture (Figure 14-4C)**

Characterized by a decreased lumbosacral angle, a decreased lumbar lordosis, hip extension, and a posterior tilting of the pelvis.

a. Potential sources of pain
   (1) lack of the normal physiologic lumbar curve which reduces the shock-absorbing effect of the lumbar region and predisposes the person to injury.
   (2) stress to the posterior longitudinal ligament
   (3) increase of the posterior disk space which allows the nucleus pulposus to imbibe extra fluid, and under certain circumstances, may protrude posteriorly when the person attempts extension (see Chapter 15)

b. Muscle imbalances observed
   (1) tight trunk flexor (rectus abdominis and intercostals) and hip extensor muscles.
   (2) stretched and weak lumbar extensor and possibly hip flexor muscles.

c. Common causes
   Continued slouching or flexing in sitting or standing postures; overemphasis on flexion exercises in general exercise programs

B. Thoracic Region

1. **Round back or increased kyphosis (see Figure 14-4B)**

Characterized by an increased thoracic curve, protracted scapulae (round shoulders), and usually an accompanying forward head.

a. Potential sources of pain
   (1) stress to the posterior longitudinal ligament
   (2) fatigue of the thoracic erector spinae and rhomboid muscles
   (3) thoracic outlet syndrome (see Chapter 15)
   (4) cervical posture syndromes (see Section C)

b. Muscle imbalances observed
   (1) tight muscles of the anterior thorax (intercostal muscles), muscles of the upper extremity originating on the thorax (pectoralis major and minor, latissimus dorsi, and serratus anterior), muscles of the cervical spine and head attached to the scapula (levator scapulae and upper trapezius), and muscles of the cervical region (see section C).
   (2) stretched and weak thoracic erector spinae and scapula retractor muscles (rhomboids and upper and lower trapezius).

c. Common causes
   Similar to the relaxed lumbar posture or the flat low-back posture, continued slouching, and overemphasis on flexion exercises in general exercise programs

2. **Flat upper back (Figure 14-4D)**

Characterized by a decrease in the thoracic curve, depressed scapulae, depressed clavicle, and a flat neck posture (see Section D). It is associated with an exaggerated military posture but is not a common postural deviation.

    a. Potential sources of pain

        (1) fatigue of muscles required to maintain the posture

        (2) compression of the neurovascular bundle in the thoracic outlet between the clavicle and ribs

    b. Muscle imbalances

        (1) tight thoracic erector spinae and scapular retractors, and potentially restricted scapula movement, which would decrease the freedom of shoulder elevation.

        (2) weak scapular protractor and intercostal muscles of the anterior thorax.

    c. Common cause

    Exaggerating the upright posture

3. Scoliosis

This usually involves the thoracic and lumbar regions (see Chapter 17 on Scoliosis). Typically, in right-handed individuals, there is a mild right thoracic, left lumbar S-curve, or a mild left thoracic-lumbar C-curve. There may be asymmetry in the hips, pelvis, and lower extremities.

    a. Potential sources of pain

        (1) muscle fatigue and ligamentous strain on the side of the convexity

        (2) nerve root irritation on the side on the concavity

    b. Muscle imbalances

        (1) tight structures on the concave side of the curve

        (2) stretched and weak structures on the convex side of the curve

        (3) If one hip is adducted, the adductor muscles on that side will be tight and the abductor muscles will be stretched and weak. The opposite will occur on the contralateral extremity.[16]

    c. Common causes

    Long-term asymmetrical postural and functional activities, handedness, and developmental patterns. (See also Chapter 17)

C. Cervical Region

1. Forward head posture (see Figure 14-4B)

Characterized by increased flexion of the lower cervical and the upper thoracic regions, increased extension of the occiput on the first cervical vertebra, and increased extension of the upper cervical vertebrae. There also may be temporomandibular joint dysfunction with retrusion of the mandible.[23]

    a. Potential sources of pain

        (1) stress to the anterior longitudinal ligament in the upper cervical spine and posterior longitudinal ligament in the lower cervical and upper thoracic spine

        (2) muscle tension or fatigue

        (3) irritation of facet joints in the upper cervical spine

        (4) narrowing of the intervertebral foramina in the upper cervical region, which may impinge on the blood vessels and nerve roots, especially if there are degenerative changes

        (5) impingement on the neurovascular bundle from anterior scalene muscle tightness (see also thoracic outlet syndrome in Chapter 15)

(6) impingement on the cervical plexus from levator scapulae muscle tightness

(7) impingement on occipital nerves from a tight or tense upper trapezius muscle, leading to tension headaches.

(8) temporomandibular joint pain from faulty head, neck, and mandibular alignment and associated facial muscle tension.

(9) lower cervical disk lesions from the faulty flexed posture

b. Muscle imbalances

(1) tight levator scapulae, sternocleidomastoid, scalene, and suboccipital muscles. If the scapulae are elevated, there may also be tight upper trapezius muscles. With temporomandibular joint symptoms, the muscles of mastication may have increased tension.

(2) stretched and weakened anterior throat muscles (hyoid becomes fixed because of the stretched position) and lower cervical and upper thoracic erector spinae muscles

c. Common causes

Occupational or functional postures requiring leaning forward for extended periods, relaxed postures, or the end result of a faulty pelvic and lumbar spine posture

2. Flat neck posture (Figure 14-4D)

Characterized by a decreased cervical lordosis and increased flexion of the occiput on atlas (this is an exaggeration of axial extension). It may be seen with an exaggerated military posture (flat upper back). There may be temporomandibular joint dysfunction with protraction of the mandible.

a. Potential sources of pain

(1) temporomandibular joint pain and occlusive changes

(2) decrease in the shock-absorbing function of the lordotic curve, which may predispose the neck to injury

(3) stress to the ligamentum nuchae

b. Muscle imbalances

(1) short anterior neck muscles

(2) Theoretically, the levator scapulae, sternocleidomastoid, and scalene muscles become stretched and weakened.

c. Common causes

Exaggeration of the posture for extended periods of time. This posture is uncommon.

D. Frontal Plane Deviations From Lower Extremity Asymmetries

Any lower extremity inequality will have an effect on the pelvis that, in turn, affects the spinal column and structures supporting it. When dealing with spinal posture, it is imperative to assess lower extremity alignment, symmetry, foot posture, range of motion, and strength. See Chapters 10, 11, and 12 for principles, procedures, and techniques for treating the hip, knee, and ankle.

1. Characteristic deviations when standing with weight equally distributed to both lower extremities

a. Elevated ilium on the long leg (LL) side, lowered on the short leg (SL) side

(1) This puts the LL in hip adduction and the SL in hip abduction.

        (2) The sacroiliac (SI) joint on the LL side is more vertical; on the SL side it is more horizontal.

    b. Side bending of the lumbar spine toward the LL side, coupled with rotation in the opposite direction

        (1) This compresses the intervertebral disk on the LL side and distracts the disk on the SL side, as well as causes a torsional stress.

        (2) There is extension and compression of the lumbar facets on the LL side (concave portion of curve) and flexion and distraction of the lumbar facets on the SL side (convex portion of curve).

        (3) There is narrowing of the intervertebral foramina on the LL side.

    c. The thoracic and cervical spine have a compensatory scoliosis in the opposite direction.

2. Potential sources of pain

    a. Greater shear forces occur in the hip and SI joints on the LL side, which increases stress in the supporting ligaments and decreases the load-bearing surface within the joint. Degenerative changes occur more frequently in hips on the LL side.[5]

    b. Stenosis in the lumbar intervertebral foramina on the LL side may cause vascular congestion or nerve root irritation.

    c. Lumbar facet compression and irritation on the LL side

    d. Disk breakdown from torsional and asymmetric forces (see Chapter 15)

    e. Muscle tension, fatigue, or spasm in response to asymmetric loading and response

    f. Lower extremity overuse syndromes

3. Muscle imbalances

    a. Tight hip muscles include adductors on the LL side and abductors on the SL side. There may also be asymmetric differences in the iliopsoas, quadratus lumborum, piriformis, erector spinae, and multifidus muscles; those on the concave side of the curve or LL side being tighter.

    b. Stretched and weakened muscles include hip adductors on the SL side, abductors on the LL side, and in general, muscles on the convex side of the curve.

4. Common causes

    Asymmetry in the lower extremities may result from structural or functional deviations at the hip, knee, ankle, or foot. Common functional problems include unilateral flat foot and imbalances in the flexibility of muscles. The resulting asymmetric ground reaction forces transmitted to the pelvis and back may lead to tissue breakdown and overuse, particularly as a person ages, becomes overweight, or generally deconditions from inactivity.[22]

E. Summary of Typical Clinical Problems Associated with Postural Pain Syndromes and Dysfunction

1. Pain from stress to sensitive structures and muscle tension

2. Decreased range of motion (dysfunctions)

3. Muscle strength imbalances (dysfunctions)

4. Altered kinesthetic awareness of normal alignment

5. Lack of knowledge of how to manage posture to prevent pain

F. General Treatment Goals and Plan of Care

Treatment Goals	Plan of Care
1. Relieve pain and muscle tension	1. Modalities and massage Muscle relaxation training Correct postural stress using goals 2 through 4
2. Restore range of motion	2. Specific stretching and flexibility exercises
3. Restore muscle balance	3. Specific resistive exercise External support to prevent positions of stretch
4. Retrain kinesthetic awareness and control of normal alignment	4. Reinforcement techniques
5. Teach patient how to manage posture to prevent recurrences	5. Teach proper body mechanics Educate patient in preventive exercises and mechanics for relief of mechanical stress in daily activities Teach relaxation exercises to cope with muscle tension Instruct patient on how to modify environment: bed, chairs, car seats, work area

The following section includes procedures used to meet the above goals and to fulfill the plan of care.

IV. PROCEDURES AND TECHNIQUES FOR TREATING PROBLEMS THAT OCCUR WITH POSTURAL PAIN SYNDROMES AND DYSFUNCTIONS

The procedures in this section are appropriate if, following a comprehensive assessment of the patient's history and clinical signs, it is determined that the patient is not suffering from an acute injury or disk derangement but that the presenting pain is due to the stresses of poor posture or related flexibility and strength losses. It is important to note that the following procedures are NOT listed as a protocol for treatment. Not all procedures are appropriate for all patients. A variety of exercises are described, allowing the therapist to make a careful selection of which ones best meet the goals for each patient.

A. Procedures to Relieve Pain and Muscle Tension

1. Modalities and massage (techniques not included in this text).

2. Muscle relaxation techniques

a. **Active ROM**

Whenever discomfort develops from maintaining a constant posture or from sustaining muscle contractions for a period of time, active range of motion, in the opposite direction, aids in taking stress off supporting structures, promoting circulation, and maintaining flexibility. All motions are performed slowly, through the full range, with the patient paying particular attention to the feel of the muscles. Repeat each motion several times.

(1) The cervical and upper thoracic region
Position of patient: sitting, with arms resting comfortably on the lap, or standing. Instruct the patient to
(a) bend his neck forward and backward. (Backward bending is contraindicated with symptoms of nerve root compression.)
(b) side bend the head in each direction, then rotate the head in each direction.
(c) roll his shoulders; protract, elevate, retract, then relax the scapulae (in a position of good posture).
(d) circle his arms (shoulder circumduction). This is done with the elbows flexed or extended, using either small or large circular motions, with the arms pointing either forward or out to the side. Both clockwise and counterclockwise motions should be done, but conclude the circumduction by going forward, up, around, and then back, so the scapulae end up in a retracted position. This has the benefit of helping retrain proper posture.

(2) The lower thoracic and lumbar region
Position of patient: sitting or standing. If standing, his feet should be shoulder-width apart, with the knees slightly bent. Have him place his hands at his waist with his fingers pointing backwards. Instruct the patient to
(a) extend the lumbar spine by leaning his trunk backwards (see Figure 14-16B). This is particularly beneficial when the person must sit or stand in a forward-bent position for prolonged periods.
(b) flex the lumbar spine by contracting the abdominal muscles, causing a posterior pelvic tilt; or if there are no signs of a disk problem, the patient can bend his trunk forward, dangling his arms toward the floor with his knees slightly bent. This motion is beneficial when the person stands in a lordotic or sway back posture for prolonged periods.
(c) side bend in each direction.
(d) rotate the trunk by turning in each direction while keeping the pelvis facing forward.
(e) stand up and walk around at frequent intervals when sitting for extended periods.

b. **General conscious relaxation techniques**
Relaxation for the entire body should be taught to a person who is generally tense (see Chapter 4).

c. **Conscious relaxation training for the cervical region**
As with general techniques, the specific techniques for this region develop the patient's kinesthetic awareness of a tensed or relaxed muscle and how to consciously reduce tension in the muscle. In addition, if done with posture training techniques in mind (see Section D), the therapist can help the patient recognize decreased muscular tension where the head is properly balanced and the cervical spine is aligned in mid-position.
Position of patient: sitting comfortably with arms relaxed, such as resting on a pillow placed on the lap; the eyes are closed. The therapist is

positioned next to the patient and uses tactile cues on the muscles and helps position the head as necessary. Instruct the patient to

(1) use diaphragmatic breathing. He breathes in slowly and deeply through his nose, allowing his abdomen to relax and expand, then relaxes and allows the air to be expired through the relaxed open mouth. This breathing is reinforced after each of the following activities.

(2) next, relax the jaw. The tongue rests gently on the hard pallet behind the front teeth with the jaw slightly opened. If the patient has trouble relaxing the jaw, have him click his tongue and allow the jaw to drop. Practice until the patient feels the jaw relax and tongue rest behind the front teeth. Follow with relaxed breathing as in (1) above.

(3) slowly flex the neck. As he does so, direct his attention to his posterior cervical muscles and the sensation of how they feel. Use verbal cues such as, "Notice the feeling of increased tension in your muscles as your head leans forward."

(4) then slowly raise his head to neutral, inhale slowly, and relax. Help him position the head properly and suggest that he note how the muscles contract to lift the head, then relax once the head is balanced.

(5) repeat the motion; again direct the patient's attention to the feeling of contraction and relaxation in the muscles as he moves. Imagery can be used with the breathing such as "fill your head with air and feel it lift up off your shoulders as you breath in, and relax."

(6) then go through only part of the range, noting how the muscles feel.

(7) next, just think of letting his head drop forward, then tightening the muscles (setting) and then think of bringing the head back, then relax. Reinforce to the patient his ability to influence the feeling of contraction and relaxation in the muscles.

(8) finally, just think of tensing the muscles and relaxing, letting the tension go out of the muscles even more. Point out that he feels even greater relaxation. Once the patient learns how to perceive tension in muscles, he can then consciously think of relaxing the muscles. Emphasize the fact that the position of his head also influences the muscle tension. Have him assume various head postures, then correct them until the feel is reinforced.

3. Demonstrate the relationship of faulty posture to the development of pain

See Section D 4.

B. Procedures to Increase the Range of Motion of Specific Structures

Note: To obtain an adequate stretch, apply the stretch force slowly and sustain it for at least 6 seconds. Release the force, then repeat three times. Reevaluate to determine change, and decide whether to proceed with the same technique or to modify it.

1. Cervical and upper thoracic region

a. **To stretch the anterior portion of the intercostal muscles and increase mobility of the anterior thorax**

(1) Position of patient: hook lying, with hands behind head and elbows resting on the mat. To increase the stretch, place a pad lengthwise under the thoracic spine between the scapulae. Segmental breathing (Chapter 19) can also be used by having the patient start with the elbows together in front of the face, then inhale as the elbows are brought down to the mat; hold; then exhale as the elbows are brought together again (see Figure 19-15A and B).

(2) Position of patient: hook lying with both arms elevated overhead. The patient attempts to keep his back flat on the mat while inhaling and expanding the anterior thorax.

(3) Position of patient: sitting on a firm straight-back chair, with his hands behind his head. He then brings his elbows out to the side as the scapulae are adducted and thoracic spine extended (head held neutral, not flexed). To combine with breathing, have the patient inhale as he takes his elbows out to the side, and exhale as he brings his elbows in front of his face (see Figure 19-14A and B).

b. **To stretch the pectoralis major muscles**

(1) Position of patient: sitting on a treatment table or mat, with his hands behind his head. The therapist kneels behind the patient, grasping the patient's elbows (Figure 14-5). Have the patient breathe in as he brings his elbows out to the side (horizontal abduction and scapular adduction). The therapist holds the elbows at this end-point as the patient breathes out. No forceful stretch is needed against the elbows, because the rib cage is elongating the proximal attachment of the pectoralis major muscle. As the patient repeats the inhalation, the therapist moves the elbows up and out to the end of the available range, then holds as the patient breathes out.

Note: Hyperventilation should not occur, because the breathing is slow and comfortable. If the patient does become dizzy, allow him to rest, then reinstruct for proper technique. Be sure the patient maintains the neck in the neutral position, not flexed.

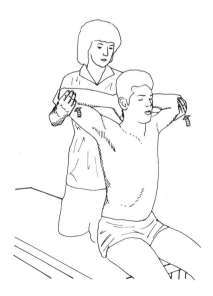

FIGURE 14-5. Active stretching of the pectoralis major muscle. The therapist holds the elbows at the end-point as the patient breathes out.

(2) Self-stretching

Position of patient: standing, facing a corner or open door, with his arms in a reverse T or a V against the wall (Figure 14-6A and B). He then leans his entire body forward from the ankles (knees slightly bent). The degree of stretch can be adjusted by the amount of forward movement.

(3) Wand exercises for stretching

Position of patient: sitting or standing. The patient grasps the wand with the forearms pronated and elbows flexed 90 degrees. He then elevates his shoulders and brings the wand behind his head and shoulders (Figure 14-7). His scapulae are adducted and elbows brought out to the side. Combine with breathing by having the patient inhale as he brings the wand into position behind the shoulders, then exhale while holding this stretched position.

c. **To isolate stretch to the pectoralis minor muscle**

Position of patient: sitting. The therapist stands on the side opposite the muscle to be stretched, places one hand posterior on the far scapula, stabilizing it against the rib cage, and the other hand anterior on the far shoulder, just above the coracoid process (Figure 14-8). The patient breathes in; the therapist fixes the scapula at the end position; then the patient breathes out. Repeat, with the therapist readjusting the end-position with each inhalation, and stabilizing as the patient exhales.

d. **To stretch the levator scapulae muscle**

Note: The muscle attaches to the superior angle of the scapula and causes it to rotate downward and elevate; it also attaches to the trans-

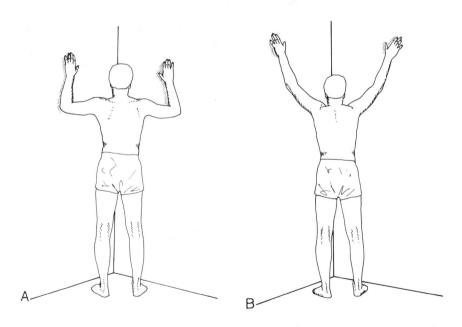

FIGURE 14-6. Self-stretching the pectoralis major muscle with the arms in a reverse T to stretch the clavicular portion (*A*), and in a V to stretch the sternal portion (*B*).

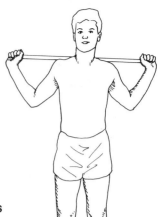

FIGURE 14-7. Wand exercises to stretch the pectoralis major muscle.

verse processes of the upper cervical vertebrae and causes them to backward bend and rotate to the ipsilateral side. Because the muscle is attached to two movable structures, both ends must be stabilized opposite to the pull of the muscle.

(1) Position of patient: sitting. The patient rotates his head opposite to the side of tightness (looks away from the tight side) and forward bends until a slight pull is felt in the posterior-lateral aspect of the neck (in the levator muscle). He then abducts the arm on the side of tightness, placing that hand behind his head to help stabilize it in the rotated position. The therapist stands behind and places one hand across the shoulder to stabilize the scapula, and the elbow of the other arm anteriorly across the patient's rotated head. The therapist's hand can then help abduct the patient's arm (Figure 14-9). With the muscle now in its stretched position, have the patient

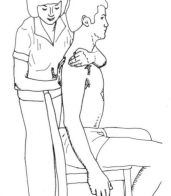

FIGURE 14-8. Active stretching of the pectoralis minor muscle. The therapist holds the scapula and coracoid process at the end-point as the patient breathes out.

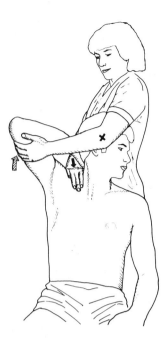

FIGURE 14-9. Active stretching of the levator scapulae muscle. The therapist stabilizes the head and scapula as the patient breathes in, contracting the muscle against the resistance. As the patient relaxes, the rib cage and scapula depress, which stretches the muscle.

breathe in, then out. The therapist holds the shoulder and scapula down to maintain the stretch as the patient breathes in again (he contracts the muscle against the resistance of the fixating hand). To increase the stretch, increase the shoulder abduction. This is not a forceful stretch but a gentle contract-relax maneuver. Do not stretch the muscle by forcing rotation on the head and neck.

(2) To do the above maneuver in a home program as a self-stretching technique, the patient assumes the same head and arm position as in (1) and then stands with his bent elbow against the wall, and if necessary, his other hand across his forehead to stabilize his rotated head. He then inhales, exhales, and moves his elbow up the wall (Figure 14-10A).

(3) Alternate self-stretching technique with the patient sitting. The head placement is the same; the head is rotated away from side of tightness, then the patient looks down until a slight pull is felt in the levator. To stabilize the scapula, the patient reaches down and back with the hand on the side of tightness and holds on to the seat of the chair. The other hand is placed on the head to gently pull it forward and to the side in an oblique direction opposite the line of pull of the tight muscle (Figure 14-10B).

e. **To stretch the scalene muscles**

Note: Because these muscles are attached to the transverse processes of the upper cervical spine and the upper two ribs, they either flex the cervical spine or elevate the upper ribs, when they contract bilaterally. Unilaterally, the scalenes side bend the cervical spine to the same side and rotate it to the opposite.

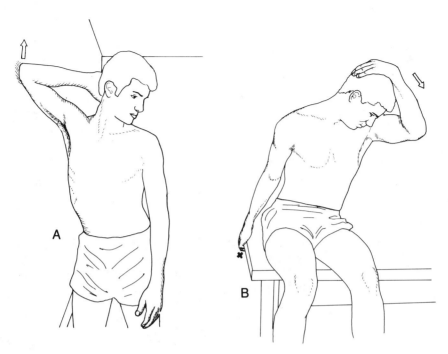

FIGURE 14-10. Self-stretching the levator scapulae muscle; (*A*) using upward rotation of the scapula, (*B*) using depression of the scapula.

(1) Position of patient: sitting. The patient first does axial extension (tucks the chin and straightens the neck), then side bends the neck opposite and rotates it toward the tight muscles. The therapist stands behind the patient and stabilizes the upper ribs, with one hand over the top of the rib cage on the side of tightness, and stabilizes the head with the other hand around the side of the patient's head and face, holding the head against her trunk (Figure 14-11). The patient inhales and exhales; the therapist then holds the ribs down as the patient inhales again. Repeat. This is a gentle contract-relax stretching maneuver.

(2) To do the above-mentioned maneuver in a home program, the patient stands next to a table and holds on to its underside. He then positions his head as in (1). To stretch, he leans away from the table, inhales, exhales, and holds the stretch position.

f. **To stretch the short suboccipital muscles**
Position of patient: sitting. The therapist identifies the spinous process of the second cervical vertebra and stabilizes it with her thumb or with the second metacarpophalangeal joint (and the thumb and index finger around the transverse process) as the patient slowly nods, doing just a tipping motion of the head on the upper spine (Figure 14-12). The therapist guides the movement by placing the other hand across the patient's forehead.

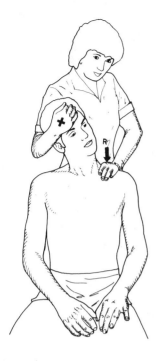

FIGURE 14-11. Unilateral active stretching of the scalenus muscles. The patient first does axial extension, then side bends the neck opposite, and rotates it towards the tight muscles. The therapist stabilizes the head and upper thorax as the patient breathes in, contracting the muscle against the resistance. As the patient relaxes, the rib cage lowers and stretches the muscle.

g. **To increase general range of motion of the cervical spine and musculature**
   (1) Inhibition techniques, as described in Chapter 4, can be used on any muscle group or motion. Suggested position for the patient is supine, with the therapist standing at the head end of the treatment table, supporting the patient's head in her hands.
   (2) Traction techniques, as described in Chapter 16, can be used for the purpose of stretching the posterior ligaments, muscles, and the facet joint capsules. This is a nonspecific form of stretching.

h. **To stretch specific joint structures in the cervical spine**
   Joint mobilization and manipulation techniques can be used by those trained in the principles and maneuvers. They require advanced training and are beyond the scope of this text.

2. **Lumbar region**
   a. **To stretch the lumbar erector spinae muscles and soft tissue posterior to the spine (to increase trunk flexion)**
      Precaution: Do not do if flexion of the spine causes a change in sensation or causes pain to radiate down an extremity (see Chapter 15).
      (1) Position of patient: hook lying. The patient first brings one knee, then the other, toward his chest, clasps his hands around the thighs, and pulls them to the chest elevating the sacrum off the mat. This may be assisted by the therapist (Figure 14-13).
      Precaution: do not grasp around the tibia; it places stress on the knee joints as the stretch force is applied.
      (2) Position of patient: cross-sitting. The patient places his hands behind his neck, adducts his scapulae, and extends his thoracic spine. This locks the thoracic vertebrae. He then leans the thorax

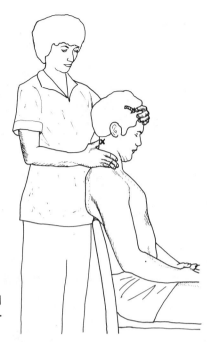

FIGURE 14-12. Stretching the short suboccipital muscles. The therapist stabilizes the second cervical vertebra as the patient slowly flexes the head.

forward onto the pelvis, flexing only at the lumbar spine. The therapist stabilizes the pelvis by pulling back on the anterior-superior iliac spines (Figure 14-14).

(3) Position of patient: on hands and knees. The patient is asked to tuck his stomach in without rounding his thorax (concentrate on flexing the lumbar spine, not the thoracic spine), hold the position, then relax (Figure 14-15). Repeat; this time bring the hips back to the feet, hold, then return to the hands and knees position.

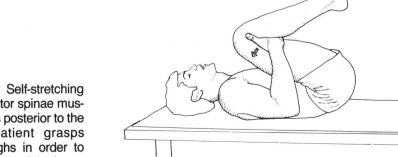

FIGURE 14-13. Self-stretching the lumbar erector spinae muscles and tissues posterior to the spine. The patient grasps around the thighs in order to avoid compression of the knee.

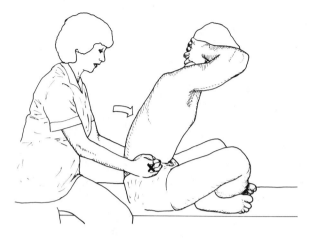

FIGURE 14-14. Stretching the lumbar spine, with the patient stabilizing his thorax in extension and the therapist stabilizing the pelvis.

    (4) Active trunk flexion exercises use the principle of reciprocal inhibition and can be used to help elongate tight lumbar extensor muscles.

  b. **To stretch soft tissue anterior to the lumbar spine (to increase trunk extension)**
    Precaution: Do not do if extension causes a change in sensation or causes pain to radiate down an extremity (see Chapter 15).
    (1) Position of patient: prone, with hands placed under the shoulders. The patient then extends his elbows and lifts his thorax up off the mat but keeps the pelvis down on the mat. This is a *prone press-up* (Figure 14-16A). To increase the stretch force, the pelvis can be strapped down to the treatment table. Hold the stretch at least 6 seconds. This exercise also stretches the hip flexor muscles and soft tissue anterior to the hip.
    (2) Position of patient: standing, with his hands placed in his low-back area. He then leans backwards and holds the stretch (Figure 14-16B).
    (3) Position of patient: on hands and knees. After the patient tucks his stomach in, have him allow his spine to sag, creating lumbar exten-

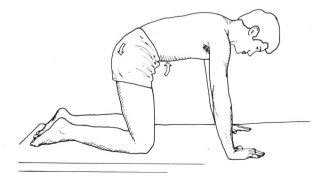

FIGURE 14-15. Active stretching of the lumbar spine. The patient tucks his stomach in without rounding his thorax.

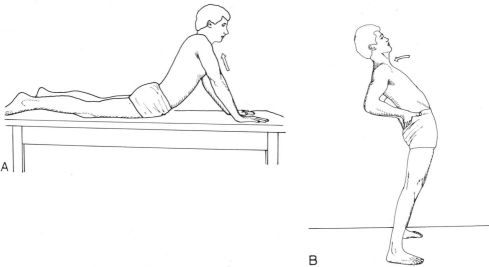

FIGURE 14-16. Self-stretching of the soft tissues anterior to the lumbar spine and hip joints with the patient prone (*A*) and standing (*B*).

sion. This can also be used to teach the patient how to control pelvic motion.

(4) Any active trunk extension exercises as described in Section C 2 b below may be used as long as the exertion does not increase symptoms.

c. **To stretch tight lower extremity musculature that affects posture**

(1) Hip muscles have a direct effect on spinal posture due to their attachment on the pelvis (see Chapter 12 for specific stretching techniques of these muscles.)

(2) Knee, ankle, and foot muscle stretching techniques are described in Chapters 10 and 11.

C. **Procedures to Train and Strengthen Muscle Balance Necessary for Postural Control of the Neck and Trunk**

Note: These exercises are listed progressively from least difficult to most difficult. Begin the patient at a level appropriate for his strength and ability to control the motion. Training follows stretching. If there is inadequate flexibility in the tight antagonistic muscles, the postural muscles cannot hold the parts in proper alignment.

1. **Cervical and upper thoracic region**

a. **To train and strengthen muscles of axial extension and thoracic extension** (these exercises also bring in the lumbar extensors as stabilizers)

(1) Position of patient: supine. The patient tucks his chin and attempts to flatten his neck against the mat while simultaneously adducting his scapulae.

(2) Position of patient: prone, with forehead on the treatment table and arms at his sides. Instruct him to lift his forehead off the plinth while

keeping his chin tucked and maintaining axial extension. This is a small motion (Figure 14-17).

(3) Progress the exercise in (2) by having the patient lift the upper portion of his chest off the plinth. He should not push with his hands.

(4) Progress by having the patient place his hands behind his head and extend so his upper chest comes off the mat; then have him hold his arms fully elevated above his head and extend his upper spine. The neck must remain in axial extension while doing these exercises.

b. **To train and strengthen the muscles of scapular adduction**

(1) Position of patient: prone. Instruct the patient to grasp his hands together behind his low back. This activity should cause scapular adduction. Then he is to hold the scapular adduction while lowering his arms to his sides. This is to help isolate control of the scapular adductors.

(2) Progress the exercise in (1) by having the patient pinch his scapulae together. This motion may be initiated while he is sitting or standing if he does not have the strength to do it prone (see Figure 14-29).

(3) Further progress the exercise by changing the position of the patient's arms, so that the weight of the arms provides varying resistance to the scapular adductor muscles. Begin with the shoulders abducted 90 degrees and the elbows flexed, then the elbows extended (Figure 14-18). Repeat with the shoulders at 145 degrees.

(4) Increased resistance can be applied by having the patient hold increments of weights appropriate to his strength and repeating the exercises in (3).

(5) Position of patient: sitting or standing. Elastic resistance material is secured in front of the patient at shoulder level. The patient flexes both shoulders to 90 degrees and holds on to the elastic material. He then horizontally abducts both arms, allowing the elbows to flex, and concentrates on adducting his scapulae (see Figure 14-25).

c. **To strengthen the cervical muscles**

A progression of manual resistive range of motion and isometric exercises are initiated at the level of strength available for each muscle group.

Position of patient: supine. The therapist stands at the head end of the treatment table, supporting the patient's head for each exercise.

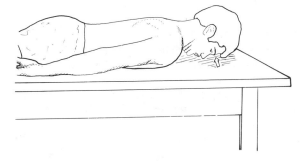

FIGURE 14-17. Axial extension exercises.

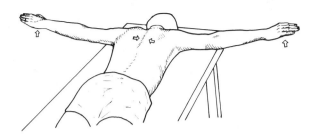

FIGURE 14-18. Scapular adduction exercises, with the arms positioned for maximum resistance from gravity. To progress the exercise further, weights can be placed in the patient's hands.

      (1) To apply manual resistive exercise, place one hand on the patient's head to resist opposite the motion. Do not resist against the mandible or the force will be transmitted to the temporomandibular joint. Resistance is given to isolated muscle actions or to general ranges of motion, whichever best gains muscle balance and function.

      (2) To provide isometric resistance, use the same procedure as in (1), except the intensity of resistance should prevent motion. The head can be placed in any position desired before applying the resistance. To avoid jerking the neck when applying or releasing the resistance, gradually build up the intensity, telling the patient to match your resistance; hold; then gradually release, and again, ask the patient to relax accordingly.

  d. **Self-resistance for isometric cervical exercises**

    Position of patient: sitting.

    (1) Flexion

      The patient places both his hands on his forehead and presses his forehead into the palms in a nodding fashion but does not allow motion (Figure 14-19).

    (2) Side bending

      The patient presses one hand against the side of his head and attempts to side bend, trying to bring his ear toward his shoulder, but not allowing motion.

    (3) Axial extension

      The patient presses the back of his head into both hands, which are placed in the back, near the top of his head (Figure 14-20).

    (4) Rotation

      The patient presses one hand against the region just superior and lateral to his eye and attempts to turn his head to look over his shoulder but does not allow motion.

  e. **Postural splints**

    If necessary, provide external support with a postural splint to prevent the extreme posture of round shoulders and protracted scapulae. It helps train correct muscle functioning by acting as a reminder for the patient to correct his posture when he slouches. Also, by preventing the position of stretch from occurring, stretch weakness can be corrected.

2. **Lumbar region**

  a. **To train and strengthen the abdominal muscles**

    (1) Pelvic tilt

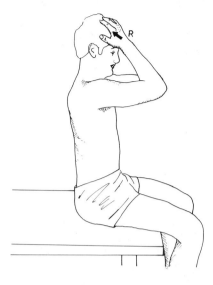

FIGURE 14-19. Self-resistance for isometric cervical flexion.

Position of patient: hook lying or supine. Teach the patient to do a posterior pelvic tilt by having him slip his hand under his low back and push his spine down on his hand. Use of the phrase "tuck your stomach in" may convey the idea for the correct motion. Have him then arch his back doing an anterior pelvic tilt, then repeat the posterior pelvic tilt until he can control the pelvic motion.

(2) Pelvic tilt; all 4's

Position of patient: on his hands and knees in the all-4's position. He practices controlling the pelvic tilt, rotating from an anterior tilt to a posterior tilt, as in Figure 14-15, being sure motion is in the pelvis and lumbar spine, not the thorax.

(3) Curl-ups

Position of patient: hook lying, with the lumbar spine flat. Begin with a posterior pelvic tilt.

First, have the patient lift his head off the mat. This will cause a stabilizing contraction of the abdominal muscles.

He progresses by lifting his shoulders until the scapulae and thorax clear the mat, keeping the arms horizontal (Figure 14-21). The patient does not come to a full sit-up, since once the thorax clears the mat, the rest of the motion is done by the hip flexor muscles. Further progress the difficulty of the curl-up by changing the arm position from horizontal, to folded across the chest, then to behind the head.

In all these activities, the low back should not arch; if it does, reduce the progression until the abdominals are strong enough to maintain lumbar flexion.

(4) Curl-downs

If the patient is unable to perform the curl-up as in (3), begin with curl-downs.

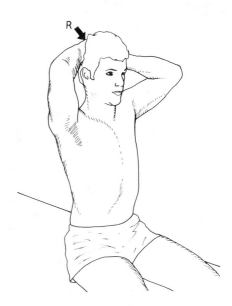

FIGURE 14-20. Self-resistance for isometric axial extension.

Position of patient: starting in the hook-sitting or long-sitting position. The patient lowers the trunk only to the point where he can maintain a flat low back; then he returns to the sitting position. Once the patient can curl-down full range, then reverse and have him do a curl-up.

(5) Diagonal curl-ups

To emphasize the external oblique muscles, the patient does a diagonal curl-up by reaching one hand toward the outside of the opposite knee as he curls up, then alternating. Reverse the muscle action by bringing one knee up toward the opposite shoulder; then repeat with the other knee.

(6) Double knee to chest

To emphasize the lower rectus abdominis and oblique muscles

Position of patient: hook lying. Have the patient set a posterior

FIGURE 14-21. The curl-up exercise to strengthen the abdominal muscles. The thorax is flexed on the lumbar spine. The arms are shown in the position for least resistance. Progress by crossing the arms across the chest, then behind the head.

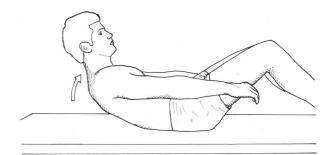

pelvic tilt, then bring both knees to his chest and return. Progress the difficulty by decreasing the angle of the hip and knee flexion (Figure 14-22).

(7) Bilateral straight leg raising (SLR)

This is a progression in difficulty of the double knee-to-chest exercise. It should be done only if the muscles are strong enough to maintain a posterior pelvic tilt. Position of patient: supine, with legs extended. The patient first does a posterior pelvic tilt, then flexes both hips, keeping the knees extended. If the hips are abducted before initiating this exercise, greater stress is placed on the oblique abdominal muscles.

(8) Bilateral straight leg lowering

This can be done if the bilateral SLR is difficult. Position of patient: supine, with the hips at 90 degrees and knees extended. The patient lowers the extremities as far as he can while maintaining a flat back, then raises the legs back to 90 degrees.

(9) Modified bicycle

Position of patient: supine. Have the patient maintain a posterior pelvic tilt, then with his back on the mat, alternately flex and extend his lower extremities. Begin with small circles with the hips and knees significantly flexed; progress by reducing the degree of hip and knee flexion (see Figure 22-2).

(10) Further progression can be accomplished by having the patient do a curl-up while simultaneously flexing his hips and knees. He can touch his elbows to his knees or his hands to his toes.

(11) Isometric elastic resistance to trunk flexors

Position of patient: sitting or standing. Secure the elastic resistance behind the patient. The patient holds on to the ends of the material with each hand, sets the abdominals, then brings the arms forward in different patterns (Figure 14-23A). For isometric training, there should be little or no motion of the trunk as the arms move except to accommodate the center of gravity. Progressively increase the resistance by using heavier grades of elastic. Vary the muscle response by changing the angle of pull or by pulling with one arm at a time.

(12) Concentric-eccentric elastic resistance to trunk flexors

Position of patient: sitting or standing. The elastic material is se-

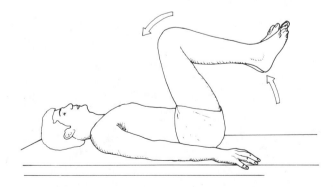

FIGURE 14-22. Strengthening the abdominal muscles by flexing the hip and pelvis on the lumbar spine. The legs are shown in the position for least resistance. Progress by decreasing the angle of hip flexion until the legs can be lifted with the knees extended.

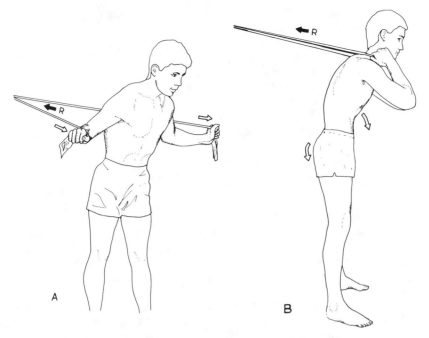

A

B

FIGURE 14-23. Using elastic resistance to train and strengthen the abdominal muscles in the upright position; (*A*) isometrically setting the abdominals while the person brings the arms forward against the resistance, (*B*) trunk flexion emphasizing posterior pelvic tilt and approximating the ribs to the pubic bone.

cured at shoulder level behind the patient. The patient holds the ends of the material with each hand. He then flexes the trunk, with emphasis on bringing the ribs down toward the pubic bone and doing a posterior pelvic tilt, rather than hip flexion (Figure 14-23B). Diagonal motions should also be done, by bringing one arm down toward the opposite knee, with emphasis on moving the rib cage down toward the opposite side of the pelvis. Repeat the diagonal motion in the opposite direction. Progress the resistance as the patient's abdominal strength increases by using a heavier grade elastic.

b. **To train and strengthen the lumbar extensor muscle groups**
   (1) Position of patient: supine, arms at his side. Instruct the patient to arch his back by touching the floor with the back of his neck and the sacrum.
   (2) Position of patient: prone, arms at his side. Have the patient tuck in his chin and lift his head. This brings in a stabilizing contraction of the lumbar extensor muscles. For greater range, have the patient lift his thorax as well as his head.
   (3) To progress resistance during the above exercise, have the patient vary his arm position from resting at his side, to placing his hands behind his head, then to placing his arms in full elevation as he

extends his spine. The lower extremities will need to be stabilized (Figure 14-24)

(4) Position of patient: prone. Begin by lifting one leg several inches off the mat (hip extension), alternate with the other leg. Progress by lifting both legs simultaneously.

(5) Further progression can be accomplished by having the patient prone and lifting both elevated arms and extended legs simultaneously.

(6) Resistance can be applied to any of the above exercises by having the patient hold weights in his hands or by strapping weights around the patient's legs.

(7) Isometric elastic resistance to trunk extensors
Training the trunk extensor muscle to function in the upright position to stabilize the trunk against resistive forces is an important goal for rehabilitation. The muscles may be trained for endurance using the principle of high repetition/low resistance, or for strength, using the principle of low repetition/high resistance. The resistance is varied by choosing the appropriate grade of elastic.
Position of patient: sitting with the elastic material secured in front of the patient. He extends or abducts the shoulders against the resistive force in various arm positions while keeping the back still (Figure 14-25A). The patient progresses the training to the standing posture (Figure 14-25B).

(8) Concentric-eccentric elastic resistance to trunk extensors
Elastic resistance can be applied for concentric-eccentric extension exercises in the upright position by securing the elastic material at shoulder level in front of the patient. He holds on to the ends of the material, sets his pelvis, and extends his spine (Figure 14-26). A boat-rowing motion with the arms also effectively stimulates the trunk extensors. Progress the exercise by increasing the grade of elastic resistance.

(9) Rotation with extension
Position of patient: standing with the elastic resistance secured under the foot or to a stable object opposite to the side being exercised. The patient pulls against the resistance, extending and rotating the back. Changing the angle of pull of the elastic material

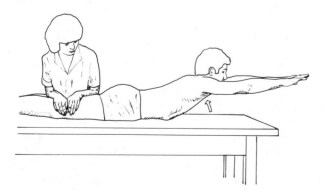

FIGURE 14-24. Strengthening the back extensors with the arms in position to provide maximum resistance. Additional resistance can be provided by holding weights in the hands.

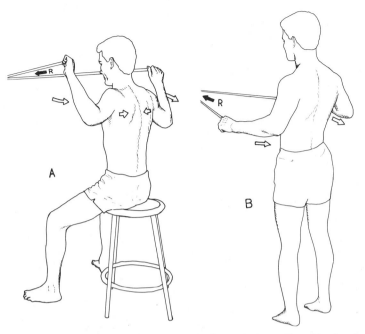

FIGURE 14-25. Using elastic resistance to train and strengthen the back extensor muscles to stabilize in the upright position; (*A*) sitting and (*B*) standing.

allows the therapist to recreate functional patterns specific to the patient's needs (Figure 14-27).

    c. **To train and strengthen muscles of the lower extremity that affect posture, see Chapters 10, 11, and 12.**

D. Procedures to Retrain Kinesthetic Awareness for Posture Correction

    1. **Improve patient awareness**

    Initially, normal alignment may be prevented because of tightness of soft tissue or malalignment of a vertebral segment, but developing patient awareness of balanced posture and its effects should begin early in the treatment program in conjunction with the stretching and muscle-training maneuvers.

    2. **Emphasize proper movement and balance by using verbal, tactile, and visual reinforcement while treating the patient**

      a. **Verbal reinforcement**

      As you interact with the patient, frequently interpret for him the sensations of muscle contraction and position that he should be feeling. This is done especially when teaching relaxation techniques (see Section IV A) and spinal control activities (see Section D 3).

      b. **Visual reinforcement**

      Use mirrors so the patient can see how he looks, what it takes to as-

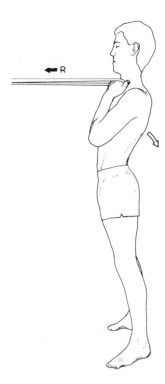

FIGURE 14-26. Using elastic resistance for concentric-eccentric back extension.

sume good alignment, and then how it feels when properly aligned. Verbally reinforce what the patient sees.

c. **Tactile reinforcement**

Help the patient position his head and trunk in correct alignment and touch the muscles that need to contract to move and hold the parts in place (see Section D 3).

3. **Teach proper movement and balance control**

Isolate each imbalanced body segment and train the patient how to move that segment. If one region is out of alignment it is likely that the entire spine is imbalanced to compensate, so total posture correction should be emphasized. Direct the patient's attention to the feel of proper movement and muscle contraction and relaxation. Use reinforcement techniques as described previously in Section 2. It may be useful to have the patient assume an extreme corrected posture, then ease away from the extreme towards mid position, then hold the corrected posture.

a. **To train axial extension to decrease a forward-head posture**

Position of patient: sitting or standing, with arms relaxed at the side. Lightly touch above his lip under the nose and ask him to lift his head up and away (Figure 14-28). Verbally reinforce the correct movement of tucking the chin in and straightening the spine, and draw his attention to the way it feels. Have him move to the extreme corrected posture, then return to mid line.

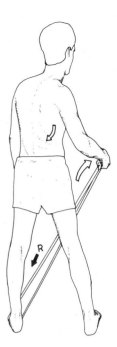

FIGURE 14-27. Rotation with extension strengthens the back extensors in functional patterns.

b. **To train scapular retraction**
   Position of patient: sitting or standing. For tactile and proprioceptive cues, gently resist movement of the inferior angle of the scapulae and ask the patient to pinch them together (retraction). The patient should not extend or elevate the shoulders (Figure 14-29).

c. **To train control of the pelvic tilt and balance of the lumbar spine**
   Position of patient: sitting, then standing with his back against a wall. After the patient has learned pelvic tilt exercises, have him practice control of movement of the pelvis and lumbar spine by moving from extreme lordosis to extreme flat back and then assuming a mild lordosis. Show him that his hand should be able to easily slip between his back and the wall, and that he can then feel his back with one side of his hand and the wall with the other side.

d. **To train control of the thorax and thoracic spine**
   Position of patient: standing. The position of the thorax affects the posture of the lumbar spine and pelvis so the feel of thoracic movement is incorporated in posture training for the lumbar spine. As the patient assumes a mild lordosis posture (as in c above), have him breathe in and lift the rib cage (extension). Guide him to a balanced posture, not an extremely extended posture.

   Note: It may be necessary to direct the patient's attention to the feel of shifting the thorax anteriorly and posteriorly and noting how it affects the lumbar spine. There is an important difference between standing with a lordotic posture (extreme lordosis in the lumbar spine with excessive anterior pelvic tilt) versus a relaxed posture (excessive extension in the lower lumbar spine with a rapid reversal into flexion in the upper lumbar spine

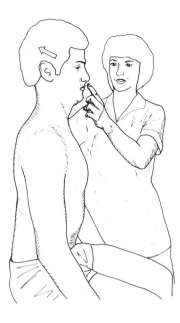

FIGURE 14-28. Training the patient to correct a forward head posture.

and thorax) (see Section III of this chapter.) It is important to recognize the difference between these two postures. Often, because the excessive extension is noted in the lower lumbar segment in patients with slouched postures, the patient erroneously is placed on a flexion exercise and training program in order to flatten the low back.[3] This approach ignores or reinforces the already flexed posture of the thorax on the upper lumbar spine and tends to accentuate that problem, particularly since curl-up exercises are emphasized in the flexion routine. In addition, our flexion-oriented society (sitting in flexion, slouching, and reclining in flexion) has produced a flat low-back syndrome that has led to further problems (see Chapter 15), including eliminating the important homeostatic mechanism of balanced spinal curves. If the reader is confused with what is described above, try the following:

(1) Stand; start with a normal lordosis. This requires elevation of the rib cage. Note that there is a mild anterior pelvic tilt and mild lumbar lordosis.

(2) Now, tilt the pelvis anteriorly and assume an increased lordosis; note the associated hip flexion. This posture is in fact extreme, and some people demonstrate this as the source of their problems.

(3) Now, again assume a midline normal lordosis posture (requiring tilting the pelvis posteriorly part way). From this normal posture, shift into a relaxed posture by allowing the pelvic segment to shift anteriorly and the rib cage to shift posteriorly and approximate the pelvis. Note, the hips are now in extension with respect to the pelvis (not an anterior pelvic tilt), but the lower lumbar spine is in extension. The thorax is, in essence, flexed on the upper lumbar spine. Often, when in this posture, a person also shifts his weight onto one leg, thus adding asymmetry to the whole picture.

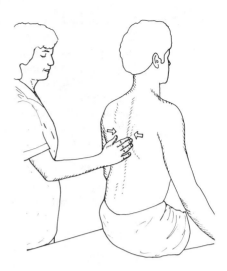

FIGURE 14-29. Training the patient to correct protracted scapulae.

The point is that this relaxed posture should NOT be corrected with a total flexion approach as would be done with a lordotic postural problem. To emphasize curl-ups only perpetuates flexing the thorax on the upper lumbar spine; instead the motion needs to be extension. In the lower lumbar spine and hips, some flexion is necessary. Here, pelvic control with pelvic tilt exercises should be done. For strengthening, active double knee-to-chest and modified bicycle exercises will emphasize flexion of the lower lumbar spine. Therefore, with this posture, a combined flexion/extension approach must be used in retraining for proper movement and control. The patient must learn to lift the rib cage and shift it anteriorly as the pelvis is shifted posteriorly, similar to taking a crooked stack of blocks and shifting it to straighten it. Telling the patient to think tall, breath in to expand the anterior thorax, and lift the head may encourage the correct response. Additional verbal prompting to help the patient imagine and then recreate the correct posture may also help.

e. **To train control of lower extremity alignment**
   If there is imbalance in the use of the lower extremities, see Chapters 10, 11, and 12 for suggestions on activities to develop muscle awareness and control. Have the patient concentrate on placement of the foot and the shifting of weight while walking.

f. **To teach awareness of the sensation of assuming a normal posture and developing spinal control**
   Position of patient: sitting. Instruct the patient to curl his entire spine by first flexing the neck, then the thorax, then the lumbar spine. Give him cues for unrolling by first touching the lumbar spine as he extends it, then the thoracic spine as he extends it and takes in a breath to elevate the rib cage. Then direct his attention to adducting the scapulae while you gently resist the motion, then lifting the head in axial extension while you give slight pressure against the upper lip. Verbally and visually reinforce the correct posture when it is obtained.

4. Demonstrate to the patient the relationship of his faulty posture to the development of pain

Have the patient assume his faulty posture and wait. When he begins to feel discomfort, point out his posture and then have him correct it and notice the feeling of relief. Many patients will not accept such a simple relationship between stress and pain, so draw their attention to noticing, throughout the day and after a night's rest, what posture they are in when pain comes on and how they can control it with the techniques they have been taught.

5. Reinforce learning

It is not possible for a person to always maintain good posture. Therefore, to reinforce learning, teach the patient to use cues throughout the day to check his posture. For example, tell him to check his posture every time he walks past a mirror, every time he waits at a red light while driving a car, every time he sits down for a meal, or every time he enters a room or begins talking with someone. Find out what daily routines the patient has that could be used for reinforcement reminders; have him practice and report the results. Provide positive feedback as the patient becomes actively involved in the relearning process.

E. Procedures to Teach Management of Posture to Avoid Recurrences of the Problem

1. Teach the patient body mechanics in lifting, stooping, and carrying

   a. Have the patient practice lifting by stooping down to the object, bringing the object close to his body, setting his back in a neutral position, then lifting with the hip and knee extensors.

      (1) Lifting with a neutral spinal posture provides greater stability to the spine[10] and uses both the ligamentous and muscular system to stabilize and control.[24]

      (2) Following back injury, the preferred lifting posture may have to be adapted depending on the type of injury and the response of the tissues when stressed.[24]

      (3) When lifting with a flexed lumbar spine (posterior pelvic tilt), support for the spine is primarily from inert structures (ligaments, lumbodorsal fascia, posterior annulus fibrosis, and facets); there is little muscle activity.

         (a) This posture may be necessary when stooping to the floor. It may also be the posture of choice for a patient who has injured his back muscles since the muscles are "quiet" when the spine is in flexion.[24]

         (b) Lifting with the lumbar spine in flexion may pose some problems. When lifting slowly with the lumbar spine in flexion, the load is maintained on the ligaments and creep of the inert tissues occurs; this increases the chance of injury if the tissue is already weakened. In addition, with the muscles lengthened and relaxed, they may be at an unfavorable length-tension relationship to quickly respond with appropriate force to resist a sudden change in load. There is greater chance of ligamentous strain when a person lifts with a flexed spine.[10]

(4) When lifting with an extended (lordotic) lumbar spine, the muscles supporting the spine are more active, which increases the compressive forces on the disk. This posture relieves stress on the ligaments, but for an individual whose back muscles fatigue quickly (in poor condition) this posture may jeopardize the spine when repeated lifts are done because the ligaments are not taut and thus are not providing support.[24]

b. Have the patient practice carrying objects close to his center of gravity so he can feel the balance. When lifting, less stress is placed on the structures on the back and hip the closer the object is held to the center of gravity.[19]

2. Educate the patient in preventive exercises and mechanics for relief of mechanical stress in daily activities

a. Review the following principles
(1) Avoid any one posture for prolonged periods. If sustained postures are necessary, take frequent breaks and do appropriate range of motion exercises at least every half hour. Finish all exercises by assuming a well-balanced posture.
(2) Avoid hyperextending the neck or being in a forward head posture or forward bent position for prolonged periods. Find ways to modify a task so it can be done at eye level or with proper lumbar support.
(3) If in a tension-producing situation, do conscious relaxation exercises.
(4) Use common sense and follow good safety habits

b. Review flexibility and strengthening exercises appropriate for the patient in order to maintain adequate range of motion and develop adequate strength for good physical conditioning.

c. Review the relationship of posture and pain; when experiencing pain, check posture.

3. Help the patient recognize environmental factors that influence his posture

a. Review the patient's work and home environment
(1) Chairs and car seats should have good lumbar support in order to maintain a slight lordosis. Use a towel roll or lumbar pillow if necessary.
(2) Chair height should allow knees to flex to take the pull off the hamstring muscles, support the thighs, and also allow the feet to rest comfortably on the floor.
(3) Desk or table height should be adequate to keep the person from having to lean over his work.
(4) Work and driving habits should allow frequent changing of posture. If normally sedentary, get up and walk every hour.

b. Review the patient's sleeping environment
(1) Mattress needs to provide firm support to prevent any exteme stresses. If it is too soft, the patient sags and stresses ligaments; if it is too firm, some patients cannot relax.
(2) Pillows should be of a comfortable height and density to promote relaxation but should not place joints at an extreme position. Foam rubber pillows tend to cause increased tension in muscles because of the constant resistance they provide.

(3) Whether the person should sleep prone, side lying, or supine is something that must be analyzed for each individual patient. Ideally, a comfortable posture is one that is mid-range and that does not place stress on any supporting structure. Pain that occurs in the morning is often related to sleeping posture; so if this is the case, listen carefully to the patient's description of postures when sleeping and see if it relates to the pain. Then attempt to modify the sleep position accordingly.

V. SUMMARY

The first section of this chapter contains a review of basic anatomy and functional relationships in the spine. The remainder of the chapter covers information on the dynamics of posture and characteristics and problems of common faulty postures and then provides guidelines for developing programs based on common problems found in postural pain syndromes and dysfunctions. Chapter 15 will cover treatment approaches for acute spinal conditions.

REFERENCES

1. Bogduk, N and MacIntosh, JE: *The applied anatomy of the thoracolumbar fascia.* Spine 9:164, 1984.
2. Bogduk, N and Twomey, LT: *Clinical Anatomy of the Lumbar Spine.* Churchill-Livingstone, New York, 1987.
3. Cailliet, R: *Low Back Pain Syndrome,* ed 3. FA Davis, Philadelphia, 1981.
4. Daniels, L and Worthingham, C: *Therapeutic Exercise for Body Alignment and Function,* ed. 2. WB Saunders, Philadelphia, 1977.
5. Friber, O: *Clinical symptoms and biomechanics of lumbar spine and hip joint in leg length inequality.* Spine 8:643, 1983.
6. Gossman, M, Sahrmann, S, and Rose, S: *Review of length-associated changes in muscle.* Phys Ther 62:1977, 1982.
7. Gracovetsky, S, Farfan, H, and Helleur, C: *The abdominal mechanism.* Spine 10:317, 1985.
8. Gracovetsky, S and Farfan, H: *The optimum spine.* Spine 11:543, 1986.
9. Gracovetsky, S: *The Spinal Engine.* Springer-Verlag Wein, New York, 1988.
10. Hart, DL, Stobbe, TJ, and Jaraiedi, M: *Effect of lumbar posture on lifting.* Spine 12:22, 1987.
11. Hellebrant, F and Fries, E: *The constancy of oscillograph stance patterns.* Phys Ther Rev 22:17, 1942.
12. Hollinshead, WJ: *Textbook of Anatomy,* ed 3. Harper & Row, Hagerstown, MD, 1974.
13. Hughes, P: *Advanced Upper Extremity Course.* Workshop Notes, St Louis, 1979.
14. Jensen, G.: *Biomechanics of the lumbar intervertebral disc: A review.* Phys Ther 60:765, 1979.
15. Kapandji, IA: *The Physiology of the Joints, Vol 3.* Churchill-Livingston, New York, 1974.
16. Kendall, F and McCreary, E: *Muscles: Testing and Function,* ed 3. Williams & Wilkins, Baltimore, 1983.
17. Lamb, C: *The neurology of spinal pain.* Phys Ther 59:971, 1979.
18. Lehmkuhl, LD and Smith, LK: *Brunnstrom's Clinical Kinesiology,* ed 4. FA Davis, Philadelphia, 1983.
19. Nemeth, G: *On hip and lumbar biomechanics, a study of joint load and muscular activity.* Scand J Rehabil Med (Suppl) 10:4, 1984.
20. Norkin, C and Levangie, P: *Joint Structure and Function: A Comprehensive Analysis.* FA Davis, Philadelphia, 1983.
21. Panjabi, MM, Goel, VK, and Takata, K: *Physiologic strains in the lumbar spinal ligaments.* Spine 7:192, 1982.
22. Porterfield, JA: *Dynamic stabilization of the trunk.* JOSPT 6:271, 1985.
23. Rocobado, M: *Temporomandibular Joint Dysfunctions.* Workshop Notes, Cincinnati, 1979.
24. Sullivan, MS: *Back support mechanisms during manual lifting.* Phys Ther 69:38, 1989.

25. Taylor, J and Twomey, L: *Sagittal and horizontal plane movement of the human lumbar vertebral column in cadavers and in living.* Rheumatol Rehabil 19:223, 1980.
26. Tesh, KM, Dunn, JS, and Evans, JH: *The abdominal muscles and vertebral stability.* Spine 12:501, 1987.
27. Twomey, T and Taylor, JR: *Sagittal movements of the human lumbar vertebral column: A quantative study of the role of the posterior vertebral elements.* Arch Phys Med Rehabil 64:322, 1983.
28. Wood, P: *Applied anatomy and physiology of the vertebral column.* Phys Ther 59:248, 1979.

CHAPTER ——————————— 15

The Spine:
Treatment of Acute Problems

Faulty posture underlies many chronic painful neck and back conditions. The reader is referred to Chapter 14 for a discussion of principles and treatment techniques directed toward managing pain and dysfunction from poor or stressful postures. The reader is also referred to Chapter 14 for a review of the anatomy and functional relationships of the spinal region.

Faulty postures may leave the structures of the spinal column vulnerable to injury or perpetuate a painful condition when normally there should be healing and recovery after an injury. Traumatic spinal injuries and acute painful conditions also occur in apparently healthy musculoskeletal systems. Acute problems that affect the neck and back will be described in this chapter by following the principles of treatment of soft-tissue and joint problems as presented in Chapter 6.

Treatment approaches for acute painful conditions in the neck and back vary considerably. With the growth of manual therapy, physical therapists have broadened their skills for managing a variety of spinal disorders[10,14,25,27,34,38] and have explored nontraditional methods for helping the patient learn to manage his own pain and to prevent future episodes from occurring.[27,28] The thinking therapist is aware that the etiology of back pain is not the same in all patients and, therefore, cannot be treated the same way in all patients.

A common approach is complete bed rest while recovering from an acute episode of back pain. In some cases this is necessary, as is resting the shoulder following an acute episode of bursitis or avoiding painful activity following an acute flare-up of tendinitis. But rest needs to be mixed with appropriately graded and controlled movement for proper healing of tissues.[44] It is a matter of transferring the same principles to the structures of the neck and back. The complicating factor in the spine is the intervertebral disk and its close proximity to the spinal cord and nerve roots. There is no simple answer to management. To define basic skills that the therapist should have in order to treat patients with acute spinal problems is the overall purpose of this chapter. It is recognized that therapists specializing in the treatment of the spine will need to develop additional skills, such as spinal mobilization, manipulation, and pain-control techniques, which are beyond the scope of this text. Every therapist should have basic skills in evaluating and identifying problems associated with back problems; this chapter is based on the assumption that those skills have already been learned.

OBJECTIVES

After studying this chapter, the reader will be able to:
1. describe intervertebral disk function and mechanical factors that influence it.
2. establish a treatment program for managing disk lesions based on the patient's response to testing procedures.
3. identify contraindications to movement during an acute disk lesion.
4. establish treatment programs for managing acute joint, muscle, and soft-tissue problems in the spinal region based on the problems identified.
5. describe the biomechanical relationship between the intervertebral disk and facet joints.
6. establish treatment programs for managing torticollis, tension headaches, thoracic outlet syndrome, and temporomandibular joint dysfunction.
7. identify safe techniques to use to meet the goals of the exercise programs.

When dealing with acute pain in the spine following trauma, fractures and instability must be ruled out before allowing movement. If these critical conditions are not present but there are symptoms of pressure against the spinal cord or a nerve root, the cause needs to be identified and treated. Causes of neurologic signs frequently seen by physical therapists include intervertebral disk protrusions, stenosis of the spinal canal or intervertebral foramina, bony impingement from degenerative changes, and nerve root entrapment. Whether the patient has symptoms of pain or has positive neurologic signs, if positioning or movement reduces the pressure against the involved tissue, mechanical techniques are attempted to treat the problem. If a disk lesion is the cause of the acute episode of back pain, treatment techniques are directed toward managing this structure first.

I.   THE INTERVERTEBRAL DISK

A. Structure and Function[5,7,12,24,26]

1. The intervertebral disk, consisting of the annulus fibrosus and nucleus pulposus, is one component of a three-joint complex between two adjacent vertebrae.
2. The *annulus fibrosus* is made up of dense layers of collagen fibers and fibrocartilage.[26] The collagen fibers in any one layer are parallel and angled around 60 to 65 degrees to the axis of the spine, with the tilt alternating in successive layers.[11,15] The orientation of the fibers provides tensile strength to the annulus when the spine is compressed, twisted, or bent and helps restrain the various spinal motions. The annulus is firmly attached to adjacent vertebrae, and the layers are firmly bound to one another. Fibers of the innermost layers blend with the matrix of the nucleus pulposus.[26] The annulus fibrosus is supported by the anterior and posterior longitudinal ligaments.
3. The *nucleus pulposus* is a gelatinous mass that normally is contained within but whose loosely aligned fibers merge with the inner layer of the annulus fibrosus. It is located centrally in the disk, but in the lumbar spine, it is situated closer to the posterior border than the anterior border of the annulus.[26] Aggregating proteoglycans, normally in high concentration in a healthy nucleus, have a great affinity for water. The resulting fluid mechanics of the confined nucleus functions to evenly distribute pressure through-

out the disk and from one vertebral body to the next under loaded conditions. Because of the affinity for water, the nucleus imbibes water when pressure is reduced on the disk and water is squeezed out under compressive loads.[12,26]

4. The *cartilaginous end-plates* cover the nucleus pulposus superiorly and inferiorly and lie between the nucleus and vertebral bodies. Each one is encircled by the apophyseal ring of the respective vertebral body. The collagen fibers of the inner annulus fibrosus insert into the end-plate and angle centrally, thus encapsulating the nucleus pulposus.[5] Nutrition diffuses from the marrow of the vertebral bodies to the disk via the end-plates.[33]

5. With flexion (forward bending) of a vertebral segment, the anterior portion of the disk is compressed and the posterior is distracted. The nucleus pulposus is displaced posteriorly, potentially to redistribute the load through the disk.[18] Asymmetric loading in flexion results in distortions of the nucleus toward the contralateral posterolateral corner where the fibers of the annulus are more stretched.[2]

B. Injury and Degeneration of the Disk[1,2,6,9,11,12,21,34]

1. Annular fiber breakdown may occur with fatigue loading over time or with traumatic rupture.[1,2]

   a. Fatigue breakdown usually occurs with repeated overloading of the spine with asymmetric forward bending and torsional stresses.[1,2,9,15]

   b. With torsional stresses, the annulus becomes distorted, most obviously at the posterolateral corner opposite the direction of rotation. The layers of the outer annulus fibrosus lose their cohesion and begin to separate from each other. Each layer then acts as a separate barrier to the nuclear material. Eventually, radial tears occur and there is communication of the nuclear material between the layers.[9]

   c. With repeated forward bending and lifting stresses, the layers of the annulus are strained; they become tightly packed together in the posterolateral corners, radial fissures develop, and the nuclear material migrates down the fissures.[1,2] Outer layers of annular fibers can contain the nuclear material as long as they remain a continuous layer.[1] Following injury, there is a tendency for the nucleus to swell and distort the annulus. Distortion is more severe in the region where the annular fibers are stretched.[2,21] If the outer layers rupture, the nuclear material may extrude through the fissures.

   d. Healing is attempted, but there is poor circulation in the disk. There may be self-sealing of a defect with the nuclear gel[26] or proliferation of cells of the annulus to seal the defect.[21] Any fibrous repair is weaker than normal and takes a long time due to the relative avascular status of the disk.

   e. Traumatic rupture of the annulus can occur as a one-time event or can be superimposed on a disk where there has been gradual breakdown of the annular rings. This is seen most commonly in traumatic hyperflexion injuries.[2]

   f. Axial overload of the disk usually results in end-plate damage or vertebral body fracture before there is any damage to the annulus fibrosus.[24]

2. Individuals are most susceptible to symptomatic disk injuries between the ages of 30 and 45 years. During this time, the nucleus is still capable of imbibing water, but the annulus weakens from fatigue loading over time

and, therefore, is less able to withstand increased pressures when there are disproportionately high stresses. The nuclear material may protrude into the tears or fissures, which most commonly are posterolateral and, with increased pressures, bulge against the outer annular fibers causing an annular distortion; or the nuclear material may extrude from the disk through complete fissures in the annulus.[1,9]

3. Any loss of integrity of the disk from infection, disease, herniation, or an end-plate defect becomes a stimulus for degenerative changes in the disk.[21]
   a. Degeneration is characterized by progressive fibrous changes in the nucleus, loss of the organization of the rings of the annulus fibrosus, and loss of the cartilaginous end-plates.[21]
   b. As the nucleus becomes more fibrotic, it loses its capacity to imbibe fluid. Water content decreases and there is an associated decrease in the size of the nucleus.[23] Acute disk protrusions caused by a bulging nucleus pulposus against the annulus or extrusions of the nucleus through a torn annulus are rare in older people.
   c. It is possible to have protrusions of the annulus fibrosus without nuclear pressure. Myxomatous degeneration with annular protrusion has been demonstrated in disk lesions in older people.[45]
4. Injury or degeneration of the disk affects spinal mechanics in general.[35] Initially there is increased mobility of the segment with greater than normal flexion-extension and forward and backward sliding of the vertebral body.[24] Force distribution through the entire segment is altered, causing abnormal forces in the facets and supporting structures[9,18] (see section II B).

C. Diskogenic Pain[38]

1. Clinical picture
   a. Symptoms may be from early stages of disk degeneration or possibly from a compression fracture of the end-plate of the vertebral body.
   b. Pain occurs without nerve root involvement, although there may be referred pain into the extremities.

2. General treatment goals and plan of care

Goals	Plan of Care
a. Relieve pain and relax muscle guarding and compression forces	a. Modalities, traction, and passive support with collar or corset
b. Restore biomechanics	b. Extension positions of the spine

D. Disk Protrusions (Derangements)

1. Terminology[24]
   a. Disk protrusion
      Any change in the shape of the annulus that causes it to bulge beyond its normal perimeter
   b. Disk herniation
      (1) Prolapse
         A protrusion of the nucleus that is still contained by the outer layers of the annulus and supporting ligamentous structures

(2) Extrusion

A protrusion in which the nuclear material ruptures through the outer annulus and lies under the posterior longitudinal ligament

(3) Free sequestration

The extruded nucleus has moved away from the prolapsed area
Note: Various authors use these terms differently. The above descriptions are from MacNab.[24] Bogduk[5] defines *prolapse* as a frank rupture of nuclear material into the vertebral canal and *herniation* as the nuclear material being partially expelled into the canal with the majority remaining in a defect in the annulus.

2. Etiology of symptoms

a. The disk is largely aneural; not all disk protrusions are symptomatic.

b. Symptoms of pain arise from pressure of the protrusion against pain-sensitive structures (ligaments, dura mater, and blood vessels around nerve roots).

c. Neurologic signs arise from pressure against the spinal cord or nerve roots. The only true neurologic signs are specific motor weaknesses and specific dermatome sensory changes. (Radiating pain in a dermatomal pattern, increased myoelectrical activity in the hamstrings, decreased straight leg-raising, and depressed deep tendon reflexes can also be associated with referred pain stimuli from spinal muscles, interspinous ligaments, the disk, and facet joints and, therefore, are not true signs of nerve root pressure.)[8,13,29]

d. Symptoms are variable depending on the degree and direction of the protrusion as well as the spinal level of the lesion.

(1) Posterior or posterolateral protrusions are most common.

(2) With a small posterior or posterolateral lesion, there may be pressure against the posterior longitudinal ligament or against the dura mater or its extensions around the nerve roots. The patient may describe a severe midline backache or pain spreading across the back into the buttock and thigh.

(3) A large posterior protrusion may cause spinal cord signs such as loss of bladder control and saddle anesthesia.

(4) A large posterolateral protrusion may cause partial cord or nerve root signs.

(5) An anterior protrusion may cause pressure against the anterior longitudinal ligament, resulting in back pain. There may be no neurologic signs.

e. Symptoms may shift if there is integrity of the annular wall, since the hydrostatic mechanism is still intact.[27]

3. Onset and behavior of symptoms[14,24,27]

a. Onset is usually between 20 and 55 years of age but most frequently from mid 30s through the 40s.

b. Except in cases of trauma, symptomatic onset is usually associated simply with bending, bending and lifting, or attempting to stand up after having been in a sitting or forward-bent posture. The person may or may not have the sensation of something tearing.

c. Many patients have a predisposing history of a faulty flexion posture (flat back or forward head postures—see Chapter 14).

    d. Pain may increase gradually when the person is inactive, such as when sitting or after a night's rest. The patient often describes the onset of pain when attempting to get out of bed in the morning.

    e. With a posterior or posterolateral protrusion, symptoms are usually aggravated with activities that increase the intradiskal pressure, such as sitting, forward bending, coughing, or straining or when attempting to stand up after being in a flexed position. Usually, symptoms are lessened when walking.

    f. During the acute phase, the pain is almost always present but varies in intensity, depending on the person's position or activity.

    g. The most common levels of protrusion are the segments between the fourth and fifth lumbar vertebrae and between the fifth lumbar vertebra and sacrum.

    h. Initially, discomfort is noticed in the lumbosacral or buttock region. Some patients experience aching that extends into the thigh. Numbness or muscle weakness (neurologic signs) are not noted unless the protrusion has progressed to a degree where there is nerve root, spinal cord, or cauda equina compression.

4. **Objective clinical findings**[14,27]

    Note: The following information relates to a posterior or posterolateral nuclear protrusion in the lumbar spine. For the less frequently seen anterior protrusion, see the brief description in Section E 4.

    a. The patient usually prefers standing and walking to sitting.

    b. The patient may have a decrease in or loss of lumbar lordosis and may have some lateral shifting of the spinal column.

    c. Forward bending is limited. When repeating the forward-bending test, the symptoms increase or peripheralize. *Peripheralization* means the symptoms are experienced further down the leg.

    d. Backward bending is limited; when repeating the backward-bending test, the pain lessens or centralizes. *Centralization* means the symptoms recede up the leg or become localized to the back. Important exceptions:[27]

      (1) If there is a lateral shift of the spinal column, backward bending increases the pain. If the lateral shift is first corrected (see Section E 3 b), then repeated backward bending lessens or centralizes the pain.

      (2) If the protrusion cannot be mechanically reduced, backward bending peripheralizes or increases the symptoms.

      (3) If there is an anterior protrusion, backward bending increases the pain and forward bending relieves the pain.

    e. Testing passive lumbar flexion when in the supine position and passive extension when in the prone position usually produces signs similar to those of the standing tests, but results may not be as dramatic because gravity is eliminated.

    f. Pain between 30 to 60 degrees of straight leg raising is considered positive for interference of dural mobility but not pathognomonic for a disk protrusion.[14,23]

    g. A contained nuclear protrusion can be influenced by movement because the hydrostatic mechanism is still intact. An extruded or sequestrated nucleus with a complete annular tear disrupts the hydrostatic mechanism and cannot be influenced by movement.[27]

5. Principles of treatment[12,14,32]

    a. Relative changes in posture and activities affect intradiskal pressure. When compared with standing, intradiskal pressure is least when lying supine, increases by almost 50 percent when sitting with hips and knees flexed, and almost doubles if leaning forward while sitting[12,32] Sitting with a back rest inclination of 120 degrees and lumbar support 5 cm in depth provides the lowest load to the disk while sitting.[3,12] Therefore, sitting with the hips and knees flexed or leaning forward should be avoided in acute disk lesions. If sitting is necessary, there should be support for the lumbar spine with the trunk reclined 120 degrees.

    b. When a person is lying down, compression forces to the disk are reduced, and with time, the nucleus potentially can absorb more water to equalize pressures. Then, upon rising, body weight compresses the disk with the increased fluid, and intradiskal pressure greatly increases. The pain or symptoms from a protrusion are accentuated. To avoid exacerbating symptoms, absolute bed rest during the acute phase should be avoided. Bed rest during the first 2 days when symptoms are highly irritable is needed to promote early healing, but it should be interspersed with short intervals of standing, walking, and appropriately controlled movement.[44]

    c. The phenomenon of imbibition during reduced pressures also occurs during periods of prolonged traction or with postures of prolonged flexion. Therefore, static traction of longer than 10 minutes should not be used during the acute stage (see Chapter 16). Similarly, sustained bed positioning with lumbar flexion should be avoided unless it is the only position that decreases symptoms.

    d. Rest in a slightly forward-bent position often lessens pain because of the space potential for the nucleus. The patient may also deviate laterally to minimize pressure against a nerve root. Movement into extension initially causes increased symptoms. In acute disk lesions in which there is protective lateral shifting and lumbar flexion, techniques that cause lateral shifting of the spine opposite to the deviation followed by passive spinal extension to mechanically compress the protrusion and shift it anteriorly have been found to relieve the clinical signs and symptoms.[16,27,28]

    e. Isometric activities (pelvic tilt exercises, straining, Valsalva maneuver) as well as active back flexion or extension exercises increase intradiskal pressures above normal and, therefore, MUST BE AVOIDED during the acute stage.

    f. Reflex muscle splinting often accompanies an acute disk lesion and adds to the compressive forces. Modalities and gentle oscillatory traction to the spine may help decrease the splinting (see Chapter 16).

6. Summary of problems during an acute disk protrusion

    a. Pain from protrusion against a pain-sensitive structure and accompanying protective muscle spasm

    b. Neurologic signs only if protrusion is against nerve root or spinal cord

    c. Abnormal spinal posture and intradiskal pressure

7. General treatment goals and plan of care during acute phase

Goals	*Plan of Care*
a. Relieve pain and promote muscle relaxation	a. Rest interspersed with periods of controlled movement Modalities, massage, traction
b. Relieve pressure against pain-sensitive neurologic structures	b. Motions that decrease the size and effect of the bulging disk. Avoid positions, exercises, and activities that increase intradiskal pressure.
c. Promote positions and movements that align the spine and reduce intradiskal pressure	c. Same as b. Patient education and involvement in the program.

8. **Precautions and contraindications during the acute stage**
   a. A patient with acute pain in the spinal region that is not influenced by changing the patient's position or by movement must be screened by a physician for signs of serious pathology.
   b. Any movement that peripheralizes the symptoms signals a movement that is contraindicated during the acute and early subacute period of treatment.
   c. Extension of the spine is contraindicated[27]
      (1) when no position or movement decreases or centralizes the described pain.
      (2) when saddle anesthesia and/or bladder weakness is present.
      (3) when a patient is in such extreme pain that he rigidly holds himself immobile with any attempted correction.
   d. Flexion of the spine should be avoided
      (1) when extension relieves the symptoms.
      (2) when flexion movements increase the pain or peripheralize the symptoms.
   e. Any form of exercise or activity that increases intradiskal pressure, such as the Valsalva maneuver, active pelvic tilt, or trunk-raising exercises, should be avoided during this stage.

E. Techniques to Mechanically Reduce a Nuclear Disk Protrusion

Note: These techniques are used only if the test movements have shown that the postures and movements used improve the symptoms.[14,27] If no test movements decrease the symptoms, the mechanical approach to treatment should not be used.

1. If symptoms are severe, bed rest is indicated with short periods of walking at regular intervals. Walking minimizes disk swelling and promotes circulation. The patient should use crutches, if he cannot stand upright, in order to help relieve the increased pressure of the forward-bent posture.[14]
2. **Posterior or posterolateral protrusion**
   If repeated flexion test movements increase the symptoms and if repeated extension test movements decrease or centralize the symptoms, all flexion activities should be avoided during this phase of treatment. Treatment begins with
   a. **passive extension**
      (1) Position of patient: prone. If the flexion posture is severe, place pillows under the abdomen for support. Gradually increase the amount of extension by removing the pillows, and then progress by

having the patient prop himself up on his elbows, allowing the pelvis to sag (Figure 15-1). When propping, pillows placed under the thorax help take strain off the shoulders. Wait 5 to 10 minutes between each increment of extension to allow for reduction of water content and size of the bulge. There should be an accompanying centralization of or decrease in symptoms. Progress to having the patient prop himself up on his hands, allowing the pelvis to sag (see Figure 14-16A).

(2) If the sustained postures are not well tolerated, have the patient do passive lumbar extension intermittently by repeating the prone press-ups (same as Figure 14-16A) rather than just propping up.

Precaution: Carefully monitor the patient's experience of symptoms. Symptoms should lessen in the thigh and buttock, but it may increase in the low back (centralize). If the symptoms progress down the leg (peripheralize), immediately stop the exercises and re-assess.[27]

b. **lateral shift**

If the patient has lateral shifting of the spine (Figure 15-2), extension alone will not reduce the nuclear protrusion until the shift is corrected. Once the shift is corrected, the patient must extend as in (a) above to maintain the correction. Methods to correct the shift include the following.

(1) The therapist stands on the side to which the thorax is shifted and places her shoulder against the patient's elbow (which is flexed against his rib cage). She then wraps her arms around the patient's pelvis on the opposite side and simultaneously pulls the pelvis toward her as she pushes the patient's thorax away (Figure 15-3). This is a gradual maneuver. Continue with the lateral shifting if centralization of the pain occurs.[28] If there is overcorrection, the pain and lateral shift may move to the contralateral side. It is corrected by shifting the thorax back. The purpose is to centralize the pain and correct the lateral shift. Once the shift is corrected, immediately have the patient backward bend (see Figure 14-16B). Again, allow time. Progress to passive extension as described in (a) above.

(2) Alternate method

Place the patient in a side-lying position, with the side to which the thorax is shifted placed downward. A small pillow or towel roll is placed under the thorax. The patient remains in this position until the pain centralizes, then rolls prone and begins passive extension as described in (a) above.

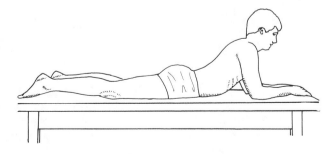

FIGURE 15-1. Passive lumbar extension accomplished by having the patient prop up on the elbows.

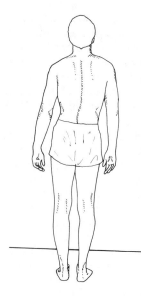

FIGURE 15-2. Patient with a lateral shift of the thoracic cage toward the right. The pelvis is shifted toward the left.

(3) Another alternate method

With the patient prone, the therapist attempts to manually side-glide the thorax and pelvis toward midline. The forces are in equal and opposite directions. Once the symptoms centralize, begin passive extension as in (a) above.

3. **Patient education**

a. Help the patient recognize what motions increase the pain and what motions decrease the pain.

b. Instruct the patient to repeat the extension activities frequently during the first couple of days.

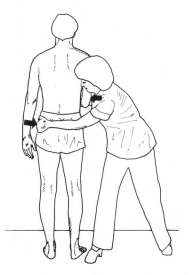

FIGURE 15-3. A lateral gliding technique used to correct a lateral shift of the thorax is applied against the patient's elbow and thoracic cage as the pelvis is pulled in the opposite direction.

    c. Instruct the patient to maintain an extended posture while the lesion is healing.

      (1) The patient should sit with lumbar support. This could be a towel roll or lumbar pillow. This is especially important when riding in a car or sitting in a soft chair.

      (2) When going to bed, he should pin a towel, folded lengthwise four times, around his waist.

    d. Teach self-correction of a lateral shift

      (1) If his spine shifts laterally, he should do self-correction before attempting extension.

      (2) To teach self-correction of the lateral shift, the patient places his hand on the side of the shifted rib cage on the lateral aspect of the rib cage and places the other hand over the crest of the opposite ilium. He then gradually pushes these regions toward the midline and holds (Figure 15-4). Eventually, he can voluntarily correct the shift.

      (3) If appropriate, the patient could also be instructed to correct the shift by side lying or prone lying as previously described.

    e. Caution the patient that if pain worsens or peripheralizes when exercising, he must immediately stop the activity.

    f. Instruct the patient to avoid flexion activities, lifting, or any other functions that increase intradiskal pressure while symptoms are acute.

4. **Anterior protrusion**

If repeated flexion tests decrease the symptoms and repeated extension tests increase the symptoms, and if the patient demonstrates an accentuated lordosis that came on suddenly, treatment begins with[27]

    a. **correction of a lateral shift if present**

Position of patient: standing and placing the leg opposite the shift on a chair so the hip is in about 90 degrees of flexion. The leg on the side of

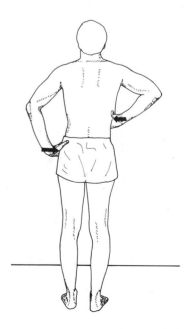

FIGURE 15-4. Self-correction of a lateral shift.

the lateral shift is kept extended. The patient then flexes his trunk onto the raised thigh and applies pressure by pulling on his ankle (Figure 15-5). Repeat several times but not to the point that the symptoms shift to the opposite side.

b. **passive flexion**
Position of patient: supine. When no lateral shift is present, the patient brings both knees to his chest and holds this position with his arms around his thighs for several minutes (see Figure 14-13). He can lower his legs part way down and pull them back up to his chest in an intermittent rhythm to create a slow oscillating motion in the spine. Progress after several days to flexion of the spine when sitting and standing.

Note: Patients with symptoms of nerve root compression from causes other than nuclear protrusion may also benefit from passive flexion exercises to relieve the symptoms because flexion of the spine widens the foramina.

5. **Traction**
Traction may be tolerated by the patient during the acute stage and has the benefit of widening the disk space and possibly reducing the nuclear protrusion by decreasing the pressure on the disk or by placing tension on the posterior longitudinal ligament[40] (see Chapter 16).

a. Time of the traction should be short; osmotic forces soon equalize. Then upon release of the traction force, there could be an increase in the disk pressure, leading to increased pain.
   (1) Less than 15 minutes of intermittent traction
   (2) Less than 10 minutes of sustained traction
b. High poundage; greater than half the patient's body weight is necessary for separation of the lumbar vertebrae.
c. If there is complete relief initially, often there will be an exacerbation of symptoms later.

F. Management when Disk Symptoms Have Stabilized

1. **Signs of improvement**
Improvement is noted with loss of spinal deformity, increased motion in the back, and negative dural mobility signs.[14] Loss of back pain with increased true neurologic signs is an indication of worsening. The patient is tested to

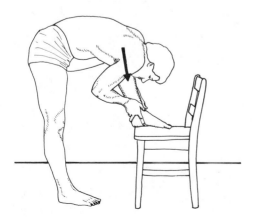

FIGURE 15-5. Self-correction of a lateral shift when there is deviation of the trunk as it flexes.

determine if the symptoms have stabilized by doing repeated flexion and extension tests with the patient standing, then lying supine and prone as done initially. The tests may be positive for dysfunction (tightness, tension) but should not cause peripheralization of the symptoms as when the condition was acute.[27]

2. Problems found in the subacute and chronic phases
a. pain when adaptively shortened structures are stretched
b. decreased range of motion
c. muscle strength imbalances
d. faulty kinesthetic awareness and control of normal spinal alignment
e. patient unaware how to prevent recurrences

3. Treatment emphasis
The emphases during this stage are *recovery of function* and *teaching the patient how to prevent recurrences of a disk protrusion.* Goals, plan of care, and suggested exercises to correct the identified problems are described in Chapter 14. The pain from adaptive shortening will decrease as normal flexibility is restored. Stretching maneuvers to increase lumbar flexion will be necessary if the patient has maintained extension while healing. Following any flexion exercises, the patient should conclude with extension exercises.[27]

4. Patient education
Teach the patient posture awareness and correction procedures to minimize predisposing his back to future painful episodes.
a. Teach the patient proper body mechanics, how to adapt his environment, and preventive exercises as described in Chapter 14.
b. Emphasize to the patient that if he must be in a flexed posture he should interrupt the flexion with backward bending at least once every hour.
c. Emphasize that if he feels the symptoms of a protrusion developing, he should immediately do press-ups in the prone position or backward bending while standing in order to prevent progression of the symptoms (see Figure 14-16A and B).

II. JOINT LESIONS IN THE SPINE

A. Characteristics of the Zygapophyseal[1] (Facet) Joints
1. Facet joints are synovial articulations that are enclosed in a capsule and supported by ligaments; they respond to trauma and arthritic changes like any peripheral joint.
2. Various types of meniscoid-like structures or invaginations of the facet capsules are present in the zygapophyseal joints of the spine. They are synovial reflections containing fat and blood vessels. In some cases, dense fibrous tissue develops as a result of mechanical stresses.[4,5] Some people describe an entrapment of these structures between the articulating surfaces with sudden or unusual movement as a source of pain and limited motion via tension on the well-innervated capsule.[17,42] Bogduk describes the *locked back mechanism* as being an extrapment of the meniscoids in the supra- or infracapsular folds, which then blocks the return to extension from the flexed position.[4,5] (It is called an extrapment since the

meniscoid fails to re-enter the joint cavity; it becomes a space-occupying lesion in the capsular folds causing pain as it impacts and stretches the capsules.)

B. Pathomechanical Relationships of the Intervertebral Disk and Facets

1. The disk and facets make up a three-joint complex between two adjoining vertebra and are biomechanically interrelated. Asymmetric disk injury affects the kinematics of the entire unit plus the joints above and below, resulting in asymmetric movements of the facets, abnormal stresses, and eventual cartilage degeneration.[35]
2. Abnormal movement caused by disk degeneration puts a stress on the supporting ligaments and paraspinal muscles, causing abnormal proprioceptive input, further affecting fine control of movement.
3. As the disk degenerates, there is a decrease in both water content and disk height. The vertebral bodies approximate and the intervertebral foramina and spinal canal narrow.[7]
   a. Initially, there is increased slack with increased mobility in the spinal segment.[24] Opposition of the facet surfaces changes and the capsules are strained, resulting in irritation, swelling, and muscle spasm.
   b. Eventually, with the repeated irritation from the faulty mechanics, there are progressive degenerative changes in the facets and vertebral bodies. Osteophyte formation along the facets and spondylitic lipping and spurring along the vertebral bodies occur and hypomobility develops.[18,30] These lead to additional narrowing of the associated foramina and spinal canal.
   c. In the cervical spine, the uncovertebral joints thicken, roughen, and distort.
4. Spinal nerve roots become involved
   a. when a protrusion of the disk compresses a nerve root.
   b. when there is decreased disk height from degenerative changes resulting in a decreased foraminal space[36] or excessive gliding of the vertebra.[24]
   c. when there is an inflammatory response from trauma, degeneration, or disease with accompanying edema and stenosis.
   d. when a facet joint subluxes and the nerve root becomes impinged between the tip of the superior articulating facet and the pedicle.
   e. when spondylosis results in osteophytic growth on the articular facets or bony spurs along the diskal borders of the vertebral bodies that impinge the nerve roots.
   f. when there is spondylolysis, spondylolisthesis, scarring, or adhesion formation following spinal surgery.
5. In all cases, the cycle of dysfunction or injury, pain, and muscle splinting leads to further restriction of movement, pain, and muscle splinting unless appropriate therapy is introduced.

C. Facet Joint Impingement (Blocking, Fixation, Extrapment)[4,5,17,38,39]

1. Clinical picture
   a. With a sudden or unusual movement, the meniscoid of a facet capsule may be extrapped, impinged, or stressed, which causes pain and mus-

cle guarding. The onset is sudden and usually involves forward bending and rotation.
b. There is loss of specific motions, and attempted movement induces
pain. At rest the individual has no pain.
c. There are no true neurologic signs, but there may be referred pain in
the related dermatome.
d. Over time, stress is placed on the contralateral joint and on the disk,
leading to problems in these structures.

2. Management of impingements

Release of the trapped meniscoid will relieve the pain and accompanying
muscle guarding. The joint surfaces need to be separated and the joint
capsules made taut.[17]
General techniques include
a. **traction.**
This may be applied manually or mechanically (see Chapter 16).
Enough force is needed to cause separation of the vertebrae, thus a
gliding-traction of the facets occurs.
b. **self-mobilization.**
(1) To treat the lumbar spine, self-mobilization may be applied by pulling both thighs to the chest (see Figure 14-13).
(2) To treat the cervical spine, the person axially extends his neck and
places his hand under the occiput to lift the weight of the head.
c. **spinal mobilization and manipulation**
These techniques require advanced training and are beyond the scope
of this text.

D. Facet Sprain, Joint Capsule Injury

1. Clinical picture

a. History of trauma
b. The joints react with effusion (swelling), the same as do peripheral
joints, and there is accompanying muscle splinting.

2. Management of acute symptoms

a. See Chapter 6 for general goals and guidelines for joint lesions.
b. Besides rest and support, techniques to relieve pain and promote relaxation include modalities and gentle intermittent manual traction. The
traction force is less than that required to separate the vertebrae, because the capsule should not be stretched when acutely injured. The
traction is applied rhythmically as a joint oscillation technique in order
to inhibit the transmission of pain stimuli and maintain movement in the
joints (see Chapter 16 for description of techniques).
c. Use passive motion techniques within the pain-free range to maintain
range of motion.
d. Muscle-setting techniques may be attempted to maintain muscle function, but they may increase pain if done too strongly since muscle contraction causes joint compression.
e. Reverse muscle action with gentle scapular motions may help maintain
muscle function without moving the spinal joints.

3. Management of subacute and chronic symptoms

     a. In order to improve the patient's function, any joint flexibility or muscle strength imbalances are treated with appropriate exercises (see Chapter 14).

     b. Techniques to relieve tension and improve posture awareness and spinal management are taught to the patient (see Chapter 14).

E. Facet Hypomobility or Hypermobility

1. Clinical picture

a. Usually there is a history of faulty posture, prolonged immobilization following injury, severe trauma, or degenerative changes in the disk.

b. In early stages of degenerative changes, as the disk height decreases from loss of hydration in the nucleus pulposus, there is greater play, or hypermobility, in the 3-joint complex. Over time, stress from the excessive motion and altered mechanics leads to osteophyte formation with spurring and lipping along the joint margins and vertebral bodies. Progressive hypomobility results.

c. Usually where there is hypomobility, compensatory hypermobility occurs in neighboring spinal segments.

d. Pain may occur from the stresses of excessive mobility or from stretch to hypomobile structures. Pain may also occur from encroachment of developing osteophytes against pain-sensitive tissue, or from swelling and irritation because of excessive or abnormal mobility of the segments.

2. Management

a. A painful hypermobile region requires stabilization with the use of passive support (collar or corset) and muscle strengthening techniques. Isometric exercises in pain-free positions may be preferred over isotonic exercises if movement is painful.

b. A hypomobile region requires stretching, but not if the techniques stress a hypermobile region. The hypermobile region should be stabilized while stretching.

c. Functional goals are established with exercises geared toward meeting the goals (see Chapter 14).

F. Osteoarthritic Changes (Degenerative Joint Disease and Spondylosis)

1. Clinical picture[7,39]

a. Symptoms of arthritis are common with degenerative disk disease or in joints continually exposed to trauma.

b. Osteophytes may develop and encroach on the spinal canal and intervertebral foramina, thereby causing neurologic signs.

c. The degenerating joint is vulnerable to facet impingement, sprains, and inflammation, as is any arthritic joint.

d. In some patients, movement relieves the symptoms; in others, movement irritates the joints and painful symptoms increase.

2. Management during periods of increased pain

a. To reduce tension

    (1) relaxation exercises

       (2) sustained traction at a force strong enough to open the intervertebral foramina and relieve pressure on nerve roots. If this causes irritation, it should not be used.

  b. To increase mobility use active range of motion and contract-relax techniques within the patient's tolerance (see Section III B 2 c).

  c. Teach the patient preventive measures and postures to relieve mechanial stress.

  d. If motion aggravates symptoms, reduce movement with passive support (collar or low-back corset) and increase muscle strength beginning with isometric exercises in the pain-free positions.

  e. **Precautions:** Because of the narrowed foramina and spinal canal, backward bending and backward bending with rotation should be avoided, since these motions narrow the foramina further.[10]

G. Rheumatoid Arthritis (RA)

1. Clinical picture

  a. Symptoms of RA can affect any of the synovial joints of the spine and ribs. There will be pain and swelling.

  b. RA in the cervical spine presents special problems including neurologic symptoms wherever degenerative changes or swelling impinge against neurologic tissue, increased fragility of tissues affected by RA such as osteoporosis with cyst formation and erosion of bone, and instabilities from ligamentous necrosis. Most common of the serious lesions are altantoaxial subluxation and C4/5 and C5/6 vertebral dislocations.[31]

  c. Pain or neurologic signs originating in the spine may or may not be related to subluxation. Therefore, these signs should be used as a precaution whenever dealing with this disease because of the potential damage to the spinal cord.

  d. X-ray examinations are important in ruling out instabilities; signs and symptoms alone are not conclusive.

2. Physical therapy management[31]

Precaution: Inappropriate movements of the spine could be life threatening or extremely debilitating because of the potential of subluxations and dislocations to cause damage to the cervical cord or vertebral artery.

  a. Follow the general guidelines and plan of care for treating rheumatoid arthritis as described in Chapter 6, section VII. Additional suggestions related to the spine follow.

  b. To relieve pain and relax the muscles modalities are appropriate. A soft cervical collar may provide support in the cervical region, or a corset may be used in the lumbar region.

  c. To decrease stiffness and increase mobility, gentle stretching using physiologic ranges and soft-tissue stretching can be done. Traction or joint mobilizations are potentially dangerous due to ligamentous necrosis and vertebral instability and, therefore, are **contraindicated**.

  d. To increase control and strength, gentle active ROM and isometric exercises are taught to the patient, staying within his tolerance. Hyperextension and circumduction motions of the spine should be avoided.

III.   MUSCLE AND SOFT-TISSUE LESIONS

A. Strains, Tears, and Contusions From Trauma or Overuse

1. Clinical picture

   a. During the acute phase, all soft-tissue injuries give a similar picture with pain, localized swelling, and tenderness on palpation. There is protective muscle guarding regardless of whether the injured tissue is inert or contractile.

      (1) A common site for injury or overuse is along the iliac crest. This is where many forces converge around the attachment of the lateral raphe of the lumbodorsal fascia, quadratus lumborum, erector spinae, and iliolumbar ligament.

      (2) Other structures commonly injured are the muscles and ligaments of the cervical spine following flexion-extension trauma.

      (3) Strain to the posterior cervical and upper thoracic muscles and fascia is common with postural and emotional stresses such as prolonged sitting at a computer terminal, drafting board, or desk.

   b. Ligamentous strains will cause pain when the ligament is stressed. If torn, there will be hypermobility of the segment.

   c. Muscle and tendon injury will cause pain when the involved muscle is stretched as well as when it contracts.

   d. Fascial tears will be painful when stressed.

   e. Often, more than one tissue may be injured as the result of trauma. The extent of involvement may not be detectable during the acute phase. As healing of the involved structures occurs, there may be adaptive shortening or scar tissue adhering to surrounding tissue.

2. Management during the acute phase

   a. Follow the guidelines and plan of care as described in Chapter 6.

   b. To relieve pain and control edema, use of modalities is appropriate.

   c. To maintain integrity of the tissue and promote circulation, use muscle-setting techniques with the muscle in the shortened range. Gradually elongate the muscle as tolerated (see technique described in Section B to follow).

   d. To maintain motion, use passive ROM techniques within the limits of pain; no stretching should be done during the acute phase.

   e. Traction techniques may aggravate a muscle or soft-tissue injury, particularly if the tissue is placed in a lengthened position during the set up or with a high dosage of pull during treatment. If the tissue is kept in a shortened position and the dosage is kept less than that which causes vertebral separation, the traction may reflexively inhibit the pain.

3. Management in the subacute and chronic stages

   a. If the muscle and soft tissue lose some flexibility while healing, they are gradually stretched by using gentle inhibition techniques or passive stretching.

   b. If there is any loss of strength, the muscle is strengthened with graded isometric and resistive dynamic exercises.

   c. Any posture abnormalities should be corrected with kinesthetic training, flexibility, and posture exercises.

   d. Often with low back problems, there are muscle imbalances in the hip region that perpetuate stresses in the low back. Refer to the muscle section in Chapter 10 for exercises to correct flexibility and strength imbalance problems in the hip.

B. Muscle Guarding (Splinting) and Spasm

1. Clinical picture

a. Muscle guarding occurs with injury to any tissue and serves the immediate purpose of immobilizing the region of the injury.

b. If the muscle contraction is prolonged, it results in the build up of metabolic waste products and sluggish circulation. This altered local environment in the muscle results in irritation of the free nerve endings so that the muscle continues to contract in response to the local painful stimulus. It becomes the source of additional pain (see Figure 6-1).

2. Management of acute muscle guarding or spasm

a. If the source of the original problem can be identified and treated early, the painful cycle that occurs with muscle spasm can be avoided. Treating only the spasm does not relieve the source of the problem.

b. Passive support to the part may be used to relieve the muscles from the job of supporting or controlling the injured part.

(1) Cervical region
   Cervical collars provide passive support. The length of time a collar is worn during the day relates to the severity of the injury and the amount of protection required. Collars often place the neck in a forward-head posture. This will cause healing in a faulty position, which will lead to future postural problems or painful syndromes. Usually, turning the collar around or cutting down the portion under the mandible will allow the neck to assume a correct alignment.

(2) Lumbar region
   Corsets provide passive support. As with the cervical region, the length of time that a corset is worn should be related to the amount of protection required. Some patients tend to become dependent on the corset and continue to wear it even after healing, when it no longer serves its intended purpose. After healing, it is better to strengthen the body's natural corset (abdominal muscles and others attached to the lumbodorsal fascia) and develop good spinal mechanics (see Chapter 14).

c. To maintain circulation and promote relaxation of the muscle, modalities and massage are helpful. In addition, muscle-setting techniques maintain muscle integrity, assist circulation, and promote relaxation. The dosage is critical; resistance is minimal; use only enough to generate a setting contraction.

(1) Cervical region
   Position of patient: supine, with the therapist at the head of the treatment table, supporting the patient's head with her hands.
   Start with the guarding muscle in its shortened position. Ask the patient to hold as a GENTLE resistance (light enough to barely move a feather) is applied. Both the contraction and the relaxation should be gradual. There should be no neck movement or jerky resistance.

   (a) If there has been muscle injury, the technique is repeated with the muscle kept in the shortened range for several days before lengthening it.

   (b) If there is no muscle injury, progress the treatment by gradually lengthening the guarded muscle after each contraction and relaxation.

Movement is done only within the patient's pain-free range; no stretching is done when there is muscle guarding.

(2) Lumbar region

Position of patient: prone, with arms resting at his side.

Have the patient lift his head. This will initiate a setting (stabilizing) contraction of the lumbar erector spinae muscles. A stronger contraction of the lumbar extensor muscles will occur if the head and thorax are extended. Alternate hip extension will also cause a setting contraction of the lumbar extensor muscles.

(a) When there is muscle injury, the muscle is kept in this shortened range for several days.

(b) For progression, if there is no muscle injury or as the muscle heals, gradually allow the muscle to elongate after each contraction by putting a pillow under the abdomen and then extending the thorax on the lumbar spine through a greater range. Elongation is done only within tolerance during the early healing phase. There should be no increase in symptoms.

(c) Alternate position: supine. The patient presses his head and neck into the bed, causing a setting contraction of the spinal extensors.

d. To maintain integrity and promote relaxation of the muscles when there is no direct trauma to them, use *reverse muscle action techniques*. These are valuable when neck motions cause pain and muscle guarding. The neck is not moved, but the muscles are called on to contract and relax through a functional range. The motions include active scapular elevation, depression, adduction, and rotation and active shoulder flexion, extension, abduction, adduction, and rotation. The shoulder motions may be done as circumduction or patterned activities, just so they do not stress the neck.

e. Passive to active range of motion is initiated within the pain-free range.

(1) Cervical region

The therapist assists the patient through the available range of motion as tolerated. When the pain and spasm are under control, the patient is taught to do the cervical motions actively in the sitting position.

(2) Lumbar region

Teach pelvic tilt exercises while the patient is supine, prone, in all 4's position, sitting, or standing, as tolerated.

Progress to forward and backward bending while standing but only in the pain-free range initially.

3. Management of subacute and chronic symptoms

When the acute symptoms begin to diminish, the intensity of the exercise program can progress.

a. Identify any muscle weakness or loss of motion and establish an exercise program as described in Chapter 14, being careful to keep the progressions within the patient's tolerance, since healing is still occurring.

b. Identify any posture problems and retrain the patient's kinesthetic awareness for correct posture.

c. Teach the patient relaxation exercises in order to reduce muscle tension as it arises.

d. Functional activities can be resumed at a safe level as soon as the patient is able, progressively increasing the level of function as ROM and strength improve. Patient education should include suggestions for adaptation of the environment as well as exercise techniques to prevent recurrences of problems.

IV. SELECTED CONDITIONS

A. Torticollis (Wryneck, Cervical Scoliosis)

This involves asymmetry in strength or functioning of the sternocleidomastoid muscle (SCM). There is cervical rotation opposite to and side bending toward the side of the contracting or shortened muscle.

1. Congenital torticollis

a. Causes

Injury *in utero* or at birth to the SCM, which then becomes fibrotic and shortens. The injury may be from a faulty position of the fetus, nerve injury, or direct trauma to the muscle.

b. Management

Gentle passive range of motion and stretching are initiated as soon as the diagnosis is made. The head is rotated toward and side bent away from the side of tightness (see Figure 14-11).

2. Asymmetric weakness (muscle imbalance)

a. Causes

A common cause is hemiplegia, in which the stronger muscle turns the head toward the side of weakness. The functional problem may develop into a static limitation if the neck is not periodically taken through full range of motion.

b. Management

If there is innervation and control of the weaker muscle, initiate strengthening exercises. Active or passive range of motion is done several times a day.

3. Hysterical torticollis

a. Causes

There may be many causes; sometimes it is described as the person turning away from an unpleasant situation.

b. Management

Physical therapy consists of resistive exercises to the opposite muscle and range of motion to maintain flexibility. Relaxation exercises may be helpful if the person tends to be tense. Close communication is maintained with the psychiatrist or psychologist working with the cause of the disorder.

B. Tension Headache

This usually involves tension in the posterior cervical muscles, pain at the attachment of the cervical extensors, and/or pain radiating across the top and side of the scalp.

1. Causes

Tension headaches may follow soft-tissue injury or may be caused by faulty or sustained postures, nerve irritation or impingement (the superior occipital nerve emerges through the neck extensor muscles where they attach at the base of the skull), or from sustained muscle contraction (from faulty posture or emotional tension) leading to ischemia. Medical causes include migraine, allergy, or sinusitis. Whatever the cause, there usually is a cycle of pain, muscle contraction, decreased circulation, and more pain, which leads to decreased function and potential soft-tissue dysfunction.

2. Management

a. Break into the cycle of pain and muscle tension using modalities, massage, and muscle-setting exercises to increase circulation to the part and carry off waste products.

b. Educate the patient in proper techniques to relieve the source or manage the irritation.

(1) If there is poor posture, teach posture correction and ways to manage posture.

(2) If the person is in tension-producing situations, teach relaxation techniques, range of motion and muscle-setting techniques, and proper spinal mechanics.

C. Thoracic Outlet Syndrome (TOS)[22,41]

1. Clinical picture

Symptoms of pain, paresthesia, numbness, weakness, discoloration, swelling, ulceration, gangrene, or in some cases, Raynaud's phenomenon may be experienced in the related upper extremity.

2. Causes

Symptoms are evoked as the blood vessels and nerves are compressed by structures in the thoracic outlet region.

a. The cervical nerve roots may be compressed in the foramina of the vertebrae. This is not a true TOS, but it causes neurologic signs in the upper extremity and should be considered in the testing procedures.

b. The proximal portion of the brachial plexus or the subclavian artery may be compressed as they course through the scalene muscles if the muscles are tight or hypertrophied or have anatomic variations.

c. The brachial plexus and subclavian artery and vein may be compressed against the first rib or a cervical rib as they course under the clavicle, particularly if the clavicle is in a depressed position, as when carrying a heavy shoulder bag or in an extreme posture. A fractured clavicle or anomolies in the region can also lead to symptoms.

d. The brachial plexus and axillary artery may be compressed against the ribs as they course under the pectoralis minor muscle if it is tight from faulty posture or if the person maintains an arm in a fully elevated position and the muscle is tight.

e. A brachial plexus stretch may occur as the plexus is pulled around the coracoid process when the arm is held in a fully elevated position.

3. Contributing factors

a. There is a wide latitude of motion in the various joints of the shoulder complex that may result in compression or impingement of the nerves or vessels.

b. Postural variations such as a forward head or round shoulders lead to associated muscle tightness in the scalene, levator, and pectoralis minor muscles.

c. Respiratory patterns that continually use the action of the scalene muscles to elevate the upper ribs lead to hypertrophy of these muscles.

d. Congenital factors such as an accessory rib or other anomaly in the region can reduce the space for the vessels. A traumatic or arteriosclerotic insult can also lead to TOS symptoms.

e. Traumatic injuries such as clavicular fracture or subacromial dislocations of the humeral head can injure the plexus and vessels, leading to TOS symptoms.

4. Management

a. If muscle, soft tissues, or joints are tight and restrict motion, use appropriate stretching techniques to the following structures
   (1) scalene muscles (see Figure 14-11)
   (2) levator scapulae muscle (see Figure 14-9)
   (3) pectoralis minor muscle (see Figure 14-8)
   (4) sternoclavicular joint (see Figure 5-22)

b. If there is a faulty forward head or round shoulder posture, increase the flexibility and strength in the related muscles, and train the proper postural muscles to function, emphasizing cervical and scapular kinesthetic training; see Chapter 14.

c. If there is faulty respiratory patterns (upper chest breathing), teach diaphragmatic breathing patterns and relaxation exercises in order to relax the upper thorax; see Chapter 19.

d. Find out what functional activities the patient does, and modify or eliminate the ones that provoke the symptoms. Functional activities frequently incriminated include carrying a heavy brief case or shoulder bag, a round shoulder and/or forward head posture, sleeping posture and pillow thickness, or faulty respiratory patterns. Tight and hypertrophied muscles in the thoracic outlet also decrease the space for the nerves and vessels.

D. Temporomandibular Joint Dysfunction (Syndrome)[19,20,37]

1. Clinical picture

Pain from a variety of sources is often cited as part of the temporomandibular joint (TMJ) syndrome.

a. Pain may occur locally in the TMJ, in the retrodiskal pad located in the posterior region of the joint, or in the ear

b. Pain from muscle spasm or myofascial pain in the massater, temporalis, or pterygoid internis or externis muscles may be described as a headache.

c. Tension in the muscles of the cervical spine may themselves be painful or cause referenced pain from irritation of the suboccipital nerve that may be described as a tension headache.

2. Causes

Imbalance occurs between the head, jaw, neck, and shoulder girdle. Causes may be

a. malocclusion, decreased vertical dimension of the bite, or other dental problems.

   b. faulty joint mechanics from inflammation, subluxation of the meniscus (disk), dislocation of the condylar head, joint contractures, or asymmetric forces from jaw and bite imbalances. Restricted motion results from periods of immobilization after reconstructive surgery or fracture of the jaw.
   c. muscle spasm in the muscles of mastication, causing abnormal or asymmetric joint forces. Muscle spasm can be the result of emotional tension, faulty joint mechanics, direct or indirect injury, or a postural dysfunction.
   d. sinus problems, resulting in the individual being a mouth breather, which indirectly affects posture and jaw position.
   e. postural dysfunctions (see Chapter 14 for related material). With a forward head posture, there is retraction of the mandible and resulting stretch on the anterior throat muscles. Consequently there is increased activity in the muscles that close the jaw to counter the changed forces. The muscles and soft tissue in the suboccipital region become tight, and the nerves and joints become compressed or irritated.
   f. trauma such as a flexion/extension accident in which the jaw forcefully opens when the head whips back into hyperextension. A direct blow from an auto accident, from boxing, from a fall or similar trauma, or sustained trauma, as occurs in prolonged dental surgery in which the mouth is held open for lengthy periods of time, may initiate symptoms in the TMJ or supporting tissue. Excessive stresses such as biting or chewing on large pieces of hard food may also traumatize the joints.

3. **Management**
   a. The approach to management will depend on the cause. In simple causes in which posture, joint dysfunction, or muscle imbalances are the source of the problem, physical therapy treatment can directly address the problems. In many cases, a dental referral, ear, nose, and throat referral, or psychologic support may be necessary to deal with primary causes. A complete evaluation is necessary prior to the initiation of any treatment.
   b. To decrease the pain and muscle guarding, use modalities, massage, and relaxation techniques.
   c. To correct muscle imbalances, relax and stretch tight postural muscles, then retrain for proper muscle control. Cervical and shoulder postural stretching and retraining exercises are described in Chapter 14.
   d. To teach control of the jaw muscles
      (1) first teach recognition of the resting position of the jaw. The lips are closed, teeth slightly apart and tongue resting lightly on the hard pallet behind the front teeth. The patient should breathe in and out slowly through the nose, using diaphragmatic breathing.
      (2) control opening and closing through the first half of the ROM of the jaw. With the tongue on the roof of the mouth, the patient opens his mouth, trying to keep the chin in midline. Use a mirror for visual reinforcement. The patient is also taught to lightly palpate the lateral poles of the condyle of the mandible bilaterally on himself and attempt to maintain symmetry between movement on the two sides when opening and closing his mouth.
      (3) if the jaw deviates while opening or closing, have the patient practice lateral deviation to the opposite side. The lateral motion should

not be excessive or cause pain.
  (4) progress to applying gentle resistance with the thumb against the chin. Do not overpower the muscles.
e. To increase range of motion if necessary
  (1) begin by placing layered tongue depressors between the central incisors. The patient can gradually work to increase the amount of tongue depressors used until he can open approximately far enough to insert the knuckles of his index and middle fingers.
  (2) placing cotton dental rolls between the back teeth while the patient bites will distract the condyle from the fossa in the joint.
  (3) joint mobilization techniques are done by using a gloved hand or hands. Determination of dosages and precautions for administration of mobilization techniques are described in Chapter 5.
    (a) Unilateral distraction (Figure 15-6A). The patient may be supine or sitting with his head supporting. Use the hand opposite the side you are working on. Place your thumb in the patient's mouth on the back molars; the fingers are outside and wrapped around the jaw. The force is in a downward (caudal) direction.
    (b) Unilateral distraction with glide (Figure 15-6B). After distracting the jaw as described in (a), pull it in a forward (anterior) direction. The other hand can be placed over the TMJ to palpate the amount of movement.
    (c) Bilateral distraction (Figure 15-7). If the patient is supine, stand at the head of the treatment table. If the patient is sitting, stand in front of the patient. Use both thumbs, placing them on the molars on each side of the mandible. The fingers are wrapped around the jaw. The force from the thumbs is equal, in a caudal direction.

V. SUMMARY

Information in this chapter was presented to help the reader to be able to design a therapeutic exercise program for common acute neck and back problems based on

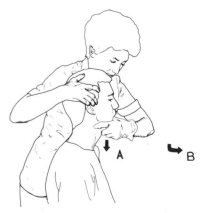

FIGURE 15-6. Unilateral mobilization of the temporomandibular joint: (*A*), distraction is in a caudal direction; (*B*) arrow indicating distraction with glide in a caudal then anterior direction.

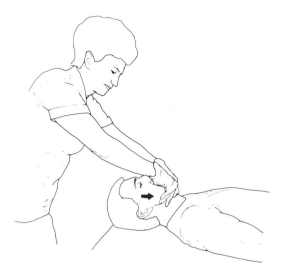

FIGURE 15-7. Bilateral distraction of the temporomandibular joint with the patient supine.

typical clinical pictures and necessary precautions. Included were intervertebral disk lesions, facet joint problems, muscle and soft-tissue lesions, and several specific problems including torticollis, tension headaches, and thoracic outlet syndrome and TMJ syndrome. Within the section on soft-tissue lesions, management techniques for muscle guarding and spasm were described. Progression of treatment was related to information presented in Chapter 14.

REFERENCES

1. Adams, MA and Hutton, WC: *Gradual disc prolapse.* Spine 10(6):524, 1985.
2. Adams, MA and Hutton, WC: *The effect of fatigue on the lumbar intervertebral disc.* J Bone Joint Surg 65B(2):199, 1983.
3. Anderson, B, Murphy, R, Ortengran, R, et al: *The influence of backrest inclination and lumbar support on lumbar lordosis.* Spine 4:52, 1979.
4. Bogduk, N and Engle, R: *The menisci of the lumbar zygapophyseal joints: A review of their anatomy and clinical significance.* Spine 9(5):454,1984.
5. Bogduk, N and Twomey, LT: *Clinical Anatomy of the Lumbar Spine.* Churchill-Livingstone, New York, 1987.
6. Burkart, S and Beresfore, W: *The aging intervertebral disk.* Phys Ther 59:969, 1979.
7. Cailliet, R: *Low Back Pain Syndrome,* ed 4. FA Davis, Philadelphia, 1988.
8. Cloward, R: *The clinical significance of the sino-vertebral nerve of the cervical spine in relation to the cervical disc syndrome.* J Neurol Surg Psychiatry 23:321, 1960.
9. Farfan, HF, et al: *The effects of torsion on the lumbar intervertebral joints: The role of torsion in the production of disc degeneration.* J Bone Joint Surg 52A(3):468, 1970.
10. Grieve, G: *Common Vertebral Joint Problems.* Churchill-Livingstone, New York, 1982.
11. Hickey, DS and Hukins, DEL: *Aging changes in the macromolecular organization of the intervertebral disc: An x-ray diffraction and electron microscopic study.* Spine 7(3):234, 1982.
12. Jensen, G: *Biomechanics of the lumbar intervertebral disc: A review.* Phys Ther 60:765, 1980.
13. Kellegren, J: *Observations on referred pain arising from muscle.* Clin Sci 3:175, 1983.
14. Kessler, R: *Acute symptomatic disk prolapse.* Phys Ther 59:978, 1979.
15. Klein, JA and Hukins, DWL: *Collagen fiber orientation in the annulus fibrosus of intervertebral disc during bending and torsion measured by x-ray defraction.* Biochim Biophys Acta 719:98, 1982.

16. Kopp, JR, et al: *The use of lumbar extension in the evaluation and treatment of patients with acute herniated nucleus pulposus.* Clin Orthop Rel Res 202:211, 1986.

17. Kos, J and Wolf, J: *Intervertebral menisci and their possible role in intervertebral blockage* (translated by Burkart, S). Bull Orthop Sports Med Sec 1(4):8, 1976.

18. Krag, MH, Seroussi, RE, Wilder, DG, and Pope, MH: *Internal displacement distribution from in vitro loading of human thoracic and lumbar spinal motion segments: Experimental results and theoretical predictions.* Spine 12:1001, 1987.

19. Kraus, SL: *TMJ Craniomandibular Cervical Complex: Physical Therapy and Dental Management.* Clinical Education Associates, Atlanta, 1986.

20. Kraus, SL: *Temporomandibular joint and dentistry.* Workshop notes, Detroit, 1987.

21. Lipson, SJ and Muir, H: *Proteoglycans in experimental intervertebral disc degeneration.* Spine 6(3):194, 1981.

22. Lord, J and Rosati, LM: *Thoracic outlet syndromes.* CIBA 23:1971.

23. Lyons, G, Eisenstein, SM, and Sweet, MBE: *Biochemical changes in intervertebral disc degeneration.* Biochim Biophys Acta 673:443, 1981.

24. MacNab, I: *Backache.* Williams & Wilkins, Baltimore, 1977.

25. Maitland, G: *Vertebral Manipulation,* ed 4. Butterworth, Boston, 1977.

26. Markolf, LK and Morris, JM: *The structural components of the intervertebral disc.* J Bone Joint Surg 56A(4):675, 1974.

27. McKenzie, R: *The Lumbar Spine: Mechanical Diagnosis and Therapy.* Spinal Publications, New Zealand, 1981.

28. McKenzie, R: *Manual Correction of Sciatic Scoliosis.* N Z Med J 89:22, 1979.

29. Mooney, V and Robertson, J: *The facet syndrome.* Clin Orthop 115:149, 1976.

30. Mooney, V: *The syndromes of low back disease.* Orthop Clin North Am 14(3):505, 1983.

31. Moneur, C and Williams, HJ: *Cervical spine management in patients with rheumatoid arthritis.* Phys Ther 68:509, 1988.

32. Nachemson, A: *The lumbar spine: An orthopaedic challenge.* Spine 1:59, 1976.

33. Ogata, K and Whiteside, LA: *Nutritional pathways of the intervertebral disc.* Spine 6(3):211, 1981.

34. Paris, S: *Spinal Dysfunction: Etiology and Treatment of Dysfunction Including Joint Manipulation.* Manual of Course Notes, Atlanta, 1979.

35. Penjabi, MM, Krag, MH, and Chung, TQ: *Effects of disc injury on mechanical behavior of the human spine.* Spine 9:707, 1984.

36. Porter, RW, Hibbert, C, and Evans, C: *The natural history of root entrapment syndrome.* Spine 9:418, 1984.

37. Rocobado, M: *Temporomandibular joint dysfunction.* Workshop notes, Columbus, 1982.

38. Saunders, JD: *Evaluation and Treatment of Musculoskeletal Disorders.* Minneapolis, 1982.

39. Saunders, JD: *Classification of musculoskeletal spinal conditions.* JOSPT 1:3, 1978.

40. Saunders, JD: *Lumbar traction.* JOSPT 1:36, 1978.

41. Smith, K: *The thoracic outlet syndrome: A protocol of treatment.* JOSPT 1:89, 1979.

42. Taylor, JR and Twomey, LT: *Age changes in lumbar zygapophyseal joints.* Spine 11(7):739, 1986.

43. Urban, L: *The straight-leg-raising test: A review.* JOSPT 2:117, 1981.

44. Waddell, G: *A new clinical model for the treatment of low back pain.* Spine 12:632, 1987.

45. Yasuma, T, Makino, E, Saito, S, and Inui, M: *Histological development of intervertebral disc herniation.* J Bone Joint Surg 68A(7):1066, 1986.

CHAPTER ——————— 16

The Spine: Traction Procedures

Traction is the "process of drawing or pulling."[20] When traction is used to draw or pull on the spinal column, it is called spinal traction. Traction is a therapeutic tool that falls in the realm of exercise because of its effects on the musculoskeletal system and use in stretching and mobilizing techniques.[11] Its mode of application is often through machines, although a therapist can apply traction to the joints of the spinal column through carefully applied manual and positional techniques. Its uses and applications are varied and subject to the patient's clinical response more than objective scientific argument for its success in decreasing symptoms.

Goals and plans of care for various posture and spinal problems are described in Chapters 14 and 15. In many instances, traction is a recommended procedure in the plan of care; therefore, the information in this chapter should be studied concurrently with the information in the previous two chapters for completeness.

OBJECTIVES

After studying this chapter, the reader will be able to:
1. identify the effects of spinal traction.
2. define the types of traction and how they are applied.
3. identify the indications, limitations, contraindications, and precautions for the use of spinal traction.
4. relate traction techniques for use within a total therapeutic exercise program.
5. describe safety rules and procedures for mechanical and manual traction techniques.
6. apply basic mechanical, positional, and manual traction techniques to the spine.

I. EFFECTS OF SPINAL TRACTION

    A. Mechanical Elongation of the Spine[8]—

Separation of the Vertebrae

1. **Mechanical separation of the vertebrae**[18]
   a. stretches the spinal muscles.
   b. tenses the ligaments and facet joint capsules.
   c. widens the intervertebral foramina.
   d. straightens the spinal curves.
   e. slides the facet joints.
   f. flattens a nuclear disk protrusion.[13]

2. **Factors that influence the amount of vertebral separation**
   a. **spinal position.**
      The greater the angle of flexion that the spine is placed in prior to the administration of traction, the greater the vertebral separation, especially the posterior aspect of the vertebral body.[4,17]
   b. **angle of pull.**
      The angle of pull of the traction force affects the amount of flexion of the spine.
      (1) In the cervical spine, the angle of pull creating the greatest posterior elongation is 35 degrees.[3]
      (2) In the lumbar spine, a harness that pulls from the posterior aspect of the pelvis rather than primarily from the sides is necessary to cause flexion of the spine.[18]
   c. **amount of force.**
      The effective force is influenced by the body position, weight of the part, friction of the treatment table, method of traction used, amount of patient relaxation, and the equipment itself. Generally, for vertebral separation:
      (1) In the cervical spine, under friction-free circumstances, a force of approximately 7 percent of the total body weight will separate the vertebrae.[5] A minimum force of 11.25 to 13.5 kg (25 to 30 pounds) is necessary to lift the weight of the head when sitting and to counteract the resistance of muscle tension. The greatest amount of separation occurs during the first few minutes of treatment at a given force.[8]
      (2) In the lumbar spine, a minimum friction-free force of half the body weight is necessary for mechanical separation.[5,10]
   d. **comfort and relaxation.**
      These are necessary for greatest benefit of vertebral separation.

B. Zygapophyseal (Facet) Joint Mobilization

1. **Effects of mobilization from various positions and forces on the spine**
   a. sliding or translation of the facet surfaces.
   b. distraction or a separation of the facet surfaces.
   c. compression or an approximation of the facet surfaces.

2. **Factors that influence the direction the facet surfaces move**
   a. **flexion of the spine.**
      Positioning the person in flexion causes a sliding of the articular surfaces between the facet joints. A longitudinal traction force reinforces the sliding effect and increases the amount of stretching that can be accomplished.

b. **side bending of the spine.**
Positioning the person in a side bending position causes a sliding force between the articular facets on the convex side of the curve. Adding a longitudinal traction force increases the amount of stretching that can be accomplished on the convex side.

c. **rotation of the spine.**
Positioning the person in rotation causes a distraction of the facets on the side toward which the body of the superior vertebra is rotating and compression on the opposite side.[16,18]

C. Muscle Relaxation

1. **With relaxation there will also be**
   a. decreased pain from muscle guarding or spasm.
   b. greater vertebral separation.

2. **Factors that influence the amount of relaxation include**
   a. **position of patient.**
   Subjectively, many patients report feeling more relaxed supine than sitting for cervical traction, and they have less tendency to deviate from the set position.[5,8] The patient needs to feel secure and well supported.[18]

   b. **spinal position.**
   Electrical activity in the upper trapezius muscle increases as the angle of application of cervical traction toward flexion increases; a lesser angle of pull results in greater relaxation.[6]

   c. **duration of application.**
   Both intermittent and continuous traction initially cause increased activity in the sacrospinalis muscles, but after 7 minutes, there is return of activity to near resting level.[9] In concluding a review of the literature, Harris states that 20 to 25 minutes of traction is necessary for muscle relaxation.[8]

   d. **force.**
   Muscle relaxation can be achieved at levels less than those needed for mechanical separation (4.5 to 6.75 kg or 10 to 15 pounds) in the cervical spine.[8]

D. Reduction of Pain

1. **Inhibition or reduction of pain may occur from**
   a. **mechanical effects.**
   (1) Movement of the region assists circulation and may help reduce stenosis from circulatory congestion, thus relieves pressure on dura, blood vessels, and nerve roots in the intervertebral foramina. Improving circulation may also help decrease the concentration of noxious chemical irritants.
   (2) Separation of the vertebrae temporarily increases the size of the intervertebral foramina, which decreases pressure on an impinged nerve root.
   (3) Tension on the facet joint capsule or distraction of the facet surfaces should release a meniscoid from an entrapment or extrapment.
   (4) Mechanical stretching of tight tissue should increase the mobility of

the segment, thus decreasing pain from restricted movement or strain on tight tissues.

b. **neurophysiologic effects.**
   (1) Stimulation of mechanoreceptors may block the transmission of nociceptive stimuli at the spinal cord or brainstem level.
   (2) Inhibition of reflex muscle guarding will decrease the discomfort from the contracting muscles.

2. **Factors that influence the amount of pain reduction include**

   a. **position of the patient.**
   The patient is positioned for comfort and ease of application of the desired technique.

   b. **spinal position.**
   (1) Acute stage: Usually the involved region of the spine is positioned so that the injured tissue is on a slack or in a pain-free position.
   (2) Subacute and chronic problems: Usually the spine is positioned with the involved segment, or the soft tissues related to the segment, on a stretch.

   c. **force and duration.**
   (1) Acute stage: With injury and inflammation, only low-intensity oscillations (no stretch) for a short period of time should be used.
   (2) Subacute and chronic stage: The amount of force and duration of treatment can be progressively increased, depending on the goal for treatment, type of traction, condition being treated, and tolerance of the patient.
   (3) If a meniscoid is blocking motion, a stretch force is necessary to release the meniscoid tissue.

II. DEFINITIONS AND DESCRIPTIONS OF TRACTION

A. Types of Application Defined

1. **Static or constant traction**

   A steady force is applied and maintained for an extended time interval.

   a. *Continuous or prolonged*
   A static traction in which the force is maintained for several hours to several days. Often it is applied in bed.
   (1) Only small amounts of weight can be tolerated.
   (2) It is ineffective in separating spinal structures and is primarily used for immobilization.

   b. *Sustained*
   A static traction in which the force is maintained from a few minutes up to one-half hour.
   (1) It is useful as a prolonged stretch to spinal structures.
   (2) Stronger poundage than that used for continuous traction can be tolerated.

2. **Intermittent**

   The force is alternately applied and released at frequent intervals, usually in a rhythmic pattern. Greater forces than that used for sustained traction can be tolerated by the patient.

B. Modes of Application

1. Mechanical

Various types of equipment are available for hospital, clinic, or home use. They usually have some form of objective indicator for measuring the amount of force applied.

2. Manual

Through positioning and handling, the therapist applies the traction force to the desired spinal segment. An objective measure of the amount of force cannot be made.

3. Positional

Through positioning, a sustained force on specific segments of the spinal column can be obtained. It may be asymmetric or symmetric.[16,18,19]

III. INDICATIONS FOR SPINAL TRACTION[18]

A. Spinal Nerve Root Impingement

1. From a herniated nucleus pulposus.

This condition requires enough traction force to cause vertebral body separation. The separation may have several effects on the bulging disk, including making the annular fibers and posterior longitudinal ligament taut, thus flattening the protrusion, or decreasing the intradiskal pressure, thus the pressure on the bulge.[13] Traction time must be short because the pressure soon equalizes and there will be increased pressure when the traction is released. To avoid the adverse effect from increased intradiskal pressure on release, the treatment times should be less than 10 minutes for sustained traction and less than 15 minutes for intermittent traction. Often in the acute phase, intermittent traction is not well tolerated. Progression depends on the patient's response. When the symptoms are less irritable, higher forces applied intermittently are tolerated.

2. From spinal or foraminal stenosis caused by ligament encroachment, spondylosis, edema, or spondylolisthesis.

Symptoms from these conditions can be temporarily relieved by applying enough force to separate the vertebrae and increase the size of the intervertebral foramina. If symptoms are highly irritable and large weights exacerbate the symptoms, gentle sustained traction may be tolerated initially (less than that required to separate the vertebrae for no more than 10 minutes). Progression depends on the patient's response. Change to intermittent traction when the patient's symptoms become predictable; greater forces can then be tolerated allowing for vertebral separation.

B. Hypomobility of the Joints from Dysfunction or Degenerative Changes

Whenever there is limited range of motion, spinal traction can be used to mobilize the joints, since the longitudinal force causes gliding of the facet surfaces. The primary disadvantage is that longitudinal spinal traction affects more than one joint, so it is a nonspecific form of stretching.

1. **To potentially localize the stretch force in the cervical spine**[11]
   a. put the cervical spine in neutral to affect the upper segments.

    b. put the cervical spine in flexion to affect the lower segments.

  2. **To potentially localize the stretch force in the lumbar spine**[1]

    a. put the lumbar spine in neutral to affect the lower segments.

    b. put the lumbar spine and knees into flexion to affect the upper segments and lower thoracic region.

  3. **To obtain unilateral effects**

    Position the spinal segment in a side bending position or side bending with slight rotation before the traction force is applied. Positional traction is also used for this purpose.

    a. For maximum distraction of the facets on one side of the neck, the neck is side bent opposite and then rotated toward the side to be affected.

    b. For maximum sliding of the facets on one side, the neck is side bent and rotated opposite the side to be affected.

    c. For maximum sliding and distraction of the lumbar spine, the trunk is side bent opposite and then rotated toward the side to be affected.

  4. **To achieve a stretch force**

    Vertebral separation must occur. Progress treatments depending on the patient's response.

  5. *Precaution:* Use caution with degenerating joints; too much movement may increase their irritability. If traction causes increased pain or decreased range of motion, either too much traction force was used or it is inappropriate to continue as a method of treatment. Traction should not be used when there are potential instabilities from ligamentous necrosis in rheumatoid arthritis[15] or conditions in which there has been prolonged use of steroids.

C. Joint Pain from Symptomatic Facet Joints

  1. **Acute stage**

    Small movements within the normal range of motion are believed to stimulate mechanoreceptors and block pain perception at the spinal level[7,21] as well as to help maintain normal fluid exchange.[7,14] Gentle forces of intermittent traction may relieve pain; the forces should not cause vertebral separation.

  2. **Chronic stage**

    Pain from hypomobility will require dosages that apply a stretch force to the limiting tissues. Patient tolerance will dictate whether to use higher dosages of intermittent or lower dosages of sustained or positional traction.

D. Muscle Spasm or Guarding

  1. If the cause of the spasm or guarding is protrusion of the nucleus pulposus or is related to a facet problem, the cause of the problem should be treated, not just the muscle spasm.

  2. With a soft-tissue injury or torn muscle, the injured area should be kept in a shortened position during the acute phase of healing then gradually lengthened as the scar becomes stable (see Chapter 6).

    a. Flexion of the spine places a stretch force on the posterior soft-tissue structures and muscles of the spine and increases the amount of muscle contraction;[6] therefore, flexion should be avoided during the acute stage of healing.

    b. The spine is placed in a pain-free position.

c. Usually a gentle intermittent traction is preferred following any acute injury when the extent of soft-tissue injury is not known.

d. If there is any exacerbation of symptoms, traction should not be given.

E. Meniscoid Blocking

A trapped meniscoid will block motion; frequently the patient is in a forward-bent position and cannot return to the upright position. Longitudinal traction will slide the facets and put tension on the joint capsule; positional traction will distract the joint surfaces as well as put tension on the joint capsule. Either one, applied at a high enough dosage to effect the desired facet motion, should release a trapped meniscoid.

F. Diskogenic Pain, Postcompression Fracture, and Other Conditions of the Spine

These conditions may respond to spinal traction. Begin with the spinal segment in a neutral or pain-free position. The symptoms should be monitored and adaptations made in the technique, depending on the patient's response.

IV. LIMITATIONS, CONTRAINDICATIONS, AND PRECAUTIONS

A. Limitations of Traction

1. The effect of vertebral separation is temporary, although the temporary relief may be enough to help break into a reflex pain cycle.

2. No consistent protocols exist; rationale is hypothetical with inconsistent clinical results.[8] Personal experience and the patient's response dictate method, force, duration, and frequency of treatment.[2]

3. The longitudinal traction force is nonspecific as to vertebral level. It affects the entire region.

B. Contraindications[18]

1. Any spinal condition or disease process in which movement is contraindicated.

2. Acute strains, sprains, and inflammation aggravated by initial traction treatments.

3. Stretch forces to areas of spinal hypermobility.

4. Increased pain or decreased range of motion.

5. Rheumatoid arthritis of the cervical spine, where there is potential necrosis of supporting ligaments that could cause instability and subluxation or dislocation of a vertebra with spinal cord damage.[15]

C. Precautions

1. Temporomandibular joint (TMJ) pain may be provoked with use of cervical halters, particularly when the chinstrap places a lot of force on the mandible. This occurs more often when the head is slightly flexed.[6] If pain increases in the TMJ, several alternatives are suggested:

   a. Use manual traction, thereby avoiding pressure under the mandible.

   b. Place cotton dental rolls between the back teeth; pressure under the chin from the traction strap will then cause a distraction of the TMJ.

   c. Use a cervical traction unit that does not require a chinstrap. Fixation comes from a strap secured across the patient's forehead and distraction from a pad under the occiput.

2. Patients wearing dentures should not remove them, because the TMJ is forced into an abnormal resting position and can be traumatized with pressure from the chinstrap.
3. Osteoporosis
4. Patients with respiratory problems or those who develop claustrophobia when placed in the traction apparatus

V. GENERAL PROCEDURES

A. Determine Appropriateness for Choice of Traction by Testing with Manual Traction First
(SEE SECTIONS VI AND VII FOR TECHNIQUES).
1. If the test traction relieves or reduces the symptoms, an initial treatment is given.
2. Conversely, if the test traction aggravates the symptoms, traction treatments should probably not be applied.
3. When evaluating, apply the traction force in various positions of flexion, extension, side bending, and rotation to find which position best reduces or relieves the symptoms. Use that position, if possible, for the initial treatment.
4. Re-evaluate the patient immediately afterward as well as the next day to determine whether traction should be modified or continued.

B. Determine if Manual, Positional, or Mechanical Traction Will Be Used

C. Position the Patient for Maximum Comfort and Relaxation
If using mechanical traction, secure the harnesses or halter to the patient and then attach it to the machine. Check to see that the rope pull is at the appropriate angle.

D. Determine Dosage and Duration
Refer to Section III for guidelines based on the patient's problem. To avoid treatment soreness:
1. The *dosage* chosen for the *initial treatment* should be less than that which would cause vertebral separation. Progression of poundage should be determined by the patient's response and the problem being treated.
2. The *duration* will depend on the type of traction (intermittent or sustained), the poundage used, the clinical condition of the patient, and the goals of the treatment.

E. Safety Rules for Mechanical Traction
1. Use only cables and ropes that are in good repair.
2. Secure the equipment so it will not move when the traction force is applied.
3. Check to see that the poundage dial is turned down to zero before setting up the patient or turning on the machine.
4. Periodically check the poundage calibration.
5. Use disposable tissue or gauze wherever the halters touch the patient's face, mouth, or hair. Disposable halters are available but are not easily adjusted to all patients.

6. Never leave the patient unattended while receiving traction unless he has some mechanism for deactivating the unit and some means to signal for assistance.

VI. CERVICAL TRACTION TECHNIQUES

A. Manual Traction

1. Position of patient: Supine on the treatment table. The patient should be as relaxed as possible.
2. Position of therapist: Standing at the head of the treatment table, supporting the weight of the patient's head in her hands. Hand placement depends on comfort. Suggestions include
   a. place the fingers of both hands under the occiput (Figure 16-1A).
   b. place one hand over the frontal region and the other hand under the occiput (Figure 16-1B).
   c. place the index fingers around the spinous process above the vertebral level to be moved. This hand placement provides a specific traction only to the vertebral segments below the level where the fingers are placed. A belt around the therapist's hips can be used to reinforce the fingers and increase the ease of applying the traction force (Figure 16-1C).
3. When manual traction is used for evaluation, vary the patient's head position in flexion, extension, side bending, and side bending with rotation and apply a traction force in each position; note the patient's response.
4. When administering treatment, use the position that most effectively reduces or relieves the symptoms.
5. The therapist applies the force by fixing her arms isometrically, assuming a stable stance, and then leaning backwards in a controlled manner. If a

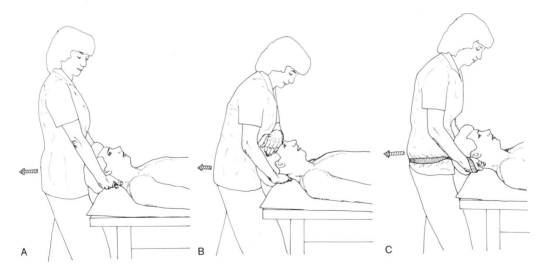

FIGURE 16-1. Manual cervical traction; (A) with the fingers of both hands under the occiput, (B) with one hand over the frontal region and the other hand under the occiput, and (C) using a belt to reinforce the hands for the traction force.

belt is used, the force is transmitted through the belt. If just the arm muscles are used to apply the force, the therapist tires quickly.

6. The force is usually applied intermittently, with a smooth and gradual building and releasing of the traction force. The intensity and duration are usually limited by the therapist's strength and endurance.

7. Value of manual traction
   a. The angle of pull and head position can be controlled by the therapist.
   b. By placing the index fingers around specific spinous processes, the level of traction can be controlled to some degree.
   c. No stress is placed on the temporomandibular joint as is frequently done with mechanical traction.

B. Positional Traction

1. Position of patient: Supine on the treatment table.
2. Position of therapist: Standing at the head of the treatment table, supporting the patient's head in her hands. Determine the segment to receive the majority of traction force and palpate the spinous process at that level.
3. Procedure:[16] Flex the head until motion of the spinous process just begins at the determined level. Support the head with folded towels at that level of flexion. Then side bend the head away from the side to be distracted until movement of the spinous process is felt at the desired level. Finally, rotate the head a few degrees toward the side to be distracted. Adjust the towel support to maintain this position for a low-intensity, sustained traction stretch to that facet joint and surrounding soft tissue.
4. Value of positional traction: The primary traction force can be isolated to a specific facet. This may be beneficial when selective stretching is necessary, as when the segment above or on the contralateral side is hypermobile and should not be stretched.

C. Mechanical Traction

1. Become familiar with the unit available by reviewing the manufacturer's directions. Learn the capabilities, limitations, and adjustments possible for the equipment.
2. Position the patient for comfort
   a. Sitting
      (1) This position uses less clinical space but requires more force to overcome muscle tension and accomplish separation of the vertebrae than the supine position.[5]
      (2) Use a comfortable chair with arm rests, or place a pillow on the patient's lap for the arms to rest on.
      (3) The height of the chair should support the thighs and allow the feet to rest comfortably on the floor or on a foot stool.
   b. Supine (Figure 16-2)
      (1) This position requires less force to overcome muscle tension than sitting.
      (2) This position tends to reduce the lordotic curve due to the force of gravity on the vertebrae.[5]
      (3) Support the patient with pillows for maximum comfort.
      (4) Depending on the angle of pull, friction of the head on the surface of the treatment table must be considered.
   c. Semi-reclining
      (1) Use of a reclining chair or tilt table provides alternate positions to

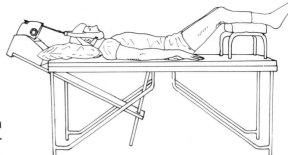

FIGURE 16-2. Mechanical traction to the cervical spine, with the patient supine.

sitting or lying supine.
(2) Gravity may or may not have an influence, depending on angle of pull.
3. Head position for the patient is determined by the evaluation as well as the condition being treated
   a. To obtain separation of the vertebrae, the head should be positioned in flexion up to 35 degrees; the greater the angle of neck flexion, the greater is the posterior elongation.[3]
   b. To obtain greater muscle relaxation, position the head closer to neutral.[6]
   c. To obtain unilateral effects, position the head in a side-bent position, or in a position of side bending with slight rotation (as described in the positional traction section) before the traction force is applied. Secure the patient's thorax with a strap so he does not realign himself with the pull of the rope.
4. Apply the head halter
   a. First, line the head halter with gauze or tissue.
   b. Adjust the halter to fit the patient comfortably. The major traction force must be against the occiput, not the chin, in order to minimize compression of the temporomandibular joint. Gauze may be placed between the teeth or padding under the chin to help absorb pressure.
   c. Do not remove dentures if the patient wears them or stress may be placed on the temporomandibular joints.
   d. Eye glasses should be safely set aside.
5. Attach the halter to the spreader bar of the traction unit; check that the patient is aligned for proper pull.
6. Set controls
   a. The poundage dial should be set at zero before activating the unit.
   b. If the unit has off-on timers for intermittent traction, these should be set for the desired time intervals.
      (1) Only 7 seconds is needed for maximum separation at any one cycle, but such frequency tends to be irritating.
      (2) Suggested starting intervals are 30 seconds on, 30 seconds off; or 1 minute on, 30 seconds off.
7. Activate the unit and gradually increase the force of traction.
   a. To avoid treatment soreness, the first treatment should not exceed 10 to 15 pounds.

      b. Progression of dosage at succeeding treatments will depend on the goals and the patient's reaction.

   8. Duration of treatment may be from 10 to 30 minutes for sustained or intermittent traction, depending on the patient's condition and goals for treatment.

   9. Demonstrate to the patient how to turn the unit off if his symptoms get worse.

  10. At the completion of treatment, turn all controls off and turn dial indicators back to zero. Remove the halter from the spreader bar, then remove the head halter.

  11. Re-evaluate the patient's condition. Be sure he does not feel dizzy or nauseated before leaving the treatment area.

  12. If the patient complains of headache, nausea, fainting, or increased symptoms during or following treatment, reduce the weight or length of treatment time at the next visit, or discontinue treatments if the condition warrants.

D. Home Traction—Mechanical

1. Have the patient practice the traction set up under your supervision. Be sure he understands:
   a. what position and neck posture to use
      (1) With an over-the-door pulley system, sit facing the weight if the flexed position is to be used.
      (2) Sit facing away from the weight if the neutral or extended position is to be used. For the neutral position, the head should be directly under the pulley; for extension, the chair is moved forward.
      (3) If a supine position is desired, the head is usually positioned in flexion with the cervical halter attached to the pulley system; the weight of the body provides the counter force.
   b. how to get comfortable
   c. how to apply and release the weights safely
2. Weight application varies.
   The most common method is with a weight pan or bag on a pulley system (Figure 16-3). If the patient uses weights, have them on a chair or table next to him. Have him practice applying the weights so it is done smoothly and safely.
3. Sustained traction (up to 30 minutes) using small amounts of weight (10 pounds) is easiest to apply. Intermittent traction requires that the patient lift the weight to take the force off the neck at frequent intervals. Assess both techniques to determine which one provides greater relaxation and relief of symptoms.

E. Self-Traction

1. The patient is sitting or lying down. He is taught to place his hands behind his neck with the fingers interlocking; the ulnar border of his fingers and hands are under the occiput and mastoid processes. He then gives a lifting motion to his head. The head may be placed in flexion, extension, side bending, or rotation for more isolated effects. He may apply the traction intermittently or in a sustained manner.
2. Positional traction can also be used for self-traction. The patient learns to assume the position determined by the therapist as described in Section VI B.

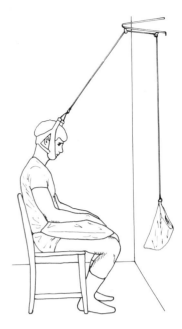

FIGURE 16-3. Home traction for the cervical spine using a bag of weights on a pulley system for the traction force with the patient positioned in flexion. For the neutral or extended position, the patient should sit under the pulley and face away from the weight.

VII. LUMBAR TRACTION TECHNIQUES

A. Manual Traction

1. Manual traction in the lumbar region is not as easily applied as in the cervical region because at least half the body weight must be moved and the coefficient of friction of the part to be moved must be overcome.
2. Position of patient: Supine on a treatment table.
3. Position of therapist: Varies with the position of the patient's hips and lower extremities.
   a. With the lower extremities extended and the lumbar spine in extension, the therapist can exert a pull at the ankles.
   b. With the hips flexed to 90 degrees and the lumbar spine in flexion, the patient's legs are draped over the therapist's shoulders. The therapist then exerts the force with her arms wrapped across the patient's thighs.
4. When manual traction is used for evaluation, vary the amount of flexion, extension, or side bending and note the patient's response.
5. During treatment, use the spinal position that best reduces the patient's symptoms.
6. The therapist must use her entire body weight to effect any traction force. Place the patient on a split traction table to minimize the resistance from friction. When applying a high-dosage traction force, the thorax is stabilized. Put a countertraction harness around the patient's rib cage and secure it to the head end of the table, or have a second person stabilize the patient by standing at the head end of the table and holding onto the patient's arms.

B. Positional Traction[16,18]

1. Position of patient: Side-lying, with the side to be treated uppermost. A rolled blanket is placed under the spine at the level where the traction force is desired; this causes side bending away from the side to be treated and therefore an upward gliding of the facets (Figure 16-4A).
2. Position of therapist: Standing at the side of the treatment table facing the patient. Determine the segment to receive the majority of the traction force, and palpate the spinous processes at that level and the level above.
3. Procedure:[16] The patient relaxes in the side-bent position. Rotation is added to isolate a distraction force to the desired level. Rotate the upper trunk by gently pulling on the arm the patient is lying on while at the same time palpating the spinous processes with your other hand to determine when rotation has arrived at the level just above the joint to be distracted. Then flex the patient's uppermost thigh, again palpating the spinous processes until flexion of the lower portion of the spine occurs at the desired level. The segment where these two opposing forces meet now has a maximum positional distraction force (Figure 16-4B).
4. Value of positional traction: The primary traction force can be directed to the side on which symptoms occur or can be isolated to a specific facet and is therefore beneficial for selective stretching.

C. Mechanical Traction (Figure 16-5)

1. Become familiar with the unit available by reviewing the manufacturer's operating instructions. The most effective traction is applied via a split-traction table, thus eliminating the need to overcome the coefficient of friction of half the patient's body weight.
2. Apply the traction and countertraction harnesses
   a. Saunders recommends a heavy duty traction harness made with a vinyl material that is attached directly to the patient's skin to avoid slippage.[18]
   b. The traction harness is applied over the pelvis so that the upper portion is secured above the crest of the ilium.

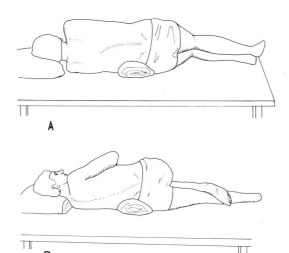

A

B

FIGURE 16-4. Positional traction for the lumbar spine; (A) side bending over a 6-8 inch roll causes a longitudinal traction to the segments on the upward side; (B) side bending with rotation adds a distraction force to the facets on the upward side.

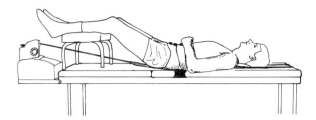

FIGURE 16-5. Mechanical traction to the lumbar spine in flexion using a split traction table with the patient supine.

    c. The countertraction harness is used to keep the patient from slipping. It is attached around the lower rib cage.
3. Position the patient either supine or prone.
    a. The thorax should be on the stationary part of the table and the pelvis on the movable part (the movable part is kept locked until ready to activate the unit) so that the lumbar spine is positioned over the split in the table.
    b. Whether the spine is in flexion, extension, or side bending is determined by the evaluation and the patient's comfort and condition as well as the goals of the treatment.
    c. To obtain posterior separation of the vertebrae, the lumbar spine should be flexed (flattened).
       (1) When supine, the hips are flexed and the thighs rest on a padded stool.
       (2) When prone, several pillows are placed under the patient's abdomen.
4. Attach the anchor straps
    a. The countertraction or stabilizing harness is secured to the head end of the traction table.
    b. The straps from the traction harness may attach to a spreader bar, which is attached to a traction rope.
    c. If unilateral traction is to be applied, attach only one anchor strap from the pelvic harness directly to the traction rope.[19]
    d. Check that the patient is aligned for proper pull, then take all the slack out of the straps.
5. Set the controls
    a. Be familiar with the type of unit. Computer models may have options such as a progressive phase that will gradually increase the traction force at programmed intervals. Other units should be set at zero before activating the unit.
    b. If the unit has off-on timers for intermittent traction, set them for the desired time intervals.
    c. Set the duration of treatment. Duration may be up to 30 minutes for most mechanical units. The duration depends on the goals and the patient's condition and reaction to the traction.
6. Unlock the split traction table so it will separate when the unit is activated.
7. Activate the unit and gradually increase the force (if the unit has not been preprogrammed to do so automatically).
    a. To avoid treatment soreness, the first treatment should not exceed half the patient's weight.

      b. Progression of dosage at succeeding treatments will depend on goals and the patient's reaction.

8. Demonstrate to the patient how to turn the unit off if his symptoms worsen while the unit is on. Make sure he has a signaling device to call for help if necessary.

9. At the completion of the treatment
    a. Turn all controls off and turn indicators back to zero.
    b. Lock the split on the table before the patient attempts to get off.
    c. Re-evaluate the patient; note any change in symptoms or range of motion.

D. Home Traction—Mechanical

1. A number of home traction units are available on the market. Choose one that best meets the goals for the patient. Set-up and instructions are specific to the design of each unit. Have the patient practice the traction set-up under your supervision. Be sure he understands:
    a. position.
    b. how to get comfortable.
    c. how to apply and release the traction force safely.

2. Since most of the home units use body weight and position within a pulley system for the distraction force, sustained traction is most easily used. Determine a safe duration for the patient compatible with the goals for treatment.

E. Self-Traction—Manual

1. To separate the posterior segment of the lumbar spine, the patient is positioned supine. He then draws both his knees up to his chest and holds them (grasping around the thighs). This can be done intermittently by releasing the hold and bringing the legs part way down, then pulling them back up again (see Figure 14-13).

    Precaution: Flexing the spine in this manner increases the intradiskal pressure; therefore, this technique should not be used to treat symptoms of an acute disk protrusion.

2. Positional traction can be used for self-traction. The patient learns to assume the position determined by the therapist as described in Section VII B (see Figure 16-4).

VIII. SUMMARY

The basic concepts, indications, contraindications, and precautions of spinal traction were described in this chapter, followed by procedural guidelines and techniques for applying cervical and lumbar traction with manual, positional, or mechanical techniques. Because spinal traction is just one technique for managing spinal and back problems, it was suggested that this material be studied concurrently with the material in Chapters 14 and 15.

REFERENCES

1. Broden, J: *Manuell Medicin och Manipulation.* Lakartidningen 63:1037, 1966. (As reported by Saunders, HD: *Lumbar traction.* JOSPT 1:36, 1979.)
2. Cailliet, R: *Neck and Arm Pain,* ed 2. FA Davis, Philadelphia, 1981.
3. Colachis, S and Strohm, B: *A study of tractive forces and angle of pull on vertebral interspaces in the cervical spine.* Arch Phys Med Rehabil 46:220, 1965.

4. Colachis, S and Strohm, B: *Effects of intermittent traction on separation of lumbar vertebrae.* Arch Phys Med Rehabil 50:251, 1969.
5. Deets, D, Hands, K, and Hopp, S: *Cervical traction: A comparison of sitting and supine positions.* Phys Ther 57:255, 1977.
6. DeLacerda, F: *Effect of angle of traction pull on upper trapezius muscle activity.* JOSPT 1:205, 1980.
7. Grieve, G: *Manual mobilizing techniques in degenerative arthrosis of the hip.* Bull Orthop Sec APTA 2/1:7, 1977.
8. Harris, P: *Cervical traction: Review of literature and treatment guidelines.* Phys Ther 57:910, 1977.
9. Hood, C, Hart, D, et al: *Comparison of electromyographic activity in normal lumbar sacrospinalis musculature during continuous and intermittent pelvic traction.* JOSPT 2:137, 1981.
10. Judovich, B: *Lumbar traction therapy.* JAMA 159:549, 1955.
11. Maitland, GD: *Vertebral Manipulation,* ed 5. Butterworth & Co, London, 1986.
12. Mathews, J: *Dynamic discography: A study of lumbar traction.* Ann Phys Med 9:275, 1968.
13. Mathews, J: *The effects of spinal traction.* Physiotherapy 58:64, 1972.
14. McDonough, A.: *Effect of immobilization and exercise on articular cartilage: A review of literature.* JOSPT 3:2, 1981.
15. Moneur, C and Wiliams, HF: *Cervical spine management in patients with rheumatoid arthritis.* Phys Ther 68:509, 1988.
16. Parris, S: *Spinal Dysfunction: Etiology and Treatment of Dysfunction Including Joint Manipulation.* Manual of Course Notes, Atlanta, 1979.
17. Reilly, J, Gersten, J, and Clinkingbeard, J: *Effect of pelvic-femoral position on vertebral separation produced by lumbar traction.* Phys Ther 59:282, 1979.
18. Saunders, H: *Lumbar traction.* JOSPT 1:36, 1979.
19. Saunders, H: *Unilateral lumbar traction.* Phys Ther 61:221, 1981.
20. *Taber's Cyclopedic Medical Dictionary,* ed 16. FA Davis, Philadelphia, 1989.
21. Wyke, B: *Neurological aspects of pain for the physical therapy clinician.* PT Forum '82, Columbus, 1982.

CHAPTER ——————— 17

Scoliosis

Scoliosis is a general term used to describe any lateral curvature of the spine. The etiology, severity, age of onset, and progression of the deformity vary.[13,28,33,41] This deformity, which most often develops in childhood, can lead to structural abnormalities of the pelvis, vertebrae, and thoracic cage. The curvature may occur in the cervical, thoracic, or lumbar regions of the spine.

Scoliosis, if undetected and untreated during the growth years, can lead to severe deformity, drastically affecting appearance and possibly shortening life expectancy. The key to preventing severe curvatures of the spine is early identification and early treatment.

This chapter provides background and descriptions of scoliosis for those therapists involved with either screening and early detection of scoliosis or the treatment of a child with scoliosis. An overview of nonoperative and operative treatment is discusssed, with an emphasis on how therapeutic exercise enters into the overall plan of care for the child with scoliosis.

OBJECTIVES

After studying this chapter, the reader will be able to:
1. define terminology related to scoliosis.
2. explain the possible causative factors that lead to the development of scoliosis.
3. describe the major components of evaluation and screening for scoliosis.
4. explain the goals of nonoperative and operative treatment of scoliosis.
5. describe the most common and successful nonoperative and operative methods of treatment of scoliosis.
6. discuss the appropriate use of therapeutic exercise in the treatment of scoliosis.
7. describe specific exercises that are used in conjunction with other methods of treatment of scoliosis.

I.   DEFINITIONS RELATED TO SCOLIOSIS

A. Structural and Nonstructural Scoliosis

1. Structural scoliosis[13,28,33,41]

a. An irreversible lateral curvature of the spine with fixed rotation of the vertebrae (Figure 17-1A)

    (1) The vertebral bodies rotate toward the convex side of the curve, and the spinous processes rotate away from the convex side of the curve.

    (2) The greatest rotation of the vertebrae occurs at the apex of the curve.

    (3) As the curve increases, the amount of rotation increases.

b. Forward bending of the trunk produces a posterior rib hump in the thoracic region on the convex side of the curve because of the rotation of the vertebrae and rib cage (Figure 17-1B).

    (1) Compression of the ribs occurs on the concave side of the curve, and separation of the ribs occurs on the convex side.

    (2) The net result, which is accentuated with forward bending, is prominence of the ribs and scapula posteriorly on the convex side of the curve.

c. Prominence of the rib cage can also be noted along the anterior aspect of the chest on the concave side of the curve.

d. Associated structural changes in the spine may include[23]

    (1) lateral displacement of the nucleus pulposus in the intervertebral disk space.

    (2) eventual wedging of the vertebral body on the concave side of the curve because of pressure on epiphyseal plates, particularly in curves of 25 degrees or greater.

e. Structural scoliosis cannot be corrected by positioning or voluntary effort.

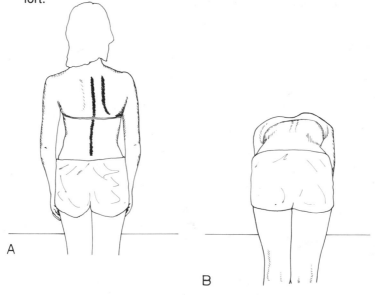

FIGURE 17-1. (*A*), Mild right thoracic left lumbar structural scoliosis with prominence of the right scapula. (*B*), Forward bending produces a slight right posterior rib hump, indicating fixed rotation of the vertebrae and rib cage.

2. Nonstructural (functional) scoliosis

a. A reversible lateral curve of the spine that tends to be positional or dynamic in nature[13,23,41]

b. There are no structural or rotational changes in the alignment of the vertebrae.

c. Correction of the lateral curve is possible by
(1) forward or side bending.
(2) positional changes and alignment of the pelvis or spine.
(3) muscle contraction.

d. The curve also disappears when the patient is supine or prone.

e. This type of curve is also called a *postural scoliosis.*[28]

B. Descriptions of Curves

1. The direction of the curve is always identified by the convexity.

For example, if a patient has a right thoracic scoliosis, the convexity of the curve will be on the patient's right and the concavity of the curve on the patient's left.

2. The major curve is the most significant curve of the scoliotic deformity.[41]

a. The major curve usually occurs in the thoracic region and has structural changes in the vertebrae.

b. The term major curve is used by the Scoliosis Research Society of North America and is preferable to the term primary curve.[41]

c. The major curve in idiopathic scoliosis is usually a right thoracic curve occurring between T-4 and T-12.

3. Compensatory curve[28,35,41]

a. A minor, compensatory curve that is less severe may develop in the opposite direction above and/or below a major curve.

b. The compensatory curve may be nonstructural or structural.

c. This compensatory curve produces a *compensated* scoliosis in which the shoulders are level and positioned directly over the pelvis.

d. If the sum of degrees of the compensatory curve(s) does not equal the degrees of deformity of the major curve, the scoliosis is said to be *decompensated.*
(1) The shoulders are not level.
(2) There is a lateral shift of the trunk (a list) to one side.

4. Double major curve[13,41]

a. If two major curves develop of equal severity and significance, a double major curve is said to be present.

b. Both curves of a double major curve are usually structural.

5. Transitional vertebra

This is the neutral vertebra at each end of the curve that makes the transition from one curve to another.

6. Apex of the curve

The apex is identified by the vertebra that is the greatest distance from the midline of the spine. It is referred to as the apical vertebra.

C. Sites and Shapes of Curves[6,13,28,41]

Note: The site and shape of the scoliosis are important factors to include when considering prognosis and treatment.

1. Sites of the curve

A lateral curvature of the spine may develop in the cervical, thoracic, lumbar, or multiple areas of the spine.

2. Shapes of curves

a. Long C-Curve
  (1) Usually extends the length of the thoracic and lumbar spine.
  (2) Is often uncompensated, leading to a high shoulder on the convex side of the curve and high pelvis on the concave side.
  (3) May be due to long-term asymmetric positioning, muscle weakness, or inadequate control of sitting balance.

b. S-Curve
  (1) The most common type of curve seen in idiopathic scoliosis; it is usually a right thoracic, left lumbar curve.
  (2) Involves a major curve and compensatory curve(s).
  (3) Usually is associated with structural changes in the vertebrae of the major curve.

D. Severity of Scoliosis[13,42]

1. The severity of scoliosis is determined by the angle of the curvature and rotation of the spine.

a. The more severe the lateral curvature, the greater the rotation of the vertebrae.

b. The more severe the curve, the greater the impact and secondary changes in the cardiopulmonary systems.[5,24,30,32,37] These changes include
  (1) decreased vital capacity and total lung capacity.
  (2) hypertrophy of the right ventricle and atrium from pulmonary hypertension.

2. Measurement techniques

a. X-ray measurements of the lateral curvature of the spine[13,24,28,41]
  (1) There are two accepted forms of measurement—the Cobb method and the Risser-Ferguson method.
  (2) The Cobb method has been found to be more reliable and is recommended by the Scoliosis Research Society of North America[13,33] (Figure 17-2).

b. Measurement of the rotational deformity[13,24,28,41]
  (1) Position of the pedicles is noted on a posterior-anterior x-ray.
    (a) Normally, the pedicles are symmetrically positioned on either side of each spinous process.
    (b) In scoliosis, the pedicles and spinous process of each vertebra are asymmetrically positioned toward the side of the concavity.
  (2) The degree of rotation of the pedicles is noted on x-ray by a 0 to +4 grading system.
    (a) 0 indicates no vertebral rotation.
    (b) Grade I (+) and Grade II (+ +) indicate minimal rotation.

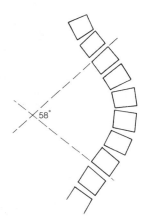

FIGURE 17-2. The Cobb method of measurement of scoliosis. A line is drawn perpendicular to the upper margin of the vertebra that inclines most toward the concavity. A line is also drawn on the inferior border of the lower vertebra with greatest angulation toward the concavity. The angle of these transecting lines is noted and recorded. (From Cailliet, R: Scoliosis. FA Davis, Philadelphia, 1975, with permission.)

         (c) Grade III (+ + +) when both pedicles are still visible indicates significant rotation in which only one pedicle is visible.
         (d) In a Grade IV (+ + + +) rotation, the one visible pedicle is rotated beyond the midline of the body.

3. Classification of severity of the curvature[41,42]
   a. Mild scoliosis
     (1) Curves of less than 20 degrees.
     (2) Curves of less than 10 degrees are considered by some to be within the limits of normal in the general population and do not warrant treatment.[41]
   b. Moderate scoliosis
     (1) Curves from 20 to 40 or 50 degrees.
     (2) Moderate scoliosis is associated with early structural changes in the vertebrae and rib cage.
   c. Severe scoliosis
     (1) Curves of 40 to 50 degrees or greater.
     (2) Severe scoliosis involves significant rotational deformity of the vertebrae and ribs.
     (3) In adults, curves of 40 degrees or greater are associated with pain and degenerative joint disease (DJD) of the spine.
     (4) Curves of 60 to 70 degrees or greater are associated with significant cardiopulmonary changes and decreased life expectancy.[30,32]

II. CLASSIFICATION OF SCOLIOSIS BY ETIOLOGY[15,16,23–26,28,35,40]

A. Etiology of Structural Scoliosis

1. Idiopathic
   a. About 75 to 85 percent of all scoliosis develops without any known cause in otherwise normal, healthy children and progresses with skeletal growth.
   b. Age of onset
     (1) Adolescent scoliosis is the most common type of idiopathic scolio-

sis and develops most often in young girls from age 10 to the end of skeletal growth (about 15 or 16).
  (2) Juvenile scoliosis occurs between ages 4 and 9 and is seen more often in girls than boys.
  (3) Infantile scoliosis develops from birth to age 3 and occurs more often in boys than girls.
  c. Theories of causes of idiopathic scoliosis
    (1) Possible bone malformation during development.[35]
    (2) Asymmetric muscle weakness.[36,45]
    (3) Abnormal postural control because of possible dysfunction of the vestibular or proprioceptive system.[16,24,29]
    (4) Abnormal distribution of muscle spindles in paraspinal musculature.[25,26]
    (5) *Note:* To date there is no known specific cause of idiopathic scoliosis. Muscle weakness, proprioceptive dysfunction, and abnormal muscle spindle distribution have all been found in patients with adolescent idiopathic scoliosis. It has not been determined whether these findings may be the *cause* or the *result* of idiopathic scoliosis.[16,25,26]

2. **Neuromuscular**
  a. About 15 to 20 percent of structural scoliosis occurs as the result of congenital or acquired neuropathic or myopathic diseases or disorders.
  b. Neuropathic causes
    (1) Congenital
       Cerebral palsy, myelomeningocele, neurofibromatosis
    (2) Acquired
       Anterior horn cell disease, traumatic paraplegia
  c. Myopathic causes
    (1) Congenital
       Amyotonia congenita, arthrogryposis
    (2) Acquired
       Muscular dystrophy

3. **Osteopathic**
  a. Congenital
     Secondary to hemivertebra (a failure of one half of the vertebra to form).
  b. Acquired
     Osteomalacia, rickets, fracture, and dislocation of the spine.

B. Etiology of Nonstructural Scoliosis
  1. **Leg length discrepancy**
    a. True
       Actual difference in bony length.
    b. Apparent
       Measurable difference because of a dislocated hip, asymmetric leg or foot postures, or rotated innominate.
    c. Congenital or acquired deformities can cause asymmetric variations that lead to pelvic obliquity (high pelvis on one side) and a compensatory lateral curvature of the spine.

2. Spasm in back muscles
a. Splinting of the back muscles may occur in response to injury of any tissue in the back.
b. Sciatic scoliosis often accompanies a posterolateral disk protrusion in the lumbar spine. The deviation (lateral shifting of the thorax) usually occurs away from the painful side.

3. Habitual asymmetric postures
a. Sitting with weight shifted onto one hip or standing with weight primarily supported on one leg results in asymmetric flexibility and tightness in soft tissue of the trunk and hips.
b. In children, continued asymmetric postures may affect remodeling of bone and adaptation of soft tissue.

III. EVALUATION OF SCOLIOSIS

Early recognition and diagnosis of scoliosis ideally leads to early treatment of this progressive spinal deformity. Since idiopathic scoliosis accounts for the greatest incidence of curvature of the spine in adolescents, an increasing emphasis on early identification has occurred. School screening programs have become more common in recent years. It is important to periodically examine a child for the presence of scoliosis, particularly during growth spurts. If a lateral curvature is noted, the child should be referred to an orthopedist for diagnosis and early treatment.

A. Evaluation Procedures
1. Postural assessment
a. Anterior, posterior, and lateral postural assessments are done with the child standing.
b. A plumb line is used to note any deviations in alignment.
c. In scoliosis, the following deviations are often noted:
   (1) Asymmetric shoulder level
   (2) Prominence of the scapula on the side of the convexity
   (3) Protrusion of the hip on one side
   (4) Pelvic obliquity
   (5) Increased lumbar lordosis

2. Flexibility of the curve
If a lateral curvature is noted, the following tests should be done to detect any early structural changes.
a. Lateral Bending Test[24,30]
   (1) This test is done to determine whether the curve corrects or reverses as the child side bends (laterally flexes the trunk) toward the convex side of the curve.
   (2) Asymmetric side bending is an early sign that structural changes may have already begun to develop in the spine.
b. Forward Bending Test[13]
   (1) This test is done to determine whether the curve straightens out as the child bends forward and to identify a visible, rotational deformity of the rib cage.

(2) If structural changes are present, the examiner will see a posterior rib hump on the side of the convexity of the thoracic curve when the child bends forward.

(3) In the lumbar spine, prominence of the erector spinae muscles may be evident on the side of the convexity. This is due to the posterior rotation of the transverse processes of the vertebrae on the side that pushes the muscles outward. This should not be misinterpreted as muscle hypertrophy on the side of the convexity.

(4) Procedure (Figure 17-3)

(a) Sit in front or in back of the child. Ask the child to bend forward to a 90-degree angle and allow the arms to hang loosely.

(b) Examine the thoracic and lumbar spine and note any asymmetry or prominence of the ribs or scapula on the convex side of the curve.

c. The following structures may be limited if asymmetry is noted during flexibility testing[24]

(1) Muscles

Erector spinae; oblique abdominals, intercostals, and quadratus lumborum. Hip muscles may also be involved if there is faulty pelvic posture.

(2) Ligaments

Anterior and posterior longitudinal, ligamentum flavum, and interspinous.

3. Evaluation of muscle strength[24,25]

a. Musculature on the convex side of the lateral curve weakens.

b. In addition, the abdominals and trunk extensors also weaken.

c. Hip muscles may also weaken if there is faulty pelvic posture.

B. Related Diagnostic Information[23,24,28,41]

1. Complete medical history and physical examination

2. X-ray series

a. Standing (posterior and lateral views from occiput to sacrum): to determine the location and severity of the curve.

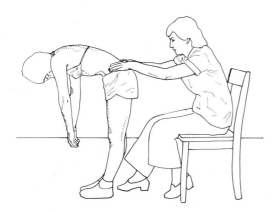

FIGURE 17-3. The examiner has the child perform a forward bending test for identification of a structural scoliosis.

b. Side bending (in both directions): to determine the flexibility of the curve.

c. Hand and wrist: to determine the skeletal maturity of the child.

3. Moiré topography[1,40]

a. Moiré topography is a form of photography that detects asymmetry on opaque surfaces. Shadows are produced on the opaque surface by light shining through a screen of thin parallel strings.

b. Moiré topography has been used in scoliosis screening and has been shown to be more sensitive than the Forward Bending Test.[1]

4. Pulmonary function tests[30,32]

A decrease in vital capacity and total lung capacity are often seen in patients with moderate and severe curves.

IV. NONOPERATIVE TREATMENT OF SCOLIOSIS

A. Background

If a diagnosis of scoliosis is made early, prior to a child reaching full skeletal growth, mild and moderate idiopathic scoliosis can be successfully treated by nonoperative methods of correction.[7,8,20,24,33,35] The number of otherwise healthy children who require treatment for idiopathic scoliosis is very low. For example, in a screening program of adolescent girls 12 to 14 years of age, only 0.3 percent were found to have curves significant enough to warrant treatment.[11,12,39,41]

The general goal of treatment is to allow the child with scoliosis to attain osseous maturity with as straight and as stable a spine as possible. Appropriate early treatment will prevent or halt the progression of the deformity and, in some instances, partially correct the existing deformity.[8,35]

The decision to initiate treatment is based on the etiology, type, and location of the scoliosis; the severity of the deformity at the time of identification, the age of the child; and the rate of progression of the deformity as noted with subsequent evaluation.[8,23,28] Treatment, usually nonoperative, is almost always indicated for curves between 18 and 40 degrees.[23]

B. Overview of Nonoperative Treatment Methods

1. Exercise[6,13,42,44]

a. The use of exercise alone for the treatment of idiopathic scoliosis has been suggested for many years. Although exercise has traditionally been used to stretch tight trunk and hip musculature and strengthen muscles of the trunk, it has been shown that exercise alone will not halt the progression of or correct an existing moderate or severe structural scoliosis. Exercise alone *may* be beneficial as a treatment for patients with very mild idiopathic scoliosis, but this has yet to be substantiated.[6,13,32,42]

b. Exercise used in conjunction with other methods of correction, such as bracing or traction, has been shown to be beneficial.[7,8,13,23,31]

2. Casts[13,23,30,38]

a. The concept of the turn-buckle cast was developed in the 1930s.

b. Later the localizer cast was developed by Risser,[38] using pressure pads localized over the apices of the curves.

    c. Both body casts are a form of cephalopelvic traction and provide passive correction of the scoliosis.

      (1) The cast is applied while the child is supported supine on a scoliosis frame.

      (2) The spine is elongated and the ribs are derotated as much as possible during the application of the cast.

    d. Since the development of the Milwaukee and Boston braces, body casts are rarely used as a sole nonoperative method of treatment because

      (1) casts must be worn for many years and must be reapplied many times.

      (2) casts are not as cosmetically acceptable as braces.

      (3) significant muscle weakness can occur over the years; exercises to maintain the strength of trunk musculature cannot be done in the cast.

    e. Today, casts are primarily used for preoperative correction or postoperative control of the trunk after spinal fusion.

3. Traction[13,23]

    a. Passive correction of scoliosis with traction requires prolonged positioning, usually supine on a frame, and gives no better correction of moderate curves than bracing.

    b. Cotrel traction[13,17,30,31]

      (1) Cotrel traction is primarily used to gain the greatest flexibility possible prior to spinal fusion but has also been used with limited success as a nonoperative method of treatment of moderate curves.

      (2) Procedure

        (a) Spinal traction is applied nightly and for specified periods of time during the day while the child is in bed. The traction consists of a removable head halter and pelvic girdle, which are attached to a weight and pulley system.

        (b) A rigorous routine of exercises, consisting of elongation, derotation, and lateral flexion of the spine, is performed several times during the day while the child is out of traction.

        (c) After several weeks of traction and exercise, a Risser body cast is applied and worn for several more weeks.

        (d) This cycle of traction, exercise, and casting is repeated until maximum correction of the scoliosis is achieved.

    c. Skeletal traction[13,30]

      (1) Prolonged skeletal traction, usually up to 3 weeks, is used preoperatively with severe or resistent curves to elongate the spine as much as possible prior to spinal fusion.

      (2) The specific types of skeletal traction will be discussed in Section V of this chapter—Operative Treatment of Scoliosis.

4. Spinal bracing

    a. The major goal of bracing patients with scoliosis is to prevent the progression of a curve or give some permanent correction and stabilization of the curve.

    b. The Milwaukee brace[7,8,14,23–35] (Figure 17-4A and B)

      (1) Since the mid-1950s, the Milwaukee brace combined with daily exercise has been the most common form of treatment of mild and

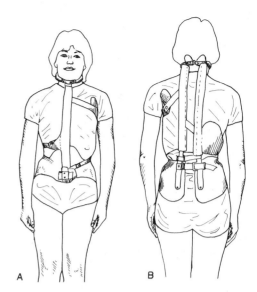

FIGURE 17-4. The Milwaukee Brace: (*A*) anterior and (*B*) posterior view.

A   B

moderate idiopathic scoliosis in patients with two or more years of remaining skeletal growth.

(2) The Milwaukee brace is also used for patients with paralytic or congenital scoliosis and children under age 10 with severe curves who are not yet candidates for spinal fusion.

(3) It is a high-profile brace that fits closely to the body. It has adjustable metal uprights attached to a molded plastic pelvic girdle and a metal neck ring and throat mold (formerly a chin rest) (Figure 17-5).

(4) The Milwaukee brace is based on the 3-point principle of fixation. A dorsal pad is placed at the apex of the thoracic curve on the convex side to decrease the rotational deformity.

(5) The brace is primarily used for high thoracic and high magnitude curves.

(6) The Milwaukee brace is designed using the concept of *dynamic (active) correction* of the scoliosis.

    (a) The brace affords correction by encouraging the patient to assume an erect posture.

    (b) Exercises are done daily, in and out of the brace, to prevent weakness of postural muscles.

    (c) Specific exercises done with the Milwaukee brace will be described later in this chapter.

(7) The brace is worn 23 to 24 hours per day for several years until the patient approaches full skeletal growth and the correction is stable Recent studies have suggested that wearing the brace 12 hours per day is equally effective in halting the progression of the curve.[20]

(8) Expected results of treatment of idopathic scoliosis with the Milwaukee brace and exercise[3,14,30,35]

    (a) The progression of the deformity has been halted in 70 percent of mild and moderate curves.

    (b) Up to 50 percent correction of a curve can be attained by wearing the brace.

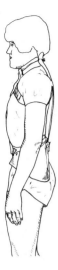

FIGURE 17-5. The anterior and posterior uprights of the Milwaukee brace are fitted close to the child's trunk.

        (c) Younger patients with milder curves have the best chance for correction.

        (d) Some curves (malignant curves) progress despite the brace and require surgical stabilization.

    (9) Long-term results

        (a) Experience has shown that some corrected curves may regress to a pre-bracing magnitude or even slightly worse.

        (b) If bracing is never used, moderate curves will usually progress to severe curves, and the patient will then require spinal fusion.

  c. The Boston brace[8,24,35,43,44] (Figure 17-6)

    (1) This is a low-profile spinal brace with no metal suprastructure.

    (2) It is a molded plastic jacket that extends from the axillas over the pelvis and can be entirely covered by the patient's clothing.

    (3) It is used for low thoracolumbar and lumbar curves and is not recommended for curves with apices above T-8.[43]

    (4) The brace is considered to be a form of passive and active correction; exercises done in conjunction with this form of bracing are similar to those done in the Milwaukee brace.

5. Electrical stimulation[2,3,9,10,22]

  a. A recent nonoperative development in the treatment of mild and moderate scoliosis is electrical stimulation of the trunk muscles on the convex side of the curve.

  b. Originally intramuscular electrodes were implanted in the paraspinal muscles. A subcutaneous neuromuscular stimulator provided intermittent electrical stimulation, caused the paraspinal muscles to contract, and alternately forced the vertebrae in and out of alignment. This form of electrical stimulation was successful in halting the progression of the major curve in more than 80 percent of the mild and moderate curves but involved the risks of surgery.[9,10]

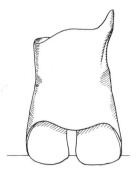

FIGURE 17-6. The low-profile Boston brace made of polypropylene.

    c. An alternative to surgical implantation of electrodes called *lateral electrical surface stimulation* (LESS) was later developed. Lateral placement of the surface electrodes on the convex side of the curve over the midaxillary line provides the greatest correction of the curve. As intermittent stimulation is applied, the lateral trunk muscles contract and the appropriate ribs move toward each other. Because the ribs articulate with the vertebrae, the corrective force is transferred to the spine, which causes straightening of the curve. LESS has been shown to be successful in halting the progression of more than 80 percent of the moderate curves treated.[2,3,22]

    d. Nighttime, intermittent neuromuscular stimulation using lateral placement of electrodes has been shown to be as effective as bracing in the treatment of moderate adolescent idiopathic scoliosis.

V. OPERATIVE TREATMENT OF SCOLIOSIS

A. Background

Surgical intervention is usually the treatment of choice for correction of curves greater than 40 to 50 degrees, for curves resistant to correction with nonoperative measures, for decompensated and cosmetically unacceptable curves, and for deformity causing considerable back pain.[13,20,23,28,30,33] Severe scoliosis leads to a decrease in cardiopulmonary function, putting the child's health at risk. Curves of this magnitude can continue to increase even into adult life and are associated with degenerative joint disease and pain. Surgical intervention will usually improve curves by approximately 50 percent and will provide the patient with a stable, pain-free spine.

    The therapist may be involved in the treatment of the patient with severe scoliosis pre- or postoperatively. Exercise may be indicated prior to surgery. The patient may wear a Milwaukee brace preoperatively and require instruction in exercises. The patient may be placed in skeletal traction pre- or postoperatively and may require daily exercise. Postoperatively, the patient may benefit from progressive ambulation and exercise to return to full activity. All of these situations require that the therapist have a general understanding of the most common surgical procedures used in the treatment of scoliosis.

B. Overview of Operative Procedures

1. **Preoperative correction**[13,30,41]
   a. Goal
      To elongate the spine and decrease the severity of the deformity prior to surgery, particularly in curves of 60 degrees or more.
   b. Traction or casts may be used preoperatively to maximize correction prior to spinal fusion.
      (1) Halo-femoral traction
          (a) This is a form of skeletal traction attached to a weight and pulley system and applied while the patient is prone or supine on a bed frame.
          (b) The halo is attached directly to the skull with pins, and the counter-traction is applied through skeletal pins at the distal femurs.
          (c) Maximum correction is usually attained in several weeks.
      (2) Halo-pelvic (DeWald)[18] traction
          (a) Upright bars are attached to a halo superiorly and to a pelvic hoop inferiorly.
          (b) The pelvic hoop is held in place by rods that penetrate the iliac crests.
          (c) The upright bars can be lengthened to elongate the spine.
          (d) With this form of skeletal traction, the patient can be ambulatory prior to surgery.
      (3) Cotrel traction and localizer (Risser) casts, which have been previously discussed in this chapter, have also been used successfully for presurgical correction.
   c. Considerations for exercise
      (1) If the patient is confined to a bed frame in halo-femoral traction for several weeks, normal range of motion should be maintained in as many joints as possible.
      (2) These patients are at risk for developing knee extension and plantarflexion contractures because of prolonged positioning in supine and prone and restriction of movement of the femurs.

2. **Spinal fusion with or without Harrington rod instrumentation**[20,28,30,33,41]
   a. Usually, a posterior approach is used for spinal fusions, but occasionally an anterior approach is indicated.[21] Most incisions extend from the thoracic region and into the lumbar region so that all rotated vertebrae can be stabilized.
   b. Harrington rod[27,28] instrumentation may or may not be done prior to a posterior spinal fusion.
      (1) The rods are used to achieve the best correction possible of late rigid curves that otherwise would be difficult to correct.
      (2) A distraction rod may be placed on the concave side of the curve and occasionally a compression rod on the convex side.
   c. An anterior spinal fusion with Luque sublamina wiring is another approach that is sometimes used. This procedure is called *segmental spinal instrumentation*.[34]

3. **Postoperative management of spinal fusions**[23,28]
   a. After most posterior spinal fusions, a body cast or brace must be worn for 6 to 9 months or for as long as 12 months.
   b. During this time, ambulation is usually permitted, although in some in-

stances the patient may be nonambulatory or may be allowed only limited ambulation for several months.

    c. No bracing or cast is necessary after the Luque segmental spinal instrumentation procedure (anterior approach) or after the relatively new Cotrel-Dubousett procedure (posterior approach). Although immobilization is not required after these procedures, physical exertion during the first year after surgery should be no more strenuous than walking.

VI. APPROPRIATE USE OF EXERCISE IN SCOLIOSIS

As previously mentioned, exercise alone cannot halt the progression of or correct an existing scoliosis. Experience has shown that there is no significant improvement or retardation of the progression of scoliosis despite a rigorous routine of exercises.[13,42] In patients with curves of 18 to 20 degrees or greater, it is clear that other methods of treatment such as bracing, electrical stimulation, or surgery must be implemented.

    There are three situations in which exercise has either been shown to be or may be of value in the treatment of scoliosis:

    1. Exercise with the Milwaukee brace.
    2. Preoperative exercise prior to spinal fusion.
    3. Exercise for the treatment of mild idiopathic scoliosis.

    It must be emphasized here that research studies must continue in order to determine the effectiveness of exercise in scoliosis.

A. Exercise With the Milwaukee Brace[7,8]

1. Rationale for exercise

    a. The Milwaukee brace is a form of dynamic correction of scoliosis in which the patient must actively participate in the correction of the deformity with a daily routine of exercises.

    b. The effectiveness of the brace depends on the patient's both wearing the brace 23 hours a day *and* carrying out a specific set of exercises daily.

2. Goals of exercise

    a. Strengthen the muscles that provide stability to the trunk.

    b. Actively decrease and correct the spinal curves and related deformities (increased lumbar lordosis and rotation of the vertebrae).

3. Specific exercises to be done daily in and out of the brace[7,8]

    a. Exercises performed out of the brace
        (1) Posterior pelvic tilt in supine with hips and knees flexed
        (2) Posterior pelvic tilt in supine with hips and knees extended
        (3) Partial sit up with knees flexed
        (4) Posterior pelvic tilt while standing
        (5) Trunk extension in the prone position
        (6) Deep-breathing exercises

    b. Exercises performed in the brace (Figure 17-7)
        (1) The same exercises are repeated in the brace as were done out of the brace.
        (2) Also included is active distraction from the thoracic pad at the posterior rib hump.
            (a) The patient shifts the trunk laterally away from thoracic pad to correct the major thoracic curve.

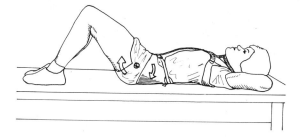

FIGURE 17-7. Exercises such as the posterior pelvic tilt are performed daily, both in and out of the Milwaukee brace.

        (b) If a lumbar pad is present, the patient also shifts away from that pad.
    (3) The patient actively distracts from the throat mold and attempts to become taller in the brace and elongate the spine.

  4. Physical activity
    a. The child should be encouraged to participate in a variety of physical activities and recreational sports.
    b. Only contact sports are contraindicated.

B. Preoperative Exercise Prior to Spinal Fusion

  1. Rationale for exercise
  By increasing the flexibility of the trunk with exercise prior to surgery, the best possible correction at the time of surgery can be achieved.

  2. Goals of exercise
    a. Increase the mobility of structures of the spine that have become tight because of the spinal curvature.
    b. Improve pulmonary function as much as possible prior to surgery.
    c. Improve postural control with general strengthening of trunk musculature.

  3. Exercise has been used in conjunction with Cotrel traction[31] prior to spinal fusion to minimize the curve.
    a. Cotrel has suggested that, prior to surgery, exercise and traction are done for
      (1) elongation.
      (2) derotation.
      (3) (lateral) flexion of the spine.
    b. This concept has been referred to as EDF.

  4. Pre-operative stretching
  Although the efficacy of pre-operative exercise alone has not been proved, stretching the following structures may be useful in improving the flexibility of the trunk in order to achieve the best correction possible at the time of surgery:

    a. Tight structures on the concave side of the curve

b. Tight hip flexors that can contribute to an increased lumbar lordosis commonly seen in scoliosis
c. Tight erector spinae
d. Tight hamstrings

5. Deep-breathing exercises

Instruction in deep-breathing exercises prior to surgery has been shown to decrease postoperative pulmonary complications. Emphasis is placed on expanding lung segments and improving chest mobility on the concave side of the major curve.

C. Exercise for Mild Idiopathic Scoliosis[42]

1. Rationale for exercise

a. In the past decade, school screening programs are identifying adolescents between the ages of 11 and 14 with mild (less than 20 degrees) curves.
b. Each of these children must be monitored for several months to determine whether their idiopathic scoliosis will increase or stabilize.
c. It has been suggested,[42] although not yet proved, that by placing the adolescent on a structured and supervised exercise program during the period of monitoring, exercise may have a positive effect on halting the progression of the curve or even improving it. It may also decrease the likelihood that these children will be lost to necessary orthopedic follow-up and later treatment if needed.

2. Goals of exercise

a. Improve the strength and postural control of trunk musculature
b. Increase the mobility of any tight structures of the trunk
c. Improve the overall posture of the child

3. Specific exercises should include

a. strengthening the abdominals and trunk extensors.
b. stretching structures on the concave side of the curve.
c. strengthening lateral trunk flexors on the convex side of the curve.
d. stretching tight hip flexors and erector spinae muscles associated with an increased lumbar lordosis.
e. posture training.

VII. SPECIFIC EXERCISES FOR TREATING SCOLIOSIS

Many of the exercises used in the treatment of scoliosis have already been explained and illustrated in Chapters 10 and 14. Those exercises will simply be mentioned here. New and additional exercises will be explained and illustrated in this chapter. Remember, exercise alone will not correct or halt the progression of scoliosis. These exercises, as well as the exercises used in conjunction with bracing, may be used to increase or maintain range of motion or strength of trunk musculature or to reduce low back pain.

A. Exercises to Increase the Flexibility of Tight Structures and Elongate the Trunk

Note: When stretching the trunk, it is necessary to stabilize the spine above and below the curve. If the patient has a double curve, one curve must be stabilized while the other is stretched.

1. **To stretch tight structures on the concave side of the curve**

   Shift the apex of the curve to the midline and passively overcorrect the curve

   a. Patient prone
      (1) Stabilize the patient at the iliac crest on the side of the concavity.
          (a) Have the patient reach toward the knee with the arm on the convex side of the curve while stretching the opposite arm up and overhead (Figure 17-8A).
          (b) Have the patient, with hands behind the head, lift the head and trunk and bend the trunk laterally away from the concavity (Figure 17-8B).
      (2) Patient stabilizes the upper trunk (thoracic curve) by holding onto the edge of the mat table with the arms. (No shoulder motion should occur.) The therapist lifts the hips and legs and laterally bends the trunk away from the concavity (Figure 17-9).
   b. Patient heel-sitting (to stabilize the lumbar curve)
      (1) The patient leans forward so the abdomen rests on the anterior thighs (Figure 17-10A).
          (a) Arms are stretched overhead bilaterally.
          (b) Hands are flat on the floor.

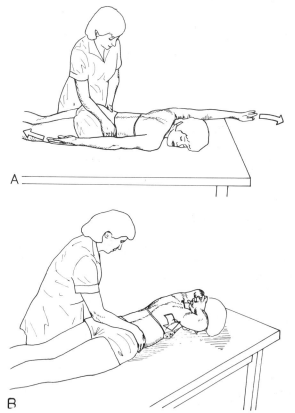

A

B

FIGURE 17-8. (*A*), Stretching tight structures on the concave side of the thoracic curve. The patient has a right thoracic left lumbar curve. (*B*), The therapist stabilizes the pelvis and lumbar spine.

FIGURE 17-9. Stretching tight structures on the concave side of a left lumbar curve. The patient stabilizes the upper trunk and thoracic curve as the therapist passively stretches the lumbar curve.

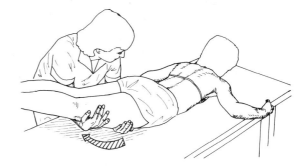

      (2) Have the patient laterally bend the trunk away from the concavity by walking the hands to the convex side of the curve. Hold the position for a sustained stretch (Figure 17-10B).

  c. Patient side-lying on the convex side of the curve

  Note: Stabilize the patient at the iliac crest. Do not allow the patient to roll forward or backward during the stretch.

      (1) Have the patient lie on a mat, top arm stretched overhead, with a rolled towel at the apex of the curve to neutralize the curve. Hold this position for a sustained period of time (Figure 17-11).

      (2) Have the patient lie over the edge of a mat table, with a rolled towel at the apex of the curve and the top arm stretched overhead. Hold this head-down position as long as possible (Figure 17-12).

2. To elongate the trunk

  a. Patient should be standing, with feet 6 inches from the wall. Stretch the arms overhead, keeping hands on the wall and heels on the floor (Figure 17-13).

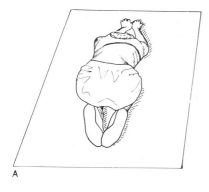
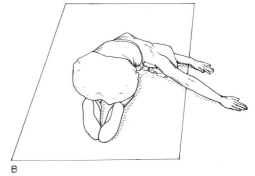

A   B

FIGURE 17-10. (A) Heel-sitting to stabilize the lumbar spine; (B) tight structures on the concave side of a right thoracic curve are stretched by having the patient reach her arms overhead and then walk her hands to the right.

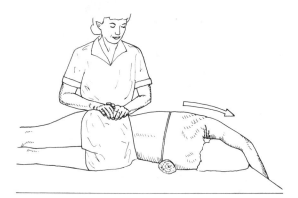

FIGURE 17-11. Stretching tight structures on the concave side of a right thoracic curve. The patient is positioned side-lying with a rolled towel at the apex of the convexity; the lumbar spine is stabilized by the therapist.

    b. Hang by the hands from stall bars so feet are off the floor (Figure 17-14).

  3. To stretch tight neck, shoulder, or hip musculature
    a. Use the stretching procedures discussed and illustrated in Chapters 10 and 14.
    b. The following muscle groups may be tight in the scoliotic patient:
      (1) Sternocleidomastoids or scalenes (see Figure 14-11)
      (2) Pectoralis (see Figures 14-5 and 14-6A and B)
      (3) Erector spinae (see Figures 14-13, 14-14, and 14-15)
      (4) Hip flexors (see Figure 10-2)
      (5) Hamstrings (see Figures 10-3A and B and 10-4)

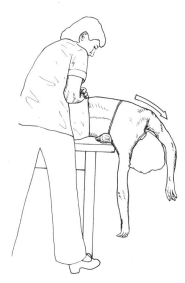

FIGURE 17-12. Side-lying over the edge of a mat table to stretch tight structures of a right thoracic scoliosis. The therapist stabilizes the pelvis.

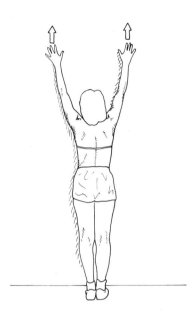

FIGURE 17-13. Elongation of the spine while standing and reaching up a wall.

B. **Exercises to Symmetrically Strengthen Trunk Muscles Necessary for Postural Control and Trunk Stability**

Note: As in Chapter 14, the exercises are listed progressively from least to most difficult. Begin the patient at the appropriate level consistent with initial strength and ability to control the motion.

The majority of these exercises have been explained in Chapter 14 and will simply be noted here.

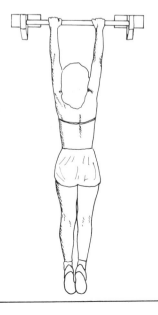

FIGURE 17-14. Elongation of the spine by hanging from stall bars.

1. To strengthen abdominal muscles
   a. Patient supine
      (1) posterior pelvic tilt with knees flexed (see Figure 17-7)
      (2) posterior pelvic tilt with knees extended
      (3) partial sit-up with a posterior pelvic tilt and arms at the patient's sides (see Figure 14-21)
      (4) progress the difficulty of the curl-up by placing arms across the chest and then clasping hands behind the head.
      (5) bilateral leg lowering from 90 degrees of hip flexion as long as a posterior pelvic tilt can be maintained (see Figure 14-22)
   b. Patient standing
      (1) posterior pelvic tilt standing, with back against the wall
      (2) posterior pelvic tilt, while standing away from the wall

2. To strengthen the thoracic and lumbar extensors
   a. Patient prone (with the chin tucked)
   Note: First have the patient shift the apex of the curve toward the midline to actively decrease the curve. Then proceed with the following exercises
      (1) trunk extension with arms at the sides
      (2) trunk extension with arms in reverse T position
      (3) trunk extension with hands clasped behind the head
      (4) trunk extension with arms reaching out over the head (see Figure 14-24)
   b. Patient supine, with lower arm at the side: have the patient arch the back (Figure 17-15).

3. To strengthen the hip extensors
   a. With the patient prone, begin by repeatedly lifting one leg, then the other.
   b. Progress by lifting both legs simultaneously and holding.

4. To strengthen the hip and back extensors simultaneously
   a. With arms at the side, lift both legs and arms simultaneously (Figure 17-16).
   b. With the arms stretched overhead, lift both legs, trunk, and arms simultaneously.

C. Exercises to Strengthen Trunk Musculature on the Convex Side of the Curve

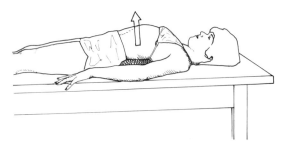

FIGURE 17-15. To strengthen the back extensors, have the patient arch her back while supine.

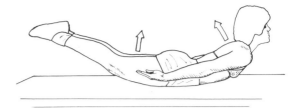

FIGURE 17-16. To strengthen the trunk and hip extensors, have the patient lift her trunk and legs off the mat simultaneously.

1. Patient side-lying on the concave side of the curve
   a. The therapist should stabilize the patient at the iliac crest.
   b. With lower arm across the chest, have the patient derotate the trunk, lift up the head and shoulders (lateral trunk bending), and slide the top arm down to the knee (Figure 17-17).
2. Patient side-lying
   Progress the difficulty of the above-mentioned exercise by having the patient clasp hands behind the head and then laterally flex the trunk against gravity (Figure 17-18).

D. **Deep-Breathing Exercises to Improve Pulmonary Function**

   Note: The specific procedures for teaching breathing exercises are found in Chapter 19. Emphasis should be placed on
   1. Diaphragmatic breathing during abdominal strengthening exercises
   2. Segmental breathing to expand the lungs on the concave side of the curve during unilateral stretching of the trunk
   3. Deep breathing with bilateral stretch to the pectoralis muscles

E. **Derotation of the Trunk**

   1. By combining deep-breathing exercises and lateral flexion of the trunk (to stretch the concave side of the curve), it has been suggested that derotation of the vertebrae can be achieved in a structural scoliosis.[20]
   2. Rib motion during deep breathing is used to create a derotation force on the thoracic vertebrae.

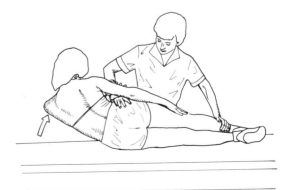

FIGURE 17-17. To strengthen weak structures on the convex side of a right thoracic curve, have the patient lie on her left side and lift her upper trunk off the mat.

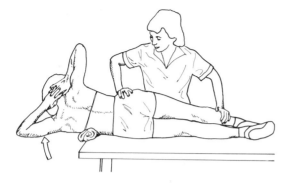

FIGURE 17-18. Progress the difficulty of strengthening the trunk on the convex side of a right thoracic curve. Have the patient lie on her left side, hands behind her head, and lift her trunk.

VIII. SUMMARY

A brief description of terminology related to scoliosis and classifications of scoliosis by type, severity, and etiology were first reviewed in this chapter. Criteria for screening, evaluation, and diagnosis of scoliosis were then outlined. An overview of nonoperative and operative methods of treatment was also covered.

The value and rationale for exercise as part of the treatment of scoliosis was then discussed. Specific exercises commonly used in the treatment of scoliosis were described and illustrated.

REFERENCES

1. Adair, IV, VanWijk, MC, and Armstrong, GWD: *Moiré topography in scoliosis screening.* Clin Orthop 129:165, 1977.
2. Axelgaard, J and Brown, JC: *Lateral electrical surface stimulation for the treatment of progressive idiopathic scoliosis.* Spine 8:242, 1983.
3. Axelgaard, J, Nordwall, A, and Brown, JC: *Correction of spinal curvature by transcutaneous electrical muscle stimulation.* Spine 8:463, 1983.
4. Axelgaard, J, Brown, JC, Nordwall, A, et al: *Transcutaneous electrical muscle stimulation for the treatment of idiopathic scoliosis—Preliminary results.* J Bone Joint Surg 4A(1):29, 1980.
5. Bates, DV, MacKeems, PT, and Christie, RV: *Respiratory Function in Disease.* WB Saunders, Philadelphia, 1971.
6. Bennett, RL: *Recognition and care of early scoliosis.* Arch Phys Med Rehabil 42:211, 1961.
7. Blount, WP and Bolinske, J: *Physical therapy in the nonoperative treatment of scoliosis.* Phys Ther 47:919, 1967.
8. Blount, WP and Moe, JH: *The Milwaukee Brace.* Williams & Wilkins, Baltimore, 1980.
9. Bobechko, WP: *Scoliosis spinal pacemaker.* J Bone Joint Surg 56:442, 1974.
10. Bobechko, WP, Herbert, MA, and Friedman, HG: *Electrospinal instrumentation for scoliosis: Current status.* Orthop Clin North Am 10:927, 1979.
11. Brooks, HL, Azen, SP, Gerberg, E, et al: *Scoliosis: A prospective epidemiological study.* J Bone Joint Surg 57:963, 1975.
12. Brooks, HL, Gerberg, E, Mazur, H, et al: *The epidemiology of scoliosis: A prospective study.* Orthop Rev 1(5): 17, 1972.
13. Cailliet, R: *Scoliosis.* FA Davis, Philadelphia, 1975.
14. Carr, WH, et al: *Treatment of idiopathic scoliosis in the Milwaukee brace.* J Bone Joint Surg (Am) 62:599, 1980.
15. Connolly, BH and Michael, BT: *Early detection of scoliosis: A neurological approach using the asymmetrical tonic neck reflex.* Phys Ther 64:304, 1984.

16. Cook, SD, et al: *Upper extremity proprioception in idiopathic scoliosis.* Clin Orthop 213:118, 1986.
17. Cotrel, Y: *Traction in the treatment of vertebral deformity.* J Bone Joint Surg 57:260, 1975.
18. Dewald, RL and Ray, R: *Skeletal traction for the treatment of severe scoliosis.* J Bone Joint Surg 52:233, 1970.
19. DiRamando, CV, Green, NE, and MacLean, WE: *Brace compliance in adolescent idiopathic scoliosis.* Scoliosis Research Society, Orlando, Fl, September, 1984.
20. Donaldson, WF: *Scoliosis.* In Ferguson, AB (ed): *Orthopedic Surgery in Infancy and Childhood,* ed 5. Baltimore, Williams & Wilkins, 1981.
21. Dwyer, AF, Newton, NC, and Sherwood, AA: *An anterior approach to scoliosis: A preliminary report.* Clin Orthop 62:192, 1969.
22. Eckerson, L and Axelgaard, J: *Lateral electrical surface stimulation as an alternative to bracing in the treatment of idiopathic scoliosis: Treatment, protocol and patient acceptance.* Phys Ther 64:483, 1984.
23. Engler, GL: *Scoliosis.* In Nickel, VL: (ed) *Orthopedic Rehabilitation.* Churchill-Livingstone, New York, 1982.
24. Farady, JA: *Current principles in the nonoperative management of structural adolescent idiopathic scoliosis.* Phys Ther 63:512, 1983.
25. Ford, DM, et al: *Paraspinal muscle imbalance in adolescent idiopathic scoliosis.* Spine 9:373, 1984.
26. Ford, DM, et al: *Muscle spindles in the paraspinal musculature of patients with adolescent idiopathic scoliosis.* Spine 13:461, 1988.
27. Harrington, PR: *Treatment of scoliosis: Correction and internal fixation by spinal instrumentation.* J Bone Joint Surg 44(A):591, 1962.
28. James, JIP: *Scoliosis,* ed 2. Churchill-Livingstone, London, 1976.
29. Jensen, GM and Wilson, KB: *Horizontal postrotatory nystagmus response in female subjects with adolescent idiopathic scoliosis.* Phys Ther 59:1226, 1979.
30. Keim, HA: *Scoliosis.* Clin Symp 24:1, Ciba Pharmaceutical Co, Summit, NJ, 1972.
31. Labreche, B, Levangie, P, and Sharby, N: *Cotrel traction: A new approach to the preoperative management of idiopathic scoliosis.* Phys Ther 54:837, 1974.
32. Levine, DB: *Influence of spinal deformities on chest function.* Phys Ther 48:968, 1968.
33. Lovell, WW and Winter, RB (eds): *Pediatric Orthopedics,* ed 2. Philadelphia, JB Lippincott, 1986.
34. Luque, ER: *Segmental correction of scoliosis with rigid internal fixation: A preliminary report.* Orthop Trans 1:136, 1977.
35. Moe, JH and Kettleson, DN: *Idiopathic scoliosis.* J Bone Joint Surg 52A(8):1509, 1970.
36. Riddle, H and Roaf, R: *Muscle imbalance in the causation of scoliosis.* Lancet 1:1245, 1955.
37. Riseborough, EJ: *The effect of scoliotic deformities in pulmonary function.* In Robin, GC (ed): *Scoliosis.* Academic Press, New York, 1973.
38. Risser, JC: *Scoliosis: Past and present.* J Bone Joint Surg 46:167, 1964.
39. Rogala, EJ, Drummond, DS, and Gar, J: *Scoliosis: Incidence and natural history: A prospective epidemiologic study.* J Bone Joint Surg 60(A):173, 1978.
40. Ruggerone, M and Austin, JHM: *Moiré topography in scoliosis: Correlations with vertebral lateral curvature as determined by radiography.* Phys Ther 66:1072, 1986.
41. Salter, RB: *Textbook of Disorders and Injuries of the Musculoskeletal System,* ed 2. Williams & Wilkins, Baltimore, 1983.
42. Stone, B, Beckman, C, Hall, V, et al: *The effect of an exercise program on change in curve in adolescents with minimal idiopathic scoliosis: A preliminary study.* Phys Ther 59:759, 1979.
43. Uden, A, Wilner, S, and Pettersson, H: *Initial correction with the Boston thoracic brace.* Acta Orthop Scand 53:907, 1982.
44. Watts, HG, Hall, JE, and Stanish, W: *The Boston brace system for treatment of low thoracic and lumbar scoliosis by the use of a girdle without suprastructure.* Clin Orthop 126:87, 1977.
45. Zuk, T: *The role of spinal and abdominal muscles in the pathogenesis of scoliosis.* J Bone Joint Surg 44:102, 1962.

PART ——————————— 3

Special Areas of Therapeutic Exercise

CHAPTER ——————————————— 18

Principles of Exercise for the Obstetric Patient

Cathy J. Konkler, B.S., P.T.

Pregnant women and postpartum women present a unique opportunity for the physical therapist. Pregnancy is a time of tremendous musculoskeletal, physical, and emotional change and yet is a condition of wellness. The physical therapist evaluates and monitors physical changes, with the focus on maintaining wellness rather than on correcting illness or deformity. This chapter does not present a specific protocol of exercise for use with the pregnant or postpartum client; rather, it provides the reader with basic information about the physical changes of pregnancy and creates a good foundation for the development of safe and effective exercise programs. The chapter also discusses modification of general exercises to meet the needs of the obstetric client. The exercises discussed in this chapter are not exclusive, and many other appropriate exercises are not covered. The information provided here is meant to assist the reader in making wise decisions about exercises to include in an uncomplicated pregnancy exercise program. Cesarean delivery, high-risk pregnancy, and the special needs of clients with these conditions are discussed separately at the end of the chapter.

OBJECTIVES

After studying this chapter, the reader will be able to:
1. identify the major stages and characteristics of pregnancy, labor, and delivery.
2. describe the normal physiologic changes of pregnancy in the organ systems and musculoskeletal system.
3. identify the common postural adjustments to pregnancy.
4. define diastasis recti and its significance in pregnancy.
5. describe the evaluation procedure for diastasis recti and corrective exercise for the condition.
6. identify other pathologies of the musculoskeletal system caused by pregnancy.
7. describe the structure, function, and significance of the pelvic floor.

8. describe rehabilitation techniques for the pelvic floor.
9. summarize the goals and guidelines of an obstetric exercise program for an uncomplicated pregnancy.
10. identify absolute and possible contraindications to exercise in pregnancy.
11. establish a safe therapeutic exercise program that addresses or corrects the changes of pregnancy and aids in preparation for labor.
12. describe the maternal and fetal responses to exercise.
13. define cesarean childbirth and high-risk pregnancy.
14. identify exercise and rehabilitative goals for cesarean and high-risk clients.
15. describe modifications or additions to exercise programs for the cesarean or high-risk client.

I.   OVERVIEW OF PREGNANCY, LABOR, AND DELIVERY[4,14,18,28,30]

A. Pregnancy (40 Weeks from Conception to Delivery)
Pregnancy is divided into three trimesters

1. **Changes during the first trimester:**[4,14,30] **weeks 0 to 12 of pregnancy**
   a. Implantation of the fertilized ovum in the uterus occurs 7 to 10 days after fertilization.
   b. The mother may be nauseated or may vomit, is very fatigued, and will urinate more frequently due to pressure from the growing uterus.
   c. The breast size may increase.
   d. There is a relatively small weight gain of 0 to 1455 g (0 to 3 lb is normal).
   e. Emotional changes may occur.
   f. By the end of the twelfth week, the fetus is 6 to 7 cm long and weighs approximately 20 g (2 oz). The baby now can kick, turn its head, and swallow, and has a beating heart, but these movements are not yet felt by the mother.

2. **Changes during the second trimester:**[4,14,30] **weeks 13 to 26 of pregnancy**
   a. The pregnancy now becomes visible to others.
   b. The mother begins to feel movement at around 20 weeks.
   c. During this trimester, most women feel very good. Nausea and fatigue have usually disappeared.
   d. By the end of the second trimester, the fetus is 19 to 23 cm (14 in) in length and weighs approximately 600 g (1 to 2 lb)
   e. The baby now has eyebrows, eyelashes, and fingernails and would have a slight chance of surviving if born prematurely.

3. **Change during the third trimester:**[4,14,30] **weeks 27 to 40 of pregnancy (38 to 42 weeks is considered full term).**
   a. The uterus is now very large and has regular contractions, although these may only occasionally be felt.
   b. Common complaints during the third trimester are frequent urination, back pain, leg edema and fatigue, round ligament pain, shortness of breath, and constipation.
   c. By the time of birth, the baby will be 33 to 39 cm long (16 to 19 in) and will weigh approximately 3400 g (7 lb, although a range from 5 to 10 lb is normal).

B. Labor[4,28,30]
1. **Onset of labor**
   a. The exact mechanism for labor induction is not known.
   b. Regular and strong involuntary contractions of the smooth muscles of the uterus are the primary symptom of labor.
   c. True labor will produce palpable changes in the cervix:
      (1) *Effacement*—shortening or thinning of the cervix from a thickness of 5 cm or 2 in before onset of labor to the thickness of a piece of paper (Figure 18-1).
      (2) *Dilatation*—opening of the cervix from the diameter of a fingertip to approximately 10 cm or 4 in (Figure 18-1).

2. **Labor—Stage 1**
   a. This is the cervical dilatation and effacement stage. At the end of this stage, the cervix is fully dilated and the baby is ready to be expelled from the uterus.

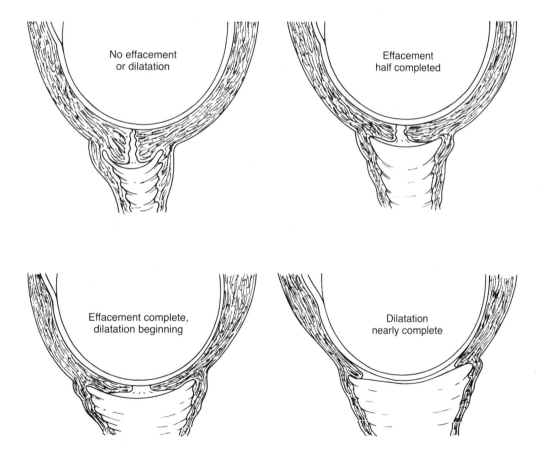

FIGURE 18-1. Effacement and dilatation of the cervix. (From Sandberg, E: Synopsis of Obstetrics, ed 10. CV Mosby, St. Louis, 1978, p. 192, with permission.)

b. Stage 1 of labor is divided into three major phases:
   (1) *Cervical dilatation phase.* The cervix dilates from 0 to 3 cm (0 to 1 in) and will almost completely efface. Uterine contractions occur from the top down, causing the cervix to open and pushing the fetus downward.
   (2) *Middle phase.* The cervix dilates from 4 to 7 cm (1 to 3 in). Contractions are stronger and more regular.
   (3) *Transition phase.* The cervix dilates from 8 to 10 cm (3 to 4 in) and dilatation is complete. Uterine contractions are very strong and close together.

3. Labor—Stage 2 (expulsion of the fetus)

a. Intra-abdominal pressure is the primary force expelling the fetus. This pressure is produced by voluntary contraction of the abdominals and diaphragm.
b. Fetal descent
   Position changes (cardinal movements) by the fetus allow it to pass through the pelvis and be born (Figure 18-2).
   (1) *Engagement.* The greatest transverse diameter of the fetal head passes through the pelvic inlet (the superior opening of the minor pelvis).
   (2) *Descent.* Continued downward progression of the fetus occurs.
   (3) *Flexion.* The fetal chin is brought closer to its thorax; this occurs when the descending head meets resistance from the walls and floor of the pelvis and the cervix.
   (4) *Internal rotation.* The fetus turns its occiput toward the mother's symphysis pubis when the fetal head reaches the level of the ischial spines.
   (5) *Extension.* The flexed fetal head reaches the vulva; the fetus extends its head, bringing the base of the occiput in direct contact with the inferior margin of the maternal symphysis pubis; this phase ends when the fetal head is born.
   (6) *External rotation.* The fetus rotates its occiput toward the mother's sacrum to allow the fetal shoulders to pass through the pelvis.
c. Expulsion
   The fetal anterior shoulder passes under the symphysis pubis, and the rest of the body follows.

4. Labor—Stage 3

a. Placental stage (expulsion of the placenta)
   (1) The uterus continues to contract and shrink following delivery; as the uterus decreases in size, the placenta detaches from the uterine wall, blood vessels are constricted, and bleeding slows. This can occur 5 to 30 minutes after fetal expulsion.
   (2) A hematoma forms over the uterine placental site to prevent further significant blood loss; mild bleeding persists for 3 to 6 weeks after delivery.
b. Uterine involution
   The uterus continues to contract and decrease in size for 3 to 6 weeks following delivery; the uterus always remains a bit enlarged over its pre-pregnant size.

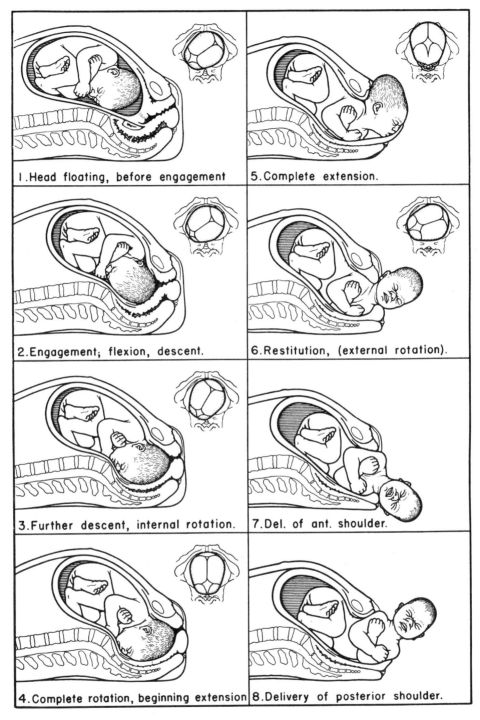

FIGURE 18-2. Principal movements in the mechanism of labor and delivery, left occiput anterior position. (From Pritchard, J and MacDonald, P: Williams Obstetrics, ed 16., Appleton-Century Crofts, Norwalk, CT, 1980, with permission.)

II. ANATOMIC AND PHYSIOLOGIC CHANGES OF PREGNANGY.[3,4,5,18,22,25,26,28,30,35]

A. Pregnancy Weight Gain.

A 25 percent increase in total weight is normal. This is necessary to nourish the fetus. Weight gain is produced by (average figures):

Fetus	3.63–3.88 kg	(7.5–8.0 lb)
Placenta	.48– .72 kg	(1.0–1.5 lb)
Amniotic fluid	.72– .97 kg	(1.5–2.0 lb)
Uterus and breasts	2.42–2.66 kg	(5.0–5.5 lb)
Blood and fluid	1.94–3.99 kg	(4.0–7.0 lb)
Muscle and fat	.48–2.91 kg	(1.0–6.0 lb)
	9.70–14.55 kg	(20.0–30.0 lb)

B. Organ Systems

1. Reproductive system

a. The uterus increases from a pre-pregnant size of 5 cm by 10 cm (2 in by 4 in) to 25 cm by 36 cm (10 in by 14 in).

b. The uterus increases 5 to 6 times in size, 3000 to 4000 times in capacity, and 20 times in weight by the end of pregnancy.

c. By the end of pregnancy, each muscle cell in the uterus has increased approximately 10 times its length prior to pregnancy.[35]

d. Once the uterus expands upward and leaves the pelvis, it becomes an abdominal organ rather than a pelvic organ.

2. Urinary system

a. The kidneys increase in length by 1 cm (0.5 in).

b. Ureters enter the bladder at a perpendicular angle due to uterine enlargement. This may result in a reflux of urine out of the bladder and back into the ureter; therefore, there is an increased chance of developing urinary tract infections in pregnancy due to urinary stasis.

3. Pulmonary system

a. Edema and tissue congestion of the upper respiratory tract occur early in pregnancy, due to hormonal changes.

b. There is upper respiratory hypersecretion (hormonally stimulated).

c. The subcostal angle progressively increases; the ribs flare up and out.

d. The anterior-posterior and transverse chest diameters each increase by 2 cm (1 in).

e. Total chest circumference increases by 5 to 7 cm (2 to 3 in) and does not always return to the pre-pregnant state.

f. Changes in rib position are hormonally stimulated and occur prior to uterine enlargement.

g. The diaphragm is elevated by 4 cm (1.5 in); this is a passive change caused by the change in rib position.

h. The respiration rate is unchanged, but the depth of respiration increases.[28]

i. Tidal volume and minute ventilation increase, but total lung capacity is unchanged or slightly decreased.[28,35]

j. There is a 15 to 20 percent increase in oxygen consumption; a natural

state of hyperventilation exists throughout pregnancy. This occurs to meet the oxygen demands of pregnancy.[28,35]
  k. The work of breathing increases due to hyperventilation; dyspnea is present with mild exercise as early as 20 weeks into the pregnancy.[28,35]

4. Cardiovascular system
  a. Blood volume progressively increases 35 to 50 percent (1.5 to 2 l) throughout pregnancy and returns to normal by 6 to 8 weeks post-pregnancy.
  b. Plasma increase is greater than red blood cell increase, leading to "physiologic anemia" of pregnancy, which is not a true anemia but is representative of the greater increase of plasma volume. The increase in plasma volume occurs as a result of hormonal stimulation in order to meet the oxygen demands of pregnancy.
  c. Venous pressure in the lower extremities increases when standing as a result of increased uterine size and increased venous distensibility.
  d. Pressure in the inferior vena cava rises in late pregnancy especially in the supine position due to compression by the uterus just below the diaphragm. The aorta is partially occluded in the supine position.
  e. The heart size increases, and the heart is elevated due to the movement of the diaphragm.
  f. Heart rhythm disturbances are more common in pregnancy.
  g. Heart rate usually increases 10 to 20 beats per minute by full term and returns to normal levels within 6 weeks post-pregnancy.
  h. Cardiac output increases 30 to 60 percent in pregnancy and is most significantly increased when side-lying on the left. In this position, the uterus places the least pressure on the aorta.
  i. Blood pressure decreases early in the first trimester. There is a slight decrease of systolic pressure and a greater decrease of diastolic pressure. Blood pressure reaches its lowest level approximately midway through pregnancy, then rises gradually from mid-pregnancy to reach the pre-pregnant level approximately 6 weeks post-delivery. Although cardiac output increases, blood pressure decreases due to venous distensibility.

5. Musculoskeletal system[22,26,35]
  a. Abdominal muscles are stretched to the point of their elastic limit by the end of pregnancy.
  b. Hormonal influence on the ligaments is profound, producing a systemic decrease in ligamentous tensile strength and an increase in mobility of structures supported by ligaments.
  c. Joint hypermobility occurs as a result of ligamentous laxity and may predispose the patient to joint injury, especially in the weight-bearing joints of the back, pelvis, and lower extremities.
  d. The pelvic floor muscles must withstand the weight of the uterus; the pelvic floor drops as much as 2.5 cm (1 in).[26]
  e. The pelvic floor may be stretched or incised or both during the birth process.

6. Posture[22,26,35]
  a. The shoulders are rounded with scapular protraction and upper ex-

tremity internal rotation due to breast enlargement and postpartum positioning for infant care.

b. Cervical lordosis increases in the upper cervical spine, and forward head posture develops to compensate for the shoulder alignment.

c. The body's center of gravity shifts upward and forward due to the increase in weight of the uterus and its contents.

d. Lumbar lordosis increases to compensate for the shift in the center of gravity and the knees hyperextend, probably due to the change in the line of gravity.

e. Weight shifts toward the heels to bring the center of gravity to a more posterior position.

f. Changes in posture do not usually correct spontaneously after childbirth, and pregnant posture may be maintained as a learned posture. Carrying the infant in the arms can also perpetuate faulty posture.

III. PREGNANCY-INDUCED PATHOLOGY

A. Diastasis Recti.[2,6,16,22,26,28,35]

1. Definition

Separation of the rectus abdominis muscles in the midline at the linea alba. The etiology of pathology is unknown, but the continuity of the abdominal wall is disrupted (Figure 18-3).

2. Incidence

Any separation larger than 2 cm is considered significant.[2,22]

a. The condition is not exclusive to childbearing women but is seen frequently in this population.

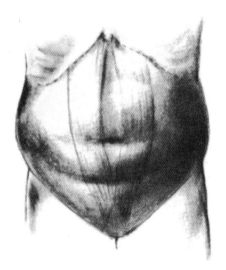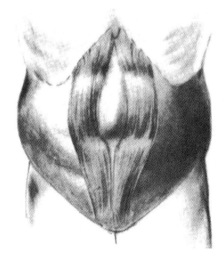

FIGURE 18-3. Diagramatic representations of diastasis recti. (From Biossonnault, JS and Kotarinus, RK: Diastasis recti. In Wilder, E (ed): Obstetric and Gynecologic Physical Therapy. Churchill-Livingstone, New York, 1988, p. 397 with permission).

b. Diastasis recti possibly occurs in pregnancy as a result of hormonal effects on the connective tissue and the biomechanical changes of pregnancy. It causes no discomfort.[22]

c. It is relatively uncommon in the first trimester, but the incidence increases as the pregnancy progresses, reaching a peak in the third trimester.

d. It does not always spontaneously resolve following childbirth and may continue past the 6-week postpartum period.

e. It can occur above, below, or at the level of the umbilicus but appears to be less common below the umbilicus.

f. It appears to be less common in women with good abdominal tone prior to pregnancy.[2]

3. Significance

a. The condition of diastasis recti may produce musculoskeletal complaints (e.g., low back pain) possibly as a result of decreased ability of the abdominal musculature to control the pelvis and lumbar spine.

b. In severe separations, the anterior segment of the abdominal wall is composed only of skin, fascia, subcutaneous fat, and peritoneum.[2,6,28] The lack of abdominal support provides less protection for the fetus.

c. Severe cases of diastasis recti may progress to herniation of the abdominal viscera through the separation in the abdominal wall.

4. Diastasis recti test[2,5,6,8,22,35]

Patient position: hook-lying. Have the patient slowly raise her head and shoulders off the floor, reaching her hands toward the knees, until the spine of the scapula leaves the floor. The therapist places the fingers of 1 hand horizontally across the mid-line of the abdomen at the umbilicus (Figure 18-4). If a separation exists, the fingers will sink into the gap. The diastasis is measured by the number of fingers that can be placed be-

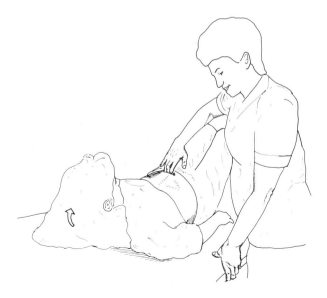

FIGURE 18-4. Diastasis recti test.

tween the rectus muscle bellies. A diastasis can also present as a longitudinal bulge along the linea alba. Since a diastasis recti can occur above, below, or at the level of the umbilicus, it should be tested at all three areas.

5. Treatment of diastasis recti
   a. Test all pregnant clients for the presence of diastasis recti prior to performing abdominal exercises.
   b. Perform corrective exercise for diastasis recti exclusive of other abdominal exercise until the separation is decreased to 2 cm or less (see Section IV).[22] At that time, abdominal exercise can be resumed, but the integrity of the linea alba should be monitored to make sure the separation continues to decrease.

B. Low back pain[1,5,10,11,22,26,28,35]

1. Postural
   a. Pain commonly occurs due to the postural changes of pregnancy, increased ligamentous laxity, and decreased abdominal function.
   b. The symptoms of low back pain usually worsen with muscle fatigue, static postures, or as the day progresses; symptoms are usually relieved with rest or change of position.
   c. Low back symptoms can be treated effectively with proper body mechanics and posture instructions (see Chapter 14; see also section IV of this chapter). The use of deep-heating agents, electrical stimulation, traction, and other treatment options is generally contraindicated during pregnancy.
   d. Usually back symptoms disappear following pregnancy if proper body mechanics are used during child care and daily activities.

2. Sacroiliac (SI) back pain
   a. The incidence of SI back pain is unknown but appears to be fairly common in pregnancy. It is caused by ligamentous laxity coupled with postural adaptations.
   b. Symptoms of SI dysfunction include pain with prolonged sitting, standing, or walking; pain when climbing stairs; unilateral standing or torsion activities; pain that is not relieved by rest and frequently worsens with activity. There also may be pubic symphysis discomfort, subluxation, or both.[27]
   c. The problems may be treated with gentle mobilization or muscle energy techniques, followed by the use of external stabilization such as belts or corsets designed for use by pregnant women. These techniques are beyond the scope of this chapter.
   d. Exercise must be modified so as not to aggravate the condition. Single-leg weight bearing should be avoided. Other activities may need to be modified to minimize stresses on the symptomatic tissues; for example, sitting in the car, side-lying with a pillow between the legs, sexual activities.

C. Varicose Veins[28]
   1. Varicosities are aggravated in pregnancy by the increased uterine weight, venous stasis in the legs, and increased venous distensibility.
   2. Occasionally, there may be a range of mild discomfort to severe pain in the lower extremities.

3. Exercises may need to be modified so that minimal weight bearing is required.
4. Elastic support stockings should be worn to provide an external pressure gradient against the distended veins, and the women should be encouraged to elevate the lower extremities as often as possible.

D. Pelvic Floor Dysfunction[7,15,22,28,33–36]

1. **Structure of the pelvic floor (Figure 18-5A):**

    The pelvic floor is a multilayered sheet of muscle stretched between the pubis and coccyx, forming the inferior support to the abdominopelvic cavity. The pelvic floor is pierced by the urethra, vagina, and rectum. The major muscle of the pelvic floor is the pubococcygeus muscle.

2. **Functions of the pelvic floor**
    a. Provides support for the pelvic organs and their contents
    b. Withstands increases in intra-abdominal pressure
    c. Provides sphincter control of the perineal openings
    d. Functions in reproductive and sexual activities

3. **Dysfunction**
    a. Muscle and soft-tissue laxity
        (1) The pelvic organs drop from their normal alignment due to increased pressure on the pelvic floor musculature, and organ prolapse may occur (Figure 18-5B).
        (2) Urinary stress incontinence (involuntary urine loss with increases in abdominal pressure) may occur and worsen with subsequent pregnancies, increases in weight, or aging.
    b. Pelvic floor disruption
        (1) Episiotomy—an incision in the pelvic floor made during childbirth to enlarge the vaginal opening and allow faster delivery. It can produce prolonged pain, cause scarring, or become infected.
        (2) Tears and lacerations may occur during childbirth, particularly if the baby is large or if a forceps delivery is necessary.
    c. Hypertonicity—an increase in muscle tension or fascial tightness of the pelvic floor significant enough to impair normal sexual and elimination functions. This problem may occur as a result of improper postpartum healing and may be quite painful.[35]

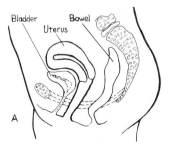
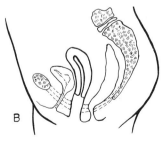

FIGURE 18-5. Good pelvic floor support with a firm base, organs in place (*A*); inadequate support and the hammock stage, contents descended (*B*).

    4. Symptoms of pelvic floor dysfunction may be treated with

      a. therapeutic exercise techniques to improve for control and relaxation of the muscles (see Section IV).

      b. modalities such as superficial heat, ice, and massage prenatally. Postpartum transcutaneous electrical stimulation or electrical muscle stimulation could also be used.

E. Joint Laxity[5,10,11,22,26,28,35]

1. Significance

    a. All joint structures are at increased risk of injury during pregnancy and the immediate postpartum period.

    b. The ligamentous support is decreased and, therefore, injury can occur if women are not educated regarding joint protection.

2. Treatment of joint laxity

    a. The woman is taught safe exercises to perform during the childbearing year, including modification of exercises to decrease excessive joint stress (see Section IV) and posture training.

    b. Non–weight bearing or less stressful aerobic activities such as swimming, walking, or biking may be suggested, particularly for women who were exercising minimally before pregnancy.

IV. PREGNANCY AND POSTPARTUM EXERCISE[11,12,22,25–27,35]

A. Potential problems summarized

1. Development of faulty postures
2. Upper extremity stresses caused by the physical changes of pregnancy and the muscular requirements of infant care
3. Changing body image
4. Altered circulation, varicose veins, lower extremity edema
5. Pelvic floor stress or trauma
6. Abdominal muscle stretch and trauma, and diastasis recti
7. Decrease in cardiovascular fitness due to lack of knowledge about adequate and safe forms of exercise
8. Lack of knowledge about physical changes in pregnancy and childbirth, possibly increasing the chance that injury-inducing behaviors will occur
9. Inadequate relaxation skills, necessary for labor and delivery
10. Improper body mechanics
11. Development of musculoskeletal pathologies (described in section III) associated with pregnancy
12. Lack of physical preparation (strength, endurance, relaxation) necessary for labor and delivery
13. Unsafe progression of postpartum exercise

B. General Goals and Plan for the Exercise Program

Goals	*Plan of Care*
1. Promote improved posture before and after pregnancy	1. Posture evaluation Exercises to stretch, train, and strengthen postural muscles Posture awareness training
2. Increase awareness of correct body mechanics	2. Teach correct body mechanics in sitting, standing, lifting,

3. Prepare the upper extremities for the demands of infant care

4. Promote increased body awareness and a positive body image

5. Prepare the lower extremities for the demands of increased weight bearing and circulatory compromise

6. Improve awareness and control of the pelvic floor musculature

7. Maintain abdominal function and prevent or correct diastasis recti pathology

8. Promote or maintain safe cardiovascular fitness

9. Provide information about the changes of pregnancy and birth

10. Improve relaxation skills

11. Prevent problems associated with pregnancy (i.e., low back pain, pelvic floor weakness, decreased circulation)

12. Prepare physically for labor, delivery, and postpartum activities

13. Provide education on safe postpartum exercise progression

and lying as well as transitions from one position to another

3. Resistive exercises to appropriate muscles

4. Body awareness and proprioception activities
Posture reinforcement

5. Evaluation of lower extremity status
Use of elastic support stockings
Stretching exercises to reduce cramping
Resistive exercises to appropriate muscles for strengthening
Evaluation for proper footwear

6. Teach awareness of pelvic floor muscle contraction and relaxation
Train and strengthen for muscle control

7. Evaluate and monitor diastasis recti
Teach appropriate exercises
Teach safe abdominal-strengthening exercises

8. Instruct safe progression of aerobic exercise according to American College of Obstetricians and Gynecologists (ACOG) and American Physical Therapy Association (APTA) guidelines

9. Childbirth education classes

10. Teach relaxation techniques

11. Education about potential problems of pregnancy
Teach prevention techniques and appropriate exercises

12. Strengthen muscles needed in labor and delivery

13. Postpartum exercise instruction

C. Guidelines for Exercise Instruction[1,10,11,19,21,22,25,26,32]

1. Suggest each participant have a physical examination by a physician prior to engaging in an exercise program.
2. Each person should then be individually evaluated prior to participation in order to screen for pre-existing musculoskeletal problems, posture, and fitness level. Exercise levels should not exceed pre-pregnancy levels.
3. Stretching exercises should be specific to a single muscle or muscle group and should not involve several groups at once. Asymmetric stretching or stretching multiple muscle groups can promote joint instability. Ballistic movements should be avoided.
4. No joint should be taken beyond its normal physiologic range.
5. Hamstring and adductor stretches should be used with caution. Overstretching of these muscle groups can increase pelvic instability or hypermobility.
6. Limit activities in which balancing or single-leg weight bearing are required. These activities can promote sacroiliac or pubic symphysis discomfort.
7. The maximal heart rate during exercise should not exceed 140 beats per minute and 15 minutes duration at that heart rate. The pulse should be monitored frequently.[1,10,11,25]
8. It is suggested that supine positioning not exceed 5 minutes at any one time after the fourth month of pregnancy to avoid vena cava compression by the uterus. When supine, a small wedge or rolled towel placed under the right hip will lessen the effects of uterine compression on abdominal vessels and improve cardiac output by turning the patient slightly toward the left (Figure 18-6).[1,25]
9. To avoid the effects of postural hypotension, rising from the floor to standing should be done slowly.[11]
10. Discourage breath holding and avoid activities that increase the tendency toward the Valsalva maneuver, because this may lead to undesirable downward forces on the uterus and pelvic floor.
11. Break frequently for fluid replenishment. The risk of dehydration during exercise is increased in pregnancy.
12. Encourage complete bladder emptying prior to exercise. A full bladder will place increased stress on an already weakened pelvic floor.
13. Include appropriate warm-up and cool-down activities.
14. Adapt or discontinue any exercise that causes pain.
15. When prone, avoid the knee-chest position with buttocks elevated above the chest level, especially in the postpartum client, due to the risk of air embolism.[19,21,32] A pregnant woman is at risk only if bleeding or other

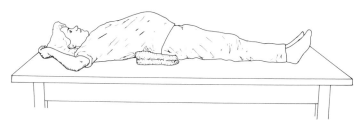

FIGURE 18-6. To prevent vena cava compressions when lying supine, a folded towel can be placed under the right side of the pelvis so patient is tipped slightly to the left.

symptoms of early placental detachment are present. An air embolism can occur when the buttocks are elevated and the uterus moves superiorly. The pressure change causes air to be sucked into the vagina and uterus, where it can enter the circulatory system through the open placental wound.

16. Observe participants closely for signs of overexertion or complications. The following signs are reasons to discontinue exercise and contact a physician:[11]

   a. Pain.
   b. Bleeding.
   c. Shortness of breath.
   d. Irregular heart beat.
   e. Dizziness.
   f. Faintness.
   g. Tachycardia.
   h. Back or pubic pain.
   i. Difficulty in walking.

D. Contraindications to Exercise[1,3,10,11,23,25,26,35]

1. Absolute contraindications (see Section VI for more detail)

   a. Incompetent cervix—early dilatation of the cervix before the pregnancy is full term.
   b. Vaginal bleeding of any amount.
   c. Placenta previa—placenta is located on the uterus in a position where it may detach before the baby is delivered.
   d. Rupture of membranes—loss of amniotic fluid prior to the onset of labor.
   e. Premature labor—labor beginning prior to the 37th week of pregnancy.
   f. Maternal heart disease.
   g. Maternal diabetes or hypertension.[10,11,35]

2. Precautions to exercise.

The woman with one or more of the following conditions may participate in exercise program under close observation by physician[1,3,11,23,25] and therapist as long as no complications arise. Exercises may require modification.

   a. Multiple gestation (These infants are frequently born prematurely. Since some exercises may precipitate uterine contractions, these patients must be watched closely.[23])
   b. Anemia—reduction in the number of red blood cells, the amount of hemoglobin, or both (causes a reduction in the oxygen-carrying capacity of the blood).
   c. Systemic infection.
   d. Extreme fatigue.
   e. Musculoskeletal complaints and/or pain.
   f. Overheating.
   g. Phlebitis.
   h. Diastasis recti.
   i. Uterine contractions (lasting several hours after exercise).

E. Suggested Sequence for Exercise Class[1,26,35]

1. Warm-up activities and stretches.

2. Upper extremity activities for cardiovascular warm-up.
3. Aerobic activity for cardiovascular conditioning (15 minutes or less).
4. Upper and lower extremity strengthening.
5. Cool-down activities.
6. Abdominal exercises.
7. Pelvic floor exercises.
8. Relaxation techniques.
9. Educational information (as appropriate).
10. Postpartum exercise instruction (e.g., when to begin exercises, how to safely progress, precautions), since client may not attend a postpartum class.

F. **Critical Areas of Emphasis and Selected Exercise Techniques**[1,10,12,22,25,26]
  1. **Postural correction**
     a. **Strengthening** (see Chapters 9, 10, 11, 12, and 14)
        (1) Upper neck flexors, lower neck and upper thoracic extensors.
        (2) Scapular retractors and depressors.
        (3) Shoulder external rotators.
        (4) Trunk flexors (abdominals).
        (5) Hip extensors.
        (6) Knee extensors.
        (7) Ankle dorsiflexors.
     b. **Stretching** (with caution).
        (1) Upper neck extensors, scalenes, and levator scapulae.
        (2) Pectoral muscles (major and minor).
        (3) Low back extensors.
        (4) Hip adductors (do not overstretch in women with pelvic instabilities).
        (5) Knee flexors (do not overstretch in women with pelvic instabilities).
        (6) Ankle plantarflexors.

  2. **Abdominal muscle strengthening**[2,5,6,8,9,16,20,22,29,35]
     As pregnancy progresses, the abdominals will not tolerate strenuous exercise. Therefore, exercise must be adapted to meet the needs of each individual. A check for diastasis recti must always be performed before initiating abdominal exercise. The following exercises progress from least to most strenuous.
     a. **Corrective exercises for diastasis recti** (Figure 18-7)[5,22]
        (1) Head lift.
            Position of woman: Supine hook-lying with her hands crossed over midline at the diastasis to support the area. As she exhales, she lifts only her head off the floor or until the point just before a bulge appears. Her hands should gently pull the rectus muscles toward midline. Then have the woman lower her head slowly and relax. This exercise emphasizes the rectus abdominus muscle and minimizes the obliques.
        (2) Head lift with pelvic tilt.
            Patient position: Supine hook-lying. If diastasis recti is present, the arms are crossed over the diastasis and pulled toward midline. She slowly lifts her head off the floor while simultaneously performing a posterior pelvic tilt (see Chapter 14), then slowly lowers her head

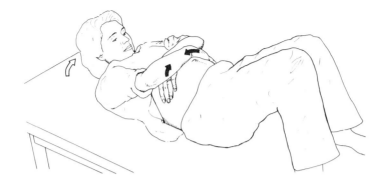

FIGURE 18-7. Corrective exercise for diastasis recti. The patient pulls with arms toward midline.

and relaxes. All abdominal contractions should be performed with an exhalation so that intra-abdominal pressure is minimized. Only this exercise and/or the head lift should be used until the separation is corrected to 2 cm or 2 finger widths.[22]

b. **Leg sliding** (Figures 18-8A and B)[22]
   (1) Patient position: Hook-lying with pelvis in posterior tilt. The woman holds the pelvic tilt as she first slides one foot along the floor until it is straight. She stops sliding the foot at the point when she can no longer hold the pelvic tilt. Slowly she lifts the leg and brings it back to the starting position, then repeats with the other leg. Breathing should be coordinated with the exercise so that abdominal contraction occurs with exhalation.
   (2) This exercise can be done with both legs at the same time if abdominal muscles can maintain the pelvic tilt through the entire exercise.

c. **Prone abdominal exercise**[5,8,9,20]
   (1) Patient position: All-4s position on hands and knees. Instruct her to do a posterior pelvic tilt. While keeping her back straight, she sucks the abdomen in and holds. Then she releases and performs an anterior tilt through partial range.
   (2) For additional exercise, while holding the abdomen in and the back straight, laterally flex the trunk to the right (side bend to the right), looking at the right hip, then reverse to the left.

d. **Curl-downs** (see Chapter 14)
e. **Curl-ups** (see Chapter 14)
f. **Leg lowering—postpartum only** (see Chapter 14)

3. **Pelvic floor awareness training and strengthening**
   a. **Isometric exercises**
      (1) Patient position: Supine or side-lying positions are the easiest in which to begin; progress to sitting or standing
      (2) Instruct the woman to tighten the pelvic floor as if attempting to stop urine flow. Hold for 3 to 5 seconds and relax.[22,31] The bladder should be empty when performing this exercise.

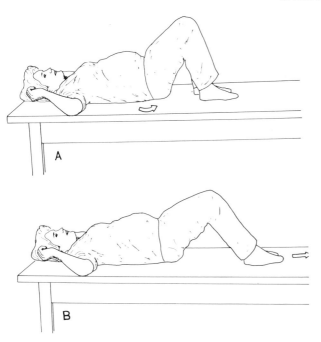

FIGURE 18-8. Leg sliding: supine hook-lying with posterior pelvic tilt (*A*). Maintain pelvic tilt as the feet slide along the floor away from the body (*B*).

(3) The pelvic floor muscles are highly fatigable. Contractions should not be held longer than 5 seconds and with a maximum of 10 repetitions per session.[22,31] When fatigued, substitution of the gluteals, abdominals, or hip adductors may occur.

b. **"Elevator" (graded isometric) exercise**
(1) Instruct the woman to visually imagine riding in an elevator. As the elevator goes from one floor to the next, contract the pelvic floor muscles a little more.
(2) Relax the muscles gradually, as if the elevator were descending one floor at a time.

4. **Upper and lower extremity strengthening**

As the abdomen enlarges it becomes impossible to comfortably assume the prone position. Exercises that are usually performed in prone position must be modified.

a. **Standing push-ups**[9,29]
Patient position: Standing facing a wall, feet pointing straight forward, a shoulder-width apart and approximately an arm-length way from wall. The palms are placed on the wall at shoulder height. Have the woman slowly bend the elbows, bringing her face close to wall, maintaining pelvic tilt, and keeping heels on the floor. Her elbows should be shoulder height. She then slowly pushes with her arms, bringing body back to original position.

b. **Hip extension**[8,9,22]
(1) Supine bridging (see Figure 10-12).
(2) All-4s leg raising (Figure 18-9A and B)

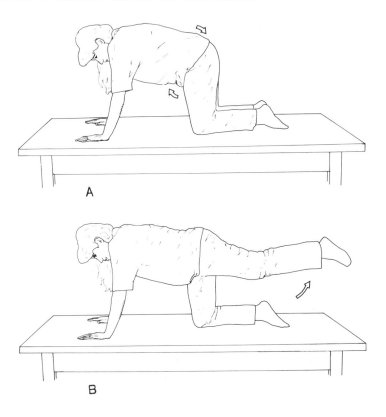

FIGURE 18-9. All-4s leg raising: Patient assumes quadriped position with posterior pelvic tilt (*A*). Leg is raised only until it is in line with the trunk (*B*).

Patient position: On hands and knees (hands may be in fists or palms open and flat). Instruct the woman to first do a posterior pelvic tilt then slowly lift one leg, extending the hip to a level no higher than the spine while keeping the back straight. She then slowly lowers the leg and repeats on with opposite side. The knee may remain flexed or can be straightened throughout the exercise. Monitor this exercise for stress on the SI joint or ligaments.

c. **Scapular retraction**
Patient position: Sitting, arms flexed to shoulder height, elbows may be flexed; arms should be together in midline. The woman slowly abducts her arms horizontally, pinching the scapulae together, then brings her arms slowly back to the original position, keeping her arms at shoulder height.

5. **Activities to promote pelvic proprioception and awareness**
   a. **Pelvic clock**[13,20]
      (1) Patient position: Supine hook-lying.
      (2) Instruct the woman to imagine her pelvis as the face of a clock. The top of the clock (12 o'clock) is the pubic symphysis and the bottom

(6 o'clock) is the sacrum. She slowly rotates the pelvis in a clockwise motion, keeping the movement smooth, then reverses and rotates the pelvis smoothly in a counterclockwise direction.

b. **Pelvic clock progressions**
The exercise, once mastered, can also be done in side-lying, all-4s, sitting, or standing positions.

6. **Activities to prepare for labor and delivery**
  a. **Relaxation**[22,26,35]
    (1) Muscle setting
      (a) Have the woman lie in a comfortable position.
      (b) Have her begin with the lower body. Instruct her to gently tighten and then relax first the muscles in the feet; then progress to the legs, thighs, pelvic floor, and buttocks.
      (c) Next progress to the upper extremities and trunk, then to the head.
      (d) Reinforce the importance of remaining awake and aware of sensations of the muscles contracting and relaxing.
      (e) Add deep, slow, relaxed breathing to the routine.
    (2) Selective tension.
      Progress her to the awareness of muscles contracting in one part of the body while remaining relaxed in other parts.
    (3) Mental imagery.
      Using music or verbal guidance, instruct the woman to concentrate on a relaxing mental image.
  b. **Breathing exercises** (see Chapter 19)
  c. **Squatting**[5,8,22,26]
    (1) This exercise prepares the legs and pelvis for childbirth and also promotes good body mechanics for lifting. It can be done supine, side-lying, or sitting on a small stool and then may progress to the more difficult standing position when comfortable. A woman with knee problems may do a partial squat or support herself by holding on to a counter or bar.
    (2) Supine: Instruct the woman to abduct the hips and pull the knees toward the chest.
    (3) Side-lying: Instruct the woman to pull the knees toward the chest with the hips abducted.
    (4) Sitting: Have the woman sit on a small stool with the hips abducted and feet flat on the floor.
    (5) Standing: Instruct the woman to stand with feet shoulder-width apart or wider, facing a counter, chair, or wall on which she can rest her hands. She slowly squats as far as is comfortable, keeping feet flat (no pronation), knees apart and over the feet, and back straight. This exercise can be done using pillows or a therapeutic ball for support until she becomes accustomed to the exercise.
  d. **Pelvic floor awareness.**[5,15,22]
    (1) The woman is instructed to contract the pelvic floor as in the strengthening exercise, then allow total voluntary release and relaxation of pelvic floor.
    (2) This activity is coordinated with breathing.

G. Exercises That Are Contraindicated During Pregnancy

1. Bilateral straight leg raising

This exercise typically places more stress on the abdominal muscles than they can tolerate. It can cause back injury or diastasis recti.

2. "Fire hydrant" exercise

This exercise is done on hands and knees. With the hip and knee flexed, the hip is abducted. If the leg is elevated too high, compression of the SI joint can occur. The exercise can be done safely if hip abduction remains within the physiologic range (see Figure 22-3). It should be avoided by any woman who has pre-existing SI joint symptoms.

3. All-4s hip extension

This exercise can be performed safely as explained earlier in this chapter (Figure 18-9). It becomes unsafe and can cause low back pain when the leg is elevated beyond the physiologic range of hip extension.

4. Unilateral weight bearing activities

Weight bearing on one leg (which includes slouched standing with the majority of weight shifted to one leg and the pelvis tilted down on the opposite side) during pregnancy can cause SI joint irritation and should be avoided by women with pre-existing SI joint symptoms. Unilateral weight bearing also can cause balance problems due to the increasing body weight and shifting of the center of gravity.

H. Maternal Response to Aerobic Exercise[1,10,11,35]

1. Aerobic exercise does not reduce blood flow to the brain and heart. It does, however, cause a redistribution of blood flow away from the internal organs and toward the working muscles.
2. The maternal respiration rate appears to adapt to mild exercise but does not increase proportionately with moderate and severe exercise when compared with a nonpregnant state. The pregnant woman reaches a maximum exercise capacity at a lower work level than a nonpregnant woman due to the increased oxygen requirements of exercise.
3. The maternal hematocrit level during pregnancy is lowered; however, it rises up to 10 percentage points within 15 minutes of beginning vigorous exercise. This condition continues for up to 4 weeks postpartum. As a result, cardiac reserve is decreased during exercise.[11]
4. Compression of the inferior vena cava by the uterus can occur after the fourth month of pregnancy, altering venous return and cardiac output. This has been suggested as a possible cause of *abruptio placenta* or premature detachment of the placenta from the uterus.
5. A caloric intake of an additional 500 calories per day is necessary to support the energy needs of pregnancy and exercise, as opposed to only a 300-calorie-per-day increase for the sedentary pregnant woman, who does not participate in any aerobic conditioning program.[1]
6. Vigorous physical activity and dehydration through perspiration can cause body core temperature to increase. This occurs in anyone who exercises but is significant to the pregnant woman because of the relationship of elevated core temperature to neural tube defects of the fetus. An increase above 39°C has rarely been found, however.

7. Hypoglycemia may occur with prolonged or strenuous exercise. This occurs more rapidly in pregnancy as a result of the elevated blood insulin level.

8. Norepinephrine and epinephrine levels increase with exercise. Norepinephrine increases the strength and frequency of uterine contractions. This may pose a problem for the woman at risk of developing premature labor.

I. Fetal Response to Maternal Aerobic Exercise[1,10,11,35]

1. No conclusive human research has proved a detrimental fetal response to mild- or moderate-intensity maternal exercise. The risk of fetal injury is probably low, but conservative levels of exercise are nonetheless recommended.

2. A 50 percent or greater reduction of uterine blood flow is necessary before fetal well-being is affected (based on animal research). This significant a decrease is unlikely to occur with mild or moderate exercise of short duration (i.e., 15 minutes) but is more likely to occur with strenuous and prolonged exercise.[1,11]

3. The fetal heart rate (FHR) usually will increase 10 to 30 beats per minute at the onset of maternal exercise but may occasionally progress to bradycardia, indicating fetal asphyxia. Following mild to moderate maternal exercise, the FHR usually returns to normal levels within 15 minutes, but in some cases the FHR may remain elevated as long as 30 minutes following strenuous maternal exercise.

4. The healthy fetus appears to be able to tolerate brief episodes of asphyxia with no detrimental results.

5. The fetus has no mechanism such as perspiration or respiration by which to dissipate heat. Therefore, an increase in maternal core temperature over 39°C as a result of exercise could produce a dangerous increase in fetal core temperature. This has been associated with the increased incidence of birth defects (based on animal studies and human reports).[1]

J. Exercise Critical to the Postpartum Period[1,22,35]

1. Uncomplicated vaginal delivery

Exercise can be started as soon after delivery as the woman feels able to exercise. All prenatal exercises can be done safely in the postpartum period. Some exercises should be initiated as soon as possible after delivery.

a. Pelvic floor strengthening. Exercises should be initiated as soon after the birth as possible. This exercise may increase circulation and aid healing.[22]

b. Diastasis recti correction. Exercises should begin approximately 3 days after delivery and continue until correction to 2 cm is achieved. At that time, more vigorous abdominal exercise can be initiated. Until 3 days post-delivery, the abdominal musculature is too stretched to accurately test for diastasis recti. Therefore, the test should not be done until 3 days post-delivery.[22]

c. Aerobic and strengthening exercises. As soon as the woman feels able, exercise can be resumed. A physical examination is suggested prior to the onset of vigorous exercise.

2. Cesarean delivery

Following a cesarean section, the woman should wait at least 6 to 8 weeks before resuming vigorous exercise. A health care professional should be consulted prior to beginning a postpartum exercise program.

3. Exercise precautions
a. If bleeding increases or turns bright red, exercise should be postponed. The woman should rest more and allow a longer recovery time.
b. Joint laxity may be present for some time after delivery, especially if the woman is breastfeeding. Precautions should be taken to protect the joints as described previously.
c. Adequate warm-up and cool-down time is important.
d. The prone knee-chest position should be avoided for at least 6 weeks postpartum due to the risk of air embolism (see Section IV).

V. CESAREAN CHILDBIRTH[5,16,22–24,28,30]

A. Definition
Delivery of a baby through an incision in the abdominal wall and uterus rather than through the pelvis and vagina. General, spinal, or epidural aesthesia may be used.

B. Significance to Physical Therapists
1. Cesarean section is the single most common operation performed in the United States.[24]
2. The cesarean birth rate in the United States is 22.7 per 100 live births (1985); therefore, for those dealing with an obstetric population, the likelihood of treating a post-cesarean patient is high.[24]
3. Women who have had cesarean deliveries still require pelvic floor rehabilitation. Many woman experience a lengthy labor and trial pushing before a cesarean section is deemed necessary. Therefore, the pelvic floor musculature and tissues are not spared the stress of labor. Also, pregnancy itself creates significant stress on the pelvic floor musculature and tissues.
4. Rehabilitation of the patient who had cesarean delivery is essentially the same as that of the patient who has had a vaginal delivery. However, a cesarean section is major abdominal surgery with all the risks and complications of such surgeries. The patient with a cesarean section will also require general postsurgical rehabilitation.
5. Many childbirth preparation classes do not adequately educate and prepare couples for the experience of a cesarean delivery. As a result, the patient with a cesarean section frequently feels as if her body has failed her, causing her to have more emotional changes than a woman who has experienced a more traditional delivery.

C. General Treatment Goals and Plan of Care

Goals	Plan of Care
1. Improve pulmonary function and decrease the risk of pneumonia	1. Breathing instruction Coughing and/or huffing[16,22]
2. Decrease incisional pain associated with coughing, movement, or breastfeeding	2. Postoperative TENS Support incision with pillow when coughing or breastfeeding

	Incisional support with pillow or hands when exercising Education regarding incisional care and risk of injury
3. Prevent postsurgical vascular complications	3. Active leg exercises to promote circulation and decrease venous stasis Early ambulation
4. Enhance incisional circulation healing; prevent adhesion formation	4. Gentle abdominal exercise with incisional support Scar mobilization and friction massage
5. Decrease postsurgical discomfort from flatulence, itching, or catheter	5. Positioning instruction, massage, and supportive exercises
6. Correct posture	6. Posture instruction
7. Protected activities of daily living (ADL) to prevent injury	7. Instruction in incisional splinting and positioning for ADL Body mechanics instruction
8. Musculoskeletal rehabilitation	8. Postpartum exercises (see Section IV)
9. Prevent pelvic floor dysfunction	9. Pelvic floor exercises (see Section IV)

D. Suggested Activities for the Patient with a Cesarean Section[16,22]

1. All prenatal and postpartum exercises should be performed by the woman.

Abdominal exercises will need to be progressed more slowly (check for diastasis). Protect the area of incision as with diastasis.

2. Coughing or huffing

a. Coughing is difficult due to pain. An alternative is huffing.[22] A huff is a forceful outward breath using the diaphragm rather than the abdominals to push air out of the lungs. The abdominals are pulled up and in, rather than pushed out, causing decreased pressure in the abdominal cavity and less strain on the incision.

b. Huffing must be done quickly to generate sufficient force to expel mucus.

c. Patient instructions

(1) Support the incision with a pillow or the hands.

(2) Say "ha" forcefully while pulling in the abdominal muscles.

3. Exercise to relieve intestinal gas pains[16,22]

a. Abdominal massage or kneading while lying on the left side

b. Pelvic tilting and/or bridging (can be done in conjunction with massage)

c. Bridge and twist.[22] Maintain a position of bridging while twisting hips to the right and left. This position may also facilitate air embolism and should be used with caution in the early postpartum period.

d. Partial abdominal curl-up

4. Scar mobilization

Cross friction massage should be initiated as soon as sufficient healing has occurred. This will minimize adhesions that may contribute to postural problems and back pain.

VI. HIGH-RISK PREGNANCY[3,17,18,26,28]

A. Definition

A pregnancy that is complicated by disease or problems that put the mother or fetus at risk for illness or death. Conditions may be pre-existing, be induced by pregnancy, or be an abnormal physiologic reaction during pregnancy.[17] The goal of medical intervention is to prevent preterm delivery usually through use of bed rest, restriction of activity, and medications when appropriate.

B. Conditions Considered High Risk

1. Preterm rupture of membranes

The amniotic sac breaks and amniotic fluid is lost prior to onset of labor. This can be dangerous to the fetus if it occurs before fetal development is complete. Labor may begin spontaneously after the membranes rupture. The chance for fetal infection also increases when the protection of the amniotic sac is lost.

2. Premature onset of labor

Labor that begins prior to 37 weeks of gestation or before completion of fetal development. Fetal life is endangered if delivery occurs too early.

3. Incompetent cervix

Painless dilatation of the cervix that occurs in the second trimester (after 16 weeks' gestation) or early third trimester of pregnancy. This leads to premature membrane rupture and delivery of a fetus too small to survive.

4. Placenta previa

The placenta attaches too low on the uterus, near the cervix. As the cervix dilates, the placenta begins to separate from the uterus and may present before the fetus, thus endangering fetal life. Symptoms are intermittent, recurrent, painless bleeding, increasing in intensity.

5. Pregnancy-related hypertension or pre-eclampsia

Characterized by hypertension, protein in the urine, and severe fluid retention. This can progress to maternal convulsions, coma, and death if it becomes severe (eclampsia). It usually occurs in the third trimester and disappears following birth. The cause is not understood.

6. Multiple gestation

More than one fetus forms. Complications of multiple gestation include premature onset of labor and birth, increased incidence of perinatal mortality, lower birth weight infants, and increased incidence of maternal complications (e.g., hypertension).

7. Diabetes

Maternal diabetes can be present before pregnancy or may occur as a result of the physiologic stress of pregnancy. Gestational diabetes (caused by pregnancy) usually disappears following pregnancy, but a greater tendency for development of the disease at some future time remains.

C. Complaints or Complications of the Bed-Bound Patient[26]

1. Joint stiffness and muscle aches
2. Muscle weakness and atrophy
3. Vascular complications
4. Decreased proprioception in distal body parts
5. Constipation due to lack of exercise
6. Postural changes
7. Boredom
8. Emotional stress—patient may be at risk of losing the baby
9. Guilt from the belief that some activity caused the problem or that the patient did not take good enough care of herself
10. Anxiety about her home situation or the impending birth

D. General Goals and Plan for Treatment of the Bed-Bound High-Risk Client[26]

Goal	Plan
1. Decrease stiffness	1. Positioning instructions Facilitation of joint motion in available range
2. Maintain muscle length and bulk and improve circulation	2. Stretching and strengthening exercises within limits imposed by the physician
3. Improve proprioception	3. Movement activities for as many body parts as possible
4. Improve posture within available limits	4. Posture instruction, modified as necessary based on allowed activity level Bed mobility and transfer techniques if able
5. Relieve boredom	5. Vary activities and positioning for exercises
6. Stress management and enhanced relaxation	6. Relaxation techniques
7. Prepare for delivery	7. Childbirth education, breathing training, and exercises to assist and prepare for labor
8. Enhance postpartum recovery	8. Exercise instruction and home program for postpartum period Body mechanics instruction

E. Guidelines and Precautions[26]

1. All exercise programs for high-risk populations should be individually established based on diagnosis, limitations, physical therapy evaluation, and consultation with the physician. Activities must address patient needs but should not further complicate the condition.
2. The therapist should re-evaluate the patient after each treatment and note any changes.

3. The patient must be closely monitored during all activities.
4. Some exercises, especially abdominal exercises, may stimulate uterine contractions and, therefore, may need to be modified or discontinued.
5. A full bladder may stimulate uterine contractions. The patient should be encouraged to empty her bladder frequently.
6. Any uterine contractions, bleeding, or amniotic fluid loss must be monitored and reported.
7. No Valsalva maneuvers should be allowed. Any increases in intra-abdominal pressure should be avoided.
8. Exercises should be slow, smooth, and simple and should require minimal exertion.
9. It is necessary to develop good rapport with the patient; she must trust the therapist.
10. Many high-risk pregnancies result in cesarean deliveries, so the patient should be educated about cesarean delivery rehabilitation.
11. Incorporate maximum muscle activities into each movement.
12. Teach the patient self-monitoring techniques.

F. Suggestions for Exercise Programs[26]

1. Positioning instructions
   a. Left side-lying to prevent vena cava compression, enhance cardiac output, and decrease lower extremity edema
   b. Pillows to support body parts and enhance relaxation
   c. Supine positioning for short periods, with a wedge placed under the right hip to decrease inferior vena cava compression (see Figure 18-6).
   d. Modified prone positioning (side-lying, partially rolled toward prone, with pillow under abdomen) to decrease low back discomfort and pressure

2. Range of motion instructions
   a. Active range of motion (ROM) of all joints should be included.
   b. Motions should be slow, nonstressful, and through the full range if possible.
   c. Teach in a gravity-neutral position if antigravity ROM is too stressful.
   d. The number of repetitions and frequency needs to be individualized to the woman's condition.

3. Suggested exercises
   a. **Lying**
      (1) Supine or side-lying alternate knee to chest
      (2) Ankle pumping
      (3) Shoulder, elbow, and finger flexion and extension; reach to ceiling; arm circles
      (4) Unilateral straight leg raise in supine or side-lying position
      (5) Bilateral active ROM in diagonal patterns for the upper and lower extremities
      (6) Lower extremity abduction and adduction
      (7) Pelvic tilt, bridging, gluteal setting
      (8) Abdominal exercises (check for diastasis); these should be very mild and closely monitored
      (9) Pelvic floor exercises

b. **Sitting (may not be allowed)**
   (1) Feet dangling over edge of bed
   (2) Hip adductor and internal rotator stretch; tailor sitting
   (3) Upper extremity push-ups
   (4) Active ROM through diagonal patterns for upper and lower extremities
   (5) Ankle-pumping exercises
   (6) Alternate active ROM knee flexion and extension
   (7) Knee extension with ankle dorsiflexed to stretch hamstrings and heel cords
   (8) Arms reaching toward ceiling, then out to the side; arm circles added
   (9) Scapular retraction, with hands behind the head
   (10) Cervical ROM emphasizing flexion and lateral bending
c. **Ambulation (almost always contraindicated; when allowed, usually will be only to use bathroom)**
   (1) Good posture in ambulation
   (2) Tip-toe or heel-walking
   (3) Gentle, partial-range squatting to stretch quadriceps
   (4) Lower extremity rotation

3. **Relaxation techniques (see Section IV)**

4. **Bed mobility and transfer activities**
   a. Moving up, down, side-to-side in bed.
   b. Rolling—incorporate neck and upper and lower extremities to aid movement.
   c. Supine to sitting, assisted by arms.

5. **Preparation for labor**
   a. Relaxation techniques.
   b. Modified squatting—supine, sitting, or side-lying with knees to chest (see section IV).
   c. Pelvic floor relaxation.
   d. Breathing exercises.

6. **Postpartum exercise instruction (see Section IV)**

VII. SUMMARY

This chapter provided an overview of pregnancy, labor, and delivery for the' apists working with the obstetric patient. Specific anatomic and physiologic changes that occur during pregnancy were enumerated. They included weight gain, changes in the organ systems, and postural changes. Certain pregnancy-induced pathologies including diastasis recti, low back pain, varicose veins, pelvic floor dysfunction, and joint laxity were also discussed and guidelines for treatment were described.

Specific exercises for pregnancy and the postpartum period were outlined. Critical areas of emphasis for exercise, contraindications to exercise, and sequencing of exercise classes were covered. The maternal and fetal responses to aerobic exercise were discussed. Exercise guidelines and precautions for high-risk pregnancy and cesarean childbirth were covered separately.

REFERENCES

1. Artal, R and Wiswell, R: *Exercise in Pregnancy.* Williams & Wilkins, Baltimore, 1986.
2. Boissonnault, J and Blaschak, M.: *Incidence of diastasis recti abdominis during the childbearing years.* Phys Ther 68:1082, 1988.
3. Boston Children's Medical Center and Feinbloom, R: *Pregnancy, Birth and the Newborn Baby,* ed 1. New York, Dell Publishing, 1979.
4. Boston Women's Health Book Collective: *Our Bodies, Our Selves,* ed 2. Simon & Schuster, New York, 1979.
5. Brewer, G: *The Pregnancy After 30 Workbook,* ed 1. Emmaus, Pa, Rodale Press, 1978.
6. Bursch, S: *Interrater reliability of diastasis recti abdominis measurement.* Phys Ther 67:1077, 1987.
7. Chiarelli, P and O'Keefe, D: *Physiotherapy for the pelvic floor.* Aust J Physiother 27:4, 1981.
8. Dale, B and Roeber, J: *The Pregnancy Exercise Book.* New York, Pantheon Books, 1982.
9. De Lyser, F: *Jane Fonda's Workout Book for Pregnancy, Birth and Recovery.* Simon & Schuster, New York, 1982.
10. *Exercise During Pregnancy and the Postnatal Period.* ACOG: Pregnancy, Work and Disability (Technical Bulletin No 58). Washington, DC, ACOG, 1980.
11. *Exercise During Pregnancy and the Postnatal Period.* ACOG Home Exercise Programs, Washington, DC, 1985.
12. Feigel, D: *Evaluating Prenatal and Postpartum Exercise Classes.* Bulletin of Section on Obstetrics and Gynecology, American Physical Therapy Association, 7:12, 1983.
13. Feldenkrais, M: *Awareness Through Movement: Health Exercises for Personal Growth,* ed 1. Harper & Row, New York, 1972.
14. Flanagan, G: *The First Nine Months of Life,* ed 2. Simon & Schuster, New York, 1962.
15. Frahm, J: *Strengthening the Pelvic Floor.* Clinical Management in Physical Therapy 5:30, 1985.
16. Gent, D and Gottlieb, K: *Cesarean Rehabilitation.* Clinical Management in Physical Therapy 5:14, 1985.
17. Gilbert, E and Harman, J: *High-Risk Pregnancy and Delivery,* ed 1. CV Mosby, St Louis, 1986.
18. Ingalls, A and Salerno, M: *Maternal and Child Health Nursing,* ed 5. CV Mosby, St Louis, 1983.
19. *Knee-Chest Exercises and Maternal Death: Comments.* Med J Aust 1:1127, 1973.
20. Mandelstam, D: *The pelvic floor,* Physiotherapy 64:8, 1978.
21. Markowiz, E and Brainen, H: *Baby Dance: A Comprehensive Guide to Prenatal and Postpartum Exercise.* Prentice-Hall, Englewood Cliffs, NJ, 1980.
22. Nelson, P: *Pulmonary Gas Embolism in Pregnancy and the Puerpurium.* Obstet Gynecol Surv 15, 1960.
23. Noble, E: *Essential Exercises for the Childbearing Years,* ed 2. Houghton Mifflin, Boston, 1982.
24. Noble, E: *Having Twins,* ed 1. Houghton Mifflin, Boston, 1980.
25. Norwood, C: *Cesarean Variations: Patients, Facilities or Policies.* International Journal of Childbirth Education 1:4, 1986.
26. *Perinatal Exercise Guidelines.* Section on Obstetrics and Gynecology, American Physical Therapy Assocation, 1986.
27. *Physical Therapy Assessment and Treatment of the Female Patient.* Obstetrical and Gynecological Implications, March 15–21, 1986. Sponsored by Programs in Physical Therapy Northwestern University Medical School and Section on Obstetrics and Gynecology, American Physical Therapy Assocation.
28. *Position Paper.* Section on Obstetrics and Gynecology: Bulletin of Section on Obstetrics and Gynecology, American Physical Therapy Association 8:6, 1984.
29. Pritchard, J and MacDonald, P (eds): *Williams' Obstetrics,* ed 16. Appleton-Century-Crofts, New York, 1976.
30. Prudden, S and Sussman, J: *Pregnancy and Back-to-Shape Exercise Program.* Workman Publishing, New York, 1980.
31. Sandberg, E: *Synopsis of Obstetrics,* ed 10. CV Mosby, St Louis, 1978.
32. Santiesteban, A: *Electromyographic and dynamometric characteristics of female pelvic floor musculature.* Phys Ther 68:344, 1988.

33. Shrock, P, Simkin, P and Shearer M: *Teaching prenatal exercise: Part II—Exercises to think twice about.* Birth Fam J 8:3, 1981.
34. Tchow, D, et al: *Pelvic-floor musculature exercises in treatment of anatomical urinary stress incontinence.* Phys Ther 68:652, 1988.
35. Wilder, E (ed): *Obstetric and Gynecologic Physical Therapy: Clinics in Physical Therapy,* Vol 20, ed 1. New York, Churchill-Livingstone, 1988.
36. Zacharin, RF: *Pelvic Floor Anatomy and the Surgery of Pulsion Enterocele.* Springer-Verlag/ Wien, New York, 1985.

CHAPTER —————————————— 19

Chest Physical Therapy

Chest physical therapy is a multifaceted area of professional practice that deals with the evaluation and treatment of patients of all ages with acute or chronic lung disorders. It employs a wide range of therapeutic exercise and related modalities to effectively evaluate and treat the patient with cardiopulmonary dysfunction.[7]

The goals of chest physical therapy are to:[7,12,14]
1. prevent airway obstruction and accumulation of secretions that interfere with normal respiration.
2. improve airway clearance and ventilation through mobilization and drainage of secretions.
3. improve endurance and general exercise tolerance.
4. reduce energy costs during respiration through breathing retraining.
5. prevent or correct postural deformities associated with respiratory disorders.
6. promote relaxation.
7. maintain or improve chest mobility.
8. improve cough effectiveness.

Treatment settings vary widely. Inpatients may be treated in intensive care, chronic care, and postsurgical units; outpatients may be seen at home or followed in pulmonary clinics or rehabilitation centers.

OBJECTIVES

After studying this chapter, the reader will be able to:
1. define chest physical therapy.
2. identify the goals of chest physical therapy.
3. summarize evaluation procedures pertinent to the assessment of the pulmonary patient.
4. describe specific evaluation procedures.
5. identify the goals, indications, and basic principles of breathing exercises and retraining.
6. describe the procedures and a sequence for teaching a patient specific breathing exercises.

7. describe the purpose and techniques of chest mobilization exercises.
8. describe the normal cough mechanism.
9. summarize factors that impair the cough mechanism.
10. explain the procedure for teaching a patient an effective cough.
11. summarize the goals, indications, and principles of postural drainage.
12. describe the procedure, positions, and techniques of postural drainage.
13. identify the precautions for and contraindications to postural drainage.

I. REVIEW OF RESPIRATORY STRUCTURE AND FUNCTION

A. The Thorax

1. **Function**
   a. The main function of the thoracic cage is to protect the internal organs of respiration, circulation, and digestion.
   b. The thoracic cage provides the site of attachment for the muscles of respiration to mechanically enlarge the thorax for inspiration or compress the thorax for expiration.
   c. It is also the site of attachment for upper extremity muscles, which function during lifting, pulling, or pushing activities. These activities are usually done in conjunction with inspiratory effort.

2. **Skeletal Structure**[9,30]
   a. Posterior
   The dorsal portion of the ribs articulate with the 12 thoracic vertebrae at the costotransverse and costovertebral joints.
   b. Anterior
   (1) 1st–7th ribs articulate directly with the sternum via the costal cartilage.
   (2) 8th–10th ribs have cartilaginous attachments to the rib above.
   (3) 11th and 12th are floating ribs.

B. Muscles of Respiration[6,9,12,14,26,30]

1. **Inspiration**
   a. Diaphragm
   (1) The diaphragm is the major muscle of inspiration. During relaxed inspiration, it is the primary muscle responsible for movement of air.
   (2) As it contracts, it moves caudally to increase the capacity of the thoracic cage.
   (3) Nerve supply: phrenic nerve (C-3, C-4, C-5).
   b. Intercostals
   (1) The external intercostals act on inspiration. The internal and transverse intercostals participate minimally.
   (2) Their function is to maintain the spaces between the ribs and to provide tone between the ribs with changes in intrathoracic pressure. During inspiration, the external intercostals also lift the ribs and increase the dimensions of the thoracic cavity in anteroposterior and transverse directions.
   (3) Nerve supply: T-1–T-12, respectively.

c. Accessory muscles of inspiration
The sternocleidomastoid (SCM), upper trapezius, and scalene muscles do not directly participate to move the ribs during resting inspiration. These muscles become increasingly active with greater inspiratory effort, which occurs frequently during strenuous physical activity. The accessory muscles of inspiration may become the primary muscles of inspiration when the diaphragm is ineffective or weak as the result of chronic lung or neuromuscular diseases.

(1) The SCM muscles elevate the sternum to increase the anteroposterior (A-P) diameter of the thorax. In patients with weakness of the diaphragm, the SCM muscles act as the primary muscles of inspiration. The nerve supply is cranial nerve XI and C-2–C-3.

(2) The upper trapezius muscles elevate the shoulders and, indirectly, the rib cage during labored inspiration. They also fixate the neck so the scalenes have a stable attachment. Their nerve supply is cranial nerve XI.

(3) The scalenes participate minimally in normal resting inspiration to stabilize the first rib. During deep or pathologic breathing, the scalenes elevate the first two ribs and increase the size of the thoracic cavity if their superior attachments on the neck are fixed.

(4) During deep breathing, other muscles, such as the serratus anterior and the pectoralis major and minor, also act as muscles of inspiration by either elevating the ribs or pulling the ribs toward the arms through reverse muscle action when the upper extremities are fixed.

2. Expiration

a. Relaxed expiration
Expiration is a passive process when a person is at rest. When the diaphragm relaxes after a contraction, the diaphragm rises and the ribs drop. The elastic recoil of tissues decreases the intrathoracic area and increases intrathoracic pressure, which causes exhalation.

b. Active expiration (forced, prolonged)
Contraction of muscles, specifically the abdominals and the internal intercostals, causes active expiration.

(1) Abdominals
  (a) The rectus abdominis, the internal and external obliques, and the transverse abdominis contract to force down the thoracic cage and force the abdominal contents superiorly into the diaphragm. When the abdominals contract, the intrathoracic pressure increases and air is forced out of the lungs.
  (b) Nerve supply: T-10–T-12.

(2) Internal intercostals
  (a) The internal intercostals primarily function during forceful expiration by depressing the ribs.
  (b) Nerve supply: T-1–T-12, respectively.

C. Mechanics of Respiration[6,9,12,27,30,37,38]

1. Movements of the thorax during respiration

Each rib has its own pattern of movement, but generalizations can be made. The ribs attach anteriorly to the sternum (except 11 and 12), and posteriorly to the vertebral bodies, disks, and transverse processes, making a closed kinematic chain. The thorax enlarges in all three planes during inspiration.

   a. Increase in the A-P diameter

      (1) There is a forward and upward movement of the sternum and upper ribs. This is described as a *pump-handle* motion.

      (2) The thoracic spine extends (straightens), enabling greater excursion of the sternum.

   b. Increase in the transverse (lateral) diameter

      (1) There is an elevation and outward turning of the lateral (midshaft) portions of the ribs. This is described as a *bucket handle* motion.

      (2) The lower ribs (8–10), which are not attached directly to the sternum, also flair or open outward, increasing the subcostal angle. This is described as *caliper* motion.

      (3) The angle at the costochondral junction also increases, making the rib segments longer during inspiration.

   c. Increase in vertical dimension

      (1) The central tendon of the diaphragm descends as the muscle contracts. This is described as a *piston action*.

      (2) Elevation of the ribs increases the vertical dimension of the thorax and improves the effectiveness of the diaphragm.

   d. At the end of inspiration, the muscles relax; elastic recoil causes the diaphragm to move superiorly. The ribs return to their resting position.

2. Movement of air

   a. External respiration (ventilation)

      (1) Ventilation is the mass exchange of gases to and from the body.

      (2) During inspiration as the thorax enlarges, the pressure inside the lungs (alveolar pressure) becomes lower than the atmospheric pressure, and air rushes into the lungs.

      (3) At the end of inspiration, the muscles relax and the elastic recoil of the lungs pushes the air out, resulting in expiration.

      (4) The movement of air can be affected by breathing exercises.

   b. Internal respiration

      (1) This involves the blood transport to tissues and gaseous exchange between blood and cells.

      (2) Breathing exercises can make adequate gases available but cannot change the physiology of gas exchange.

3. Compliance of the lungs

   a. Compliance refers to the distensibility (elastic recoil) of lung tissue or how easily the lungs inflate during inspiration.

   b. Normal lungs are very distensible (compliant).

   c. Compliance changes with age and the presence of disease.

4. Airway resistance

   a. The amount of resistance to the flow of air depends on

      (1) the bifurcation and branching of airways.

      (2) the size (diameter) of the lumen of the airway. The diameter of the lumen can be decreased by:

         (a) mucus or edema in the airways.

         (b) contraction of smooth muscles.

b. Normally, the airways widen during inspiration and narrow during expiration.

c. As the diameter of the airway decreases, the *resistance* to airflow increases.

d. In diseases that cause bronchospasm (asthma) or increased mucus production (chronic bronchitis), airflow resistance will be even greater than normal during expiration. Patients with these conditions will have great difficulty getting air out of their lungs during respiration.

D. Anatomy and Function of the Respiratory Tracts

1. **Upper respiratory tract**[9,12,14,30]

   a. Nasal cavity

   b. Pharynx

      (1) Function

          (a) Warms air to body temperature.

          (b) Filters and removes particles. Mucosal lining has cells that secrete mucus and cells that are ciliated.
          Cilia and mucosa trap particles. A sneeze removes large particles.

      (2) With illness and elevated body temperature

          (a) The mucus membrane tends to dry out, so the body secretes more mucus. This mucus dries out, and a cycle begins.

          (b) Action of the cilia is inhibited by drying of mucus.

          (c) The patient tends to breathe by mouth, which decreases the humidification of mucus and increases its viscosity.

   c. Larynx

      (1) Extends from C-3–C-6.

      (2) Controls airflow and, when it contracts rapidly, prevents food, liquids, or foreign objects from entering the airway.

2. **Lower respiratory tract structure**[9,12,14,30]**—Tracheobronchial tree (Figure 19-1)**

   There are 23 generations (branchings) within the tracheobronchial tree.

   a. Trachea

      (1) Extends from C-6 to the sternal angle (2nd rib, T-5) where the trachea bifurcates.

      (2) Passes in an oblique downward direction.

      (3) Oval-shaped, flexible, cartilaginous tube.

          (a) Supported by semicircular rings of cartilage.

          (b) The posterior wall is smooth muscle.

      (4) Contains an equal number of ciliated epithelial cells and mucus-containing goblet cells.

   b. Mainstem bronchi: 2

      (1) Right—almost vertical

      (2) Left—more oblique

   c. Lobar bronchi: 5

      (1) Two mainstem bronchi divide into five lobar bronchi: three on the right and two on the left.

      (2) Mainstem and lobar bronchi have a great amount of cartilage.

   d. Segmental bronchi: 18

      (1) Lobar bronchi divide into 10 right segmental bronchi and 8 left segmental bronchi.

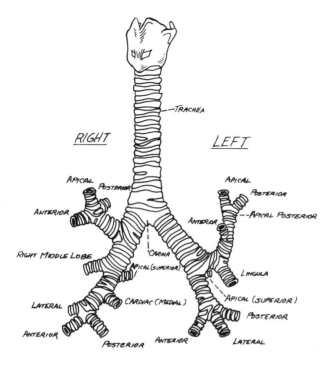

FIGURE 19-1. Lower respiratory tract—Tracheobronchial tree. (From Frownfelter, DL: Chest Physical Therapy and Pulmonary Rehabilitation. Year Book Medical Publishers, Chicago, 1987, with permission.)

    (2) Segmental bronchi have scattered cartilage, smooth muscle, elastic fibers, and a capillary network.
    (3) The mainstem, lobar, and segmented bronchi have a mucous membrane essentially the same as the trachea.
  e. Bronchioles
    (1) Segmental bronchi divide into subsegmental bronchi and bronchioles, which have less and less cartilage and ciliated epithelial cells. These bronchioles divide into the *terminal bronchioles*, which are distal to the last cartilage of the tracheobronchial tree. Terminal bronchioles contain no ciliated cells.
    (2) Terminal bronchioles divide into *respiratory bronchioles* and provide a transitional zone between the bronchioles and alveoli. The respiratory bronchioles divide into alveolar ducts and alveolar sacs (Figure 19-2). One duct may supply several sacs. The ducts contain smooth muscle, which narrows the lumen of the duct with contraction.
  f. Alveoli—approximately 300 million in the adult lung
    (1) Located in the periphery of the alveolar ducts and sacs.
    (2) Are in contact with capillaries (alveolar-arterial membrane).
    (3) Gas exchange occurs here.

3. Function of the tracheobronchial tree
  a. Conducts air to the alveolar system.
  b. Helps with humidification and traps small particles to clean the air with the mucosal lining.

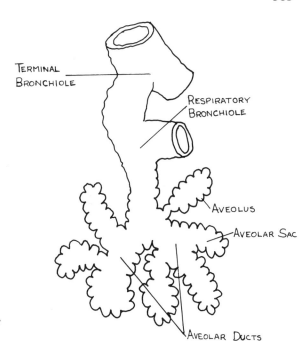

TERMINAL
BRONCHIOLE

RESPIRATORY
BRONCHIOLE

AVEOLUS

AVEOLAR SAC

AVEOLAR DUCTS

FIGURE 19-2. Bronchopulmonary segment.

     c. Traps particles and moves mucus upward with the cilia.
     d. Warms the air by the vascular supply.
     e. Elicits the cough reflex because of the action of the chemical receptors.

E. Anatomy of the Lungs (Figure 19-3)[9,12,30]
  1. Right lung
     a. 3 lobes—upper, middle, and lower.
     b. 10 bronchopulmonary segments.
  2. Left lung
     a. 2 lobes—upper and lower plus the lingula.
     b. 8 bronchopulmonary segments.
  3. Each lung is covered by the pleura.
     a. Visceral pleura—membrane that covers the lungs.
     b. Parietal pleura—membrane that covers the thoracic wall.
     c. A negative pressure in the minute space between the pleurae serves to keep the lungs inflated.
     d. Pleural fluid is found between the pleurae and lubricates the pleurae as they slide on each other during respiration.

F. Lung Volumes and Capacities[35] (Figure 19-4)
  1. Pulmonary function tests are done to evaluate the mechanical function of the lungs. A basic understanding of these tests will be useful for the therapist who is treating the patient with pulmonary dysfunction.
     a. Tidal volume (TV)
       A relaxed inspiration followed by a relaxed expiration.

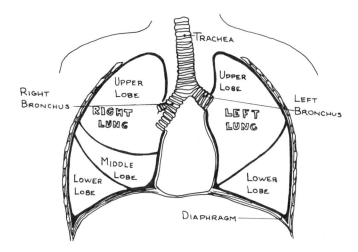

FIGURE 19-3. Structure of the right and left lungs.

    b. Inspiratory reserve volume (IRV)
       The amount of air a patient can breathe in after a resting inspiration.
    c. Expiratory reserve volume (ERV)
       The amount of air a patient can exhale after a normal resting expiration.
    d. Vital capacity (VC)
       A maximum inspiration followed by a maximum expiration (IC + ERV).
    e. Residual volume (RV)
       That amount of air left in lungs after a maximum expiration (dead air).
    f. Total lung capacity (TLC)
       Vital capacity and residual volume. This is the maximum amount of air in the lungs after a maximum inspiration.
    g. Inspiratory capacity (IC)
       The maximum amount of air a patient can breathe in after a resting expiration.
    h. Functional residual capacity (FRC)
       The amount of gas remaining in lungs after a normal expiration.
  2. Effects of aging and disease on lung volumes
    a. Vital capacity
      (1) Decreases with age
      (2) Decreases with restrictive and obstructive lung diseases
    b. Residual volume
      (1) Increases with age
      (2) Increases with obstructive lung diseases such as emphysema

G. Physiology of Respiration

Discussion of the complex nature of the physiology of respiration and pulmonary perfusion goes well beyond the scope of this text. The therapist is referred to several references for further study.[9,10,12,16,30,46]

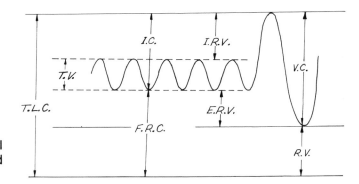

FIGURE 19-4. Normal lung volumes as measured by spirometry.

II. EVALUATION IN CHEST PHYSICAL THERAPY[7,11,12,18,33,37]

A. Purpose

1. To provide the therapist with additional information on the physical and functional status of the pulmonary patient.
2. To develop an individualized treatment plan for the patient.
3. To establish baseline information on the patient in order to measure a patient's progress and the effectiveness of the treatment.
4. To determine when to discontinue the treatment.
5. To plan and implement a home program.

B. Background and Techniques of Evaluation for the Pulmonary Patient

1. General appearance of the patient

a. Vital signs
   Check the heart rate, rate of respiration, and blood pressure of the patient prior to, during, and after treatment.

b. Observe the patient
   (1) Level of awareness (level of consciousness)
       Alert? Responsive? Lethargic? Cooperative? Oriented? Changes in levels of consciousness can occur if a patient becomes hypercarbic (increased PCO_2) or hypoxic (decreased PO_2).
   (2) Color
       Cyanotic peripherally? (nail beds) Centrally? (lips); cyanosis occurs when a patient is hypoxic.
   (3) Condition of the skin
   (4) Clubbing of the fingernails
   (5) Jugular vein engorgement (because of increased venous pressure in patients with congestive heart failure)
   (6) Hypertrophy of accessory muscles of respiration (as the result of overuse in patients with chronic lung disease) or weakness of the diaphragm.
   (7) Use of pursed-lip breathing indicates the presence of chronic obstructive pulmonary disease and difficulty with expiration.

2. Breathing pattern

a. Rate, regularity, and location of respiration are noted at rest and with activity. The normal rate of inspiration to expiration is 2:1. The normal sequence of inspiration is (1) the diaphragm contracts and descends and the abdomen (epigastric area) rises; (2) this is followed by lateral costal expansion as the ribs move up and out; finally (3) the upper chest rises.

b. In healthy individuals, the neck muscles (accessory muscles of inspiration) will only act during deep breathing.

c. Abnormal breathing patterns
   (1) *Dyspnea:* shortness of breath; distressed, labored breathing.
   (2) *Tachypnea:* rapid, shallow respiration; decreased tidal volume but increased rate.
   (3) *Hyperventilation:* deep, rapid respiration; increased tidal volume and increased rate of respiration.
   (4) *Orthopnea:* difficulty breathing in the supine position.
   (5) *Apnea:* Cessation of breathing in the expiratory phase.
   (6) *Apneusis:* Cessation of breathing in the inspiratory phase.
   (7) *Cheyne-Stokes:* cycles of gradually increasing tidal volumes, followed by a series of gradually decreasing tidal volumes, and then a period of apnea. This is sometimes seen in the patient with a severe head injury.

3. Chest mobility

a. Symmetry of chest movement
   Place your hands on the patient's chest and assess the excursion of each side of the chest during inspiration and expiration. Each of the three lobar areas can be checked.
   (1) To check upper lobe expansion, face the patient; place the tips of your thumbs at the midsternal line at the sternal notch. Extend your fingers above the clavicles. Have the patient fully exhale and then inhale deeply.
   (2) To check middle lobe expansion, continue to face the patient; place the tips of your thumbs at the xyphoid process and extend your fingers laterally around the ribs. Again, ask the patient to breathe in deeply.
   (3) To check lower lobe expansion, place the tips of your thumbs along the patient's back at the spinous processes (lower thoracic level) and extend your fingers around the ribs. Ask the patient to breathe in deeply.
   (4) As the patient inhales and exhales, check the symmetry of movement of both sides of the chest.

b. Depth of excursion
   (1) Can be measured by taking the girth of the chest at three levels (axilla, xyphoid, and subcostal) during inspiration and expiration.
   (2) Can also be measured by placing both hands on the patient's chest and back as described above. Note the amount of space between your thumbs after the patient takes a deep inspiration.

4. Analysis of posture and chest deformities

a. Symmetry of posture
   Observe anteriorly, posteriorly, and laterally and note deformities such

as scoliosis and kyphosis. These deformities restrict rib movement.
b. Mobility of the trunk
Check active movements in all directions and determine if there is any restricted spinal motion, particularly in the thoracic spine.
c. Common chest deformities
(1) *Barrel chest:* The circumference of the upper chest appears larger than that of the lower chest. The sternum appears prominent and the A-P diameter of the chest is greater than normal. Many patients with chronic obstructive pulmonary disorders, who are usually upper chest breathers, develop a barrel chest.
(2) *Pectus excavatum* (funnel breast): The lower part of the sternum is depressed and the lower ribs flare out. Patients with this deformity are diaphragmatic breathers; excessive abdominal protrusion and little upper chest movement occur during respiration.

5. Palpation
a. Definition
A procedure that involves touching the chest with the hand to feel chest movement and assess the quality of the underlying tissue.
b. Procedure
Place your hand along the lower, middle, and upper chest areas. Ask the patient to say 99. Vibration (known as *vocal* or *tactile fremitus*) should be felt if the lungs are normal.
c. Decreased fremitus indicates pathology, such as atelectasis or obstructed airways.

6. Percussion
a. Definition
An evaluation technique designed to assess the air:solid ratio in the lungs.
b. Procedure
Place several fingers flat against the patient's chest (usually posterior); tap firmly over the knuckles with two fingertips of the other hand.
c. A hollow resonant sound is normal.
d. The sound will be dull and flat if there is a greater than normal amount of solid matter (tumor, secretions) in the lungs in comparison with the amount of air.
e. The sound will be hyperresonant if there is a greater than normal amount of air (as in patients with emphysema).

7. Auscultation
a. Definition
Listening to sounds within the body, specifically to breath sounds.
b. Breath sounds, normal and abnormal, occur because of movement of air in the airways during inspiration and expiration. A stethoscope is used to magnify these sounds. Breath sounds should be evaluated
(1) to identify the areas of the lungs where congestion exists and where postural drainage should be performed.
(2) to determine the effectiveness of any postural drainage treatment.
(3) to determine whether or not the lungs are clear, and whether or not postural drainage should be discontinued.

    c. Procedure
       (1) Have the patient sit in a comfortable, relaxed position. Place the diaphragm of the stethoscope directly against the patient's skin along the anterior or posterior chest wall.
       (2) Follow a systematic pattern (Figure 19-5A and B) and place the stethoscope against specific thoracic landmarks (T-2, T-6, T-10) along the right and left sides of the chest wall.
       (3) Ask the patient to breathe in and out through his mouth, more deeply and slowly than normal, as you move the stethoscope from point to point.
    d. Normal breath sounds are classified by
       (1) location
       (2) pitch and intensity
       (3) ratio of sound heard on inspiration versus expiration.
    e. Types of normal breath sounds
       (1) *Tracheal*
       Loud, harsh, and very high pitched; heard only over the trachea.
       (2) *Bronchial*
       Loud, hollow, tubular, and high-pitched; heard along the sides of the sternum. These sounds are heard longer with the expiratory phase than with the inspiratory phase.
       (3) *Bronchovesicular*
       Softer, breezier quality; heard equally on inspiration and expiration only near the mainstem bronchi in the first and second intercostal spaces and between the scapulae, posteriorly.
       (4) *Vesicular*
       Soft, swishy, breezy sounds; heard over most of the chest, except near the trachea and bronchi, and between the scapulae. These sounds are audible much longer on inspiration than on expiration.

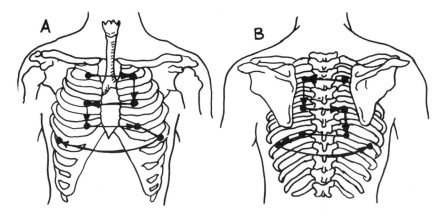

FIGURE 19-5. Pattern of specific thoracic landmarks for auscultation. The diaphragm of the stethoscope is placed along the right and left (*A*) anterior chest wall and the (*B*) posterior chest wall at T-2, T-6, and T-10. (From Frownfelter, DL: Chest Physical Therapy and Pulmonary Rehabilitation. Year Book Medical Publishers, Chicago, 1987, with permission.)

Note: It is important that the therapist practice respiratory auscultation and be able to identify these normal breath sounds in normal individuals.

f. Abnormal and adventitious (extra) breath sounds
  (1) Terminology used to describe abnormal and extra breath sounds is inconsistent.
  (2) Breath sounds may be totally absent, indicating total obstruction of airways and lack of aeration or may be diminished. This may be due to bronchospasm (in asthma) or collapse of an airway (atelectasis, emphysema) or blockage of airways with secretions (pneumonia).
  (3) *Rales*
      Fine crackling sounds (like hairs being rubbed between your fingers next to your ear) heard on inspiration. They indicate the presence of secretions in the distal airways.
  (4) *Rhonchi*
      Coarse rattles or popping sounds heard on inspiration or expiration. They indicate congestion in the proximal airways and can often be cleared with an effective cough.
  (5) *Wheezing*
      High-pitched noise heard on expiration because of narrowing of the lumen; often caused by bronchospasm; cannot be cleared by coughing.
g. Identifying and interpreting abnormal breath sounds in the patient with a respiratory condition takes a great deal of practice.

8. Cough and sputum[14,24]
  a. An effective cough is sharp and deep. In the respiratory patient it may be superficial, soft, throaty, shallow, dry, or moist. If the cough is totally ineffective, suctioning may be indicated.
  b. Sputum should be checked for
    (1) color (clear, white, yellow, green, blood streaked). Clear secretions are normal. Yellow or green secretions indicate infection. The term used to describe blood-streaked sputum is *hemoptysis*.
    (2) consistency (viscous, thin, frothy).
    (3) amount.

9. Other areas of evaluation are
  a. range of motion, particularly of the shoulders and trunk.
  b. muscle strength.
  c. general endurance (see Chapter 21).
  d. functional independence.
  e. pain.
  f. use of assistive respiratory equipment.
  g. *Note:* In addition to the chest examination, other procedures such as evaluation of blood gases, radiographs, pulmonary function studies, graded exercise testing, and bacteriologic tests must also be performed for a complete assessment of the pulmonary patient.

III. BREATHING EXERCISES

Patients with acute and chronic lung disease are taught controlled breathing activities to improve the efficiency and lessen the work of respiration. Breathing exercises are designed to retrain the muscles of respiration and improve ventilation and oxygenation. Active range of motion exercises to the shoulders and trunk also help expand the chest, facilitate deep breathing, and often stimulate the cough reflex.[12,14,33,38,45]

Research studies indicate that although breathing exercises may affect and possibly alter a patient's rate and depth of respiration, they may not necessarily have any impact on internal respiration (alveolar ventilation and oxygenation).[18,45] Therefore, breathing exercises are only part of a treatment program designed to improve pulmonary status and to improve a patient's overall endurance and function in daily living activities. Depending on the patient's clinical problem, breathing exercises are often combined with medication, postural drainage, the use of respiratory therapy devices, and a graded exercise (conditioning) program.

A. Indications for Breathing Exercises

1. Acute or chronic lung disease
   a. Chronic obstructive lung disease
   b. Pneumonia
   c. Atelectasis
   d. Pulmonary embolism
   e. Acute respiratory distress
2. Pain in the thoracic or abdominal area because of surgery or trauma
3. Airway obstruction secondary to bronchospasm or retained secretions.
4. Deficits in the central nervous system that lead to muscle weakness
   a. High spinal cord injury
   b. Acute, chronic, or progressive myopathic or neuropathic diseases
5. Severe orthopedic abnormalities, such as scoliosis and kyphosis, that affect respiratory function.
6. Stress management

B. Goals of Breathing Exercises

1. Improve ventilation.
2. Increase the effectiveness of the cough mechanism.
3. Prevent atelectasis.
4. Improve the strength, endurance, and coordination of respiratory muscles.
5. Maintain or improve chest and thoracic spine mobility.
6. Correct inefficient or abnormal breathing patterns.
7. Promote relaxation.
8. Teach the patient how to deal with shortness-of-breath attacks.

C. General Principles for Teaching Breathing Exercises

1. If possible, choose a quiet area for instruction where you can interact with the patient with a minimum of distractions.
2. Explain to the patient the aims and rationale of breathing exercises.
3. Place the patient in a comfortable, relaxed position and loosen restrictive clothing.
   a. Initially, a hook-lying position in bed, with the head and trunk elevated approximately 45 degrees, is desirable. By totally supporting the head and trunk and by flexing the hips and knees and supporting the legs with a pillow, the abdominal muscles remain relaxed.
   b. Other positions such as supine, sitting, or standing may be used initially or as the patient progresses in treatment.
4. Observe and evaluate the patient's natural breathing pattern while at rest and with activity.

a. Determine whether or not retraining is indicated.

b. Determine the emphasis, either inspiratory or expiratory, that the breathing exercise program should take.

c. Establish a baseline for assessment of change and progress in treatment.

5. If necessary, teach the patient relaxation techniques. This will relax the muscles of the upper thorax, neck, and shoulders to minimize the use of the accessory muscles of respiration. Pay particular attention to relaxation of the sternocleidomastoids, scalenes, upper trapezius and levator scapulae.

6. Demonstrate the desired breathing pattern to the patient.

7. Have the patient practice the correct breathing pattern in a variety of positions at rest and with activity.

D. Precautions[12,14,33,38]

When teaching breathing exercises, be aware of the following precautions:

1. Never allow a patient to force expiration. Expiration should be relaxed and passive. Forced expiration only increases turbulence in the airways, which can lead to bronchospasm and increased airway restriction.

2. Do not allow a patient to take a very *prolonged* expiration. This causes the patient to gasp with the next inspiration. His breathing pattern then becomes irregular and inefficient.

3. Do not allow the patient to initiate inspiration with the accessory muscles and the upper chest. Advise the patient that his upper chest should be relatively quiet during respiration.

4. Allow the patient to practice deep breathing for only three or four inspirations and expirations at a time to avoid hyperventilation.

E. Breathing Patterns and Methods of Instruction

All breathing patterns should be deep, voluntarily controlled, and relaxed, regardless of the pattern being taught to the patient.

1. Diaphragmatic breathing[12,14,15,17,18,38,45]

a. The diaphragm controls breathing at an involuntary level, but a patient can be taught breathing control by correct use of the diaphragm and relaxation of accessory muscles.

b. Diaphragmatic breathing exercises are designed to improve ventilation, oxygenation, and the excursion (descent and ascent) of the diaphragm. Diaphragmatic breathing exercises are also used to mobilize lung secretions during postural drainage.

c. Procedure:

(1) Prepare the patient in a relaxed and comfortable position, evaluate his breathing pattern, and demonstrate the correct method of diaphragmatic breathing.

(2) Place your hand(s) on the rectus abdominis just below the anterior costal margin (Figure 19-6).

(3) Ask the patient to breathe in slowly but deeply, keeping his shoulders relaxed and upper chest quiet and allowing his abdomen to rise.

(4) Then tell the patient to slowly let all the air out.

(5) Have the patient practice this three or four times and then rest. Do not allow the patient to hyperventilate.

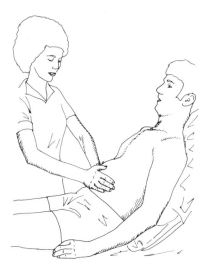

FIGURE 19-6. The semisitting position is a comfortable, relaxed position in which to teach diaphragmatic breathing.

    (6) Have the patient place his own hand below the anterior costal margin and feel the movement himself (Figure 19-7).

    (7) After the patient understands and is able to breathe using a diaphragmatic pattern, suggest that he breathe in through his nose and out through his mouth.

    (8) Practice diaphragmatic breathing in a variety of positions (sitting, standing) and during activity (walking and climbing stairs).

  d. **Note:** The effect of diaphragmatic breathing exercises on ventilation, oxygenation, and excursion of the diaphragm in normal subjects and in patients with pulmonary disorders remains unclear.[20,49] Studies have both supported[17,36,39] and refuted[5,36] the positive impact of diaphragmatic breathing exercises on each of these areas of function. Diaphragmatic breathing exercises will continue to be an integral part of most chest physical therapy programs as research on the effects of diaphragmatic breathing continues.

2. Exercises to strengthen inspiratory muscles and to increase the depth of inspiration

  a. Diaphragmatic breathing exercises can also be used to delay the onset of fatigue of the diaphragm by improving the strength and metabolic capacity of this major muscle of inspiration. In particular, clinicians suggest that patients with neuromuscular disorders that weaken the diaphragm or other muscles of inspiration can benefit from strengthening exercises for the diaphragm.[3,47]

  b. **Use of weights for strengthening the diaphragm.**[3,13,22,47]

    (1) Have the patient assume a supine or slightly head-up position.

    (2) Be sure that the patient knows how to breathe in by primarily using the diaphragm.

    (3) Place a small weight (3–5 lb) over the epigastric region of the patient's abdomen.

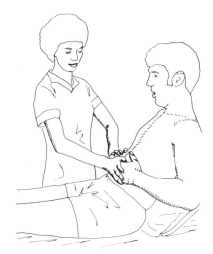

FIGURE 19-7. The patient places his own hands on his abdomen to feel the movement of proper diaphragmatic breathing. By placing his hands on his abdomen, he can also feel the contraction of the abdominals, which occurs with controlled expiration or coughing.

      (4) Tell the patient to breathe in deeply while trying to keep the upper chest quiet. The resistance should not interfere with full excursion of the diaphragm.

      (5) Gradually increase the time that the patient breathes against the resistance of the weight. The weight can be increased when the patient can sustain the diaphragmatic breathing pattern for 15 minutes.

      (6) *Note:* Although this method of strenghening the diaphragm is often suggested for patients with weakness, the results of a recent study of normal subjects indicate that this method of strengthening may be invalid.[28]

  c. **Inspiratory resistance training**[1,2,4,8,12,21,23,34,40]

      (1) Inspiratory resistance training is a recently developed method of improving the strength and endurance of the muscles of inspiration in order to improve ventilation and lessen the occurrence of inspiratory muscle fatigue. This method of strengthening has been used with patients with chronic obstructive lung disease, in those with neuromuscular disorders, and in those being weaned from mechanical ventilation.

      (2) Procedure:

         (a) The patient inhales through a handheld resistive training device that he places in his mouth. Inspiratory resistive training devices are narrow tubes of varying diameters that provide resistance to airflow during inspiration and therefore place resistance on inspiratory muscles to improve strength. The narrower the diameter of the airway, the greater the resistance.

         (b) The patient inhales through the tube for a specified period of time several times each day. The time is gradually increased to 20 to 30 minutes at each training session to increase inspiratory muscle endurance.

         (c) As the patient's strength and endurance improves, the diameter of the handheld tube is decreased. The commercially available inspiratory resistance devices have six different diameters to provide levels of resistance appropriate for each patient.

(3) The effectiveness of inspiratory resistance training continues to be investigated. Some studies have shown that ventilatory muscle strength and endurance have improved as the result of this type of training. Other studies have shown that respiratory rate decreases and exercise tolerance increases over time.[3,8,23]

d. **Incentive respiratory spirometry**[15,47]

(1) Incentive spirometry is a form of low-level resistance training that emphasizes sustained maximal inspiration. The patient inhales through a spirometer that provides visual or auditory feedback as the patient breathes in as deeply as possible. Incentive spirometry increases the volume of air inspired and has been used to prevent alveolar collapse in postoperative conditions and to strengthen weak inspiratory muscles in patients with neuromuscular disorders.

(2) Procedure:[12,47]

(a) Place the patient in a comfortable position (supine or semi-upright).

(b) Have the patient take three to four slow, easy breaths.

(c) Have the patient maximally exhale with the fourth breath.

(d) Then have the patient place the spirometer in his mouth and maximally inhale through the spirometer and hold the inspiration for several seconds.

(e) This sequence is repeated 5 to 10 times, several times per day.

e. *Precaution:* Avoid prolonged periods of resistance training for inspiratory muscles. Unlike muscles of the extremities, the diaphragm cannot totally rest to recover from a session of resistance exercises. Use of accessory muscles of inspiration (neck muscles) is a sign that the diaphragm is beginning to fatigue.

3. **Segmental breathing**[14,33,38]

It is questionable whether a patient can be taught to expand localized areas of his lung while keeping other areas quiet. It is known, however, that hypoventilation does occur in certain areas of the lungs because of pain and muscle guarding after surgery, atelectasis, and pneumonia. Therefore, there are certain instances when it will be important to emphasize expansion of problem areas of the lung and chest wall.

a. **Lateral costal expansion**

(1) This is sometimes called lateral basal expansion and may be done unilaterally or bilaterally.

(2) The patient may be sitting or in a hook-lying position.

(3) Place your hands along the lateral aspect of the lower ribs to fix the patient's attention to the areas where movement is to occur (Figures 19-8 and 19-9).

(4) Ask the patient to breathe out, and feel the rib cage move downward and inward.

(5) As the patient breathes out, place a firm downward pressure into the ribs with the palms of your hands.

(6) Just prior to inspiration, apply a quick downward and inward stretch to the chest. This places a quick stretch on the external intercostals to facilitate their contraction. These muscles move the ribs outward and upward during inspiration.

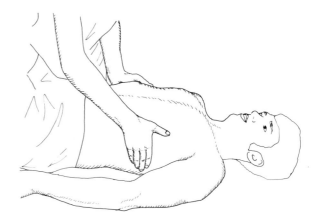

FIGURE 19-8. Bilateral lateral costal expansion—supine.

(7) Tell the patient to expand the lower ribs against your hands as he breathes in.
(8) Apply *gentle* manual resistance to the lower rib area to increase sensory awareness as the patient breathes in, and the chest expands and ribs flare.
(9) Then again, as the patient breathes out, assist him by gently squeezing the rib cage in a downward and inward direction.

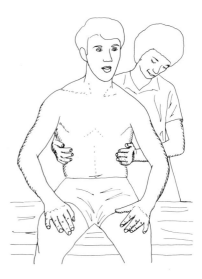

FIGURE 19-9. Bilateral lateral costal expansion—sitting.

(10) The patient may then be taught the maneuver himself. He may place his own hand(s) over his ribs (Figure 19-10), or he may apply his own resistance using a belt (Figure 19-11A and B).

b. **Posterior basal expansion**
   (1) Have the patient sit and lean forward, slightly bending his hips.
   (2) Place your hands over the posterior aspect of the lower ribs.
   (3) Follow the same procedure as described above.
   (4) This form of segmental breathing is important for the postsurgical patient who is confined to bed in a semi-upright position for an extended period of time. Secretions often accumulate in the posterior segments of the lower lobes.
   (5) By placing his hands on his abdomen, he can also feel the contraction of the abdominals, which occurs with controlled expiration or coughing.

c. **Right middle lobe or lingula expansion**
   (1) Patient is sitting.
   (2) Place your hands at either the right or the left side of the patient's chest, just below the axilla.
   (3) Follow the same procedure as described for lateral basal expansion.

d. **Apical expansion** (Figure 19-12)
   (1) Patient is sitting.
   (2) Apply pressure (usually unilaterally) below the clavicle with the fingertips.
   (3) This pattern is appropriate in an apical pneumothorax after a lobectomy.

4. **Glossopharygneal breathing**[12,19]

   a. Glossopharyngeal breathing is a means of increasing a patient's inspiratory capacity when there is severe weakness of the muscles of inspiration. It is taught to patients who have difficulty taking in a deep breath— for example, in preparation for coughing.

   b. This type of breathing pattern was originally developed to assist post-polio patients with severe muscle weakness. Today it is most frequently taught to patients with high spinal cord injuries who can easily develop respiratory problems.[12,19,29]

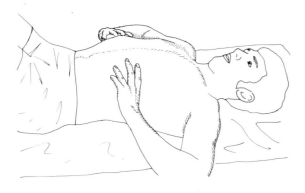

FIGURE 19-10. The patient applies his own manual pressure during lateral costal expansion.

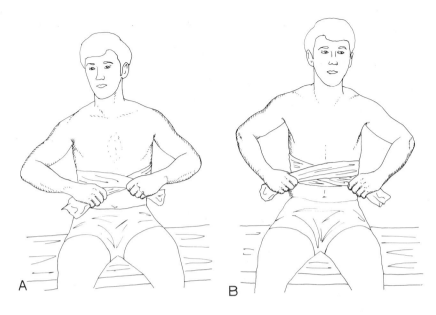

FIGURE 19-11. Belt exercises (*A*) reinforce lateral costal breathing during inspiration; and (*B*) assist with pressure along the rib cage during expiration.

    c. Procedure:

        The patient takes in several "gulps" of air. Then the mouth is closed and the tongue pushes the air back and traps it in the pharynx. The air is then forced into the lungs when the glottis is opened. This increases the depth of the inspiration and the patient's vital capacity.[31]

5. Pursed-lip breathing[8,18,31]

    a. Whether it is appropriate to teach pursed lip breathing to a patient is debatable.

        (1) Most therapists feel that gentle pursed lip breathing with passive expiration is a useful procedure to keep airways open by creating a backpressure in the airways. It is taught to help a patient with chronic obstructive pulmonary disease (COPD) deal with attacks of shortness of breath.[12,33] Studies suggest that pursed-lip breathing decreases the respiratory rate, increases the tidal volume, and improves exercise tolerance.[8,31]

        (2) Some patients spontaneously develop this pattern of breathing. If so, they should not be discouraged from using it.

        (3) *Precaution:* The use of *forced* expiration during pursed-lip breathing must be avoided. Forceful or prolonged expiration while the lips are pursed can increase the turbulence in the airways and cause further restriction of the small bronchioles. For this reason, therapists have suggested that patients may perform pursed-lip breathing inappropriately and, therefore, should not be taught this form of breathing.

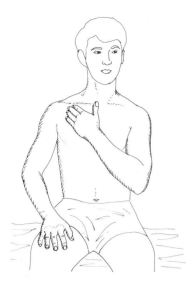

FIGURE 19-12. Segmental right upper lobe expansion.

(4) It is the opinion of the authors of this textbook that pursed-lip breathing (with passive expiration) is a valuable means of dealing with shortness-of-breath attacks (dyspnea on exertion) and *should* be taught to patients with COPD.

b. Procedure:
   (1) Have the patient assume a comfortable position and relax as much as possible.
   (2) Explain to the patient that expiration must be relaxed (passive) and that contraction of the abdominals must be avoided.
   (3) Place your hand over the patient's abdominal muscles to detect any contraction of the abdominals.
   (4) Instruct the patient to breathe in slowly and deeply.
   (5) Then have the patient loosely purse his lips and exhale.

6. **Dealing with shortness-of-breath attacks**
   a. Many patients with COPD (emphysema and asthma, for example) may suffer from periodic attacks of dyspnea (shortness of breath) particularly with physical exertion or when in contact with allergens. Whenever a patient's normal breathing pattern is interrupted, shortness of breath can occur. It is helpful to teach patients to try to prevent shortness of breath attacks with *controlled breathing* and by becoming aware of what activity or situation causes dyspnea.
   b. Procedure:
      (1) Have the patient assume a relaxed, forward-bent posture (see Figures 20-1, 20-2, and 20-3). This position stimulates diaphragmatic breathing (the viscera drops forward and the diaphragm descends more easily).
      (2) Use bronchodilators as prescribed.
      (3) Have the patient gain control of his breathing and reduce the respiratory rate by using pursed-lip breathing during expiration. Be sure

that the patient does not use forceful expiration. Have the patient emphasize the expiratory phase of breathing.

(4) After each pursed-lip expiration, have the patient breathe in diaphragmatically, avoiding the use of accessory muscles.

(5) Have the patient remain in this posture and continue to breathe in as relaxed a manner as possible.

IV. EXERCISES TO MOBILIZE THE CHEST

A. Definition

Chest mobilization exercises are any exercises that combine active movements of the trunk or extremities with deep breathing.

B. Goals

1. Maintain or improve mobility of the trunk and shoulders when it affects respiration. For example, a patient with tightness of the trunk muscles on one side of the body will not expand that part of the chest fully during inspiration. Exercises that combine stretching of these muscles with deep breathing will improve ventilation on that side of the chest.

2. Reinforce or emphasize the depth of inspiration or expiration. For example, a patient can improve expiration by leaning forward at his hips or flexing the spine as he breathes out. This pushes the viscera superiorly into the diaphragm and further reinforces expiration.

C. Specific Exercises

1. **To mobilize one side of the chest**

   a. With the patient sitting, have him bend away from the tight side to lengthen tight structures and expand that side of the chest during inspiration (Figure 19-13A).

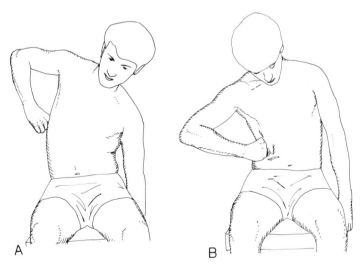

FIGURE 19-13. Chest mobilization during inspiration and expiration. To mobilize the lateral rib cage: (*A*) have the patient bend away from his right side during inspiration; and (*B*) bend toward his right side during expiration.

    b. Then, have him push his fisted hand into the lateral aspect of his chest, as he bends toward the tight side and breathes out (Figure 19-13B).

    c. Progress by having the patient place his arm on the tight side of the chest over his head and side bend away from the tight side. This will place an additional stretch on the tight tissues.

2. **To mobilize the upper chest and stretch the pectoralis muscles**

    a. With the patient sitting in a chair and his hands clasped behind his head, have him horizontally abduct his arms (elongating the pectoralis muscles) during inspiration (Figure 19-14A).

    b. Then, have him bring his elbows together and bend forward to emphasize expiration (Figure 19-14B).

    c. This may also be done with the patient supine (Figure 19-15A and B).

3. **To mobilize the upper chest and shoulders**

    a. With the patient sitting in a chair, have him reach with both arms overhead (180 degrees bilateral shoulder flexion and slight abduction) during inspiration (Figure 19-16A)

    b. Bend forward at the hips and reach for the floor during expiration (Figure 19-16B).

4. **To increase expiration during deep breathing**

    a. Have the patient breathe in while in a hook-lying position (hips and knees are slightly flexed) (Figure 19-17A).

    b. Then, have him pull both knees to his chest (one at a time to protect the low back) during expiration (Figure 19-17B and C).

5. Wand exercises (see Chapter 2) emphasizing shoulder flexion during inspiration may also be combined with breathing exercises.

D. Additional Activities

In addition to exercises specifically designed to mobilize the chest, the therapist may also instruct the patient in

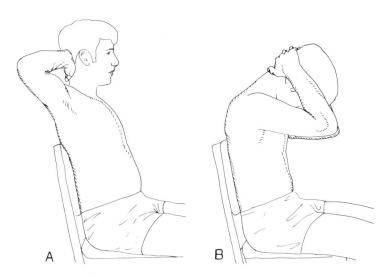

FIGURE 19-14. (*A*), A stretch is applied to the pectoralis muscles during inspiration; and (*B*), the patient brings the elbows together to facilitate expiration.

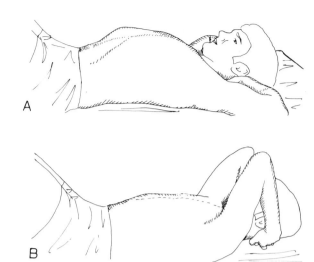

FIGURE 19-15. Stretch to the pectoralis muscles during inspiration followed by expiration with the patient supine.

1. posture correction.
2. manual stretching of the trunk.
3. range of motion exercises to maintain or increase joint motion in the extremities.

V. COUGHING

An effective cough is necessary to eliminate respiratory obstructions and keep the lungs clear. It is an important part of treatment of patients with acute or chronic respiratory conditions.

A. The Cough Mechanism[12,24,50]

The following series of actions occur when a patient coughs:
1. Deep inspiration occurs.
2. Glottis closes and vocal cords tighten.
3. Abdominal muscles contract and diaphragm elevates, which causes an increase in intrathoracic and intra-abdominal pressures.
4. Glottis opens.
5. Explosive expiration of air occurs.

B. The Normal Cough Pump

1. A cough may be reflexive or voluntary.
2. In the normal individual, the cough pump is effective to the seventh generation of bronchi. (There are a total of 23 generations of bronchi in the tracheobronchial tree.)
3. Ciliated epithelial cells are present up to the terminal bronchiole and raise secretions in normal individuals.

C. Factors that Decrease the Effectiveness of the Cough Mechanism and Cough Pump

1. **Inability of the patient to take in a deep breath because of**

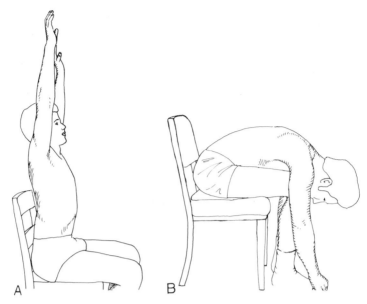

FIGURE 19-16. (*A*), Chest expansion is increased with bilateral movement of the arms overhead during inspiration. (*B*), Expiration is then increased by reaching the arms toward the floor.

    a. Pain
        (1) acute lung disease
        (2) rib fracture
        (3) trauma to the chest
        (4) recent thoracic or abdominal surgery
    b. Specific muscle weakness that affects the diaphragm or accessory muscles of inspiration.
        (1) high spinal cord injury
        (2) anterior horn cell disease (Guillain-Barré syndrome)

2. Inability of the patient to forcibly expel air as the result of
    a. spinal cord injury above T-10
    b. myopathic disease and weakness such as muscular dystrophy
    c. tracheostomy
    d. critical illness that causes excessive fatigue

3. Decrease in normal ciliary action in the bronchial tree secondary to
    a. general anesthesia and intubation.
    b. COPD (chronic obstructive pulmonary disease) such as chronic bronchitis; there is a decreased number of ciliated epithelial cells in the bronchi.
    c. smoking.

4. Increase in the amount and thickness of mucus caused by
    a. cystic fibrosis
    b. chronic bronchitis

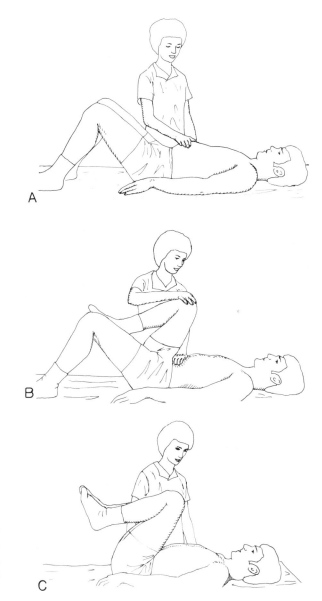

FIGURE 19-17. (*A*), Begin inspiration in hook-lying position. (*B*), Bring one knee to the chest. (*C*), Then bring the other knee to the chest to assist expiration.

      c. pulmonary infections such as pneumonia
      d. dehydration

D. Teaching an Effective Cough[12,14,33,38]

    Since an effective cough is an integral part of any chest therapy program, a patient must be taught the significance of an effective cough, how to produce an efficient, voluntary cough, and when to cough.
    1. Evaluate the patient's voluntary or reflexive cough.

2. Place the patient in a relaxed and comfortable position for deep breathing and coughing.
   a. Sitting or leaning forward is usually the best position for coughing.
   b. The patient's neck should be slightly flexed to make coughing more comfortable.
3. Teach the patient deep controlled diaphragmatic breathing.
4. Demonstrate a sharp, deep, double cough.
5. Demonstrate the proper muscle action of coughing (contraction of the abdominals).
6. Have the patient place his hands on his abdomen and do three huffs with expiration to feel the contraction of the abdominals (see Figure 19-7).
7. Have the patient practice making a K sound to experience tightening the vocal cords and closing the glottis.
8. When the patient has put these actions together, have him take a deep but relaxed inspiration, followed by a sharp double cough. The second cough during a single expiration is more productive.
9. Use glossopharyngeal breathing in selected patients to augment inspiration, if necessary.
10. *Precaution:* Never allow the patient to suck air in by gasping, because it
    a. increases the work (energy expenditure) of breathing and the patient fatigues more easily.
    b. tends to increase turbulence and resistance in the airways and may lead to increased bronchospasm (further constriction of airways).
    c. may push mucus or a foreign object deep into air passages.

E. Additional Means of Facilitating a Cough[12,14,19]

1. Manual assisted cough[19]

a. If the patient has abdominal weakness (for instance, as the result of a midthoracic or cervical spinal cord injury), manual pressure on the abdominal area will assist in developing greater intra-abdominal pressure for an effective cough. Manual pressure can be applied by either the therapist or the patient.
b. Procedure
   (1) Therapist-assisted (Figures 19-18 and 19-19)
       (a) With the patient in a supine position, the therapist places the heel of one hand on the patient's abdomen at the epigastric area. She then places her other hand on top of the first either keeping the fingers open or interlocking them.
       (b) After the patient inhales as deeply as possible, the therapist manually assists the patient as he attempts to cough. The abdomen is compressed with an inward and upward force, which pushes the diaphragm upward to cause a more forceful and effective cough.
       (c) This same maneuver can be done with the patient in a chair. The therapist or family member can stand in front of or in back of the patient and apply manual pressure during expiration.
       (d) *Precaution:* Avoid excessive pressure on the xyphoid process.
   (2) Self-assisted (see Figure 19-19)
       (a) While the patient is in a sitting position, he crosses his arms across his abdomen.
       (b) After a deep inspiration, he pushes inward and upward on the

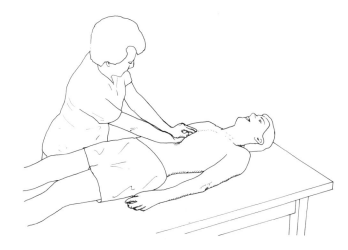

FIGURE 19-18. Therapist-assisted manual cough technique.

abdomen with his wrists or forearms and simultaneously leans forward as he attempts to cough.

2. Splinting

If incisional pain from recent surgery is restricting the cough, teach the patient to splint over the incision.

a. Have the patient press his hands or a pillow firmly over the incision to support the painful area as he coughs (Figure 19-20).

b. If the patient cannot reach the incision, the therapist should assist (Figure 19-21).

3. Humidification

If secretions are very thick, work with the patient after humidification of secretions with intermittent positive-pressure breathing (IPPB) therapy or ultrasonic nebulizer (USN) therapy.

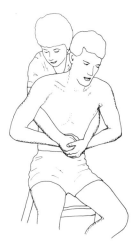

FIGURE 19-19. Therapist-assisted or self-assisted manual cough technique.

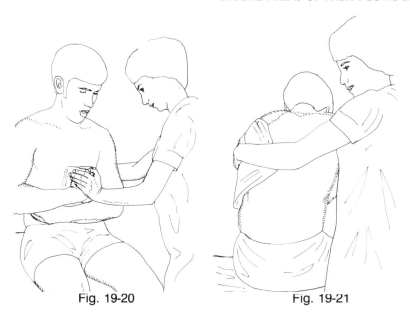

Fig. 19-20   Fig. 19-21

FIGURE 19-20. Splinting over an anterior surgical incision.
FIGURE 19-21. Splinting over a posterior lateral incision.

4. Tracheal trickle
A tracheal tickle may be used with infants or disoriented patients who cannot cooperate in the treatment.
   a. This is a somewhat uncomfortable maneuver, done to elicit a reflexive cough.
   b. The therapist places two fingers at the sternal notch and applies a circular motion with pressure downward into the trachea to facilitate a reflexive cough.

F. Precautions
1. Avoid uncontrolled coughing spasms (paroxysmal coughing).
2. Avoid forceful coughing with patients who have a history of cerebrovascular accident or aneurysm. Have these patients *huff* several times to clear the airways.
3. Be sure that the patient coughs while in a somewhat erect posture.

G. Suctioning—Alternative to Coughing
1. Suctioning may be the only means of clearing the airways in patients who are unable to cough voluntarily or after reflex stimulation of the cough mechanism.
2. Suctioning is indicated in all patients with artificial airways.
3. The suctioning procedure will clear only the trachea and the mainstem bronchi.
4. ***Precaution:*** Only individuals who have been instructed in proper suctioning technique should use this alternative means of clearing the airways.

Suctioning, if performed incorrectly, can introduce an infection into the airways or damage the delicate mucosal lining of the trachea and bronchi.

VI. POSTURAL DRAINAGE

A. Definition

Postural drainage (bronchial drainage) is a means of clearing the airways of secretions by placing the patient in various positions so that gravity will assist in the flow of mucus. The positions are based upon the anatomy of the tracheobronchial tree and are designed to drain specific areas of the lungs. Mucus is moved from the affected bronchioles to the larger bronchi and trachea where it can then be coughed or suctioned out.[12,14,25,33,38]

B. Goals of Postural Drainage

1. Prevent accumulation of secretions in patients at risk for pulmonary complications. This may include
   a. patients with pulmonary diseases that are associated with increased production of mucus such as chronic bronchitis and cystic fibrosis.
   b. patients who are on prolonged bed rest.
   c. postsurgical patients who have received general anesthesia and who may have painful incisions that restrict deep breathing and coughing postoperatively.
   d. any patient who is on a ventilator if they are stable enough to tolerate the treatment.
2. Remove secretions already accumulated in the lungs of
   a. patients with acute or chronic lung disease, such as pneumonia, atelectasis, acute lung infections, and COPD.
   b. patients who are generally very weak or are elderly.
   c. patients with artificial airways.

C. Contraindications to Postural Drainage

1. **Hemorrhage (severe hemoptysis)**
   a. Copious amounts of blood in the sputum.
   b. This is different from lightly blood-streaked sputum.

2. **Untreated acute conditions**
   a. Severe pulmonary edema
   b. Congestive heart failure
   c. Large pleural effusion
   d. Pulmonary embolism
   e. Pneumothorax

3. **Cardiovascular instability**
   a. Cardiac arrhythmia
   b. Severe hypertension or hypotension
   c. Recent myocardial infarction

4. **Recent neurosurgery**
   Head-down positioning may cause increased intracranial pressure.

D. Techniques Used During Postural Drainage[12,14,42,50]

In addition to the specific positions used in postural drainage designed to maximize the effect of gravity on the flow of lung secretions, a variety of techniques are used in conjunction with positioning. These techniques further assist with the clearing of secretions from the lungs. They include

1. Deep breathing

The patient should be taught deep segmental breathing exercises, which should be done while the patient is receiving postural drainage.

2. Deep coughing

An effective cough is necessary to mobilize the secretions once they reach the larger bronchial segments.

3. Percussion

   a. This technique is used to further mobilize secretions by mechanically dislodging viscous or adherent mucus from the lungs.
   b. Percussion is done with cupped hands (Figure 19-22A) over the lung segment being drained. The therapist's cupped hands alternately strike the patient's chest wall in a rhythmic fashion (Figure 19-22B). The therapist should try to keep shoulders, elbows, and wrists loose and mobile during the maneuver.
   c. Percussion is continued for several minutes or until the patient needs to alter his position to cough.
   d. This procedure should not be painful or uncomfortable. To prevent irritation to sensitive skin, have the patient wear a lightweight gown or shirt.
   e. **Contraindications**
      Percussion should *not* be applied
      (1) over bony prominences.
      (2) over breast tissue in women.

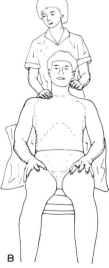

FIGURE 19-22. (*A*), Hand position for applying percussion. (*B*), The therapist alternately percusses over the lung segment being drained.

(3) over fractures, spinal fusion, or osteoporotic bone.

(4) over tumor area.

(5) if a patient has a pulmonary embolus.

(6) if a patient has a condition in which hemorrhage could easily occur, such as in the presence of a low platelet count, or if a patient is receiving anti-coagulation therapy.

(7) if a patient has unstable angina.

(8) if a patient has chest wall pain—for example, after thoracic surgery.

4. **Vibration**

   a. The technique is used in conjunction with percussion in postural drainage. It is applied only during expiration as the patient is deep breathing to move the secretions to the larger airways.

   b. Vibration is applied by placing both hands on the chest wall (or one hand on top of the other) and gently compressing and rapidly vibrating the chest wall as the patient breathes out (Figure 19-23).

   c. Pressure is applied in the same direction as that in which the chest is moving.

   d. The vibrating action is achieved by the therapist's isometrically contracting (tensing) the muscles of the upper extremities from shoulders to hands.

5. **Other techniques that may be used with postural drainage are**

   a. Shaking

   A slower form of vibration, applied to the chest wall with wide movement of the therapist's hands.

   b. Rib springing

   A more vigorous form of vibration with greater pressure to the chest wall. A springing action is applied to the chest wall several times during exhalation.

E. **Postural Drainage Positions**

   1. Positions are based on the anatomy of the lungs and the tracheobronchial tree (see Figures 19-1 and 19-3).

   2. Each segment of each lobe is drained using the positions demonstrated in

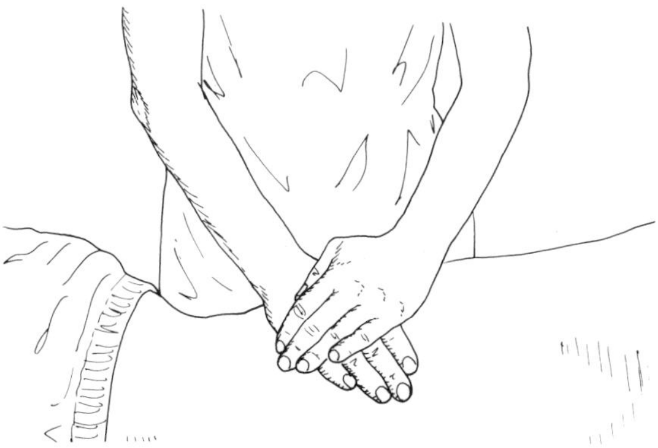

FIGURE 19-23. Hand placement for vibration during postural drainage.

Figures 19-24 to 19-35. The shaded area in each illustration indicates the area of the chest wall where percussion or vibration is applied.

   3. The patient may be positioned on a
     a. postural drainage table that can be elevated at one end.
     b. tilt table.
     c. reinforced padded table with a lift.
     d. hospital bed.
   4. A small child can be positioned on the therapist's lap.

F. Treatment Procedures for Postural Drainage

1. General considerations

   a. Time of day
     (1) Never administer postural drainage directly after a meal.
     (2) Coordinate treatment with IPPB and aerosol therapy. The philosophy varies.
       (a) Some therapists feel that IPPB combined with humidification prior to postural drainage will help loosen secretions and increase the likelihood of productivity.
       (b) Others believe that IPPB is best after postural drainage when the patient's lungs are clearer and maximum benefit can be gained from medication administered through IPPB therapy.
     (3) Choose a time (or times) of day that will be of benefit to the patient.
       (a) A patient's cough tends to be very productive in the early morning because of accumulation of secretions from the night before.
       (b) Postural drainage in the early evening will clear the lungs prior to sleeping and help the patient rest more easily.
   b. Frequency of treatments will depend upon the pathology of the patient's condition.
     (1) Thick copious mucus: 2 to 4 times per day until lungs are clear.
     (2) Maintenance: 1 to 2 times per day to prevent further accumulation of secretions.

2. Prepare the patient

   a. Loosen tight or bulky clothing. It is not necessary to expose the skin. The patient may wear a lightweight shirt or gown.
   b. Have a sputum cup or tissues available.
   c. Have sufficient pillows for positioning and comfort.
   d. Explain the treatment procedure to the patient.
   e. Teach the patient deep breathing and an effective cough prior to beginning postural drainage.
   f. If the patient is producing copious amounts of sputum, ask him to cough or have him suctioned prior to positioning.
   g. Make any adjustments of tubes and wires, such as chest tubes, ECG wires, or catheters, so they remain clear during positioning.

RIGHT AND LEFT UPPER LOBES

Anterior apical segments   Posterior apical segments

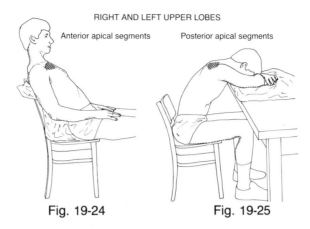

Fig. 19-24   Fig. 19-25

FIGURE 19-24. Percussion is applied directly under the clavicle.

FIGURE 19-25. Percussion is applied above the scapulae. Your fingers curve over the top of the shoulders.

Anterior segments

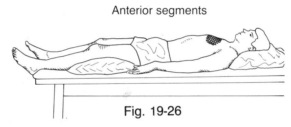

Fig. 19-26

FIGURE 19-26. Percussion is applied bilaterally, directly over the nipple or just above the breast.

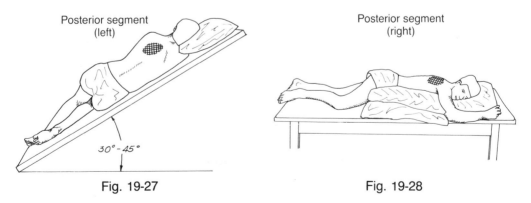

Posterior segment (left)

Posterior segment (right)

30° – 45°

Fig. 19-27   Fig. 19-28

FIGURE 19-27. Patient lies one-quarter turn from prone and rests on his right side. Head and shoulders are elevated 45 degrees or approximately 18 inches if pillows are used. Percussion is applied directly over the left scapula.

FIGURE 19-28. Patient lies flat and one-quarter turn from prone on his left side. Percussion is applied directly over the right scapula.

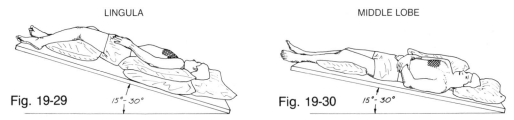

LINGULA   MIDDLE LOBE

Fig. 19-29   15°-30°   Fig. 19-30   15°-30°

FIGURE 19-29. Patient lies one-quarter turn from supine on the right side, supported with pillows, and in a 30 degrees head-down position. Percussion is applied just under the left breast.

FIGURE 19-30. Patient lies one-quarter turn from supine on left side, supported with pillows behind his back, and in a 30-degree head-down position. Percussion is applied under the right breast.

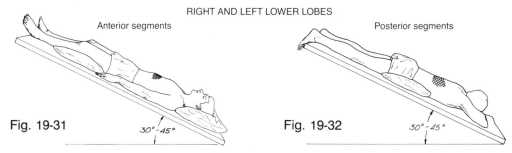

RIGHT AND LEFT LOWER LOBES

Anterior segments   Posterior segments

Fig. 19-31   30°-45°   Fig. 19-32   30°-45°

FIGURE 19-31. Patient lies supine, pillow under knees, in a 45-degree head-down position. Percussion is applied bilaterally over the lower portion of the ribs.

FIGURE 19-32. Patient lies prone, pillow under abdomen in a 45-degree head-down position. Percussion is applied bilaterally over the lower portion of the ribs.

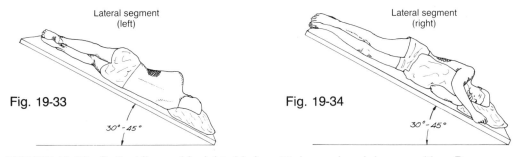

Lateral segment   Lateral segment
(left)   (right)

Fig. 19-33   30°-45°   Fig. 19-34   30°-45°

FIGURE 19-33. Patient lies on his right side in a 45-degree head-down position. Percussion is applied over the lower lateral aspect of the left rib cage.

FIGURE 19-34. Patient lies on his left side in a 45-degree head-down position. Percussion is applied over the lower lateral aspect of the right rib cage.

Superior segments

FIGURE 19-35. Patient lies prone, pillow under his abdomen to flatten his back. Percussion is applied bilaterally, directly below the scapulae.

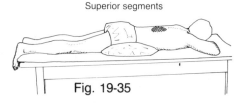

Fig. 19-35

3. Treatment sequence

a. Evaluate the patient (as outlined in section II of this chapter) to determine which segments of the lungs should be drained.
   (1) Some patients with chronic lung diseases, such as cystic fibrosis, will need to be drained in all positions.
   (2) Other patients may require drainage of only a few segments in which secretions have accumulated.
   (3) Check the patient's chart daily to determine his status.
   (4) Check the patient's vital signs, such as respiratory rate and pulse.
b. Position the patient in the correct position for drainage. See that he is as comfortable and relaxed as possible.
c. Stand in front of the patient, whenever possible, in order to observe his color.
d. Maintain the desired position for at least 5 to 10 minutes if the patient can tolerate it, or as long as the position is productive.
e. Have the patient breathe deeply in a relaxed manner during drainage. Do not allow the patient to hyperventilate or become short of breath.
f. Apply percussion over the segment being drained while the patient is in the correct position.
g. Encourage the patient to take a deep, sharp double cough whenever necessary. It may be more comfortable for the patient if he momentarily assumes a semi-upright position (resting on one elbow) as he coughs.
h. If the patient does not cough spontaneously during positioning with percussion, have him take several deep breaths and apply vibration during expiration. This may help elicit a cough.
i. If the patient's cough is not productive after 5 to 10 minutes of positioning, go on to the next position. Secretions that have been mobilized during a treatment may not be coughed up by the patient until 30 minutes to 1 hour after treatment.
j. IPPB may occasionally be used during postural drainage if the patient has difficulty taking deep breaths.
k. The total duration of any one treatment should not exceed 40 to 45 minutes, as the procedure is quite fatiguing for the patient.
   (1) Many patients need to be seen two or four times a day.
   (2) Schedule several treatment times if lungs are very productive or if any or all segments of both lungs must be drained.

4. Concluding the treatment

a. Have the patient sit up slowly and rest for a short while after the treatment. Watch for signs of postural hypotension when the patient rises from a supine position or a head-down position to sitting.
b. Advise the patient that even if his cough was not productive during treatment, it may be productive a short while after treatment.
c. Assess the effectiveness of the treatment and make appropriate notations in the patient's chart.
   (1) Note the type, color, consistency, and amount of secretions produced.
   (2) Note how the patient tolerated the treatment.
   (3) Check the patient's vital signs after treatment.
   (4) Auscultate over the segments that were drained and note changes in breath sounds.

(5) Observe the patient's breathing pattern to determine whether it is deeper, less rapid, more relaxed, or less labored.

(6) Check the symmetry of chest wall expansion.

G. Modified Postural Drainage[12,14,48]

1. Some patients who require postural drainage cannot assume or cannot tolerate the positions that are optimal for treatment. For example

   a. The patient with congestive heart failure may develop orthopnea (shortness of breath caused by lying flat).

   b. The postneurosurgery patient may not be allowed to assume a head-down position because this position causes increased intracranial pressure.

   c. The postthoracic or postcardiac surgery patient may have chest tubes and monitoring wires that may limit positioning.

2. The positions in which postural drainage is done are modified to meet the patient's medical or surgical problems. This compromise is better than not administering postural drainage at all.

H. Home Program of Postural Drainage

1. Postural drainage may have to be carried out on a regular basis at home for patients with chronic lung disease.

2. Patients need to be shown how to position themselves using inexpensive aids.

   a. An adult may place pillows over hard wedges or stacks of newspapers to achieve the desired head-down positions in bed, or he may lean his chest over the edge of the bed, resting with the arms on a chair or stool.

   b. A child may be positioned on an ironing board propped up against a couch.

3. A family member should be instructed in positioning and percussion to assist the patient when needed.

4. Guidelines and precautions, previously discussed, should be followed.

I. Discontinue Postural Drainage If

1. **Chest x-ray is relatively clear.**

2. **Patient is afebrile for 24 to 48 hours.**

3. **Normal or near-normal breath sounds are heard with auscultation.**

4. **Patient is on a regular home program.**

VII. SUMMARY

In Chapter 19, a brief review of respiratory structure and function was outlined. A review of the anatomy of the thorax, upper and lower respiratory tracts, and lungs was followed by a discussion of the mechanics of breathing. Emphasis was placed on discussing the musculature, chest movements, and mechanics of airflow that the therapist may affect during treatment. Evaluation procedures in chest physical therapy and an explanation of tests specific to chest assessment were discussed. Overall goals of chest physical therapy were summarized. Goals, procedures of and precautions for breathing exercises, chest mobility exercises, effective cough training, and postural drainage were then discussed. The application of these chest physical therapy procedures will be presented in

Chapter 20 in conjunction with a discussion of common acute and chronic pulmonary disorders.

REFERENCES

1. Aldrich, T: *The application of muscle endurance training to the respiratory muscles in COPD.* Lung 163:15, 1985.
2. Aldrich, T and Karpel, J: *Inspiratory muscle resistive training in respiratory failure.* Am Rev Respir Dis 131:461, 1985.
3. Alvarez, SE, Peterson, M, and Lunsford, BA: *Respiratory treatment of the adult patient with spinal cord injury.* Phys Ther 61:1737, 1981.
4. Asher, MI, et al: *The effects of inspiratory muscle training in patients with cystic fibrosis.* Am Rev Respir Dis 126:855, 1982.
5. Brach, BB, et al: *Xenon washout patterns during diaphragmatic breathing: Studies in normal subjects and patients with COPD.* Chest 71:735, 1977.
6. Campbell, E, Agostoni, E, and Davis, J: *The Respiratory Muscles.* WB Saunders, Philadelphia, 1970.
7. Cardiopulmonary Section, American Physical Therapy Association: *A Statement: A Definition of Chest Physical Therapy.* Cardiopulmonary Sect Quarterly 4:15, Spring 1983.
8. Casiari, RJ, et al: *Effects of breathing retraining in patients with chronic obstructive pulmonary disease.* Chest 79:393, 1981.
9. Cherniak, RM and Cherniak, L: *Respiration in Health and Disease,* ed 3. WB Saunders, Philadelphia, 1983.
10. Comroe, JH, et al: *Physiology of Respiration.* Year Book Medical Publishers, Chicago, 1974.
11. Crane, LD: *The chest examination.* Phys Ther Health Care 1:11, 1987.
12. Frownfelter, DL: *Chest Physical Therapy and Pulmonary Rehabilitation,* ed 2. Year Book Medical Publishers, Chicago, 1987.
13. Gaynard, P, et al: *The effects of abdominal weights on diaphragmatic position and excursion in man.* Clin Sci 35:589, 1968.
14. Glaskell DV and Webber, BA: *The Brompton Hospital Guide to Chest Physiotherapy,* ed 4. CV Mosby, St Louis, 1981.
15. Gross, D: *The effect of training on strength and endurance of the diaphragm in quadriplegia.* Am J Med 68:27, 1980.
16. Harper, RW: *A Guide to Respiratory Care: Physiology and Clinical Application.* JB Lippincott, Philadelphia, 1981.
17. Hughes, RC: *Does abdominal breathing affect regional gas exchange?* Chest 76:258, 1979.
18. Humberstone, N: *Respiratory assessment and respiratory treatment.* In Irwin, S and Tecklin, J: *Cardiopulmonary Physical Therapy.* CV Mosby, St Louis, 1985.
19. Imle, PC: *Physical therapy and respiratory care for the patient with acute spinal cord injury.* Phys Ther Health Care 1:45, 1987.
20. Kigin, CM: *Chest physical therapy for the postoperative or traumatic injury patient.* Phys Ther 61:1724, 1981.
21. Kim, MJ: *Respiratory muscle training: Implications for patient care.* Heart Lung 13:333, 1984.
22. Lane, C: *Inspiratory muscle weight training and its effect on vital capacity of patients with quadriplegia.* Cardiopulmonary Quarterly 2:13, 1982.
23. Leith, D and Bradley, M: *Ventilatory muscle strength and endurance training.* J Appl Physiol 41:508, 1976.
24. Leith, DE: *Cough.* Phys Ther 48:439, 1968.
25. Lough, M, Doershuk, C, and Stern, R (eds): *Pediatric Respiratory Therapy.* Year Book Medical Publishers, Chicago, 1974.
26. Luce, C: *Respiratory muscle function in health and disease.* Chest 81:82, 1982.
27. Mead, J and Martin, H: *Principles of respiratory mechanics.* J Am Phys Ther Assoc 48:478, 1968.
28. Merrick, J and Axen, K: *Inspiratory muscle function following abdominal weight exercise in healthy subjects.* Phys Ther 61:651, 1981.
29. Metcalf, VA: *Vital capacity and glossopharyngeal breathing in traumatic quadriplegia.* Phys Ther 46:835, 1966.

30. Moore, K: *Clinically Oriented Anatomy.* Williams & Wilkins, Baltimore, 1980.
31. Meuller, RE, et al: *Ventilation and arterial blood gas changes induced by pursed lip breathing.* J Appl Physiol 28:784, 1970.
32. Nunn, K: *Applied Respiratory Physiology.* Butterworth, London, 1971.
33. Reinisch, E: *Functional approach to chest physical therapy.* Phys Ther 58:972, 1978.
34. Rochester, DF and Goldberg, SK: *Techniques of respiratory physical therapy.* Am Rev Respir Dis 122:133, 1980.
35. Ruppell, G: *Manual of Pulmonary Function Testing.* CV Mosby, St. Louis, 1975.
36. Sackner, MA, et al: *Distribution of ventilation during diaphragmatic breathing in obstructive lung disease.* Am Rev Respir Dis 109:331, 1974.
37. Shaffer, T, Wolfson, M, and Bhutoni, VK: *Respiratory muscle function: Assessment and training.* Phys Ther 61:1711, 1981.
38. Sinclair, JD: *Exercise in pulmonary disease.* In Basmajian, JV (ed): *Therapeutic Exercise,* ed 3. Williams & Wilkins, Baltimore, 1978.
39. Shearer, MC, et al: *Lung ventilation during diaphragmatic breathing.* Phys Ther 52:139, 1972.
40. Sobush, D, Dunning, M, and McDonald, K: *Exercise prescription components for respiratory muscle training.* Respir Care 34:30, 1985.
41. Sonne, L and Davis, J: *Increased exercise performance in patients with severe COPD following inspiratory resistive training.* Chest 81:436, 1982.
42. Sutton, P, et al: *Assessment of percussion vibratory shaking and breathing exercises in chest physiotherapy.* Europ J Respir Dis 66:147, 1985.
43. Visich, R: *Knowing what you hear: A guide to breath and heart sounds.* Nursing 81:64, 1981.
44. Warren, A: *Mobilization of the chest wall.* In Hislop, H (ed): *Chest Disorders in Children.* Proceedings of a Symposium, American Physical Therapy Association, Washington, DC, 1968.
45. Watts, N: *Improvement of breathing patterns.* In Hislop, H (ed): *Chest Disorders in Children.* Proceeding of a Symposium, American Physical Therapy Association, Washington, DC, 1968.
46. West, JB: *Respiratory Physiology: The Essentials.* Williams & Wilkins, Baltimore, 1974.
47. Wetzel, J, et al: *Respiratory rehabilitation in the patient with spinal cord injury.* In Irwin, S and Tecklin, J (eds): *Cardiopulmonary Physical Therapy.* CV Mosby, St Louis, 1985.
48. White, J and Mawdsley, R: *Effects of selected bronchial drainage positions on blood pressure of healthy human subjects.* Phys Ther 63:325, 1983.
49. Zadai, CC: *Physical therapy for the acutely ill medical patient.* Phys Ther 61:1746, 1981.
50. Zausmer, E: *Bronchial drainage: Evidence supporting the procedure.* J Am Phys Ther Assoc 48:586, 1968.

CHAPTER ——————————— 20

Management of Obstructive and Restrictive Pulmonary Conditions

The intent of this chapter is to provide an overview of the clinical problems and the goals and techniques of management of common pulmonary conditions. The two general types of pulmonary disorders that will be discussed in this chapter are obstructive lung diseases and restrictive pulmonary disorders. The specific techniques of management of these conditions such as evaluation procedures, breathing exercises, postural drainage, coughing, and mobility exercises for the trunk and thorax have all been explained and illustrated in Chapter 19. Guidelines for general conditioning and endurance training can be found in Chapter 21.

OBJECTIVES

After studying this chapter, the reader will be able to:
1. define obstructive lung disease and restrictive lung disease.
2. identify common causes of obstructive and restrictive lung disease.
3. summarize the general clinical problems found in patients with obstructive and restrictive lung disease.
4. identify general treatment goals and plan of care in obstructive and restrictive lung diseases.
5. describe the clinical picture, summarize the clinical problems, and explain the goals and techniques of treatment of the following obstructive lung diseases: chronic bronchitis, emphysema, asthma, cystic fibrosis, and bronchiectasis.
6. describe the clinical picture, summarize the clinical problems, and explain the goals and techniques of treatment of the following restrictive lung problems: post-thoracic surgery, post-open heart surgery, atelectasis, and pneumonia.
7. describe specific precautions in the treatment of each condition discussed.

I.   OVERVIEW OF OBSTRUCTIVE LUNG DISEASE

A. Definition

Obstructive lung disease is a general term that refers to a number of chronic pulmonary conditions. All obstructive lung diseases are characterized by[1,7,10]
1. increased retention of pulmonary secretions.
2. narrowing and obstruction of airways.
3. structural deterioration of alveoli.

B. Several Terms Are Used to Describe Obstructive Lung Disease. They Include

1. COLD: chronic obstructive lung disease.
2. COAD: chronic obstructive airway dysfunction.
3. COPD: chronic obstructive pulmonary disease.
   The term COPD will be used in this chapter for purposes of consistency.

C. Diseases Classified as COPD

1. Chronic bronchitis
2. Emphysema
3. Asthma
4. Other diseases such as cystic fibrosis and bronchiectasis usually lead to chronic obstructive dysfunction and therefore will be discussed in this section.

D. Characteristics of Patients with Obstructive Lung Disease

1. Patients exhibit persistent resistance of airflow, which causes prolonged and often forced expiration.
2. Vital capacity is decreased.
3. Exercise tolerance is markedly diminished. Patients with COPD become dyspneic with minimal physical exertion.

E. General Clinical Problems[4,7,10]

1. Frequent episodes of shortness of breath (dyspnea on exertion).
2. Prolonged and labored expiration. Air gets trapped as airways narrow during expiration.
3. Chronic accumulation of pulmonary secretions.
4. Decreased endurance and capacity for exercise.
5. Associated postural defects.

A more detailed explanation of several obstructive lung diseases follows. Chronic bronchitis and emphysema, asthma, cystic fibrosis, and bronchiectasis will be discussed. The treatment goals and appropriate plan of care will then be outlined.

II. SPECIFIC OBSTRUCTIVE PULMONARY CONDITIONS

A. Chronic Bronchitis and Emphysema

Chronic bronchitis and emphysema are both classified as chronic obstructive pulmonary diseases (COPD). Since these diseases are often closely related and often seen in conjunction with each other, the underlying goals and principles of treatment are similar.

1. Chronic bronchitis—Clinical picture

a. Chronic bronchitis is an inflammation of the bronchi that causes an

        irritating and productive cough that lasts at least 3 months and recurs over at least 2 consecutive years.[1,7,10]
  b. This condition usually develops in heavy smokers.
  c. The pathologic changes that occur in chronic bronchitis are[1]
    (1) an increase in the number of mucus-producing goblet cells in the lining of the bronchial tree.
    (2) a decrease in the number and action of the ciliated epithelial cells which mobilize secretions.
    (3) a narrowing of airways because of chronic inflammation of the bronchial tree.
  d. General appearance of the patient
    (1) cyanotic because of hyoxemia.
    (2) short of breath.
    (3) bloated because of venous stasis.
    (4) often overweight.

2. **Emphysema—Clinical picture**[1,4,5,8,9]
  a. Emphysema is a chronic inflammation, narrowing, thickening, and destruction of the respiratory bronchioles and alveoli. These airways become scarred, distorted, and kinked, and the alveoli lose their elastic recoil, then weaken and rupture. As a result, the patient experiences difficulty during expiration, and air remains trapped in the lungs (residual volume increases). Over a period of years, severe chronic bronchitis and emphysema often lead to congestive heart failure and death.
  b. Emphysema is usually a condition that develops secondary to chronic bronchitis. Although not as common, emphysema can also be a primary disease that can occur in nonsmokers.[1,10]
  c. The pathologic changes that occur in emphysema are[1]
    (1) an overinflation of the lungs and formation of pockets of air known as *bullae*. This causes an increase in the air space in the lungs.
    (2) destruction of lung tissue and loss of area where effective gas exchange can occur.
  d. General appearance of the patient
    (1) pink and thin
    (2) abnormal posture—forward head, rounded and elevated shoulders
    (3) clubbing of fingers
    (4) excessive use and hypertrophy of accessory muscles and diminished diaphragmatic breathing during inspiration.
    (5) use of pursed-lip breathing during expiration.
    (6) increase in the A-P diameter of the chest (barrel chest).

3. **Clinical problems of chronic bronchitis and emphysema summarized**[1,4,10,18]
  a. An increase in the amount and viscosity of mucus production
  b. A chronic, often productive cough
  c. Attacks of shortness of breath (dyspnea)
  d. An abnormal breathing pattern that results in
    (1) increased respiratory rate (tachypnea).
    (2) use of accessory musculature and decreased diaphragmatic excursion.
    (3) upper chest breathing.
    (4) poor exchange of air in the lower lobes.

    e. Most difficulty during expiration; use of pursed-lip breathing

    f. Changes in pulmonary function

       (1) increased residual volume

       (2) decreased vital capacity

    g. Decreased mobility of the chest wall—a barrel chest deformity develops.

    h. Abnormal posture—forward head and rounded and elevated shoulders.

    i. Decrease in general endurance during daily activities.

4. General treatment goals and plan of care

Treatment Goals	*Plan of Care*
a. Decrease the amount and viscosity of secretions.	a. Administration of bronchodilators, antibiotics, and humidification therapy. If the patient smokes, he should be strongly encouraged to stop.
b. Remove or prevent the accumulation of secretions. (This is an important goal if emphysema is associated with chronic bronchitis or if there is an acute respiratory infection.)	b. Deep and effective cough. Postural drainage to areas where secretions are identified. *Note:* Drainage positions may need to be modified if the patient is dyspneic in the head-down position.
c. Promote relaxation of the accessory muscles of inspiration to decrease reliance on upper chest breathing and to decrease muscle tension associated with dyspnea.	c. Positioning for relaxation.[7] Relaxed head-up position in bed—trunk, arms, and head are well supported. Sitting—leaning forward, resting forearms on thighs (Figure 20-1)

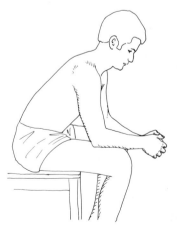

FIGURE 20-1. To relieve shortness of breath, the patient assumes a relaxed sitting position, leaning forward, resting his forearms on his thighs or on a pillow in his lap.

d. Improve the patient's breathing pattern and ventilation.
Emphasize *relaxed* expiraton; decrease the work of breathing, rate of respiration, and the use of accessory muscles.
Carry over controlled breathing to functional activities.

e. Minimize attacks of shortness of breath.

Sitting—leaning forward against pillows on a table (Figure 20-2)
Standing—leaning forward on an object, with hands on the thighs (Figure 20-3) or leaning backward against a wall.
Relaxation exercises for shoulder musculature.
Active shoulder shrugging followed by relaxation.
Shoulder and arm circles.
Horizontal abduction and adduction of the shoulders.

d. Breathing exercises.
Relaxed diaphragmatic breathing with minimal upper chest movement.
Lateral costal breathing
Pursed-lip breathing (careful to *avoid forced* expiration).
Inspiratory resistance exercises.
Practice controlled breathing during standing, walking, climbing stairs, and so on.

e. Have the patient assume a relaxed position (see Figures 20-1 through 20-3) so the upper chest is relaxed and the lower chest is as mobile as possible.
Emphasize relaxed and controlled diaphragmatic breathing.

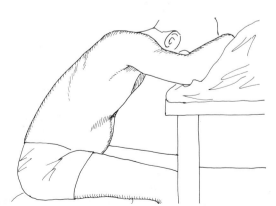

FIGURE 20-2. The patient can sit and lean forward on a pillow to relax and relieve a shortness-of-breath attack.

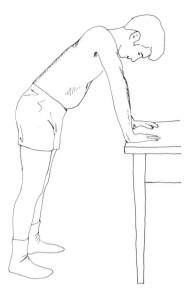

FIGURE 20-3. A patient can lean forward and support some of his weight on his arms while standing to relieve shortness of breath.

Have the patient breathe out as rapidly as possible *without forcing* expiration.

Note: Initially, the rate of respiration will be rapid and shallow. As the patient gets control of his breathing, he will slow down the rate.

Administer supplemental oxygen in a severe attack, if needed.

f. Improve the mobility of the lower thorax.

f. Exercises for chest mobility, emphasizing movement of the lower rib cage during deep breathing.

g. Improve posture.

g. Exercises to decrease forward head and rounded shoulders (see Chapter 14).

h. Increase exercise tolerance.

h. Graded endurance and conditioning exercises (see Chapter 21).

Note: The efficacy of general conditioning and its effect on lung function and respiratory muscle function in the patient with COPD is questionable. Little quantitative data are available to indicate that breathing retraining, abdominal muscle strengthening, or general conditioning exercises increase lung function. Patients with COPD who participate in a pulmonary rehabilitation program that includes aerobic conditioning exercises report a better level of general well-being, fewer episodes of dyspnea, and a higher functional capacity. Chest physical therapy and a reconditioning program for the patient with COPD will not arrest the disease process or change lung function. Patients with mild to moderate COPD will benefit more from a conditioing program than will patients with late stage disease.[3,4,10,18,22,23] Appropriate quantitative assessment prior to and after a patient has been involved in general conditioning will help to determine the effectiveness of the program.

B. Asthma

Asthma is an obstructive lung disease seen in young patients. It is related to hypersensitivity of the trachea and bronchi and causes difficulties with respiration because of bronchospasm and increased mucus production.[1,7,10,19]

1. Clinical picture
a. The majority of patients with asthma are children.
b. Asthmatic attacks involve severe shortness of breath when the patient comes in contact with a specific allergen. The patient has a very rapid rate of respiration and primarily uses accessory muscles for breathing. There are audible wheezes and rhonchi, and the patient feels severe tightness in his chest. The expiratory phase of respiration is prolonged.
c. Pathologic changes[1,10]
    (1) Severe spasm of smooth muscle of the bronchial tree
    (2) Narrowing of airways
    (3) Inflammation of the mucosal lining of the tracheobronchial tree and hypersecretion of mucus, which is usually sticky and therefore obstructive because of an increase in the size and number of goblet cells.
    (4) Severe asthma over a prolonged number of years can lead to emphysema.
d. General appearance of the patient
    (1) chronically fatigued
    (2) often thin
    (3) poor posture—rounded shoulders, forward head, and hypertrophy of accessory muscles

2. Clinical problems of asthma summarized
a. Severe attacks of shortness of breath
b. Cough—usually unproductive during an asthmatic attack, but productive later
c. Abnormal breathing pattern; overuse of accessory muscles, resulting in upper chest breathing and increased respiratory rate
d. Poor posture—rounded shoulders, forward head

3. General treatment goals and plan of care

Treatment Goals[7,10,19]	Plan of Care
a. Decrease bronchospasm.	a. Removal of allergen(s); bronchodilators with IPPB.
b. Minimize attacks of shortness of breath and gain control of breathing.	b. Relaxation of upper chest and accessory muscles by positioning (see Figures 20-1 through 20-3). Diaphragmatic breathing, emphasizing relaxed expiration.

Use of pursed-lip breathing as needed.
Use of controlled rate of breathing.

c. Mobilize and remove secretions *after* attack of shortness of breath.

c. Humidification of secretions with aerosol therapy.
Effective coughing.
Postural drainage (after, not during, the asthmatic attack, since it may increase bronchospasm).

d. Correct posture to decrease rounded shoulders and forward head.

d. Postural training (see Chapter 14).

e. Gradually increase exercise tolerance and endurance.

e. Avoid prolonged, vigorous physical activities.
Encourage mild to moderate activities for short periods of time, followed by rest.
Use controlled breathing during exertion.

C. Bronchiectasis

Bronchiectasis is an obstructive lung disease characterized by dilation of the medium-sized bronchioles, usually the fourth to the ninth generations, and repeated infections in these areas.[1,7,10]

1. Clinical picture
   a. Severe infection of dilated obstructed bronchioles
   b. Productive cough with purulent sputum and hemoptysis
   c. Pathologic changes
      (1) Repeated infections of the lower lobes of the lungs
      (2) Destruction of ciliated epithelial cells in infected areas
   d. If the infections are localized, a lobectomy may be indicated.

2. Clinical problems of bronchiectasis summarized[7,10]
   a. Repeated infections of the affected lung area
   b. Accumulation of purulent secretions
   c. Productive cough

3. General treatment goals and plan of care

Treatment Goals	*Plan of Care*
a. Clear the airways of secretions	a. Effective, controlled cough Postural drainage BID to QID during acute episodes.
b. Prevent recurrent infections	b. Home program of postural drainage to be carried on throughout life.

4. Precautions
   a. If *mild hemoptysis* (blood-streaked sputum) occurs, continue postural

drainage but omit percussion for at least 24 hours.
  b. If *severe hemoptysis* (hemorrhage) occurs, discontinue postural drainage until advised by physician.

D. Cystic Fibrosis

Cystic fibrosis is a genetically based disease (autosomal recessive) that involves malfunction of the exocrine glands, leading to abnormal secretions in the body. The disease is characterized by a very high concentration of sodium in the sweat, diffuse lung disease, and malfunction of the pancreas.[20] The disease must be managed throughout life with diet, medication, and preventive chest physical therapy as soon as any symptoms are noted in the young child.

1. Clinical picture[20,25,27]
  a. These children are usually small for age because of malabsorption of foods.
  b. The exocrine gland dysfunction leads to increased production of viscous mucus, which obstructs the airways. Chronic obstruction of the airways and pooling of secretions leave the child vulnerable to pulmonary infection.
  c. Prognosis for survival has improved in the past 25 years. The average patient now survives into the late 20s or early 30s. The digestive involvement can be managed by diet; pulmonary complications are eventually the cause of death.

2. Clinical problems of cystic fibrosis summarized
  a. Increased production of viscous mucus throughout the lungs
  b. Periodic pulmonary infections
  c. Possible problems of compliance with a life-long regimen of home postural drainage and prevention of lung infections

3. General treatment goals and plan of care

Treatment Goals[7,25,26,27]	*Plan of Care*
a. Prevent accumulation of secretions and pulmonary infection	a. Daily home program of postural drainage, usually BID, if no acute pulmonary problems exist
b. Decrease viscosity of secretions	b. Humidification therapy with mist tent or IPPB
c. Prevent use of accessory muscles of respiration	c. Diaphragmatic breathing and lateral costal expansion Daily practice and use of deep breathing during postural drainage is important. Emphasize *relaxed* expiration so bronchospasm and air trapping does not occur.
d. Removal of secretions during an acute infection	d. Postural drainage QID or for longer periods of time, as needed Appropriate use of antibiotics

e. Increase exercise tolerance and functional capacity

e. Graded endurance and conditioning exercises (see Chapter 21)

Note: The key to successful preventive treatment of the complications of cystic fibrosis over many years is a consistent home program of postural drainage. This requires a supportive and cooperative family atmosphere.

III. OVERVIEW OF RESTRICTIVE LUNG DISORDERS

A. Definition[9]

Restrictive lung disorders are characterized by the inability of the lungs to fully expand as the result of an extrapulmonary or pulmonary restriction.
1. Tidal volume, inspiratory and vital capacities, and total lung capacity are all diminished.
2. The rate of respiration is usually increased (tachypnea).
3. In restrictive lung disease, it is extremely difficult for the patient to take a deep inspiration.

B. Causes of Restrictive Lung Disease[9]
1. Extrapulmonary restrictions
   a. Pleural disease (pleural effusion)
   b. Chest wall injury or stiffness
      (1) Chest wall pain, secondary to trauma or rib fracture or to pulmonary or cardiac surgery
      (2) Structural abnormality (scleroderma, pectus excavatum)
      (3) Postural deformities (scoliosis, kyphosis, ankylosing spondylitis)
   c. Respiratory muscle weakness
      (1) Neuromuscular disease or dysfunction (muscular dystrophy, anterior horn cell disease, parkinsonism)
      (2) CNS depression or injury (drug overdose, very high spinal cord injury)
   d. Insufficient excursion of the diaphragm because of obesity or ascites.

2. Pulmonary restrictions
   a. Tumor
   b. Pneumonia
   c. Atelectasis
   d. Heart disease

C. General Clinical Problems
1. Inability to inspire deeply
2. Tachypnea—The patient *must* breathe at an increased rate.
3. Ineffective cough
4. Decreased thoracic mobility (primary or secondary)
5. Postural deviations
6. General weakness and fatigue

IV. SPECIFIC RESTRICTIVE PULMONARY CONDITIONS

A. Post-Thoracotomy
Patients with pulmonary or cardiac conditions that require surgical intervention are at high risk for restrictive pulmonary complications, such as atelecta-

sis and pneumonia, after chest surgery. A *thoracotomy,* an incision into the chest wall, is required in a variety of pulmonary and cardiac surgeries. In addition to pulmonary complications, a thoracotomy predisposes the patient to postsurgical postural deviations. It has been recognized for many years that effective pulmonary hygiene, particularly in the early days after surgery, is an important adjunct to surgery. A carefully planned program of *preoperative* and *postoperative* chest physical therapy can minimize postsurgical complications and restore normal function for these patients.[7,21]

1. **Pulmonary surgery**
   a. Reasons for surgery
      (1) Malignant or benign tumors
      (2) Lung abscess
      (3) Bronchiectasis
      (4) Tuberculosis
      (5) Abnormalities of the pleura
   b. Types of surgery
      (1) Lobectomy
          Removal of one or more lobes of the lungs, usually as the result of carcinoma
      (2) Pneumonectomy
          Removal of an entire lung
      (3) Segmental resection
          Removal of a segment of a lobe of the lung, usually for benign tumors, or diseased tissue secondary to bronchiectasis or tuberculosis
      (4) Pleurectomy
          An incision into the pleura

2. **Cardiac surgery (open heart surgery)[7,15,16,19]**
   a. Reasons for surgery
      (1) Coronary artery disease
      (2) Cardiac valve insufficiency and stenosis
      (3) Aneurysm
      (4) Congenital abnormalities of the heart
          (a) Atrial or ventricular septal defects (ASD or VSD)
          (b) Patent ductus arteriosus (PDA)
   b. Types of surgery
      (1) Open heart procedures, which have been performed since the 1950s, require extracorporeal perfusion (total cardiopulmonary bypass using the heart-lung bypass pump). Open heart surgery procedures include
          (a) aortocoronary bypass surgery, which constitutes 50 percent of all open heart surgical procedures.
          (b) replacement of the mitral, aortic, or tricuspid valves of the heart.
          (c) repair of artrial and ventricular septal defects and patent ductus arteriosis.
          (d) Commissurotomy: Splitting or cutting of the commissures of a valve secondary to valvular stenosis.
          (e) Aneurysmectomy: Cutting, approximation, and resuturing of a cardiac aneurysm.
      (2) Heart transplantation surgery

3. **Factors that increase the risk of pulmonary complications and restrictive lung dysfunction after pulmonary or cardiac surgery**[2,8,14,17]

   The post-thoracotomy patient experiences considerable chest pain, which leads to chest wall immobility, poor lung expansion, and an ineffective cough. Pulmonary secretions also tend to be greater than normal postoperatively. Therefore, the patient is more likely to accumulate pulmonary secretions and develop secondary pneumonia or atelectasis. The factors that increase postoperative pulmonary complications are

   a. General anesthesia
      (1) decreases the normal ciliary action of the tracheobronchial tree.
      (2) depresses the respiratory center of the central nervous system, which causes a shallow respiratory pattern (decreased tidal volume).
   b. Intubation (insertion of an endotracheal or nasogastric tube)
      (1) causes muscle spasm and immobility of the chest.
      (2) irritates the mucosal lining of the tracheobronchial tree, which causes an increase in mucus production.
      (3) decreases the normal action of the cilia in the pulmonary tree, which leads to pooling of secretions.
   c. Incisional pain
      (1) causes the patient to take shallow breaths. Lung expansion is restricted and secretions are not adequately mobilized.
      (2) restricts a deep and effective cough. The patient usually has a weak, shallow cough that does not effectively mobilize secretions.
   d. Pain medication
      Although pain medication administered postoperatively tends to diminish incisional pain, it also
      (1) depresses the respiratory center of the central nervous system.
      (2) decreases the normal ciliary action in the bronchial tree.
   e. General inactivity and bed rest postoperatively cause secretions to pool, particularly in the posterior basalar segments of the lower lobes.
   f. General weakness and fatigue decrease the effectiveness of the cough.
   g. Other risk factors, not directly related to the surgery include:[17]
      (1) the patient's age (over age 50).
      (2) history of smoking.
      (3) history of COPD or restrictive pulmonary disorder due to neuromuscular weakness.
      (4) obesity.
      (5) poor mentation and orientation.
   h. **Note:** Patients who undergo abdominal surgery also have a high risk of developing postoperative pulmonary complications. Postoperative pain is often greater after upper abdominal surgery than after thoracic surgery, which results in hypoventilation, an ineffective cough, and a higher incidence of postoperative pulmonary complications.[17]

4. **Clinical problems of the post-thoracotomy patient summarized**[2,5,7,15,16,21,28]

   a. Poor lung expansion or an inability to take a deep inspiration because of incisional pain
   b. Decreased effectiveness of the cough because of incisional pain and irritation of the throat from intubation

    c. Possible accumulation of pulmonary secretions either preoperatively or postoperatively

    d. Decreased chest wall and upper extremity mobility

    e. Poor postural alignment because of incisional pain or chest tubes

    f. Increased possibility of thrombophlebitis because of extracorporeal perfusion (in the open heart surgery patient) or bed rest and inactivity postoperatively

    g. General weakness, fatigue, and disorientation

5. Preoperative evaluation and treatment

A thorough presurgical evaluation of the patient who is to have either pulmonary or cardiac surgery is essential.[15,16,21,24]

    a. Preoperative evaluation of

        (1) breathing pattern, respiratory rate, and heart rate.

        (2) effectiveness and productivity of the cough.

        (3) accumulation of secretions and the possible need for postural drainage.

        (4) range of motion, particularly of the shoulders.

        (5) posture and alignment of the trunk.

    b. Preoperative treatment and patient education

The preoperative period is an ideal time to prepare the patient physically and psychologically for surgery and to teach the patient activities that will be carried out in the early postoperative days. Instructions should include

        (1) a general explanation of what to expect postoperatively, such as the location of the incision, incisional pain, the placement and function of chest tubes, endotracheal intubation, intravenous tubes, Foley catheter, an arterial line, or cardiac electrodes and monitor.

        (2) breathing exercise instruction with an emphasis on deep inspiration using

            (a) diaphragmatic breathing.

            (b) lateral and posterior basal breathing.

        (3) incentive spirometry or inspiratory resistance training as an adjunct to deep breathing exercises.

        (4) effective cough instruction and an explanation of splinting techniques.

        (5) removal of any accumulated secretions with full or modified postural drainage.

        (6) lower extremity exercise to maintain circulation and prevent thrombophlebitis.

        (7) postural alignment in bed.

6. Thoracic surgery—Postoperative considerations[2,5,7,8,14,15,17,21,28]

The patient who has undergone a thoracotomy for a pulmonary or cardiac condition will usually be hospitalized for 1 week or longer. In addition to the primary pulmonary or cardiac problem such as a malignant tumor, lung abscess, or coronary artery disease, the patient may also have related cardiopulmonary problems such as angina, congestive heart disease, chronic bronchitis, or emphysema. The patient with a long history of cardiac disease may also have preoperative pulmonary conditions such as hypoxemia, dyspnea on exertion, orthopnea, or pulmonary congestion. If this is the case, the postoperative rehabilitation may be longer and more complicated.

Most patients undergoing pulmonary surgery will have a large posterolateral or anterolateral chest wall incision. A standard posterolateral approach (Figure 20-4), for example, is performed by incising the chest wall along the intercostal space that corresponds to the location of the lung lesion. The incision divides the trapezius and rhomboid muscles posteriorally and the serratus anterior, latissimus dorsi, and external and internal intercostals laterally.

Postoperatively, the incision is quite painful, and the potential for pulmonary complications is significant. Many patients, quite understandably, complain of a great deal of shoulder soreness on the operated side. Loss of range of shoulder motion and postural deviations are possible because of the disturbance of the large arm and trunk musculature during surgery.

The most common incision used with cardiac surgery is a *median sternotomy*. A large incision extends along the anterior chest from the sternal notch to the xyphoid. The sternum is then split and retracted so that the chest cavity can be exposed.

Extracorporeal perfusion by means of a heart-lung bypass pump is required during open heart surgery. Although development of the heart-lung bypass pump in the 1950s has revolutionized cardiac surgery, extracorporeal circulation also puts the patient at further risk of developing postoperative pulmonary or circulatory complications. Pulmonary hypoxia occurs as circulation to the heart and lungs is bypassed. Microemboli in the pulmonary vascular system occur more frequently with extracorporeal perfusion.

During cardiac surgery, an endotracheal tube is put in place and remains in place 1 day postoperatively so that the patient can be mechanically ventilated for the first 24 hours. The patient's cardiac status is constantly monitored postoperatively by an ECG.

During most thoracotomies that involve a lateral incision, two chest drainage tubes are put in place at the time of surgery to prevent a pneumothorax or a hemothorax. While these tubes are in place, crimping, clamping, or traction on the tubes must be avoided during postoperative treatment.

The patient will fatigue easily in the first few postoperative days, so treatment sessions should be short but frequent, usually QID. The dura-

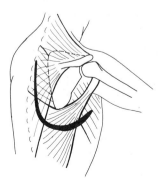

FIGURE 20-4. A posterolateral approach commonly used in thoracic surgery incises the trapezius, rhomboid, latissimus dorsi, serratus anterior, and internal and external intercostal muscles.

tion and intensity of treatment should be slowly and gradually increased during the patient's hospital stay.

Check the patient's chart regularly to note any day-to-day changes in vital signs, temperature, and laboratory test results. Always monitor vital signs such as heart rate and rhythm, respiratory rate, and blood pressure prior to, during, and after every treatment session.

7. General treatment goals and plan of care

Postoperative Goals	*Plan of Care*
a. Ascertain the status of the patient before each treatment.	a. Evaluate color, respiratory rate, heart rate, breath sounds, sputum, drainage into chest tubes, and orientation.
b. Maintain adequate ventilation and re-expand lung tissue to prevent atelectasis and pneumonia.	b. Begin deep-breathing exercises on the day of surgery as soon as the patient is conscious. Diaphragmatic breathing. Apical expansion. Lateral costal and posterior basal expansion. Add incentive spirometry or inspiratory resistance exercises to improve inspiratory capacity. Continue deep-breathing exercises QID postoperatively until the patient is ambulatory.
c. Assist in the removal of secretions.	c. Begin deep, effective coughing as soon as the patient is alert and can cooperate. *Precaution:* Adequately splint over the incision with your hand or a pillow to minimize incisional pain (see Figures 19-20 and 19-21). Initiate modified postural drainage, *if necessary;* modified postural drainage may be necessary several days after surgery if secretions accumulate. If x-ray examinations and breath sounds are normal and if the patient can breathe deeply and cough effectively, postural drainage will not be necessary. *Precautions:* Modify the postural drainage positions in which the patient is placed to minimize stress to the incision. The head-down position

should be avoided until the chest tubes are removed. Take great care when turning the patient (use a log-roll). Be sure to avoid traction or pressure on chest tubes and avoid percussion near the site of the incision.

d. Maintain adequate circulation in the lower extremities to prevent thrombophlebitis.

d. Begin active exercises to the lower extremities, with emphasis on ankle pumping exercises, on the first day after surgery.

Continue leg exercises until the patient is allowed out of bed and is ambulatory.

e. Maintain range of motion in the shoulders.

e. Begin relaxation exercises to the shoulder area on the first postoperative day. These can include shoulder shrugging or shoulder circles.

Initiate active-assistive range of motion to the shoulders, being careful not to cause pain.

Note: Reassure the patient that gentle movements will not injure the incision.

Progress to active shoulder exercises on the succeeding postoperative days to the patient's tolerance until full active range of motion has been achieved.

Precaution: In a patient with a lateral incision, in order to prevent dislodging a chest tube, limit shoulder flexion on the operated side to 90 degrees for several days until the chest tube is removed.

f. Prevent postural defects.

f. Reinforce symmetric alignment and positioning of the trunk on the first postoperative day when the patient is in bed.

Note: The patient will tend to lean toward the side of the incision.

Instruct the patient in symmetric sitting posture when he is allowed to sit up in a chair or at the side of the bed by the third or fourth postoperative day.

g. Restore exercise tolerance.

g. Begin a progressive and graded ambulation program as soon as chest tubes are removed, and the patient is allowed to be ambulatory.

B. Pneumonia

Pneumonia is an inflammation of the lungs, characterized by consolidation and exudation and caused by a bacterial or viral infection.[7,11] Chest physical therapy, when applied appropriately and in conjunction with antibiotics and respiratory modalities, can be an important aspect of the overall treatment of the patient with pneumonia. Patients with obstructive lung disease, such as chronic bronchitis, emphysema, and cystic fibrosis; patients who have recently undergone surgery; comatose patients; and patients with artificial airways are at particular risk for developing pneumonia. Whenever possible, chest physical therapy should be used to *prevent* pneumonia in these patients.

1. Classifications of pneumonia

a. By anatomic location

(1) *Bronchopneumonia*
Inflammation of the bronchial tree
(a) Common in the postoperative patient, especially those with a history of chronic bronchitis
(b) Characterized by a productive cough and copious amounts of purulent sputum. There is usually no pain with deep inspirations or cough and no consolidation or pleural effusion.
(c) Early and vigorous chest physical therapy is indicated.

(2) *Acute lobar pneumonia*
Inflammation of an entire lobe or lobes of the lung, often caused by a pneumococcal infection.
(a) Not common today because of effective chemotherapy
(b) Characterized by fever and pulmonary consolidation; dyspnea; a nonproductive cough in the early stages; and acute and localized chest pain with deep inspiration or cough. In the later stage when pain and fever subside and consolidation decreases, the cough becomes productive and rust-colored sputum is produced.
(c) In the early acute stage, chest physical therapy should consist of deep, relaxed breathing, localized to the area of involvement, to mobilize secretions. The patient may be assisted with IPPB therapy during breathing exercises. Percussion should not be done because of pain.
(d) In the later stages, when the cough becomes productive and pain decreases, postural drainage with percussion may be performed over the affected areas.

(3) *Segmental pneumonia*
Localized to one or two small segment(s) of a lobe

b. By causal organism

(1) *Viral pneumonia*
(a) Fever, dyspnea, and a chronic, nonproductive cough
(b) Chest physical therapy includes deep breathing exercises.

(c) Postural drainage with percussion is not done, because secretions are not present.

(2) *Bacterial pneumonia*

Often named by the organism: pneumococcus, streptococcus, or staphylococcus organisms.

(a) Fever, dyspnea, tachypnea and a productive cough with rust-colored sputum are present.

(b) Chest physical therapy is initiated early and vigorously, with emphasis on deep breathing, postural drainage with percussion, and frequent positional changes.

2. General treatment goals and plan of care

Treatment Goals	*Plan of Care*
a. Control the infection.	a. Use of appropriate medications, usually antibiotics.
b. Maintain or improve ventilation.	b. Deep-breathing exercises, localized to the area of involvement. Use of IPPB Frequent positional changes of the patient in and out of bed.
c. Mobilize secretions when consolidation and pain decrease and the cough becomes productive.	c. Postural drainage with percussion and vibration to the affected areas. Effective cough—ensure that the cough is deep and controlled.

3. Precautions:

a. Postural drainage should only be used for patients with increased mucus production, accumulated secretions, and a productive cough.

b. Percussion and vibration should not be used in patients who are experiencing a great deal of pleural pain with coughing or with deep inspirations.

C. Atelectasis

Atelectasis is a restrictive lung dysfunction in which lobes or segments of a lobe of a lung have collapsed. Lung tissue can collapse due to an increase in pressure on the lungs from a pneumothorax, hemothorax, or increased pleural fluid. Airway obstructions from abnormal secretions and tumor can cause collapse of lung tissue distal to the obstruction.[10,29]

1. Clinical picture and problems summarized

a. Absent breath sounds over the collapsed lung area

b. Tachypnea; cyanosis

c. Decreased chest movement over the affected area

d. Atelectasis prone to develop in patients with accumulated secretions and a poor cough after intubation and thoracic surgery

2. General treatment goals and plan of care

Treatment Goals	*Plan of Care*
a. Reinflate collapsed areas of the lung.	a. Postural drainage with percussion and vibration for removal of secretions. Initiate effective coughing.
b. Increase inspiratory capacity.	b. Segmental breathing with emphasis over collapsed areas. Splinting to decrease pain if present.

V. SUMMARY

This chapter provided general information on obstructive and restrictive lung diseases. The causes and clinical problems associated with obstructive diseases, such as chronic bronchitis, emphysema, asthma, cystic fibrosis, and bronchiectasis, were outlined. The causes and clinical problems of selected restrictive lung disorders and dysfunction were also discussed. Particular emphasis was placed on the respiratory and physical problems of the patient who has undergone thoracic or cardiac surgery.

An outline of the goals of treatment and guidelines and precautions for therapeutic management were also given. The reader was referred to Chapter 19 for specific details of chest physical therapy procedures, such as breathing exercises, postural drainage, and exercises for thoracic mobility.

REFERENCES

1. American Lung Association: *Chronic Obstructive Pulmonary Diseases: Manual for Physicians,* ed 3. New York, 1972.
2. Berendt, DM and Austen, GW: *Patient Care in Cardiac Surgery.* Little, Brown and Co, Boston, 1985.
3. Busch, AJ and McClements, JD: *Effects of supervised home exercise program on patients with severe chronic obstructive pulmonary disease.* Phys Ther 68:469, 1988.
4. Casciari, RJ, et al: *Effects of breathing retraining in patients with chronic obstructive pulmonary disease.* Chest 79:393, 1981.
5. Clough, P: *Physical therapy management of the post-thoracotomy shoulder.* Cardiopulmonary Section Quarterly, American Physical Therapy Association 3:7, 1982.
6. DeCesare, J and Babchyck, B: *Radionuclide assessment of the effects of chest physical therapy on ventilation in cystic fibrosis.* Phys Ther 62:820, 1982.
7. Glaskell, DV and Webber, BA: *The Brompton Hospital Guide to Chest Physiotherapy,* ed 4. CV Mosby, St. Louis, 1981.
8. Gless Williams, et al: *Thoracic and Cardiovascular Surgery,* ed 4. Appleton-Century-Crofts, New York, 1983.
9. Gold, W: *Restrictive lung disease.* J Am Phys Ther Assoc 48:455, 1968.
10. Hammon, WE: *Pathophysiology in chronic pulmonary disease.* In Frownfelter, D: *Physical Therapy and Pulmonary Rehabilitation,* ed. 2. Year Book Medical Publishers, Chicago, 1987.
11. Hobson, L: *Viral and bacterial pneumonia.* In Frownfelter, D: *Chest Physical Therapy and Pulmonary Rehabilitation,* ed 2. Year Book Medical Publishers, Chicago, 1987.
12. Hodgkins, JE: *The scientific status of chest physiotherapy.* Respir Care 26:657, 1981.
13. Hollis, M: *Practical Exercise Therapy,* ed 2. Blackwell Scientific Publications, Oxford, 1981.
14. Horwath, PT: *Care of the Cardiac Surgery Patient.* John Wiley & Sons, New York, 1984.

15. Howell, S and Hill, JD: *Acute respiratory care in the open heart surgery patient.* Phys Ther 52:253, 1972.
16. Howell, S and Hill, JD: *Chest physical therapy procedures in open heart surgery.* Phys Ther 58:1205, 1978.
17. Kigin, CM: *Physical therapy for the postoperative or traumatic injury patient.* Phys Ther 61:1724, 1981.
18. Lane, C: *COPD: The effects of training.* Cardiopulmonary Section Quarterly, American Physical Therapy Association, 1:2, 1980.
19. Lough, M, Doershuk, C, and Stern, R (eds): *Pediatric Respiratory Therapy.* Year Book Medical Publishers, Chicago, 1974.
20. National Cystic Fibrosis Research Foundation: *Guide to Diagnosis and Management of Cystic Fibrosis.* Atlanta, 1971.
21. Perlstein, MF: *Cardiovascular and thoracic surgery.* In Frownfelter, D: *Chest Physical Therapy and Pulmonary Rehabilitation.* Year Book Medical Publishers, Chicago, 1978.
22. Shaffer, T, Wolfson, M, and Bhutoni, VK: *Respiratory muscle function, assessment and training.* Phys Ther 61:1711, 1981.
23. Simpson, L: *Effect of increased abdominal muscle strength on forced vital capacity and forced expiratory volume.* Phys Ther 63:334, 1983.
24. Stein, M and Cassara, FL: *Preoperative pulmonary evaluation and therapy for surgery patients.* JAMA 211:787, 1962.
25. Tecklin, J and Holsclaw, D: *Cystic fibrosis and the role of the physical therapist in its management.* Phys Ther 53:386, 1973.
26. Tecklin, J and Holsclaw, DS: *Evaluation of bronchial drainage in patients with cystic fibrosis.* Phys Ther 55:1081, 1975.
27. Tecklin, J: *Physical therapy for children with chronic lung disease.* Phys Ther 61:1774, 1981.
28. Vraciu, JK and Vraciu, R: *Effectiveness of breathing exercises in preventing pulmonary complications following open heart surgery.* Phys Ther 57:1367, 1977.
29. Wohl, ME: *Atelectasis.* J Am Phys Ther Assoc 48:472, 1968.

CHAPTER ——————————— 21

Principles of Aerobic Exercise
Carolyn N. Burnett, M.S., P.T.

There are numerous sources from which to obtain information on training for endurance in athletes and healthy young people and in individuals with coronary heart disease. But there is little information or emphasis on endurance training and the improvement of fitness in the individual who has other types of chronic disease or disability. This chapter uses information from well-known sources to demonstrate that the physical therapist can use aerobics when working with either healthy individuals or patients with a variety of problems. In addition, some fundamental information about cardiovascular and respiratory parameters in children and the elderly, as well as the young or middle-aged adult, is presented so the physical therapist can be prepared to treat individuals of all ages.

OBJECTIVES

After studying this chapter, the reader will be able to:
1. define fitness, endurance, conditioning, adaptation, cardiac output, $\dot{V}O_2$ max, A-VO_2 difference, training stimulus threshold, MET, telemetry, and efficiency.
2. describe the determination of fitness and/or endurance levels in humans.
3. discuss the factors influencing the transport of oxygen.
4. identify the changes that occur with deconditioning and the implications of these changes.
5. compare the characteristics of the three energy systems.
6. describe the determination of energy expenditure.
7. differentiate high-level and low-level activity in terms of energy cost.
8. differentiate between stress testing and fitness testing.
9. identify the end points used to determine if $\dot{V}O_2$ max is achieved.
10. list the signs and symptoms that determine cessation of the stress test or the exercise session.
11. identify the appropriate guidelines for determining the intensity, duration, and frequency of an exercise program.

12. calculate the maximum heart rate for an individual of a certain age and determine the safest way to calculate the target heart rate for individuals of differing physical capacities, using the maximum heart rate or the heart rate reserve.
13. discuss the overload principle in endurance training or conditioning.
14. differentiate between high- and low-level exercise programs (characteristics, activities, and energy expenditure).
15. identify some special considerations that need to be taken into account when setting up an exercise program.
16. list the cardiovascular and biochemical changes that occur with endurance training and the mechanisms for their occurrence.
17. compare cardiovascular and respiratory parameters and $\dot{V}O_2$ max in the child, young adult, and aged.

I. KEY TERMS

A. Fitness

Fitness is a general term indicating a level of cardiovascular functioning that results in heightened energy reserves for optimum performance and well being. Optimum strength and flexibility may also be included in the use of the term.

1. Fitness means different things to different people.
   a. For the athlete, it may mean running long distances against the clock.
   b. For the nonathletic college student, it may mean participating in both mental and physical extracurricular activities throughout a long day.
   c. For the middle-aged adult, it may mean pursuing relaxing sedentary or physical activities at the end of the work day or work week.
   d. For the elderly, it may mean functioning independently at home, climbing a flight of stairs, gardening, or biking and swimming (at a reduced pace), if previously accomplished.
2. Fitness levels are designated on a continuum from very poor to superior.[2,13]
   a. They are influenced by age, gender, heredity, inactivity, and disease.
   b. They can be measured using a variety of screening methods.
      (1) One test determines the time to run 1.5 miles (most suited for the untrained).
      (2) A second test determines the distance run in 12 minutes.
   c. Level of fitness is dependent on endurance.

B. Endurance

Endurance (a measure of fitness) is the ability to work for prolonged periods of time and the ability to resist fatigue. It includes muscular endurance, which is local or specific endurance, and cardiovascular endurance, which is more general total body endurance.[29,42] It is dependent on the transport of oxygen, which is influenced by pulmonary function, the oxygen-binding capacity of the blood, cardiac function, oxygen extraction capabilities, and muscular oxidative potential.[6,39]

C. Maximum Oxygen Consumption

Maximum oxygen consumption ($\dot{V}O_2$ max) is a measure of the capacity of the aerobic or oxygen system of the total body and is the maximum volume of oxygen consumed per minute.[17,18,24,29,39,42,46]

1. It is also referred to as *maximum aerobic capacity, maximum aerobic power* or *oxygen uptake,* and *cardiovascular endurance capacity.*
2. $\dot{V}O_2$ max is mathematically defined as $\dot{V}O_2$ max (ml/min) = heart rate (bpm) × stroke volume (ml) × A-$\dot{V}O_2$ difference (ml/dl blood).
   a. The heart or the individual's cardiovascular capacity appears to be the major limiting factor to $\dot{V}O_2$ max, although the enzymatic capabilities of the working muscle to extract oxygen from the blood supply is also critical.
   b. If the pulmonary system is functioning within normal limits, it is not a determining factor of $\dot{V}O_2$ max.[39,46]
3. The $\dot{V}O_2$ max is influenced by gender, heredity, and the presence of disease.
4. $\dot{V}O_2$ max is the best single measure of cardiovascular reserve and physical fitness. It can be increased by conditioning exercises.

D. Conditioning

Conditioning is an augmentation of the energy capacity of the muscle through an exercise program.[18]
1. Conditioning is dependent on exercise of sufficient intensity, duration, and frequency.
2. Conditioning produces adaptation of the organism and is reflected in the individual's level of endurance.

E. Adaptation

Adaptation occurs over a long period of time in the cardiovascular system and muscle as a result of endurance exercises or training.[20]
1. Adaptation results in increased efficiency of the cardiovascular system and the active muscles and performance of work with less fatigue.
2. Adaptation is dependent on:
   a. the ability of the organism to change. The person with a low level of fitness will have more room to improve than the one who has a high level of fitness.[29]
   b. the training stimulus threshold (the stimulus that elicits a training response).[20,42]
      (1) Training stimulus thresholds are variable.
      (2) The higher the initial level of fitness the greater the intensity of exercise needed to elicit a significant change.

F. Maximum Myocardial Oxygen Consumption

Maximum myocardial oxygen consumption (m$\dot{V}O_2$) is a measure of the oxygen consumed by the myocardial muscle.[17,23,39]
1. The need or demand for oxygen is determined by heart rate, systemic blood pressure (afterload), myocardial contractility, and left ventricular wall tension. Left wall tension is influenced by left ventricular end-diastolic pressure and left ventricular end-diastolic volume, and, to a small degree, basal oxygen requirements, activation energy, and fiber shortening.
2. The ability to supply the myocardium with oxygen is dependent on the arterial oxygen content (blood substrate), hemoglobin oxygen dissociation, and coronary blood flow, which is determined by aortic diastolic pressure, duration of diastole, coronary artery resistance, and collateral circulation.
3. In a healthy individual, a balance between myocardial oxygen supply and

demand is maintained during maximal exercise. When the demand for oxygen is greater than the supply, myocardial ischemia results.

4. Since the myocardial muscle extracts 70 to 75 percent of the oxygen from the blood during rest, its main source of supply during exercise is through an increase in coronary blood flow.

G. Deconditioning

Deconditioning occurs with prolonged bed rest, and its effects are frequently seen in the patient who has had an extended illness. These effects are also seen, although possibly to a lesser degree, in the individual who has spent a period of time on bed rest without any accompanying disease process, and in the individual who is sedentary because of life-style and increasing age.

II. ENERGY SYSTEMS, ENERGY EXPENDITURE, AND EFFICIENCY

A. Energy Systems

Energy systems are metabolic systems involving a series of chemical reactions resulting in the formation of waste products and the manufacture of adenosine triphosphate (ATP). Only from the energy released by the breakdown of this compound can the cell perform work. There are three energy systems.[18,27,29] The intensity and duration of activity determine when and to what extent each of the metabolic systems contribute.

1. The ATP-PC system

The ATP-PC system (adenosine triphosphate-phosphocreatine) has the following characteristics:
a. Phosphocreatine and ATP are stored in the muscle cell.
b. Phosphocreatine is the chemical fuel source.
c. No oxygen is required.
d. When muscle is rested, the supply of ATP-PC is replenished.
e. The maximal capacity of the system is small (0.7 moles ATP).
f. The maximal power of the system is great (3.7 moles ATP per min).
g. The system provides energy for short quick bursts of activity.
h. It is the major source of energy during the first 30 seconds of intense exercise.

2. The anaeorobic glycolytic system

The anaerobic glycolytic system has the following characteristics:
a. Glycogen (glucose) is the food fuel source.
b. No oxygen is required.
c. ATP is resynthesized in the muscle cell.
d. Lactic acid is produced.
e. The maximal capacity of the system is intermediate (1.2 moles, ATP).
f. The maximal power of the system is intermediate (1.6 moles ATP per min).
g. The systems provide energy for activity of moderate intensity and short duration.
h. It is the major source of energy from the 30th to 90th second of exercise.

3. The aerobic system

The aerobic system has the following characteristics:

a. Glycogen, fats, and proteins are food fuel sources.
b. Oxygen is required.
c. ATP is resynthesized in the mitochondria of the muscle cell. The ability to metabolize oxygen and other substrates is related to the number and concentration of the mitochondria and cells.
d. The maximal capacity of the system is great (90.0 moles, ATP).
e. The maximal power of the system is small (1.0 mole ATP per min).
f. The system predominates over the other energy systems after the second minute of exercise.

4. **Recruitment of motor units**

Recruitment of motor units is dependent on rate of work. Fibers are recruited selectively during exercise.[29,42]
a. Slow twitch fibers (type I) are characterized by a slow contractile response, are rich in myoglobin and mitochondria, have a high oxidative capacity and a low anaerobic capacity, and are recruited for activities demanding endurance. These fibers are supplied by small neurons with a low threshold of activation and are used preferentially in low-intensity exercise.
b. Fast twitch fibers (type IIb) are characterized by a fast contractile response, have a low myoglobin content and few mitochondria, have a high glycolytic capacity, and are recruited for activities requiring power.
c. Fast twitch fibers (type IIa) have characteristics of both type I and type IIb fibers and are recruited for both anaerobic and aerobic activities.

B. Functional Implications[6]

1. Bursts of intense activity (seconds) develop muscle strength and stronger tendons and ligaments. ATP is supplied by the phosphagen system.
2. Intense activity (1 to 2 minutes), repeated after 4 minutes of rest or mild exercise provides anaerobic power. ATP is supplied by the phosphagen and anaerobic glycolytic system.
3. Activity with large muscles, which is less than maximal intensity for 3 to 5 minutes repeated after rest or mild exercise of similar duration, may develop aerobic power and endurance capabilities. ATP is supplied by the phosphagen, anaerobic glycolytic, and aerobic systems.
4. Activity that is of submaximal intensity lasting 30 minutes or more taxes a high percentage of the aerobic system and develops endurance.
5. Prolonged exercise progresses on a pay-as-you-go basis, with more than 99 percent of the energy requirement generated by aerobic reactions.

C. Energy Expenditure

Energy is expended by individuals engaging in physical activity. Activites can be categorized as light or heavy by determining the energy cost. Most daily activities are light activity and are aerobic, since they require little power but occur over prolonged periods.[29] Heavy work is usually aerobic and anaerobic.
1. Energy expenditure can be determined easily by open-circuit spirometry or telemetry.
a. *Open-circuit portable spirometry* requires that the individual breathe into and out of a mouthpiece with a valve.[29]
(1) The air expired passes directly through an automatic gas analyzer that measures volume and analyzes the oxygen and carbon dioxide

composition of the expired air. This occurs automatically on a breath-by-breath basis.

(2) The energy expenditure is computed from the amount of oxygen consumed.

b. *Telemetry,* or physiologic radio transmission, allows the individual to move freely without the encumbrance of a portable spirometer.[18] The heart rate of the individual is picked up through the air by a radio transmitter which can be connected to a graphic printout system, producing an electrocardiographic strip.

(1) Heart rate is linearly related to the work performed.[18,29,42]

(2) Heart rate is therefore also linearly related to the amount of oxygen consumed per minute.

2. Energy expended is computed from the amount of oxygen consumed. Units used to quantify energy expenditure are kilocalories and METs.

a. A *kilocalorie* (large calorie) is a measure expressing the energy value of food. It is the amount of heat necessary to raise 1 kilogram (kg) of water 1° C. A kilocalorie (Kcal) can be expressed in oxygen equivalents. Five kilocalories equal approximately one liter of oxygen consumed (5 Kcal = 1 liter O_2).

b. A *MET* is defined as the oxygen consumed (milliliters) per kilogram of body weight per minute (ml/kg/min). It is equal to approximately 3.5 ml/kg/min.[18]

c. Activities are classified as light or heavy according to energy expended or oxygen consumed while accomplishing them.[3,29]

(1) Strolling 1.6 km/hr, or 1.0 mph, requires 4 to 7 ml O_2/kg/min and is considered to be light work. The energy expended is equivalent to 2 to 2½ Kcal/min or 1½ to 2 METs.

(2) Jogging 8.0 km/hr, or 5.0 mph, requires 25 to 28 ml O_2/kg/min and is considered heavy work. The energy expended is equivalent to 8 to 10 Kcal/min or 7 to 8 METs.

3. A large body (heavy) will expend more energy than a smaller one.

4. The energy expenditure necessary for most industrial jobs requires less than 3 times the energy expenditure at rest.[29]

5. Energy expenditure of certain physical activity can vary, depending on factors such as skill, pace, and fitness level.[29]

6. As mentioned previously, most daily activities are aerobic.

D. Efficiency

Efficiency is usually expressed as a percentage.[18]

$$\text{Percent efficiency} = \frac{\text{useful work output}}{\text{energy expended or work input}} \times 100$$

1. Work output equals force times distance (W = F × D). It can be expressed in power units or work per unit of time (P = ^{w}/t).[18]

a. On a treadmill, work equals the weight of the subject times the vertical distance the subject is raised walking up the incline of the treadmill.

b. On a friction type bicycle, work equals the distance (which is the circumference of the flywheel times the number of revolutions) times the bicycle resistance.

2. Work input equals energy expenditure and is expressed as the net oxygen consumption per unit of time.

   a. With aerobic exercise, the resting volume of oxygen used per unit of time ($\dot{V}O_2$ value) is subtracted from the oxygen consumed during 1 minute of the steady state period.
      (1) Steady state is reached within 3 to 4 minutes after exercise has started.
      (2) In the steady state period, $\dot{V}O_2$ remains at a constant (steady) value.
   b. Total net oxygen cost is multiplied by the total time in minutes that the exercise is performed.
3. The higher the net oxygen cost, the lower the efficiency in performing the activity.
4. Efficiency of large muscle activities is usually 20 to 25 percent.[18]
5. Submaximal aerobic exercise is more efficient than higher intensity anaerobic exercise.[31]

III. PHYSIOLOGIC RESPONSE TO AEROBIC EXERCISE

The rapid increase in energy requirements during exercise requires equally rapid circulatory adjustments to meet the increased need for oxygen and nutrients to remove the end products of metabolism such as carbon dioxide and lactic acid and to dissipate excess heat. The shift in body metabolism occurs through a coordinated activity of all the systems of body; neuromuscular, respiratory, cardiovascular, metabolic, and hormonal. Oxygen transport and its utilization by the mitochondria of the contracting muscle are dependent on the coupling of blood flow and ventilation to cellular metabolism.[39,40]

A. Cardiovascular Response to Exercise[17,23,39,40]

1. **The exercise pressor response.**
   Stimulation of small myelinated and unmyelinated fibers in skeletal muscle involves a sympathetic nervous system (SNS) response. The central pathways are not known.
   a. The SNS response includes a generalized peripheral vasoconstriction and increased myocardial contractility, an increased heart rate, and hypertension. This results in a marked increase and redistribution of the cardiac output.
   b. The degree of the response equals the muscle mass involved and the intensity of the exercise.

2. **Cardiac effects**
   a. Frequency of sinoatrial node depolarization increases and heart rate increases; there is a decrease in vagal stimuli as well as an increase in SNS stimulation.
   b. There is an increase in the force development of the myofibers; a direct inotropic response of the SNS increases myocardial contractility.

3. **Peripheral effects**
   a. Generalized vasoconstriction occurs that allows blood to be shunted from the nonworking muscles, kidneys, liver, spleen, and splanchnic area to the working muscles.
   b. A locally mediated reduction in resistance in the working muscle arterial vascular bed, independent of the autonomic nervous system, is produced by metabolites such as K^+, H^+, and PCO_2.

    c. The veins of the working as well as the nonworking muscles remain constricted.

    d. A *net* reduction in total peripheral resistance results.

4. **The cardiac output increases because of the:**

    a. increase in myocardial contractility.

    b. increase in heart rate.

    c. increase in the blood flow through the working muscle.

    d. increase in the constriction of the capacitance vessels on the venous side of the circulation in both the working and nonworking muscles raising the peripheral venous pressure.

    e. net reduction in the total peripheral resistance.

5. **The increase in the systolic blood pressure is the result of the augmented cardiac output.**

B. Respiratory Response to Exercise

1. Respiratory changes occur rapidly with an increased gas exchange by the first or second breath. Of several possibilities, we do not know which stimulates increased ventilation during exercise. During exercise there is a decrease in venous O_2 saturation, an increase in PCO_2 and H^+, an increase in body temperature, increased epinephrine, and an increased stimulation of receptors of the joints and muscles; any of these factors, alone or in combination, may stimulate the respiratory system. Baroreceptor reflexes, protective reflexes, pain, emotion, and voluntary control of respiration may also contribute to the increase in respiration.

2. Minute ventilation increases as respiratory frequency and tidal volume increase.

3. Alveolar ventilation, occurring with the diffusion of gases across the capillary-alveolar membrane, increases 10- to 20-fold in heavy exercise to supply the additional oxygen needed and excrete the excess carbon dioxide produced.

C. Responses Providing Additional Oxygen to Muscle

1. **The increased blood flow to the working muscle previously discussed provides additional oxygen.**

2. **There is also extraction of more oxygen from each liter of blood. There are several changes that allow for this.**

    a. A decrease of the local tissue PO_2 occurs due to the use of more oxygen by the working muscle. As the partial pressure of oxygen decreases, the unloading of oxygen from hemoglobin is facilitated.

    b. The production of more carbon dioxide causes the tissue to become acidotic (the hydrogen-ion concentration increases) and the temperature of the tissue to increase. Both situations increase the amount of oxygen released from hemoglobin at any given partial pressure.

    c. The increase of red blood cell 2,3-diphosphoglycerate (DPG) produced during glycolysis during exercise also contributes to the enhanced release of oxygen.

3. **Factors determining how much of the oxygen is consumed are:**

    a. the vascularity of the muscles.

b. the fiber distribution.

c. the number of mitochondria.

d. the oxidative mitochondrial enzymes present in the fibers.

The oxidative capacity of the muscle is reflected in the A-$\dot{V}O_2$ difference, which is the difference between the oxygen content of arterial and venous blood.

IV. TESTING AS A BASIS FOR EXERCISE PROGRAMS

Testing for physical fitness of normal individuals should be distinct from graded exercise testing of convalescing patients,[20] individuals with symptoms of coronary heart disease, or individuals who are age 35 years or older but asymptomatic. Regardless of the type of testing, the level of performance is based on the submaximal or maximal oxygen uptake ($\dot{V}O_2$ max) or the symptom-limited oxygen uptake. The capacity of the individual to transport and utilize oxygen is reflected in the oxygen uptake.

A. Fitness Testing of Healthy Subjects

1. Field tests for the determination of cardiovascular fitness include time to run 1.5 miles or distance run in 12 minutes. These correlate well with $\dot{V}O_2$ max, but their use is limited to young persons or middle-aged individuals who have been carefully screened and have had recent experience in jogging or running.[13,28,46]

2. Multistage testing can provide a direct measurement of $\dot{V}O_2$ max. Testing is done in 4 to 6 stages, with each stage being approximately 3 to 6 minutes. Electrocardiographic (ECG) monitoring is warranted during the testing. There are several end points that can be considered to determine if $\dot{V}O_2$ max is achieved.[18,46]

   a. The individual is exhausted.

   b. The oxygen uptake does not increase with an increase in the workload.

   c. The heart rate is greater than 190 beats/min.

B. Stress Testing for Convalescing Individuals and Individuals at Risk is Multistage Testing

Individuals undergoing stress testing should have a physical examination, be monitored by the ECG, and be closely observed at rest, during exercise, and during recovery.

1. **The *principles of stress testing* include:**[3,17,18,24,29,39]

   a. the need for several thresholds of workload.

   b. an initial workload that is low in terms of the individual's anticipated aerobic threshold.

   c. maintenance of each workload for 2 to 6 minutes.

   d. termination of the test at the onset of symptoms or a definable abnormality of the ECG.

2. **In addition to serving as a basis for determining exercise levels or the exercise prescription, the stress test:**[3]

   a. establishes a diagnosis of overt or latent heart disease.

   b. evaluates cardiovascular functional capacity, as a means of clearing individuals for strenuous work or exercise programs.

   c. determines the physical work capacity in kilogram-meters per minute (kg-m/min) or the functional capacity in METs.
   d. evaluates responses to conditioning and/or preventive programs.
   e. assists in the selection and evaluation of appropriate modes of treatment.
   f. increases individual motivation for entering and adhering to exercise programs.
   g. is used clinically to evaluate patients with chest sensations or a history of chest pain to establish the probability that such patients have coronary disease. It can also evaluate the functional capacity of patients with chronic disease.

2. **All individuals who are taking a stress test should:**
   a. have had a physical examination.
   b. be monitored by the ECG and closely observed at rest, during exercise, and during recovery.
   c. sign a consent form.

3. *Precautions* **to be taken are applicable for both stress testing and the exercise program.**[3]
   a. Pulse increases with exercise.
   b. Blood pressure increases with exercise approximately 7 to 10 millimeters (mm) of mercury (Hg) per MET of physical activity.[3,39]
      (1) Systolic pressure should not exceed 220 to 240 mm Hg.[42]
      (2) Diastolic pressure should not exceed a 20 mm Hg increase with arm exercises.[5] It usually stays the same with leg work.
   c. Rate and depth of respiration increase with exercise.
      (1) Respiration should not be labored.
      (2) The individual should have no perception of shortness of breath.
   d. The increase in blood flow while exercising, which regulates core temperature and meets the demands of the working muscles, results in changes in the skin of the cheeks, nose, and earlobes. They become pink, moist, and warm to the touch.[5]

4. **End points requiring termination of the test period are:**
   a. an abnormal heart rate response.
   b. abnormal blood pressure responses.
   c. labored respiration.
   d. facial pallor or signs of distress.
   e. signs of excessive fatigue, with complaints of nausea and dizziness.
   f. problems with coordination and equilibrium.

      (1) The diabetic patient may become hypoglycemic. Orange juice will minimize symptoms of incoordination and dysequilibrium.
      (2) A patient may develop cerebral ischemia. If this is a transient episode, rest will reduce the symptoms.
   g. any electrocardiographic abnormalities.

C. Multistage Testing

Each of 4 to 6 stages is approximately 3 to 6 minutes. Differences in protocols involve the number of stages; magnitude of exercise (intensity); equipment used (bicycle, treadmill); duration of stages; end-points; position of body; muscle groups exercised; and types of effort.

1. Protocols have been developed for multistage testing. Two examples of protocols are the Bruce protocol and the modified Astrand protocol.
   a. The Bruce protocol[11]
      (1) Speed and gradient are changed at 3-minute intervals.
      (2) Speed and gradient change from 1.7 mph at 10 percent grade, to 2.5 mph at 12 percent, to 3.4 mph at 14 percent, to 4.2 mph at 18 percent, and 5.0 mph at 20 percent grade.
   b. The modified Astrand protocol[6]
      (1) Variation in percent grade of the treadmill is 2.5 to 10 percent at timed intervals.
      (2) Speed remains constant at 5 to 8.5 mph.
   c. A low-level protocol can be given to the patient with an uncomplicated myocardial infarction prior to discharge from the hospital (ten days to two weeks).[11] Examples include:
      (1) use of a bicycle ergometer at 50 rpm for three minutes at 0, 12, and 25 watts.
      (2) use of a treadmill at 1.2 mph for 3 minutes at 0, 3, and 6 percent gradients, until the threshold of signs and symptoms is reached. The aerobic cost is 8 to 12 ml/kg/min or 2 to 3 METs whether the bicycle or treadmill is used.
2. There are special considerations when selecting equipment to be used.
   a. Greater energy expenditure occurs with upper extremity exercises.
   b. $\dot{V}O_2$ max is greater with the treadmill than the bicycle, although this is not clinically significant.[42]
   c. Heart beat increases more when tested on a bicycle than on a tread-mill.

V. DETERMINANTS OF AN EXERCISE PROGRAM

Just as testing for fitness should be distinct from stress testing for patients or individuals at high risk, training programs for healthy individuals are distinct from the exercise prescription for patients. The intensity required for exercise programs for the healthy to achieve a conditioning response is well documented. Exercise prescription for the patient is based on less precise information.

Effective endurance training must produce a conditioning or cardiovascular response. Elicitation of the cardiovascular response is dependent on three critical elements of exercise: *intensity, duration,* and *frequency.*[18,29,39,42]

A. Intensity[6,29,39]

Determination of the appropriate intensity of exercise to use is based on the *overload principle* and the *specificity principle.*
1. The *overload principle.*
   Overload is a stress on an organism that is greater than the one regularly encountered during everyday life. To improve cardiovascular and muscular endurance, an overload must be applied to these systems. The exercise load (overload) must be above the training stimulus threshold (that stimulus that elicits a training or conditioning response) for adaptation to occur.
2. Once adaptation to a given load has taken place, in order for the individual to achieve further improvement, the training intensity (exercise load) must be increased.
3. Training stimulus thresholds are variable depending on the individual's

level of health, level of activity, age, and gender.
4. The higher the initial level of fitness, the greater the intensity of exercise needed to elicit a change.
5. A conditioning response occurs generally at 70 to 85 percent maximum heart rate (60 to 80 percent $\dot{V}O_2$ max).[42]
   a. 70 percent maximum heart rate is a minimal level stimulus for eliciting a conditioning response in healthy young individuals.
   b. 85 to 95 percent maximum heart rate is usually necessary to achieve a conditioning response for an athlete.
   c. The exercise does not have to be exhaustive to achieve a training response.
6. Determining *maximum heart rate* and *exercise heart rate* for training programs provides the basis for the initial intensity of the exercise.[1,6,18,42]
   a. When the individual is young and healthy, the *maximum heart rate* can be determined directly from a maximum performance multistage test, extrapolated from a heart rate achieved on a predetermined submaximal test, or less accurately calculated as 220 minus age.
   b. The *exercise heart rate* is determined:
      (1) as a percentage of the maximum heart rate. The percentage used is dependent on the level of fitness of the individual.
      (2) using the heart rate reserve (Karvonen's formula).[16,18,29]
         (a) It is based on the heart rate reserve (HRR), which is the difference between the resting heart rate (HR rest) and the maximal heart rate (HR max).
         (b) The exercise heart rate is determined as a percentage (usually 60 to 70 percent) of the heart rate reserve plus the resting heart rate.

Exercise heart rate $= HR_{rest} + 60\%$ to $70\% (HR_{max} - HR_{rest})$

         (c) Utilizing Karnoven's formula, the exercise heart rate is higher than when using maximum heart rate alone.
7. *Maximum heart rate* and *exercise heart rate* used for the exercise prescription for individuals at risk for coronary artery disease, individuals with coronary artery disease or other chronic disease, and for individuals who are elderly are determined from performance on the stress test.[6,18,42]
   a. *Maximum heart rate* cannot be determined in the same manner as with the young and healthy.
      (1) Assuming that an individual has an average *maximum heart rate*, using the formula 220 minus age will produce substantial errors in prescribing exercise intensity for these individuals.[45]
      (2) The symptom-limited heart rate is considered a *maximum heart rate*. At no time should the exercise heart rate exceed that of the symptom-limited heart rate achieved on the exercise test.
   b. The *exercise heart rate* as a percentage of the *maximum heart rate* varies considerably.
      (1) Use of the heart rate reserve method, which assumes a linear heart rate increment from rest to peak exercise, frequently overestimates the desired aerobic training intensity in early cardiac rehabilitation.[16]
      (2) Some low-level training can be achieved from prolonged activities that require only 25 percent of the *maximum heart rate*.[42]
8. Exercising at a high intensity for a shorter period of time appears to elicit a

greater improvement in $\dot{V}O_2$ max than exercising at a moderate intensity for a longer period of time. However, as exercise approaches the maximum limit, there is an increase in the relative risk of cardiovascular complications and the risk of musculoskeletal injury.

9. The higher the intensity and the longer the exercise intervals, the faster the training effect.[17]

10. Maximum oxygen consumption ($\dot{V}O_2$ max) is the best measure of intensity. Aerobic capacity and heart rate are linearly related and, therefore, maximum heart rate is a function of intensity.

11. The *specificity principle* as related to the specificity of training refers to adaptations in metabolic and physiologic systems depending on the demand imposed. Work load and work-rest periods can be selected so that training is directed toward:[6,30,39]

   a. muscle strength without a significant increase in total oxygen consumption.

   b. aerobic processes without mobilizing anaerobic processes.

   c. anaerobic processes without maximally effecting the oxygen transport system.

   d. both aerobic and anaerobic gains simultaneously.

B. Duration[29,33,42,46]

1. A threshold duration has not been identified as optimal for cardiovascular conditioning. It is dependent on the total work done, exercise intensity, training frequency, and fitness level.

2. Generally speaking, the greater the intensity of the exercise, the shorter the duration needed for adaptation. The lower the intensity of exercise, the longer the duration needed.

3. A 20 to 30 minute session is generally optimal at 70 percent maximum heart rate. When the intensity is below the heart rate threshold, a 45-minute continuous exercise period may provide the appropriate overload. With high-intensity exercise, 10 to 15 minute exercise periods are adequate. Three 5-minute daily periods may be effective in some deconditioned patients.

4. Exercise of longer than 45 minutes' duration increases the risk of musculoskeletal complications.

C. Frequency[18,29,33,39,42,46]

1. Like duration, there is no clear-cut information provided on the most effective frequency of exercise for adaptation to occur. Frequency may be a less important factor in exercise training than intensity or duration.

2. Frequency varies dependent on the health and age of the individual. Optimal frequency of training is generally three to four times a week. If training is at a low intensity, greater frequency may be beneficial. A frequency of two times a week does not generally evoke cardiovascular changes, although older individuals and convalescing patients may benefit from a program of that frequency.[42]

3. As frequency increases beyond the optimal range, the risk of musculoskeletal complications increases.

4. For individuals who are in good general health, exercising 30 to 45 minutes at least three times a week (2000 kcal/week) appears to protect against coronary heart disease.

D. Mode[1,18,29,39,42]

1. Many types of activities provide the stimulus for improving cardiorespiratory fitness. The important factor is that exercise involve large muscle groups that are activated in a rhythmic, aerobic nature. However, the magnitude of the changes may be determined by the mode used.

2. For specific aerobic activities such as cycling and running, the overload must use the muscles required by the activity as well as stress the cardiorespiratory system *(specificity principle)*. If endurance of the upper extremities is needed to perform activities on the job, then the upper extremity muscles must be targeted in the exercise program. The muscles trained develop a greater oxidative capacity with an increase in blood flow to the area. The increase in blood flow is due to increased microcirculation and more effective distribution of the cardiac output.

3. Training benefits are optimized when programs are planned to meet the individual needs and capacities of the participants. The skill of the individual, variations among individuals in competitiveness and aggressiveness, and variation in environmental conditions all need to be considered.

E. The Reversibility Principle[29,39]

The beneficial effects of exercise training are transient and reversible.

1. Detraining occurs rapidly when a person stops exercising. After only two weeks of detraining, significant reductions in work capacity can be measured and improvements can be lost within several months. In addition, a similar phenomenon occurs with individuals who are confined to bed with illness or disability. The individual becomes severely deconditioned, with loss of the ability to carry out normal daily activities as a result of inactivity.

2. The frequency or duration of physical activity required to maintain a certain level of aerobic fitness is less than that required to improve it.

VI. THE EXERCISE PROGRAM

A carefully planned exercise program can result in higher levels of fitness for the healthy individual, slow the decrease in functional capacity of the elderly, and recondition those who have been ill or have chronic disease. There are three components of the exercise program: (1) a warm-up period, (2) the aerobic exercise period, and (3) a cool-down period.

A. The Warm-Up Period

Physiologically, there is a time lag that exists between the onset of activity and the bodily adjustments needed to meet the physical requirements of the body.[2,18,29,34,42]

1. The purpose of the warm-up period is to enhance the numerous adjustments that must take place before physical activity. During this period there is:

   a. an increase in muscle temperature; the higher temperature increases the efficiency of muscular contraction by reducing muscle viscosity and increasing the rate of nerve conduction.

   b. an increased need for oxygen to meet the energy demands for the muscle. Extraction from hemoglobin is greater at higher muscle temperatures facilitating the oxidative processes at work.

   c. dilatation of the previously constricted capillaries with increases in the circulation, augmenting oxygen delivery to the active muscles and minimizing the oxygen deficit and the formation of lactic acid.

d. adaptation in sensitivity of the neural respiratory center to various exercise stimulants.

e. an increase in venous return; this occurs as blood flow is shifted centrally from the periphery.

2. The warm-up also prevents or decreases:

a. the susceptibility of the musculoskeletal system to injury by increasing flexibility.

b. the occurrence of ischemic ECG changes and arrhythmias.

3. The warm-up should be gradual and sufficient to increase muscle and core temperature without causing fatigue or reducing energy stores. Characteristics of the period include:

a. a 10-minute period of total body movement exercises such as calisthenics, static stretching, and running slowly.

b. the attainment of a heart rate within 20 bpm of the target heart tissue.

B. The Aerobic Exercise Period

The aerobic exercise period is the conditioning part of the exercise program. Attention to the determinants of intensity, frequency, duration, and mode of the program, as previously discussed, will have an impact on the effectiveness of the program. The main consideration when choosing a specific method of training is that the *intensity* be great enough to stimulate an increase in stroke volume and cardiac output and to enhance local circulation and aerobic metabolism within the appropriate muscle groups. The exercise period must be within the person's tolerance, above the threshold level for adaptation to occur, and below the level of exercise that evokes clinical symptoms.[2,3,6–8,11,18,26,29,42]

In aerobic exercise, submaximal, rhythmic, repetitive, dynamic exercise of large muscle groups is emphasized.

There are four methods of training that will challenge the aerobic system; continuous, interval (work-relief), circuit, and circuit-interval.

1. Continuous training[6,18,29,30,46]

a. A submaximal energy requirement, sustained throughout the training period, is imposed.

b. Once the steady state is achieved, the muscle obtains energy by means of aerobic metabolism. Stress is placed on the slow twitch fibers.

c. The activity can be prolonged for 20 to 60 minutes without exhausting the oxygen transport system.

d. Work rate is increased progressively as training improvements are achieved; overload can be accomplished by increasing the exercise duration.

e. In the healthy individual, continuous training is the most effective way to improve endurance.

2. Interval training[6,18,29,42,46]

In this type of training, the work or exercise is followed by a properly prescribed relief or rest interval. Interval training is perceived to be less demanding than continuous training. In the healthy individual, interval training tends to improve strength and power more than endurance. It is most appropriate in increasing endurance in the coronary patient, because anaerobic metabolism is less, thus, decreasing the risk of arrhythmias.

   a. The relief interval is either a rest relief (passive recovery) or a work relief (active recovery), and its duration ranges from a few seconds to several minutes. Work recovery involves continuing the exercise, but at a reduced level from the work period. During the relief period, a portion of the muscular stores of ATP and the oxygen associated with myoglobin that were depleted during the work period are replenished by the aerobic system. An increase in $\dot{V}O_2$ max occurs.

   b. The longer the work interval, the more the aerobic system is stressed. With a short work interval, the duration of the rest interval is critical if the aerobic system is to be stressed (a work:recovery ratio of 1:1 to 1:5 is appropriate). A rest interval equal to $1\frac{1}{2}$ times the work interval allows the succeeding exercise interval to begin before recovery is complete and stresses the aerobic system. With a longer work interval, the duration of the rest is not as important.[29]

   c. A significant amount of high-intensity work can be achieved with interval or intermittent work if there is appropriate spacing of the work relief intervals. The total amount of work that can be completed with intermittent work is greater than the amount of work that can be completed with continuous training.

3. Circuit training[12,29]

Circuit training employs a series of exercise activities. At the end of the last activity, the individual starts from the beginning and again moves through the series. The series of activities is repeated several times.

   a. Several exercise modes can be used involving large and small muscle groups and a mix of static or dynamic effort.

   b. Use of circuit training can improve strength and endurance by stressing both the aerobic and anaerobic systems.

4. Circuit-interval training[30]

   a. Combining circuit and interval training is effective because of the interaction of aerobic and anaerobic production of ATP.

   b. In addition to the aerobic and anaerobic systems' being stressed by the various activities, with the relief interval there is a delay in the need for glycolysis and the production of lactic acid prior to the availability of oxygen supplying the ATP.

C. The Cool-Down Period[2,18,34,42]

A cool-down period is necessary following the exercise period.

1. The purpose of the cool-down period is:

   a. to prevent pooling of the blood in the extremities by continuing to use the muscles to maintain venous return.

   b. to prevent fainting by increasing the return of blood to the heart and brain as cardiac output and venous return decreases.

   c. to enhance the recovery period with the oxidation of metabolic waste and replacement of the energy stores.

   d. to prevent myocardial ischemia, arrhythmias, or other cardiovascular complications.

2. **Characteristics of the cool-down period are similar to those of the warm-up period:**
   a. Total body exercises such as calisthenics are appropriate.
   b. The period should last 5 to 8 minutes.

VII. PHYSIOLOGIC CHANGES THAT OCCUR WITH TRAINING

Changes in the cardiovascular and respiratory systems as well as changes in muscle metabolism occur following endurance training. These changes are reflected both at rest and with exercise. It is important to note that all of the following training effects cannot result from one training program.[29]

A. Cardiovascular Changes

1. **Changes at rest**[6,18,20,22,29,31]
   a. a reduction in the resting pulse rate because of
      (1) a decrease in sympathetic drive, with decreasing levels of norepinephrine and epinephrine.
      (2) a decrease in atrial rate secondary to biochemical changes in the muscles and levels of acetylcholine, norepinephrine, and epinephrine in the atria.
      (3) an increase in parasympathetic (vagal) tone secondary to decreased sympathetic tone.
   b. a decrease in blood pressure.
      (1) This occurs with a decrease in peripheral vascular resistance.
      (2) The largest decrease is in systolic blood pressure.
      (3) This is most apparent in hypertensive individuals.
   c. an increase in blood volume and hemoglobin, which facilitates the oxygen delivery capacity of the system.

2. **Changes with exercise**
   a. a reduction in the pulse rate because of the mechanisms listed in section A 1 a.
   b. an increased stroke volume because of:
      (1) an increase in myocardial contractility.
      (2) an increase in ventricular volume.
   c. an increased cardiac output.
      (1) The increased cardiac output is a result of the increased stroke volume.
      (2) The increased cardiac output occurs with maximal exercise, but not with submaximal exercise.
      (3) The magnitude of the change is directly related to the increase in stroke volume and the magnitude of the reduced heart rate.
   d. an increased extraction of oxygen by the working muscle because of enzymatic and biochemical changes in the muscle.
   e. an increased maximum oxygen uptake ($\dot{V}O_2$ max).
      (1) Greater $\dot{V}O_2$ max results in a greater work capacity.
      (2) The increased cardiac output increases the delivery of oxygen to the working muscles.
      (3) The increased ability of the muscle to extract oxygen from the blood increases the utilization of the available oxygen.
   f. a decreased blood flow per kg of the working muscle.

(1) This occurs even though increasing amounts of blood are shunted to the exercising muscle.

(2) The increase in extraction of oxygen from the blood compensates for this change.

g. a decreased myocardial oxygen consumption (pulse rate times systolic blood pressure) for any given intensity of exercise.

(1) This results from a decreased pulse rate, with or without a modest decrease in blood pressure.

(2) The product can be decreased significantly in the healthy subject without any loss of efficiency at a specific workload.

B. Respiratory Changes

These changes are observed at rest and with exercise after endurance training.

1. Changes at rest:

a. larger lung volumes because of improved pulmonary function.

b. larger diffusion capacities because of
   (1) larger lung volumes
   (2) greater alveolar-capillary surface area.

2. Changes with exercise:

a. larger diffusion capacities for the same reasons as those listed in section 1 b. Maximal capacity of ventilation is unchanged.[37]

b. a lower amount of air ventilated at the same oxygen consumption. Maximum diffusion capacity is unchanged.[37]

c. an increased maximal minute ventilation.

d. an increased ventilatory efficiency.

C. Metabolic Changes

These changes are observed at rest and with exercise following endurance training.

1. Changes at rest:

a. muscle hypertrophy and increased capillary density.

b. an increased number and size of mitochondria increasing the capacity to generate ATP aerobically.

c. increases in muscle myoglobin concentration.[18]
   (1) Myoglobin increases the rate of oxygen transport.
   (2) Myoglobin possibly increases the rate of oxygen diffusion to the mitochondria.

2. Changes with exercise:

a. a decreased rate of depletion of muscle glycogen at submaximal work levels.
   (1) This is due to:
      (a) an increased capacity to mobilize and oxidize fat.
      (b) increased fat mobilizing and metabolizing enzymes.
   (2) Another term for this phenomenon is glycogen sparing.

b. lower blood lactate levels at submaximal work.
   (1) The mechanism is unclear.

(2) It does not appear to be related to a decrease in hypoxia of the muscles.
c. less reliance on phosphocreatine (PC) and ATP in skeletal muscle.
d. an increased capability to oxidize carbohydrate because of
(1) an increased oxidative potential of the mitochondria.
(2) an increased glycogen storage in the muscle.

3. *Note:* Ill health may influence metabolic adaptations to exercise.[24]

D. Other System Changes

Changes in other systems that occur with training include
1. a decrease in body fat.
2. a decrease in blood cholesterol and triglyceride levels.
3. an increase in heat acclimatization.
4. an increase in the breaking strength of bones, ligaments, and tendons.

VIII. APPLICATION OF PRINCIPLES OF AN AEROBIC CONDITIONING PROGRAM FOR THE PATIENT WITH CORONARY DISEASE

The use of the principles of aerobic conditioning in physical therapy has been most dominant in program planning for the individual following a myocardial infarction (MI) or following coronary artery bypass surgery.

In the past 10 to 15 years, there have been major changes in the medical management of these patients. These changes have included shortened hospital stays, a more aggressive progression of activity for the patient following MI or surgery, and earlier initiation of an exercise program based on a low-level stress test prior to discharge from the hospital. An aerobic conditioning program is a dominant part of the four phases of cardiac rehabilitation.

A. Phase I[3,23,39,42,43]

This phase of the program occurs in the hospital following stabilization of the patient's cardiovascular status after MI or coronary bypass surgery, and is 1 to 2 weeks in duration.
1. The *purpose* of the program is to:
   a. provide an orthostatic challenge to the cardiovascular system.
   b. minimize deconditioning effects. However, with early increased levels of activity for these patients, the complications of bed rest seldom are seen.
   c. minimize the psychologic effects of lessened activity.
   d. determine the effects of prescribed medications during activity.
   e. establish clinical data that contributes to the medical management of the patient.
2. *Activities* are aerobic, isotonic, submaximal and dynamic, using large muscle groups with an energy cost of less than 2 METS. The patients are monitored for heart rate, blood pressure, and electrocardiographic signs and symptoms of ischemia during the activities. Exercises include:
   a. self-care activities such as sitting up in bed and moving from bed to chair.
   b. calisthenics of varying intensity.
   c. continuous, monitored ambulation of an initial 2 to 5 minutes duration that progresses to 15 to 20 minutes. Heart rate is often limited to 20 bpm above resting heart rate or to 120 bpm.

3. Prior to discharge, a low-level exercise test is frequently performed.
   a. The exercise test can distinguish those patients at high risk for a repeat infarction or sudden death from those at low risk by determining prognosis and severity of disease and evaluating dysrhythmias. The effectiveness of medications or surgical treatment can also be established.
   b. A low-level protocol can be given to the patient with an uncomplicated MI prior to discharge from the hospital (10 days to 2 weeks). It can entail the:
      (1) use of a bicycle ergometer at 50 rpm for 3 minutes at 0, 12, and 25 watts *or*
      (2) use of a treadmill at 1.2 mph for 3 minutes at 0, 3, and 6 percent grades until the threshold of signs and symptoms is reached. The aerobic cost is 8 to 12 ml/kg/min or 2 to 3 METs whether the bicycle or treadmill is used.
4. Patient and family education plus initial psychosocial and vocational assessment also occurs in Phase I.

B. Phase II

This program is initiated upon discharge from the hospital. It is highly supervised, monitored by telemetry, based in an institution, and is 0 to 3 months in duration. Healing of the myocardium usually takes place in a minimum of 6 to 8 weeks during Phase II.

1. The purpose of the program is to:
   a. increase the person's exercise capacity in a safe and progressive manner so that adaptive cardiovascular and muscular changes occur. The early part of the program is referred to by some as "low-level" exercise training.
   b. enhance cardiac functions and reduce the cardiac cost of work. This may help eliminate or delay symptoms such as angina and ST-segment changes in the patient with coronary heart disease.
   c. produce favorable metabolic changes.
   d. determine the effect of medications on increasing levels of activity.
   e. relieve anxiety and depression.
   f. progress the patient to an independent exercise program.
2. A symptom-limited test is performed 6 to 12 weeks after hospital discharge or as early as 2 to 4 weeks following discharge.
3. *Activities* and the exercise program are predominantly aerobic, although in the second half of Phase II anaerobic exercises can be incorporated into the program. During the early part of the program, the intensity remains low (3 to 4 METs), but duration and frequency are gradually increased and during the later period of Phase II energy cost reaches 5 to 7 METs.
   a. The level of activity or training intensity can be based on a low- or moderate-level stress test with a predetermined end point. Intensity is set at a level that will not interfere with the healing process or produce cardiovascular complications and may be 80 to 95 percent of the heart rate achieved on the low-level test. Two to four evenly spaced sessions per week will increase the $\dot{V}O_2$ max and are cost effective. A maximal stress test can be given at the end of the Phase II period.
   b. If the patient has not had an exercise stress test, initial walking or cycling activities can be initiated with the heart beat not exceeding 120 to 130 bpm.

    c. Interval training may be more appropriate for the coronary patient than sustained activities because it avoids or limits the occurrence of a large oxygen debt.

    d. Continuous exercise is considered by some to be more appropriate as the cardiac patient improves. However, early activity (2 to 4 weeks) can include 10 to 15 minutes of continuous low-intensity training with a heart rate 20 to 30 beats above the resting heart rate. At this duration, for training to occur, the patient will be sweating and will have mild fatigue and slight breathlessness. In uncomplicated MI, the heart rate can be increased in 1 to 2 weeks.[23,30]

        (1) Walking may be of benefit to the recovering patient also, but the intensity is usually not great enough to elicit a training effect.

        (2) The patient progresses to 30 to 45 minutes of continuous lower extremity exercise and 10 to 15 minutes of upper extremity exercise.[30]

    e. Circuit-interval exercise is a common method used with the patient in Phase II.[30] The patient can exercise on each modality at a defined work load, compared with exercising continuously on a bicycle or treadmill. As a result, he can:

        (1) perform more physical work.

        (2) exercise at a higher intensity. Fitness may improve in a shorter period of time.

        (3) maintain lactic acid and the oxygen deficit at minimum levels.

        (4) exercise at a lower rate of perceived exertion.

    f. Circuit weight training can also be effective not only in increasing strength in the cardiac patient but in increasing aerobic endurance.[12,25] Some caution is needed with isometric components of circuit weight training because of reported increases in blood pressure and ECG changes. However, with avoidance of the Valsalva maneuver with static effort and with relatively few repetitions and a resistance less than 80 percent of maximum in weight lifting, the negative effect of arterial blood pressure and negative ECG responses can be avoided.[21]

    g. Progression of the work load occurs when there have been three consecutive sessions (every-other-day sessions) during which the peak heart rate is below the target heart rate.

C. Phase III

This phase of cardiac rehabilitation includes a supervised exercise conditioning program, which is often continued in a hospital or community setting. This phase lasts 3 to 12 months.

1. The purpose of the program is to improve fitness levels at a high level of exercise training. Few cardiac patients, however, participate in programs that increase their fitness levels past 7 METs.

2. *Recreational activities* to maintain levels gained in Phase II can include:[30,39]

    a. swimming, which incorporates both arms and legs. However, there is a decreased awareness of ischemic symptoms while swimming, especially when skill level is poor.

    b. Outdoor hiking, which is excellent if on level terrain.

3. Activities at 8 METs include:[3]

    a. jogging approximately 5 miles per hour.

    b. cycling approximately 12 miles per hour.

    c. vigorous down-hill skiing.

D. Phase IV

Cardiac rehabilitation at 12 months after discharge from the hospital concerns long-term maintenance of performance levels reached during Phase II or Phase III.[39]

E. Special Considerations

There are special considerations related to types of exercise and patient needs that must be recognized when developing conditioning programs for patients with coronary disease.[6,18,42]

1. Arm exercises elicit different responses than leg exercises.
   a. Mechanical efficiency based on the ratio between output of external work and caloric expenditure is lower than with leg exercises.
   b. Oxygen uptake at a given external work load is significantly higher for arm exercises than for leg exercises.
   c. Myocardial efficiency is lower with leg exercises than with arm exercises.
   d. Myocardial oxygen consumption (heart rate times systolic blood pressure) is higher with arm exercises than with leg exercises.
2. Coronary patients complete 35 percent less work with arm exercises than with leg exercises before symptoms occur.

F. Adaptive Changes

Adaptive changes following training of individuals with cardiac disease include:[23,39,42]

1. an increased myocardial aerobic work capacity.
2. an increased maximum aerobic or functional capacity by predominantly widening the arteriovenous oxygen (A-$\dot{V}O_2$) difference.
3. an increase in stroke volume following high intensity training 6 to 12 months into the training program.
4. a decreased myocardial demand for oxygen.
5. an increase in myocardial supply by the decreased heart rate and prolongation of diastole.
6. an increased tolerance to a given physical work load before angina occurs.
7. a heart rate significantly lower at each submaximal work load and therefore a greater heart rate reserve. When muscles are used that are not directly involved in the activity, the reduction in heart rate will not be as great.
8. An improved psychologic orientation and, over time, an impact on depression scores, scores for hysteria, hypochondriasis, and psychoasthenia on the Minnesota Multiphasic Personality Inventory.

Note: Cardiovascular complications will be prevented and/or reduced if the program includes appropriate selection of patients, continuous evaluation of each patient, medical supervision of the exercise throughout the training period, regular communication with the physician, specific instructions to patients about adverse symptoms, class size limitations to 30 patients or less, and the maintenance of accurate records related to compliance to the program.[42]

IX. GENERAL CLINICAL APPLICATIONS OF AEROBIC TRAINING

A. Chronic Illness and Deconditioning

Deconditioned individuals, including those with chronic illness and the elderly, may have major limitations in pulmonary and cardiovascular reserve that severely curtail their daily activities.[7,39]

1. Implications of the changes due to deconditioning brought on by inactivity, resulting from any illness or chronic disease, are important to remember.[18,36,42]

   a. There is a decreased work capacity, which is a result of:

      (1) a decreased maximum oxygen uptake and decreased ability to utilize oxygen and perform work.

      (2) a decreased cardiac output. Cardiac output is the major limiting factor.

   b. There is a decreased circulating blood volume that can be as much as 700 to 800 ml. For some individuals, this results in tachycardia along with orthostatic hypotension, dizziness, and episodes of syncope when initially attempting to stand.

   c. There is a decrease in plasma and red blood cells, which increases the likelihood of life-threatening embothrombolic episodes and the prolongation of the convalescent period.

   d. There is a decrease in lean body mass, which results in:

      (1) decreased muscle size.

      (2) decreased muscle strength and ability to perform activities requiring large muscle groups. For example, the individual may have difficulty walking with crutches or climbing stairs.

   e. There is an increased excretion of urinary calcium, which results:

      (1) from a decrease in the weight bearing stimulus critical in maintaining bone integrity.

      (2) in bone loss or osteoporosis.

      (3) in an increased likelihood of fractures upon falling due to the osteoporosis.

2. Through an exercise program, the negative cardiovascular, neuromuscular, and metabolic functions can be reversed. This results in:[18,36,42]

   a. a decrease in resting heart rate, heart rate with any given exercise load, and urinary excretion of calcium.

   b. an increase in stroke volume at rest, stroke volume with exercise, cardiac output with exercise, total heart volume, lung volume (ventilatory volume), vital capacity, maximal oxygen uptake, circulating blood volume, plasma volume and red blood cells, and lean body mass.

   c. a reversal of the negative nitrogen and protein balance.

   d. an increase in levels of mitochondrial enzymes and energy stores.[24]

   e. less use of the anaerobic systems during activity.[24]

B. Disability, Functional Limitations, and Deconditioning

Individuals who have a physical handicap should not be excluded from a conditioning program that will increase their fitness level. This includes individuals in wheelchairs or persons who have problems ambulating, such as the paraplegic, hemiplegic, or amputee, and patients who have an orthopedic problem, such as arthrodesis.[8]

1. Adaptations must be made in testing the physically handicapped utilizing a wheelchair treadmill or more frequently using the upper extremity ergometer (bicycle).

2. Exercise protocols may emphasize upper extremities and manipulation of the wheelchair.

3. It is important to remember that energy expenditure is increased when the

gait is altered, and wheelchair use is less efficient than walking without impairment.

C. Problems, Goals, and Plan of Care

The goals of an aerobic exercise program are dependent on the initial level of fitness of the individual and on his specific clinical needs. The general goals are to decrease the deconditioning effects of disease and chronic illness and improve the individual's cardiovascular and muscular fitness.

1. Selected clinical problems

   a. Increased susceptibility to thromboembolic episodes, pneumonia, atelectasis, and the likelihood of fractures
   b. Tachycardia, dizziness, and orthostatic hypotension when moving from sitting to standing
   c. A decrease in general muscle strength, with difficulty and shortness of breath in climbing stairs
   d. A decrease in work capacity limiting distances walked and activities tolerated
   e. Increased heart rate and blood pressure responses (rate-pressure product) to various activities
   f. A decrease in the maximum rate-pressure product tolerated with angina or other ischemic symptoms appearing at low levels of exercise

2. Measurable short-term goals

   a. Prevention of thromboembolic episodes, pneumonia, atelectasis, and fractures
   b. A decrease in the magnitude of the orthostatic hypotensive response
   c. Ability to climb stairs safely and without shortness of breath
   d. Tolerance for walking longer measured distances and completing activities without fatigue or symptoms
   e. A decrease in the heart rate and blood pressure (rate-pressure product) at a given level of activity
   f. An increase in the maximum rate-pressure product tolerated without ischemic symptoms

3. Measurable long-term goals

   a. An improved pulmonary, cardiovascular, and metabolic response to various levels of exercise
   b. An improved ability to complete selected activities with appropriate heart rate and blood responses to exercise

4. Plan of care (convalescent)

   a. Determine the exercise heart rate response that can be safely reached, based on the number of beats over the resting heart rate.
   b. Initiate a program of activities for the patient that will not elicit a cardiovascular response over the exercise heart rate (e.g., calisthenics, walking).
   c. Provide the patient with clearly written instructions about any activity he performs on his own.
   d. Initiate an educational program that provides the patient with information about effort symptoms and exercise precautions, monitoring of heart rate, and modification, when indicated, of risk factors.

5. **Plan of care (with emphasis on adaptation)**
   a. Determine the maximum heart rate or symptom-limited heart rate by multistage testing with ECG monitoring.
   b. Decide on the threshold stimulus (percentage of maximum or symptom-limited heart rate) that will elicit a conditioning response for the individual tested and that will be used as the exercise heart rate.
   c. Determine the intensity, duration, and frequency of exercise that will result in attainment of the exercise heart rate and a conditioning response.
   d. Determine the mode of exercise to be used based on the individual's physical capabilities and interest.
   e. Initiate an exercise program with the patient and provide him with clearly written instructions regarding the details of the program.
   f. Educate the patient about:
      (1) effort symptoms and the need to cease or modify exercise when these symptoms appear and to communicate with the physical therapist and/or physician about these problems.
      (2) monitoring heart rate at rest as well as during and following exercise.
      (3) the importance of exercising within the guidelines provided by the physical therapist.
      (4) the importance of consistent long-term follow-up about the exercise program so that it can be progressed within safe limits.
      (5) the importance of modifying risk factors related to cardiac problems.

X. AGE DIFFERENCES

Differences in endurance and physical work capacity among children, young adults, and middle-aged or elderly individuals are evident. Some comparisons are made between maximal oxygen uptake and the factors influencing it and between blood pressure, respiratory rate, vital capacity, and maximum voluntary ventilation in the different age categories.

A. Children[6,9,17,19,42]

Between the ages of 5 and 15 there is a threefold increase in body weight, lung volume, heart volume, and maximum oxygen uptake.

1. Heart rate
   a. Resting heart rate is on the average above 125 (126 in girls, 135 in boys) at infancy.
   b. Resting heart rate drops to adult levels at puberty.
   c. Maximum heart rate is age related (220 minus age).

2. Stroke volume
   a. Stroke volume is closely related to size.
   b. Children 5 to 16 years of age have a stroke volume of 30 to 40 ml.

3. Cardiac output
   a. Cardiac output is related to size.
   b. Cardiac output increases with increasing stroke volume.

    c. The increase in cardiac output for a given increase in oxygen consumption is a constant throughout life. It is the same in the child as in the adult.

4. Arteriovenous oxygen difference
    a. Children tolerate a larger A-$\dot{V}O_2$ difference than adults.
    b. The larger A-$\dot{V}O_2$ difference makes up for the smaller stroke volume.

5. Maximal oxygen uptake ($\dot{V}O_2$ max).[6,17]
    a. $\dot{V}O_2$ max increases with age up to 20 years (expressed as liter per minute).
    b. Before puberty, girls and boys show no significant difference in maximal aerobic capacity.
    c. Cardiac output in children is the same as in the adult for any given oxygen consumption.
    d. Endurance times increase with age until 17 to 18 years.

6. Blood pressure
    a. Systolic blood pressure increases from 40 mm Hg at birth to 80 mm Hg at age 1 month to 100 mm Hg several years before puberty. Adult levels are observed at puberty.
    b. Diastolic pressure increases from 55 to 70 mm Hg from 4 to 14 years of age, with little change during adolescence.

7. Respiration
    a. Respiratory rate decreases from 30 breaths per minute at infancy to 16 breaths per minute at 17 to 18 years of age.
    b. Vital capacity and maximum voluntary ventilation correlate with height, although the greater increase in boys than girls at puberty may be due to an increase in lung tissue.

B. Young Adult[2,18,29,42]

There are more data on the physiologic parameters of fitness for the young and middle-aged adult than for the child or the elderly.

1. Heart rate
    a. Resting heart rate reaches 60 to 65 beats per minute at 17 to 18 years of age (75 beats per minute in a sedentary young man, sitting).[42]
    b. Maximum heart rate is age related (190 beats per minute in the same sedentary young man).

2. Stroke volume
    a. The adult values for stroke volume are 60 to 80 ml (75 ml in a sedentary young man, sitting).
    b. With maximal exercise, stroke volume is 100 ml in that same sedentary young man.

3. Cardiac output for the sedentary young man at rest
    a. Cardiac output at rest is 75 beats per minute times 75 ml, or 5.6 liters per minute.
    b. With maximal exercise, cardiac output is 190 beats per minute times 100 ml, or 19 liters per minute.

4. Arteriovenous oxygen difference (A-$\dot{V}O_2$ difference)
   a. Twenty-five to 30 percent of the oxygen is extracted from blood as it runs through the muscles or other tissues at rest.
   b. In a normal young sedentary man, it increases threefold (5.2 to 15.8 ml/100 ml blood) with exercise.

5. Maximum oxygen uptake
   a. The difference in $\dot{V}O_2$ max between male and female is greatest in the adult.
   b. Differences in $\dot{V}O_2$ max between the sexes is minimal when $\dot{V}O_2$ max is expressed relative to lean body weight.
   c. In the sedentary young man, maximum oxygen uptake equals 3000 ml per minute (oxygen uptake at rest equals 300 ml per minute).

6. Blood pressure
   a. Systolic blood pressure is 120 mm Hg (average). At peak effort of exercise, values may range from as low as 190 mm Hg to as high as 240 mm Hg.
   b. Diastolic blood pressure is 80 mm Hg (average). Diastolic pressure does not change markedly with exercise.

7. Respiration
   a. Respiratory rate is 12 to 15 breaths per minute.
   b. Vital capacity is 4800 ml in a man 20 to 30 years of age.[14]
   c. Maximum voluntary ventilation varies considerably from laboratory to laboratory and is dependent on age and surface area of the body.[42]

C. Older Adult[6,26,35,38,41]

With increasing interest in the aged, data are appearing in the literature about this age group and their response to exercise.

1. Heart rate
   a. Resting heart rate is not influenced by age.
   b. Maximum heart rate is age related and decreases with age (in very general terms, 220 minus age). The average maximum heart rate for men 20 to 29 years of age is 190 beats per minute; for men 60 to 69 years of age, it is 164 beats per minute.
   c. The amount that the heart rate increases in response to static and maximum dynamic exercise (hand grip) decreases in the elderly.

2. Stroke volume
Stroke volume decreases in the aged and results in decreased cardiac output.

3. Cardiac output
Cardiac output decreases on an average of 7 liters per minute to 3.4 liters per minute from age 19 to 86 years.[35]

4. A-$\dot{V}O_2$ difference
Arteriovenous oxygen difference decreases as a result of decreased lean body mass and low oxygen-carrying capacity.[38]

5. Maximum oxygen uptake

a. According to cardiorespiratory fitness classification,[2] if men 60 to 69 years of age of average fitness level are compared with men 20 to 29 years of age of the same fitness level, the maximal oxygen uptake for the older man is lower.

20 to 29 years	31 to 37 ml/kg·min
60 to 69 years	18 to 23 ml/kg·min

b. Maximum oxygen consumption decreases on an average from 60 ml/kg·min to 25 ml/kg·min from the first to the ninth decade.[35]

6. Blood pressure

Blood pressure increases because of increased peripheral vascular resistance.

a. Systolic blood pressure of the aged is 150 mm Hg (average).

b. Diastolic blood pressure is 90 mm Hg (average).

c. If the definition of high blood pressure is 160/95, then 22 percent of men and 34 percent of women 65 to 74 years of age are hypertensive.[38]

d. Using 150/95 mm Hg as a cutoff, 25 percent of individuals are hypertensive at age 50 years and 70 percent between the ages of 85 and 95 years.

7. Respiration

a. Respiratory rate increases with age.

b. Vital capacity decreases with age. There is a 25-percent decrease in the vital capacity of the 50- to 60-year-old male compared with the 20- to 30-year-old male with the same surface area.

c. Maximum voluntary ventilation decreases with age.

XI. SUMMARY

This chapter presented the topics of fitness and endurance and ways to achieve increased performance of physical activity in the healthy individual as well as the individual with coronary heart disease, a physical handicap, or debilitating illness. Fitness, endurance, conditioning, deconditioning, and adaptation to exercise were discussed. Energy expended for different levels of physical activity is given, and the efficiency of the human being during activity is included. A differentiation of fitness and stress testing is emphasized as is the development of training programs and the exercise prescription. Changes that occur with training and the mechanisms for their occurrence are enumerated. Some basic information about comparing cardiovascular and respiratory parameters in the various age groups is given.

REFERENCES

1. American College of Sports Medicine: *Guidelines for Graded Exercise Testing and Exercise Prescription,* ed 2. Lea & Febiger, Philadelphia, 1986.
2. American Heart Association, The Committee on Exercise: *Exercise Testing and Training of Apparently Healthy Individuals: A Handbook for Physicians.* American Heart Association, 1972.
3. American Heart Association, The Committee on Exercise: *Exercise Testing and Training of Individuals with Heart Disease or at High Risk for Its Development: A Handbook for Physicians.* American Heart Association, 1975.

4. Amundsen, L: *Cardiac Rehabilitation. Clinics in Physical Therapy.* Vol 1. Churchill-Livingston, New York, 1981.

5. Amundsen, L and Nielsen, D: *Normal and abnormal cardiovascular responses to acute physical exercise.* In Amundsen, L (ed): *Cardiac Rehabilitation. Clinics in Physical Therapy.* Vol 1. Churchill-Livingston, New York, 1981.

6. Astrand, P and Rodahl, K: *Textbook of Work Physiology. Physiological Basis of Exercise, ed 3.* McGraw-Hill, New York, 1986.

7. Blocker, W, Harley, H, and Payne, R: *Rehabilitation exercise programs for the older disabled.* In Blocker, W and Cardus, D (eds): *Rehabilitation in Ischemic Heart Disease.* SP Medical and Scientific Books, New York, 1983.

8. Blocker, W and Kitowski, V: *Cardiac rehabilitation of the physically handicapped (amputee, hemiplegic, spinal cord injury patient, and obese patient).* In Blocker, W and Cardus, D (eds): *Rehabilitation in Ischemic Heart Disease.* SP Medical and Scientific Books, New York, 1983.

9. Blomqvist, CG: *Exercise physiology: Clinical aspects.* In Wenger, NK (ed): *Exercise and the Heart.* FA Davis, Philadelphia, 1978.

10. Brammel, HL: *Rehabilitation of the cardiac patient.* In DeLisa, JB (ed): *Rehabilitation Medicine, Principles and Practice.* JB Lippincott, Philadelphia, 1988.

11. Bruce, RA: *Exercise testing methods and interpretations.* Adv Cardiol 24:6, 1978.

12. Butler, RM, et al: *The cardiovascular response to circuit weight training in patients with cardiac disease.* J Cardiopulm Rehabil 7:402, 1987.

13. Cooper, KH and Robertson, JW: *Aerobics in action.* In Long, C (ed): *Prevention and Rehabilitation in Ischemic Heart Disease. Rehabilitation Medicine Library.* Williams & Wilkins, Baltimore, 1980.

14. Comroe, JH, et al: *The Lung,* ed 2. Year Book Medical Publishers, Chicago, 1962.

15. Dorossier, DL: *Principles of training and exercise prescription.* Adv Cardiol 24:67, 1978.

16. Dressendorfer, RH and Smith, JL: *Predictive accuracy of the maximum heart rate reserve method for estimating aerobic training intensity in early cardiac rehabilitation.* J Cardiac Rehabil 4:484, 1984.

17. Ellestad, MH: *Stress Testing: Principles and Practice,* ed 2. FA Davis, Philadelphia, 1986.

18. Fox, EL and Mathews, DK: *Physiological Basis of Physical Education and Athletics,* ed 3. Saunders College Publishing, Philadelphia, 1981.

19. Godfrey, S: *Exercise Testing in Children.* WB Saunders, Philadelphia, 1974.

20. Golding, LA: *Exercise physiology.* In Long, C (ed): *Prevention and Rehabilitation in Ischemic Heart Disease. Rehabilitation Medicine Library.* Williams & Wilkins, Baltimore, 1980.

21. Halam, DRS, et al: *Direct measurements of arterial blood pressure during formal weightlifting in cardiac patients.* J Cardiopulm Rehabil 8:213, 1988.

22. Haskins, TH: *Physiological effects of endurance training.* In Amundsen, L (ed): *Cardiac Rehabilitation. Clinics in Physical Therapy,* Volume 1. Churchill-Livingston, New York, 1981.

23. Irwin, S and Tecklin JS: *Cardiopulmonary Physical Therapy.* Vol 1. CV Mosby Company, St Louis, 1985.

24. Jones, NL and Campbell, EJM: *Clinical Exercise Testing,* ed 2. WB Saunders, Philadelphia, 1982.

25. Kelemen, MH, et al: *Circuit weight training in cardiac patients.* JACC 7:38, 1986.

26. Kenney, RA: *Physiology of Aging: A Synopsis.* Year Book Medical Publishers, Chicago, 1982.

27. Littell, E: *Support responses of the cardiovascular system to exercise: Part I.* Phys Ther 61:1260, 1981.

28. Long, C: *Exercise prevention and rehabilitation of ischemic heart disease.* In Long, C (ed): *Prevention and Rehabilitation in Ischemic Heart Disease. Rehabilitation Medicine Library.* Williams & Wilkins, Baltimore, 1980.

29. McCardle WD, Katch, FI, and Katch, VL: *Exercise Physiology: Energy, Nutrition and Human Performance.* Lea & Febiger, Philadelphia, 1986.

30. Meyer, GC: *The role of circuit interval and continuous conditioning in cardiac rehabilitation.* In Hall, LK (ed): *Cardiac Rehabilitation: Exercise Testing and Prescription.* Spectrum Publications, Laurel, MD, 1984.

31. Michel, T: *Physiological effects of endurance training.* In Amundsen, L (ed): *Cardiac Rehabilitation. Clinics in Physical Therapy.* Volume 1. Churchill-Livingston, New York, 1981.

32. Nielsen, DH: *Exercise physiology: An overview with emphasis on aerobic capacity and energy cost.* In Amundsen, L (ed): *Cardiac Rehabilitation. Clinics in Physical Therapy.* Volume I. Churchill-Livingston, New York, 1981.

33. Pollock, M, Gettman, L, Mileses, C, et al: *Effects of frequency and duration of training on attrition and incidence of injury.* Med Sci Sports 9:31, 1977.

34. Reith, CA: *Warm-up and cool-down cardiac rehabilitation.* In Hall, LK (ed): *Exercise Testing and Prescription.* Spectrum Publications, Laurel, MD, 1984.

35. Rowe, JW and Besdine, RW: *Health and Disease in Old Age.* Little, Brown and Company, Boston, 1982.

36. Saltin, B, et al: *Response to exercise after bed rest and after training.* Circulation, 38:5 Supplement VII, 1968.

37. Sanne, H: *Physiology of training in normals and coronary patients.* Adv Cardiol 24:57, 1978.

38. Schrier, RW: *Clinical Internal Medicine in the Aged.* WB Saunders, Philadelphia, 1982.

39. Skinner, JS: *Exercise Testing and Exercise Prescription for Special Cases. Theoretical Basis and Clinical Application.* Lea & Febiger, Philadelphia, 1987.

40. Smith, JJ and Kampine, JP: *Circulatory Physiology—the Essentials.* Williams & Wilkins, Baltimore, 1984.

41. Wells, T: *Aging and Health Promotion.* Aspen Systems Corporation, Rockville, MD, 1982.

42. Wenger, NK and Hellerstein, HK: *Rehabilitation of the Coronary Patient.* John Wiley & Sons, New York, 1984.

43. Wenger, NK: *Future directions in cardiovascular rehabilitation.* J Cardiopulm Rehabil 6:168-174, 1987.

44. Whipple, DV: *Dynamics of Development: Euthenic Pediatrics.* McGraw-Hill, New York, 1966.

45. Londeree, BR and Moeschberger, ML: *Influence of age and other factors on maximal heart rate.* J Cardiac Rehabil 4:44, 1984.

46. Pollock, ML, Wilmore, JH, and Fox, SM: *Exercise in Health and Disease: Evaluation and Prescription for Prevention and Rehabilitation.* WB Saunders, Philadelphia, 1984.

CHAPTER ———————————————— 22

Critical Analysis of Exercise Programs

When establishing a balanced exercise program, two concerns should be addressed: what goals and kinds of exercise make up a well-designed program, and do the proposed exercises safely and effectively accomplish the intended goals? The patient's condition; age; any previous injuries, deformities, or dysfunctions; and any potential risks from diseases should be taken into account.

Information about exercise routines is found everywhere: in popular magazines, in sports and health magazines and journals, on television and videotapes, and in books. These routines are designed by anyone, from the physician to the shapely movie personality, either with or without consultation from someone trained in safe exercise techniques. Well-intended people advise others in exercise routines to stretch, tone, strengthen, prepare for this or that, slim down, or build up. Most people have at one time or another become involved in a supervised exercise program, perhaps at school or at a health club or YMCA. Today, with the popularity of aerobic conditioning and exercise programs, many people with good intentions try various forms of exercising without adequate preparation or guidance only to find that they develop back, leg, or joint pain; muscle strain; or simply muscle soreness form overexercising or exercising improperly. They either become discouraged and feel defeated, or they persevere and injure themselves. Why this happens can be traced to the observation that some of the exercises chosen are not biomechanically safe for the strength, flexibility, or endurance level of the person doing the exercise, or they are the wrong exercises to accomplish the intended purpose.

This chapter is designed to help the reader critically analyze commonly used exercises in terms of how they can be used to evaluate problems, and then be adapted to accomplish a desired goal. The intent is not to describe the ideal exercise protocol—there is no such thing—but to help the reader recognize that to accomplish an exercise goal as safely as possible, exercises have to be adapted to the individual level of the person involved and must be balanced with other appropriate exercise activities.

OBJECTIVES

After studying this chapter, the reader will be able to:

1. look at specific exercises used for testing and determine if they are evaluating appropriate factors safely and correctly.
2. look at specific exercises and determine if they are safely accomplishing the intended goals.
3. identify misconceptions in common exercises and exercise programs.

I. DESIGNING AN EXERCISE PROGRAM: WHY EXERCISE?

There are many reasons for exercising. One general reason is to improve or maintain physical well-being. Other reasons could be to prepare for an upcoming athletic event, to relieve anxiety, to build up strength, to slim down the waist, or simply to enjoy the social interaction with others who also exercise. Whatever the reason, it is important to choose an exercise program that best meets the needs of the individual. The intended purpose or goals for the program need to be identified. Common goals are to:
1. increase strength (see Chapter 3).
2. increase flexibility (see Chapter 4).
3. increase endurance (see Chapter 21).
4. increase skill in an activity. This includes coordination, agility, balance, timing, and speed.

II. ESTABLISHING A BASELINE BY WHICH IMPROVEMENT CAN BE MEASURED

Realistic testing can serve as a motivational tool when progress is noted. Therapists routinely use manual muscle testing[1,4] and other objective forms of testing such as tensiometer readings and torque output readings in order to obtain a baseline of muscle strength. Goniometric measurements are taken to obtain an objective baseline of range of motion and flexibility.[8,9] These testing procedures have been standardized and are commonly accepted as reliable indicators of change and will not be discussed here. Other tests commonly used in group exercise programs are not as objective and can be misleading. Tests used for physical fitness and conditioning programs need to be scrutinized by asking the following questions:
1. Does the test in fact test the intended muscle or function?
2. Will the test grade improve as muscle function improves?
3. Is the test biomechanically safe?

A. Tc Test Strength

A method typically used is to repeat a strenuous activity until the person tires. Improvement in strength is noted as the number of repetitions increases. This is a satisfactory method of testing strength as long as it is recognized that endurance is also related to the number of repetitions performed. In addition, the test should have various grades of difficulty so that the person can be tested at a level where at least one repetition can be accomplished safely and correctly. Then, as strength improves, progess is noted first by the increased number of repetitions, then by progression to the next level of difficulty at a lower number of repetitions.
1. In popular exercise programs, strength is usually tested by having the subjects do an activity that uses the body weight as resistance.
   a. Sit-ups and straight-leg lifts are used to test abdominal muscle strength.
   b. Push-ups and chin-ups are used to test arm muscle strength.

      c. Prone-lying chest and leg lifts are used to test back muscle strength.

      d. Jumping activities are used to test leg strength.

      e. Throwing a ball is used to test arm strength.

2. If the above activities are not done correctly, they can be biomechanically unsafe, or they may not test the muscles intended. If continued as an exercise, the appropriate muscle will not be strengthened, or supporting structures will be stressed and damaged. Also, if the person is unable to do a test, progress cannot be measured in the early stages of the program; a simpler form of the test needs to be used. Other activities than the ones listed here may also be used to test strength, but just these will be analyzed to illustrate what needs to be considered when choosing an activity for testing.

    a. **Analysis of sit-ups (curl-ups) as a test of abdominal strength**

       (1) In order to isolate the abdominal muscles as trunk flexors, the person must curl the trunk, not arch the back, and needs to come up no further than clearing the thorax from the floor. Once the thorax clears the floor, the rest of the motion is hip flexion, using primarily the action of the hip flexor muscles.[3] If the back is allowed to arch, a sit-up is possible without abdominal muscle participation through reverse muscle action of the iliopsoas (hip flexor) muscles.

       (2) The hips and knees are placed in a partially flexed position to release the stretch on the iliopsoas and sartorius muscles, allowing the pelvis to rotate posteriorly as the abdominals contract.[3] Fixating the feet and sitting up through full range encourages reverse muscle action of the hip flexors rather than contraction of the abdominals to do the motion and, therefore, should not be done when testing abdominal strength.

       (3) The position of the arms and hands will vary the resistance and thus the difficulty of the activity. The easiest position is with the hands along side of the trunk; next in difficulty is with the hands across the chest; the most difficult is with the hands behind the head. If the person cannot curl up with his arms at the side, note how far he can curl (just the head, the head and shoulders, or the head, shoulders, and upper thorax).

       (4) The person should not use momentum by throwing his arms or jerking the trunk when curling up.

    b. **Analysis of bilateral straight-leg raising as a test for abdominal strength**

       (1) In order to test the strength of the abdominal muscles in this activity, the back must be kept flat and not allowed to arch.[3] If the back arches, it means the abdominal muscles are not strong enough to stabilize the pelvis and lumbar spine against the pull of the iliopsoas muscles. Raising and lowering of the legs can be accomplished purely by the iliopsoas muscles.

       (2) Maximum resistance from the legs occurs when the legs are horizontal (just off the floor).

       (3) To use this activity as a test of lower abdominal strength, begin with the resistance from the legs in the least stressful position by having both hips flexed to 90 degrees and the knees extended; instruct the person to maintain the back flat against the exercise mat as the legs are slowly lowered. When the back begins to arch, the angle of

the legs with repect to the floor should be noted as the maximum resistance tolerated by the abdominals.[3]

c. **Analysis of push-ups as a test of upper extremity strength**

   (1) In order to effectively do a push up, the individual must have not only adequate upper extremity strength but also strength in the trunk, hip, and knee muscles in order to maintain a rigid structure to lift. If the person can maintain the trunk and lower extremities in line, then the triceps and pectoralis major muscles become the prime movers in this activity. This activity can be modified to allow the knees to bend so that not as much weight needs to be lifted.

   (2) The main problem with this activity as a test is that many people cannot maintain the isometric hold in the trunk and lower extremities or do not have enough strength in the arms to do even one push-up. Therefore, it is difficult or impossible to measure progress in the weaker individual, and this becomes a test of only those who already are in a state of fitness. An easier level would be to have the subject do push-ups against a wall or a bar placed at shoulder level. To progress the difficulty (resistance), move the feet further away from the wall or lower the bar, until eventually the subject is near horizontal and can be tested by pushing up from the floor.

   (3) The position of the hands with respect to the shoulders also affects the difficulty of this activity. It is more difficult to do with the hands placed directly under the shoulders than with the hands out to the side. For consistency, the hands should always be placed in the same position.

d. **Analysis of pull-ups or chin-ups as a test of strength in the arms**

   (1) This test requires the shoulder extensor, elbow flexor, and finger flexor muscles to lift the body weight. If the activity is done with the forearms supinated, elbow flexion primarily occurs from action of the biceps brachii muscle; if done with the forearms pronated, the biceps lose their functional advantage and the flexion primarily is from action of the brachialis muscles.

   (2) Either one of these positions is difficult for the less-trained individual; for those not able to do even one pull-up, a simpler test needs to be defined. A modified pull-up requires use of an adjustable bar. The easiest position would be with the bar at the shoulder height of the subject. The person holds on to the bar and leans backward keeping his feet on the floor; then he pulls his body toward the bar until his chest touches it and then lowers himself to the starting position. To progress the difficulty of the activity, the bar is lowered and the subject hangs the extended body below the bar, his feet remaining on the floor. As strength improves, the subject can then be tested in the standard pull-up position in which the entire body weight is lifted.

e. **Analysis of prone chest lifts for testing strength of the back extensors**

   (1) With the subject lying prone and with his hands behind his head, he can extend his spine only if someone holds down his legs, or else both the legs and thorax will lift up from the floor, making it a difficult activity.

   (2) With the legs stabilized, most people are able to lift the chest off the floor; if the person is quite weak, the test is made easier by placing

the arms along side of the trunk rather than behind the head. This activity requires strength in the neck and thorax extensors as well as scapula adductors to hold the upper spine and shoulders in position while the lower back is extending. Weakness in any one of these areas will make this test difficult to do.

f. **Analysis of prone leg lifts for testing strength of the back extensors**
   (1) To do this test, someone must hold down the subject's thorax, or it too will lift up from the floor, making it a difficult activity.
   (2) This activity requires strength in the hip extensor muscles in order to keep the hip extended. It may be difficult to do if the back extensors are weak because of the long lever arm that the legs provide. For someone who could not do it, the resistance of the lever arm is reduced by flexing the knees.

g. **Analysis of vertical or broad jumping activities as a test of leg strength**
   (1) In order to jump, the subject must have strength in the ankle planterflexing gastrocnemius and soleus muscles.
   (2) Whether the subject is allowed to take a running start before jumping needs to be consistent, since running provides additional momentum to the body.

h. **Analysis of throwing a ball as a test of arm strength**
   (1) This activity requires the subject to have not only strength in the upper extremity but also coordination of trunk and lower extremity motions as well as skill for proper timing in release and follow through. Flexibility of the shoulder and trunk could also affect proper execution. As a result, measurement of the distance a ball is thrown may not give a realistic picture of arm strength.
   (2) The subject should receive training for properly coordinated execution of this activity if it is going to be used as a measure of strength.

B. **To Test Flexibility**

The motion should be done without bouncing; the subject should sustain the position for several seconds.

1. In popular exercise programs, flexibility is usually tested with one activity—forward bending and attempting to touch the toes while sitting or standing. Its purpose is to test back and hamstring muscle length. Since this activity is so commonly used both as a test and as an exercise, its faults will be discussed, with emphasis on alternative ways of measuring flexibility more accurately.
   a. Bending forward and touching the toes can be accomplished if the low back, hamstrings, or upper back is overflexible, even if one of the other regions is tight. Also, disproportionate length between arms, trunk, and legs can make this activity easier for some and more difficult for others. The only way to discern the region of tightness is to observe the contour of the back and position of the pelvis. This is usually not done in group exercise programs and usually can be done only by someone trained to recognize the variations in movement of body parts. The common criterion is how close to the floor a person can get his fingers, not which region of his back or legs is most flexible or tight. The danger is that, if toe-touching is used as an exercise, the overflexible region will continue to remain hypermobile in compensation for the tight region, so

the less flexible part may not increase in flexibility. If the subject does toe-touching while long-sitting, there is a tendency to also flex the thoracic spine excessively.

b. There is a belief that young people lose their flexibility because of a soft life and are no longer able touch their toes.[10] In a classic article, this problem is discussed by Kendall, who states:

"... there is a period between the years of ten and fourteen when a majority of children may not be able to touch the toes with knees straight. The inability to successfully perform this feat apparently results from a discrepancy between leg and trunk length during this growth period. To encourage or force children to accomplish this feat may be harmful in the sense that undue flexibility of the back may result."[3]

The long bones grow rapidly during puberty; the flexibility of muscles lags behind.[5] To excessively stretch the muscles when they are already undergoing lengthening because of the rapid growth of the bones may also lead to weakness in the overstretched muscles. Or possibly, the tendon may elongate and the muscle tissue may not adapt, resulting in a weakened muscle.[2]

c. **To realistically test the flexibility of the hamstrings**
The pelvis should be stabilized and one leg tested at a time. The subject should lie supine, keep one leg extended on the floor, and lift the other leg, keeping the knee straight to the point where pulling is felt in the posterior thigh. This is termed unilateral straight-leg raising. The ankle is allowed to plantarflex in order to minimize the pull of the gastrocnemius muscle posterior to the knee.

d. **To test the flexibility of the low-back region**
The subject stabilizes the pelvis by sitting with his legs crossed. He stabilizes the upper back in extension by placing both hands behind his head and bringing the elbows out to the side. He then bends forward, flexing only the low back, and does not allow his thorax to curl.

2. Other tests of flexibility should also be done, particularly to regions that tend to become tight from faulty postures or muscle imbalances. Suggestions include

a. **Flexibility of the scapular protractors**
Test to determine whether or not the person can lie supine with hands behind his neck and then lower his elbows to the exercise mat.

b. **Flexibility of the short upper neck extensors**
Test to determine whether or not the person can lie supine and almost flatten the cervical spine against the exercise mat.

c. **Flexibility of the trunk and hip flexors**
Test to determine whether or not the person can lie prone, then press the thorax upward (as in a push-up) while keeping the pelvis on the floor. The hands should be placed under the shoulders, not out to the side or forward.

d. **Flexibility of the ankle plantarflexors**
Test to determine how far the person can dorsiflex his ankles while sitting with the knees extended.

C. To Test Endurance

1. To test local muscle endurance

High repetitions of a movement without resistance are repeated until the muscles fatigue. The number of repetitions is counted.

2. To test cardiovascular endurance

The simplest method is to have the patient perform a controlled repetitive total body activity for a period of time and to check the heart rate. As endurance for doing that activity improves, the resting heart rate will decrease. Because of potential physical risks, the reader is referred to the complete procedures and precautions discussed in Chapter 21.

3. In some testing procedures, speed is used to measure endurance

Speed may have some effect on endurance, but skill, agility, and coordination are also necessary for doing an activity with speed, and therefore, it is not a true indicator of endurance.

D. To Test Skill

Skill encompasses coordination, agility, balance, timing, and speed. Often, speed is used as the measure of ability to do a skilled activity, implying that the faster one can do an activity, the more skillful he is. This is not easily resolved because it holds true for some skills but not others. Prior to testing, the person should have adequate instruction and should practice so that he knows what is required in the skill.

III. ESTABLISHING REALISTIC GOALS

Review the results of the testing procedures to determine the goals of the exercise program. In other words, what muscles need to be strengthened, what regions need to be stretched, does endurance need to be improved, or do skills need to be developed or improved? The goals then can give a realistic picture of what exercises need to be included in the program. Exercises used to accomplish the goals need to be scrutinized with the following questions:
1. Is the proposed exercise able to meet the goal?
2. If the exercise cannot meet the goal, what is the best and safest way to do so?
3. Are there any problems with the individual that will require special precautions or modifications of the exercises?

A. Exercises to Increase Strength

Many of the activities used to test strength can also be used as exercises to increase strength, either by increasing the number of repetitions or increasing the resistance. When weights are not available for increasing the resistance, as is the case in many group exercise classes, resistance can be increased by increasing the lever arm of the moving part. Examples of this include moving the arms further away from the axis of motion as done with the curl-up activity (Section I A 2 a) or changing the angle of the body with respect to gravity as described with the pull-up activity (Section I A 2 d).

1. Common errors in strengthening programs

a. **The activity required is too strenuous.**

Most exercises require that some muscles act as stabilizers for part of the body as other muscles do the intended motion. Either one or both muscle groups may be strengthened with the activity (the stabilizers through isometric holding; the prime movers through the isotonic activity). If any or all involved muscle groups are too weak to carry out the intended function, strain can occur. Begin exercises at a resistance level at which *all* the muscle groups can function properly. For example

(1) *Bilateral straight leg-raising*

This activity requires that the abdominal muscles be strong enough to stabilize the pelvis (keep the back flat) against the pull of the hip flexing iliopsoas muscles. The extended legs provide a long lever arm, and thus the hip flexors must contract forcefully to lift them. If the abdominals are not strong, they cannot stabilize against the strong hip flexor pull; the pelvis will be pulled anteriorly and the lumbar spine will arch. This causes back strain. If the subject cannot do the straight leg-lowering test (see Section I A 2 b) and keep the back flat, he should NOT do straight leg-lifts as an exercise. Modifications include doing the straight leg-lowering activity only to the point where the back begins to arch (as described in the testing section), or shortening the lever arm of the resistance by bending the hips and knees and doing knee-to-chest exercises. As strength in the stabilizing action of the abdominals improves, less and less bend in the hips and knees is used.

(2) *Scissors*

This activity is done with the person supine and legs held extended several inches above the exercise mat. The person then abducts and adducts the legs, mimicking a scissors motion. The mechanics of the activity are similar to straight leg-raising in that it requires a strong abdominal muscle contraction to stabilize the pelvis against the pull of the hip flexor muscles, which, in this case, must contract strongly to hold the legs up off the ground. There is no resistance to the abductor and adductor muscles, since the legs move parallel to the ground. To stabilize the pelvis, the person is often instructed to place his hands under the pelvis. Doing this defeats the intent of strengthening the abdominals, because they then do not have to work. To modify this exercise if the person does not have strength in the abdominals to stabilize the pelvis (cannot do the straight leg-lowering test), begin with the hips flexed 90 degrees and do the scissoring with the legs in this position of least resistance. Progress by gradually lowering the legs to an angle just before the back begins to arch and scissor in that position, keeping the back flat.

(3) *Curl-ups*

This activity requires that the abdominal muscles pull the thorax toward the pelvis to flex the lumbar spine. The abdominal muscles function only in the first third of the range of sitting up. Full sit-ups serve no additional benefit but may have some detrimental effects such as increasing intradiskal pressure—especially if the sit-up is done with the hips and knees flexed.[6] If the abdominal muscles are not strong enough, the person arches the back to lock the spine and lifts the trunk by flexing the pelvis on the femurs (reverse muscle action of the hip flexors).[4] If the subject cannot do a curl-up with the hands behind the head, begin at an easier level, for example, with the arms at the side. If he still cannot curl up, have him begin strengthening by just lifting the head (this sets the abdominals), progress with lifting the head and shoulders (arms at the side of the trunk), then the head, shoulders, and thorax. Eventually progress by moving the arms across the thorax, then behind the neck. Do not allow momentum to occur by jerking of the arms. The jerking of the arms could also cause neck pain. This exercise should also include diagonal motions of the trunk to recruit the oblique abdominal muscles. See Chapter 14 for additional suggestions and precautions for strengthening the abdominal muscles.

b. **There is an overemphasis on exercises that perpetuate faulty postures.**

(1) *Flexion exercises*

Examples are exercise programs that primarily consist of flexion activities (curling the trunk, flexing the hips, flexing the shoulders, and protracting the scapula) without including a comparable number of exercises to extend the trunk, hips, and shoulders and retract the scapulae. To have a well-balanced program, for every flexion exercise there should be an extension exercise in the same region. For example, for every curl-up exercise, do a lumbar extension exercise; for every push-up exercise, do a shoulder abduction, scapular retraction exercise; for every hip flexion exercise, do a hip extension exercise (see Chapter 14 for exercise suggestions).

(2) *Inverted bicycle*

This popular exercise is performed by the subject starting supine, then rolling up on to his shoulders so that his feet are up in the air. The weight of the inverted body is borne on the upper thoracic and cervical spine (Figure 22-1). Once in this position, the person attempts to balance while flexing and extending the lower extremities in a reciprocal manner. Problems with this exercise include the position itself, which places the head in a forward-head posture. The body weight becomes a strong stretch force into flexion on the upper thoracic region, a region that frequently tends to be flexed from faulty posture. The flexed and inverted position compresses the lungs and heart, decreasing their potential effectiveness. It is questionable whether the benefits of this exercise outweigh the combined negative effects on the neck and upper back posture, circulation, and respiration. To adapt this exercise to meet various goals

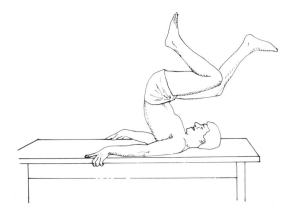

FIGURE 22-1. The inverted bicycle exercise accentuates the faulty postures of forward head and round upper back and compresses the thorax.

(a) if balance is the purpose, use of a balance beam in the upright position would be safer.

(b) if improving strength in the trunk muscles is the purpose, a number of exercises are safer and more effective, such as appropriately graded curl-ups, leg lifts, and prone extension. A *modified bicycle* exercise is another alternative. The subject lies supine and maintains a posterior pelvic tilt while the lower extremities are flexed and extended in a reciprocal pattern (Figure 22-2). The amount of hip extension allowed depends on the strength of the abdominal muscles and their ability to stabilize the pelvis and keep the back flat.

(c) if relieving circulatory stress in the legs is the purpose, lying supine with just the legs elevated is safer. Various motions of the feet and legs can be added to the elevated legs.

(d) if coordination of the lower extremities is the purpose, doing the modified bicycle is safer.

c. **Differentiation is not made between fatigue and strain.**

This may result in damage to the part that is being strained. The cliché "No pain, no gain" is often misunderstood and therefore abuse to vulnerable tissue occurs. In order to develop strength, the muscles need to be exercised to near fatigue, but once fatigued, the subject begins substituting and therefore can strain a poorly stabilized part or develop an overuse syndrome. If straining occurs, the activity is either too difficult to begin with or the muscles involved are fatigued and can no longer do the function properly.

d. **The original design of the exercise is altered or exaggerated.**

This is sometimes done with the idea of progressing the exercise by making it more difficult. The result places stresses on supporting tissues. For example:

(1) *The fire hydrant*

This exercise, if done properly, should strengthen the gluteus maximus muscle. The individual is on his hands and knees in the all-4's position, then extends and externally rotates the thigh, keeping the knee flexed. The subject should keep the pelvic tilt neutral (requiring good pelvic stability) and stop the motion at the end of the range of hip extension (Figure 22-3). Instead, individuals often challenge themselves to see how high they can kick the leg, causing locking

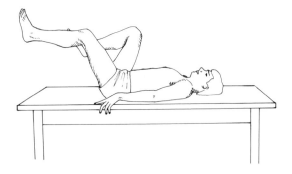

FIGURE 22-2. The modified bicycle exercise can be used to strengthen the abdominal muscles if the back is kept flat while the hips and knees are flexed and extended.

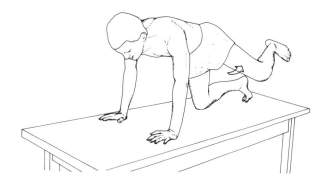

FIGURE 22-3. The fire hydrant. To do this exercise correctly, the subject must stabilize his pelvis mid range, then stop the extension, external rotation motion when the hip has completed its range. The leg should not be "kicked as high as possible" or stress to the hip, sacroiliac joint, and lumbar spine will result.

of the hip joint ligaments and capsule and the transmission of stresses to the sacroiliac (SI) joint and lumbar spine. If momentum is also a part of the exercise routine, the uncontrolled forces cause additional stress to the SI and lumbar spinal joints and supporting tissues. If a person exaggerates this motion or has SI or low back problems, he should not do this exercise.

(2) *Side-lying abduction*

For effective strengthening of the prime mover for hip abduction, the gluteus medius, the individual is side-lying, with the bottom leg flexed for stability. The top leg should be extended in line with the trunk and kept neutral to rotation; then abduction against gravity is done. The range of abduction is approximately 30 to 45 degrees.[9] To exaggerate this exercise, individuals usually roll the pelvis backward and kick the leg upward with excessive flexion and rotation while abducting the hip. This substitutes action of the tensor fascia lata muscle, which, through its attachment on the iliotibial band, can lead to increased tension in the band and lateral knee pain. Tightness in this muscle can lead to faulty mechanics when running, and therefore should not be emphasized over the gluteus medius.

e. **Some exercises are biomechanically unsafe due to the extreme forces placed on vulnerable structures.**

It is worthy to repeat that many of the aforementioned exercises, when done incorrectly or excessively, will be unsafe or at least may precipitate musculoskeletal problems. Examples of exercises that are biomechanically unsafe include

(1) *Bridging with full body weight on the head and feet*

To assume this bridging position, the individual begins supine with hips and knees flexed so that the feet are on the floor, and then lifts the body weight upward, pressing the head and feet into the floor so that only the head and feet are supporting the body. This position results in extreme pressure on the cervical spine and has the potential to cause damaging compressive forces on the disks.[7] This exercise has been safely modified by having the individual press upward with the feet and upper back (see Figure 10-12), thus keeping all forces off the vulnerable neck structures yet obtaining the benefit of strengthening the hip and spinal extensors. The neck musculature is then exercised separately.

(2) *Duck waddle and deep knee bends*

Squatting full range so that the knees are maximally flexed, then shifting weight from side to side (often done with children when mimicking animals) causes excessive stress to the structures at the knee. The ligaments are strained, the menisci are maximally compressed between the tibia and femur, and the patella is maximally compressed against the femur, predisposing the articular cartilage to damaging forces. Highly trained or elite athletes and dancers may progressively work into this activity because of the requirement for performance,[7] but for the recreational athlete or untrained individual, the structures have not been appropriately trained to respond to the excessive forces. Modification of the exercise is to do partial squats, going only through partial range of hip and knee flexion while standing, thus exercising the quadriceps femoris and hip extensor muscles through a functional range and in a functional pattern.

(3) In summary, any exercise can become biomechanically unsafe if done by an individual unprepared for the activity, or if done by an individual with predisposing musculoskeletal dysfunctions or diseases. (Refer to appropriate chapters throughout this book for detailed explanations and precautions.)

2. Suggestions for a safe strengthening program

a. First, identify which muscle groups need strengthening and choose exercises that, when properly executed, will strengthen the appropriate muscles.

b. Begin each exercise at a level safe for the individual. If straining is necessary to complete the exercise, it is probably too difficult and should be simplified with less exercise resistance.

c. When fatigue occurs do not push to the point of straining.

d. Balance each exercise between antagonistic muscle groups and include each region of the body.

e. Do each exercise in a biomechanically correct manner so that the muscles to be strengthened are doing the prime motion or stabilization.

f. If there is poor posture and flexibility, strengthen the muscles antagonistic to the tight muscles.

g. Warm up the muscles to be strengthened by stretching them first. Finish the strengthening program by again stretching each muscle group.

h. The speed of the motion can vary and will depend on the purpose of the exercise. (See Chapter 3 for discussion on specificity of exercises.)

B. Exercises to Increase Flexibility

1. Common errors in flexibility programs

a. Improper emphasis

Stretching routines may emphasize regions that are already flexible and neglect regions that are tight from faulty postures. Total body stretching, such as toe-touches, may maintain or overstretch a mobile area and not affect a tight area, and therefore will not satisfactorily meet the goal. See discussion in the testing section on toe-touching (Section I B).

b. **Flexibility imbalances**

In areas where there is a strength imbalance between antagonistic muscle groups, there tends to also be a flexibility imbalance. Just as flexion exercises tend to be overemphasized in strengthening programs, extensors tend to be overstretched in flexibility programs.

c. **Use of ballistic stretch**

Ballistic stretching can be dangerous. It can cause tearing of soft tissue and may increase tone in the muscles to be stretched.

d. **Exercise pain**

The phrase "No pain, no gain" is often used inappropriately as the guidelines for intensity of stretch. An effective stretching or flexibility routine should not cause pain or excessive stress to tissues. For an effective stretch, there should be a "pulling" sensation in the tight tissue. A low-intensity, prolonged stretch is more effective and longer lasting than a high-intensity, quick stretch. Refer to Chapter 4 for additional information.

e. **Faulty biomechanics**

Some popular stretching exercises do not respect the biomechanics of the region. Whenever abnormal stresses are placed on supporting tissue or joint structures, the exercise should be modified. Some examples include:

(1) *locking the intermediate joint with forward bending or push-ups.*
When doing any forward bending exercises, individuals have a tendency to lock their knees. This stresses the posterior capsule and anterior cruciate ligaments, and over time can lead to genu recurvatum. The knees should be slightly bent, or unlocked, whenever doing forward bending exercises. Similarly, with push-ups, locking the elbow stresses the joint.

(2) *hurdler's stretch*
When the hurdler's stretch position is assumed for the purpose of stretching the hamstrings, excessive stress is placed on the medial capsule and medial collateral ligament of the knee that is placed behind the individual. The hurdler's position can effectively be used to stretch the rectus femoris muscle as described in Chapter 10 (see Figure 10-3), but alternative positions are recommended for hamstring stretches, such as unilateral straight-leg raising. By lying supine and lifting one lower extremity to the point of stretch, the individual can support the knee with his hands. An effective stretch can occur even with the knee slightly flexed.

(3) *Gastroc-soleus stretch*
An easy and apparently effective way to stretch the plantarflexors is by standing with the leg to be stretched placed behind the individual. The individual then shifts his weight forward onto the leg in front, keeping the heel of the hind foot on the floor. If the knee is kept straight, the gastrocnemius is stretched; if the knee is bent, the soleus is stretched. The major problem occurs when this exercise is done without good arch support or barefooted, and when the foot is turned slightly outward. The forces are transmitted to the ligamentous structures supporting the arch, and may lead to a hypermobile foot. Modify this exercise by turning the foot inward prior to the stretch; this will lock the bones of the foot and provide stability for the arch. (See Chapter 12 for additional information.)

2. Suggestions for a safe flexibility program

a. If a subject is excessively mobile in a segment or region of the body, selectively stretching tight structures is safer than total body stretching. Isolate stretching of the hamstring, the low back, and the upper back muscles as described in the testing section (Section I B). Other suggestions for self-stretching techniques are found for each region of the body in Chapters 7 through 12 and in Chapter 14.

b. Maintain a balance in flexibility between antagonistic muscle groups. If there is decreased flexibility because of poor posture, emphasize stretching the tight muscles. Typically, they are the hip flexors, trunk flexors, shoulder flexors, and scapular protractors.

c. Use a sustained stretch rather than bouncing or ballistic stretches. Maintain each position approximately 10 seconds or longer.

d. Stretching (flexibility exercises) should be used prior to and after a strengthening or conditioning program.

e. Do not stress joints and ligaments at the end of the range; protect vulnerable joints.

C. Exercises to Increase Endurance

1. Suggestions for a safe muscle endurance program

a. For local muscle endurance, an exercise is performed with many repetitions and minimal resistance to the point of muscle fatigue. When signs of fatigue occur, do not push to the point of straining the supporting tissue.

b. Increased muscle endurance is a by-product of increased strength when repetitions of motion are used.

2. Suggestions for a safe cardiovascular endurance program

Chapter 21 describes aerobic conditioning principles and procedures. Specific precautions and suggestions for medical conditions are also explained.

a. Establish the target heart rate and maximum heart rate.

b. Warm up gradually for 5 to 10 minutes; include stretching and repetitive motions at slow speeds, gradually increasing the effort.

c. Increase the pace of the activity so that the target heart rate can be maintained for 20 to 30 minutes. Examples include fast walking, running, bicycling, swimming, cross-country skiing, and aerobic dancing.

d. Cool down for 5 to 10 minutes with slow, total body repetitive motions and stretching activities.

e. The aerobic activity should be done 3 to 5 times per week.

f. To avoid injuries from stress, use appropriate equipment, such as correct footware, for proper biomechanical support. Avoid running, jogging, or aerobic dancing on hard surfaces such as asphalt and concrete.

g. To avoid overuse syndromes to structures of the musculoskeletal system, proper warm-up and stretching of muscles to be used should be done. Progression of activities should be within the tolerance of the individual. Overuse commonly occurs when there is an increase in time or effort without adequate rest (recovery) time between sessions. Increase repetitions or time by no more than 10 percent per week.[7] If pain begins while exercising, heed the warning and reduce the stress.

  h. Individualize the program of exercise. Not all people are at the same fitness level and therefore cannot do the same exercises. Any one exercise has the potential to be detrimental if attempted by someone not able to execute the exercise properly. Begin at a safe level for the individual and progress as the individual meets the desired goals.

D. Exercises to Increase Skill

1. Skill includes coordination, agility, balance, timing, and speed.
2. The skill needs to be identified and analyzed and broken into the components that make up the action. The action may require strength, flexibility, and endurance as a base before the skill can be properly executed. Exercises that replicate the motion, velocity, and position then follow. Ultimately, the skill must be practiced for timing and form.

E. Re-evaluate at Frequent Intervals to See if the Baseline Has Changed.

Use the same testing procedures for consistency in interpreting the results. If there is no change, either the exercises are not being carried out properly or they are not appropriate. As improvement occurs, the satisfaction of improved function is immeasurable.

IV. SUMMARY

Popular exercise programs may be the precipitating factor in musculoskeletal complaints—not because exercising should not be done, but because the exercises are done improperly or for the wrong purpose. This chapter outlined an approach for analyzing and choosing safe testing and exercising procedures and cited several commonly misunderstood and misued tests and exercises as examples.

REFERENCES

1. Daniels, L and Worthingham, C: *Muscle Testing Techniques of Manual Examination,* ed 4. WB Saunders, Philadelphia, 1980.
2. Gossman, M, Sahrmann, S, and Rose, S: *Review of length associated changes in muscle.* Phys Ther 62:1799, 1982.
3. Kendall, F: *A criticism of current tests and exercises for physical fitness.* J Am Phys Ther Assoc 45:187, 1965.
4. Kendall, F and McCreary, E: *Muscles: Testing and Function,* ed 3. Williams & Wilkins, Baltimore, 1983.
5. Kendall, H and Kendall, F: *Normal flexibility according to age groups.* J Bone Joint Surg 30:690, 1948.
6. Liemohn, W, Snodgrass, L, and Sharpe, G: *Unresolved cotroversies in back management—A review.* JOSPT 9:239, 1988.
7. Lubell, A: *Potentially dangerous exercises: Are they harmful to all?* Phys Sports Med 17:187, 1989.
8. Minor, MD and Minor, SD: *Patient Evaluation Methods for the Health Professional.* Reston Publishing Co, Reston, VA, 1985.
9. Norken, C and White, DJ: *Measurement of Joint Motion: A Guide to Goniometry.* FA Davis, Philadelphia, 1985.
10. Schultz, P: *Flexibility: Day of the static stretch.* The Physician and Sports Medicine. 7:109, 1979.

GLOSSARY ———————————————————————

accessory movement. Movement within a joint and surrounding soft tissues that is necessary for normal range of motion but cannot be voluntarily performed

accommodating resistance exercise. A term used synonymously with isokinetic exercise

active inhibition. A type of stretching exercise in which there is reflex inhibition and subsequent elongation of the contractile elements of muscles

adaptation. The ability of an organism to change over time in response to a stimulus

adenosine triphosphate (ATP). A high-energy compound from which the body derives energy

adhesions. Abnormal adherence of collagen fibers to surrounding structures during immobilization, following trauma, or as a complication of surgery, which restricts normal elasticity of the structures involved

aerobic exercise. Submaximal, rhythmic, repetitive, exercise of large muscle groups, during which the needed energy is supplied by inspired oxygen

aerobic system. An aerobic energy system in which ATP is manufactured when food is broken down

airway resistance. The resistance to the flow of air in the lungs offered by the bronchioles

amniotic fluid. The liquid contained in the amniotic sac. The fetus floats in the fluid, which serves as a cushion against injury and helps maintain a constant fetal body temperature

anaerobic exercise. Exercise that occurs without the presence of inspired oxygen

anaerobic glycolytic system (lactic acid system). An anaerobic energy system in which ATP is manufactured when glucose is broken down to lactic acid

anemia. A decrease below normal in the number of red blood cells or hemoglobin in the blood

apnea. Cessation of breathing

arteriosclerosis obliterans (ASO). See arteriosclerotic vascular disease

arteriosclerotic vascular disease (ASVD). Progressive narrowing, loss of elasticity, fibrosis, and eventual occlusion of the large and middle-sized arteries, usually in the lower extremities

arteriovenous oxygen difference (A-VO$_2$ difference). The difference between the oxygen content of arterial and venous blood

arthritis. Inflammation of the structures of a joint

arthrodesis. Surgical fusion of bony surfaces of a joint with internal fixation such as pins, nails, plates, and bone grafts; usually done in cases of severe joint pain and instability in which mobility of the joint is a lesser concern

arthroplasty. Any reconstructive joint procedure, with or without a joint implant designed to relieve pain and/or restore joint motion

arthroscopy. Examination of the internal structures of a joint by means of an endoscopic viewing apparatus inserted into the joint

arthrotomy. Surgical incision into a joint

asthma. An obstructive lung disease seen in young patients, associated with a hypersensitivity to specific allergens and resulting in bronchospasm and difficulty in breathing

atelectasis. Collapse or incomplete expansion of the lung

ATP-PC system. An anaerobic energy system in which adenosine triphosphate (ATP) is manufactured when phosphocreatine (PC) is broken down

atrophy. The wasting or reduction of size of cells, tissues, organs, or body parts

auscultation. Listening to heart or lung sounds within the body, usually with a stethoscope

bronchiectasis. A chronic obstructive lung disease characterized by dilation and repeated infection of medium-sized bronchioles

Buerger's disease. See thromboangitis obliterans

bursitis. Inflammation of a bursa

capsular pattern. A pattern of limitation, characteristic for a given joint, that indicates that a problem exists with that joint

cardiac output. The volume of blood pumped from a ventricle of the heart per unit of time; the product of heart rate and stroke volume

cardiorespiratory endurance. The ability of the lungs and heart to take in and transport adequate amounts of oxygen to the working muscle, allowing activities that involve large muscle masses to be performed over long periods of time

cervix. The narrow lower end of the uterus, opening into the vagina

chondromalacia. Deterioration of the articular cartilage at the posterior aspect of the patella

chronic bronchitis. An inflammation of the bronchi that causes an irritating, productive cough that lasts up to 3 months and recurs over at least 2 consecutive years

chronic obstructive pulmonary disease (COPD). A term used to describe a variety of chronic lung conditions such as chronic bronchitis, emphysema, and asthma

circuit training. A training program that uses selected exercises or activities performed in sequence

clubbing. Broadening or thickening of the soft tissues of the terminal phalanges of the fingers and toes, often seen in persons with chronic pulmonary disease

compression dressing. A sterile bandage applied around or over a new surgical incision to compress the wound site and promote healing

concentric muscle contraction. An overall shortening of the muscle as it generates tension and contracts

conception. The onset of pregnancy

conditioning. An augmentation of the energy capacity of the muscle through an exercise program

continuous training. A training program that uses exercise over a given duration without rest periods

contracture. Shortening or tightening of skin, fascia, muscle, or joint capsule that prevents normal mobility or flexibility of that structure

contusion. Bruising from a direct blow, resulting in capillary rupture

coordination. Using the right muscles at the right time with correct intensity. Coordination is the basis of smooth and efficient movement, which often occurs automatically

cyanosis. A bluish appearance of skin and mucous membranes due to insufficient oxygenation of the blood

cystic fibrosis. A genetically based disease that involves malfunction of the exocrine glands and leads to chronic lung infections and pancreatic dysfunction

deconditioning. A change that takes place in cardiovascular, neuromuscular, and metabolic functions as a result of prolonged bed rest or inactivity

degenerative joint disease (DJD). See osteoarthritis

derangement (disk protrusion). Any change in the shape of the nucleus pulposus of the intervertebral disk that causes it to protrude beyond its normal limits

dislocation. Displacement of a part, usually the bony partners within a joint

distensibility. The ability of an organ or tissue to be stretched out or enlarged

distraction. A pulling apart or separation of joint surfaces

dynamometer. A device that quantitatively measures muscle strength

dysfunction. A loss of function as a result of adaptive shortening of soft tissues and loss of mobility

dyspnea. Shortness of breath; labored, distressed breathing

eccentric muscle contraction. An overall lengthening of the muscle as it develops tension and contracts to control motion performed by an outside force; negative work is done

efficiency. The ratio of work output to work input

embolus. A thrombus, or clot of material, that has been dislodged and transported in the blood stream from a larger to a smaller vessel, resulting in occlusion of the vessel

emphysema. A chronic obstructive pulmonary disease that is characterized by inflammation, thickening, and deterioration of the respiratory bronchioles and alveoli

end feel. The quality of feel the evaluator experiences when passively applying pressure at the end of the available range of motion

endurance. The ability to resist fatigue

endurance, general (total body). The ability of an individual to sustain low intensity exercises, such as walking, jogging, or climbing, over an extended period of time

endurance, muscular. The ability of a muscle to perform repeated contractions over a prolonged period of time

energy systems. Metabolic systems involving a series of chemical reactions resulting in the formation of waste products and the manufacture of adenosine triphosphate (ATP). The systems include the ATP-PC (adenosine triphosphate-phosphocreatine) system, the anaerobic glycolytic system, and the aerobic system

ergometer. An apparatus, such as a stationary bicycle or treadmill, used to quantitatively measure the physiologic effects of exercise

exercise bouts. The number of sets of a repetition maximum performed during each exercise session

exercise duration. The total number of days, weeks, or months during which an exercise program is performed

exercise frequency. The number of times exercise is done within a day or within a week

exercise load. The amount of weight used as resistance during an exercise

exercise prescription. Individualized exercise program involving the duration, frequency, intensity, and mode of exercise

expiratory reserve volume (ERV). The maximum amount of air an individual can exhale after a normal, relaxed expiration

extrapment. A tissue trapped on the outside of a structure unable to assume its normal relationship. When a meniscoid tissue becomes trapped outside a zygapophyseal joint as the surfaces slide together, the motion is blocked and tension is placed on the capsular tissue

extrusion. A protrusion of the nucleus pulposus of the intervertebral disk in which the nuclear material ruptures through the outer annulus and lies under the posterior longitudinal ligament

fast twitch (FT) fiber. A skeletal muscle fiber with a fast reaction time, which has a high anaerobic capacity and is suited for phasic muscle activity

fatigue, general (total body). The diminished response of a person during prolonged physical activity such as walking or jogging that may be due to a decrease in blood sugar (glucose) levels, a decrease in glycogen stores in muscle and liver, or a depletion of potassium, especially in the elderly

fatigue, local (muscle). A diminished response of the muscle due to a decrease in energy stores, insufficient oxygen, and a build-up of lactic acid; protective influences from the central nervous system; or a decrease in the conduction of impulses at the myoneural junction

fetus. The developing embryo in the uterus from seven to eight weeks after fertilization until birth

fitness. A general term indicating a level of cardiovascular functioning that results in heightened energy reserves for optimum performance and well being

flat low-back posture. A posture characterized by decreased lumbosacral angle, decreased lumbar lordosis, and posterior tilting of the pelvis

flexibility. The ability of muscle and other soft tissue to yield to a stretch force

flexibility exercise. A general term used to describe exercises performed by a person to passively or actively elongate soft tissues without the assistance of a therapist

forceps. A two bladed instrument with a handle for grasping and extracting the fetal head from the maternal passages

forward head posture. A posture characterized by an increased flexion of the lower cervical and upper thoracic regions, increased extension of the occiput on the first cervical vertebra, and increased extension of the upper cervical vertebrae

fremitus, vocal or tactile. The vibration that can be felt on the chest wall as a person speaks

full arc extension. Active or active-resisted extension of a joint through its full range of motion from flexion to extension

functional excursion. The distance a muscle can shorten after it has been stretched to its maximum length

ganglia. A ballooning of the wall of a joint capsule or tendon sheath

gestation. The period of development from the time of fertilization to birth (pregnancy)

glossopharyngeal breathing. A type of breathing exercise used to increase a patient's inspiratory capacity by gulping in air

glycogen. The storage form of carbohydrates in the body, found predominantly in the muscles and the liver

glycolysis. The incomplete chemical breakdown of glycogen, with the end product of pyruvic acid in aerobic glycolysis and the end product of lactic acid in anaerobic glycolysis

hemarthrosis. Bleeding into a joint, usually from severe trauma

hemoptysis. The expectoration of blood or blood-streaked sputum from the bronchial tree and lungs

hemothorax. A collection or effusion of blood in the pleural cavity

herniation. Abnormal protrusion of an organ or other body structure through a defect or natural opening in a covering membrane, muscle, or bone

hypertrophy. An increase in the cross-sectional size of a fiber or cell

hyperventilation. An increase in the rate and depth of respiration above a level necessary for normal ventilatory function

implantation. The attachment of the fertilized ovum in the lining of the uterus

inspiratory reserve volume (IRV). The maximum amount of air a person can inhale after a relaxed inspiration

inspiratory resistance training. A method of strengthening the muscles of inspiration

intermittent claudication. The cramping of muscles after short periods of exercise; often seen in patients with occlusive arterial disorders

intermittent positive-pressure breathing (IPPB). Assisted ventilation of the lungs with a mechanical apparatus; primarily used for patients who are able to breath spontaneously but have an inadequate depth of respiration

intermittent traction. A traction force that is alternately applied and released at frequent intervals, usually in a rhythmic pattern

intermittent work. Exercises performed with alternate periods of rest, as opposed to continuous work

interval training. A training program that alternates bouts of heavy work with periods of rest or light work

intrinsic muscle spasm. The prolonged contraction of a muscle in response to the local circulatory and metabolic changes that occur when a muscle is in a continued state of contraction

intubation. Insertion of a tube, such as an endotracheal or nasogastric tube, into the body

involution. The progressive contraction of the uterus following childbirth, returning the organ to near its prepregnant size

isokinetic exercise. A form of active-resistive exercise in which the speed of movement of the limb is controlled by a pre-set rate-limiting device

isometric (static) contraction. A muscle contraction in which tension is developed but no mechanical work is done. There is no appreciable joint movement, and the overall length of the muscle remains the same

isotonic (dynamic) contraction. A concentric or eccentric muscular contraction that results in movement of a joint or body part

joint mobilization. Passive traction and/or gliding movements applied to joint surfaces that maintain or restore the joint play normally allowed by the capsule, so that the normal roll-slide joint mechanics can occur as a person moves

joint play. Capsular laxity or elasticity that allows movements of the joint surfaces. The movements include distraction, sliding, compression, rolling, and spinning

labor. The physiologic process by which the uterus contracts and expels the products of conception after 20 or more weeks of gestation

load-assisting exercise. A form of exercise in which the exercise load assists a weak muscle in overcoming gravity

load-resisting exercise. Any exercise in which a load or a weight producing an external force resists the internal force generated by a muscle as it contracts

lobectomy. Surgical removal of a lobe of a lung

lordotic posture. A posture characterized by an increase in the lumbosacral angle, causing an increased lumbar lordosis, anterior pelvic tilt, and hip flexion

lung compliance. Refers to the distensibility or elastic recoil of lung tissue

lymphedema. Excessive accumulation of extravascular and extracellular fluid in tissue spaces

manipulation. A passive movement using physiologic or accessory motion, which may be applied with a thrust or when the patient is under anesthesia. The patient cannot prevent the motion

mastectomy. Removal of a breast

maximal aerobic power (max V̇O₂). The maximal volume of oxygen consumed per unit of time

maximal heart rate reserve (HRR). The difference between the resting heart rate and the maximal heart rate

membranes. The thin layer of tissue that lines the uterus and forms a sac, protecting the fetus and providing for its nutrition

meniscectomy. An intra-articular procedure at the knee by which the meniscus (fibrocartilage) is removed surgically

metabolic equivalent (MET). The amount of oxygen required per minute under quiet resting conditions; equal to 3.5 milliliters of oxygen consumed per kilogram of body weight per minute

mobilization. Passive stretching movements performed by a therapist at a speed slow enough that the patient can stop the movement

muscle-setting exercise. A form of isometric exercise but one not performed against any appreciable resistance; gentle static muscle contractions used to maintain mobility between muscle fibers and to decrease muscle spasm and pain

muscle spasm. See intrinsic muscle spasm

neural tube. The embryonic bony encasement of the spinal cord or skull

occlusion. Closure or obstruction of a vessel such as an artery or vein

orthopnea. Difficulty breathing while lying supine

osteoarthritis (degenerative joint disease). A chronic degenerative disorder primarily affecting the articular cartilage with eventual bony overgrowth at the margins of the joints

osteoporosis (bone atrophy). A condition of bone that leads to a loss of bone mass, a narrowing of the bone shaft, and widening of the medullary canal

osteotomy. The surgical cutting and realignment of bone to correct joint deformity and reduce pain

overload. Stressing the body or parts of the body to levels above that normally experienced

overstretch. A stretch beyond the normal range of motion of a joint and the surrounding soft tissues

overwork. A phenomenon that causes temporary or permanent deterioration of strength as a result of exercise, observed clinically in patients with nonprogressive, lower motor neuron diseases who participate in excessively vigorous resistance exercise programs

oxygen deficit. The time period during exercise in which the level of oxygen consumption is below that necessary to supply all the ATP required for the exercise

oxygen transport system (V̇O₂). Composed of stroke volume, heart rate, and arterial-mixed venous oxygen difference

pallor. Chalky white appearance or blanching of the skin

paresthesia. Abnormal sensation perceived as burning or prickling

pendulum (Codman's) exercises. Self-mobilization techniques that use the effects of gravity to distract the humerus from the glenoid fossa and gentle pendulum motions to move the joint surfaces

percussion. A technique used with postural drainage to mobilize secretions by mechanically dislodging viscous or adherent secretions in the lungs; also refers to a procedure used to evaluate the air:solid ratio in the lungs

perinatal. The period from the 20th week of gestation to approximately four weeks after birth

phlebitis. Inflammation of a vein

phosphocreatine (PC). Creatine phosphate; an energy-rich compound that plays a critical role in providing energy for muscular contraction

physiologic movement. Movement that a person normally can do, such as flexion, extension, rotation, abduction, and adduction

placenta. An organ formed from the fetal membranes and carrying nutrients from the mother's blood into the fetus' blood and waste products from the fetus to the mother. The placenta attaches to the interior wall of the uterus

pleural effusion. The presence of fluid in the pleural cavity

pleurectomy. An incision into the pleura

pneumonectomy. Surgical excision of lung tissue. In some instances, the term denotes removal of an entire lung

pneumonia. An inflammation of the lungs characterized by consolidation and exudation; often caused by a bacterial or viral infection

pneumothorax. The presence or accumulation of air in the pleural cavity

postpartum. With reference to the mother, occurring after childbirth

postural drainage. A means of clearing the airways of secretions by placing the patient in various positions so that gravity will assist in the flow of mucus

postural dysfunction. A faulty posture in which adaptive shortening of soft tissues and muscle weakness has occurred

postural fault (postural pain syndrome). A posture that deviates from normal alignment but has no structural limitations

posture. A position or attitude of the body, the relative arrangement of body parts for a specific activity, or a characteristic manner of bearing one's body

power. Work per unit of time (force × distance/time) or force times velocity

progressive resistance exercise (PRE). An approach to exercise whereby the load or resistance to the muscle is applied by some mechanical means and is quantitatively and progressively increased over time

prolapse. A protrusion of the nucleus pulposus that is still contained by the outer layers of the annulus

pulmonary edema. An infiltration of fluid (serum) in the lungs

pumping exercises. Active repetitive exercises, usually of the ankles or wrists, done to maintain or improve circulation in the extremities

Q-angle. The angle formed by intersecting lines drawn from the anterior-superior iliac spine through the mid-portion of the patella, and from the anterior tibial tuberosity through the midpatella. The norm is 15 degrees

rales. Abnromal breath sounds heard with a stethoscope during inspiration; caused by secretions in the small airways of the lungs

range of motion (ROM). The amount of motion allowed between any two bony levers

range of motion, active. Movement, within the unrestricted ROM for a segment, which is produced by an active contraction of the muscles crossing that joint

range of motion, active-assistive. A type of active ROM in which assistance is provided by an outside force, either manually or mechanically, because the prime mover muscles need assistance to complete the motion

range of motion, passive. Movement, within the unrestricted ROM for a segment, which is produced entirely by an external force. There is no voluntary muscle contraction

Raynaud's disease. A functional vasospasm of the small arteries, particularly in the hands, caused by an abnormality of the sympathetic nervous system

reflex muscle guarding. The prolonged contraction of a muscle in response to a painful stimulus. Guarding ceases when the pain is relieved but may progress to muscle spasm

reflux. A backward or return flow of urine back toward the kidneys from the bladder

relaxation. A conscious effort to relieve tension in muscles

relaxed (slouched) posture. Also called sway back posture. A posture characterized by a shifting of the pelvic segment anteriorly, resulting in hip extension, and shifting of the thoracic segment posteriorly, resulting in flexion of the thorax on the upper lumbar spine. An increased lordosis in the lower lumbar region, an increased kyphosis in the thoracic region, and a forward head are usually observed with relaxed posture

repetition maximum (RM). The greatest amount of weight a muscle can move through the range of motion a specific number of times in a load-resisting exercise routine

repetition minimum. The least amount of weight required to help a patient lift a body part against gravity a specified number of times

residual volume (RV). The amount of air that is left in the lungs after a maximum expiration

resistance exercise. Any form of active exercise in which a dynamic or static muscular contraction is resisted by an outside force

resistance exercise, manual. A type of active exercise in which resistance is provided by a therapist or other health professional to either a dynamic or static muscular contraction

resistance exercise, mechanical. A type of active exercise in which resistance is applied through the use of equipment or mechanical apparatus

respiration, external. The exchange of air in and out of the body; also referred to as ventilation

respiration, internal. The exchange of gases between blood and cells at the alveolar-capillary membrane

resting position. The position of the joint in which there is maximum laxity in the capsule and surrounding structures

rheumatoid arthritis. A chronic joint disease, which is often systemic; characterized by inflammation of the synovial membrane, with periods of exacerbation and remission

rhonchi. Abnormal breath sounds, usually heard on expiration; caused by congestion in the proximal airways

round back posture. A posture characterized by an increased thoracic curve, protracted scapulae, and a forward head

round ligament. A fibromuscular band attaching to the uterus anteriorly, passing through the abdominal ring, and inserting into the Labia majora

rubor. Redness of the skin associated with inflammation

scoliosis. An abnormal lateral curvature of the vertebral column

scoliosis, functional. A nonstructural reversible lateral curvature of the spine

scoliosis, structural. An irreversible lateral curvature of the spine with fixed rotation of the vertebrae

selective tension. The administration of specific tests in a systematic manner in order to determine whether the site of a lesion is in an inert structure (joint capsule, ligament, bursae, fascia, dura mater, or dural sheaths around nerve roots) or in a contractile unit (muscle with its tendons and attachments)

self-mobilizing. Techniques whereby the patient is taught to apply joint mobilization techniques to restricted joints using proper gliding techniques

self-stretching. Techniques whereby the patient is taught to stretch a joint or soft tissue passively by using another part of the body for applying the stretch force

setting exercise. See muscle-setting exercise

short arc extension (terminal extension) exercise. Active or active-resisted extension of a joint through the final degrees of its range of motion; most often applied to the knee from 35 degrees flexion to full extension

skill. Refined movement requiring coordination, agility, balance, timing, and speed

slow twitch (ST) fiber. A skeletal muscle fiber with a slow reaction time and a high aerobic capacity, suitable for tonic muscle activity

specificity of training. The principle underlying the development of a training program for a specific activity or skill and the primary energy systems involved during performance

sphincter. A circular muscle constricting a passage or closing a natural orifice

sprain. Severe stress, stretch, or tear of soft tissues such as joint capsule, ligament, tendon, or muscle

static traction. A steady traction force applied and maintained for an extended time interval. It may be continuous (prolonged) or sustained

steady state. Pertaining to the time period during which a physiologic function remains at a constant value

strain. Overstretching, overexertion, overuse of soft tissue; tends to be less severe than a sprain; occurs from slight trauma or unaccustomed repeated trauma of a minor degree

strength. The force output of a contracting muscle. It is directly related to the amount of tension a contracting muscle can produce

stress testing. A multistage test that determines the cardiovascular functional capacity of the individual

stretch weakness. The weakening of muscles that are habitually kept in a stretched position beyond their physiologic resting length

stretching. Any therapeutic maneuver designed to lengthen (elongate) pathologically shortened soft tissue structures and thereby to increase range of motion

stretching, passive. A type of mobility exercise in which manual, mechanical, or positional stretch is applied to soft tissues and in which the force is applied opposite to the direction of shortening

stretching, self: See self-stretching

stroke volume. The amount of blood pumped out of the ventricles with each contraction (systole)

subluxation. An incomplete or partial dislocation that often involves secondary trauma to surrounding soft tissue

suspension. A technique that is used to free a body part from the resistance of friction by suspending the part in a sling attached to a rope that is fixed either above the center of gravity or above the axis of the joint

sway back. See relaxed (slouched) posture

synovectomy. Surgical removal of the synovium (lining of the joint) in patients with chronic joint swelling

synovitis. Inflammation of a synovial membrane; an excess of normal synovial fluid within a joint or tendon sheath

target heart rate. A predetermined heart rate to be obtained during exercise

tendinitis. Scarring or calcium deposits in a tendon

tenosynovitis. An inflammation of the synovial sheath covering a tendon

tenovaginitis. A thickening of a tendon sheath

terminal extension. See short arc extension

thoracotomy. Any surgical cutting of the chest wall

thromboangitis obliterans (Buerger's disease). An inflammatory reaction and subsequent vasospasm of the arteries as a result of exposure to nicotine

thrombophlebitis. An inflammatory occlusion of a deep or superficial vein with a thrombus

thrombosis. The formation of a clot in a blood vessel

thrombus. A blood clot

tidal volume (TV). The amount of air that a person breathes in and breathes out during a relaxed inspiration and expiration

tight weakness. The weakening of a muscle that has been kept in a habitually shortened position. It may test strong in the shortened position but tests weak as it is lengthened

total lung capacity (TLC). The total amount of air in the lungs; the vital capacity plus the residual volume

traction. The process of drawing or pulling

umbilical cord. The structure connecting the fetus to the placenta

umbilicus. Scar marking the site of entry of the umbilical cord in the fetus

uterus. The hollow muscular organ in women in which the fertilized ovum implants and develops

Valsalva maneuver. An expiratory effort against a closed glottis

vasoconstriction. Narrowing of a blood vessel due to contraction of smooth muscle in the walls of the vessels, resulting in a decrease in blood flow

ventilation. The movement or mass exchange of air in and out of the body; also referred to as external respiration

vibration. A technique of rapid shaking with small amplitude used with postural drainage to mobilize secretions

vital capacity (VC). The greatest amount of air that a person can inspire and expire

wheezes. Abnormal breath sounds heard primarily on expiration, caused by narrowing of the airways

INDEX

A page number in *italics* indicates a figure. A "t" following a page number indicates a table.